P9-AFZ-670

PROGRESS IN BRAIN RESEARCH

VOLUME 68

COEXISTENCE OF NEURONAL MESSENGERS: A NEW PRINCIPLE IN CHEMICAL TRANSMISSION

Recent volumes in PROGRESS IN BRAIN RESEARCH

Volume 46: Membrane Morphology of the Vertebrate Nervous System. A Study with Freeze-etch Technique, by C. Sandri, J. M. Van Buren and K. Akert — *revised edition* — 1982

Volume 53: Adaptive Capabilities of the Nervous System, by P. S. McConnell, G. J. Boer, H. J. Romijn, N. E. Van de Poll and M. A. Corner (Eds.) — 1980

Volume 54: Motivation, Motor and Sensory Processes of the Brain: Electrical Potentials. Behaviour and Clinical Use, by H. H. Kornhuber and L. Deecke (Eds.) — 1980

Volume 55: Chemical Transmission in the Brain. The Role of Amines, Amino Acids and Peptides, by R. M. Buijs, P. Pévet and D. F. Swaab (Eds.) — 1982

Volume 56: Brain Phosphoproteins, Characterization and Function, by W. H. Gispen and A. Routtenberg (Eds.) — 1982

Volume 57: Descending Pathways to the Spinal Cord, by H. G. J. M. Kuypers and G. F. Martin (Eds.) — 1982

Volume 58: Molecular and Cellular Interactions Underlying Higher Brain Functions, by J.-P. Changeux, J. Glowinski, M. Imbert and F. E. Bloom (Eds.) — 1983

Volume 59: Immunology of Nervous System Infections, by P. O. Behan, V. terMeulen and F. Clifford Rose (Eds.) — 1983

Volume 60: The Neurohypophysis: Structure, Function and Control, by B. A. Cross and G. Leng (Eds.) — 1983

Volume 61: Sex Differences in the Brain: The Relation Between Structure and Function, by G. J. DeVries, J. P. C. De Bruin, H. B. M. Uylings and M. A. Corner (Eds.) — 1984

Volume 62: Brain Ischemia: Quantitative EEG and Imaging Techniques, by G. Pfurtscheller, E. J. Jonkman and F. H. Lopes da Silva — 1984

Volume 63: Molecular Mechanisms of Ischemic Brain Damage, by K. Kogure, K.-A. Hossmann, B. K. Siesjö and F. A. Welsh (Eds.) — 1985

Volume 64: The Oculomotor and Skeletal Motor Systems, by H.-J. Freund, U. Büttner, B. Cohen and J. Noth (Eds.) — 1986

Volume 65: Psychiatric Disorders: Neurotransmitters and Neuropeptides, by J. M. van Ree and S. Matthysse (Eds.) — 1986

Volume 66: Peptides and Neurological Disease, by P. C. Emson, M. N. Rossor and M. Tohyama (Eds.) — 1986

Volume 67: Visceral Sensation, by F. Cervero and J. F. B. Morrison (Eds.) — 1986

Volume 68: Coexistence of Neuronal Messengers: A New Principle in Chemical Transmission, by T. Hökfelt, K. Fuxe and B. Pernow (Eds.) — 1986

Volume 69: Phosphoproteins in Neuronal Function, by W. H. Gispen and A. Routtenberg (Eds.) — 1986

Volume 70: Aging of the Brain and Senile Dementia, by D. F. Swaab, E. Fliers, M. Mirmiram, W. A. Van Gool and F. P. A. J. Van Haaren (Eds.) — 1986

Volume 71: Neural Regeneration, by F. J. Seil, E. Herbert and B. Carlson (Eds.) — 1987

PROGRESS IN BRAIN RESEARCH

VOLUME 68

COEXISTENCE OF NEURONAL MESSENGERS: A NEW PRINCIPLE IN CHEMICAL TRANSMISSION

Proceedings of the Marcus Wallenberg Symposium, held at the Grand Hotel, Saltsjöbaden, Stockholm, on 26–28 June, 1985

EDITED BY

T. HÖKFELT

Department of Histology, Karolinska Institutet, Box 60400, S-10401 Stockholm, Sweden

K. FUXE

Department of Histology, Karolinska Institutet, Box 60400, S-10401 Stockholm, Sweden

and

B. PERNOW

Department of Clinical Physiology, Karolinska Hospital, Box 60400, S-10401 Stockholm, Sweden

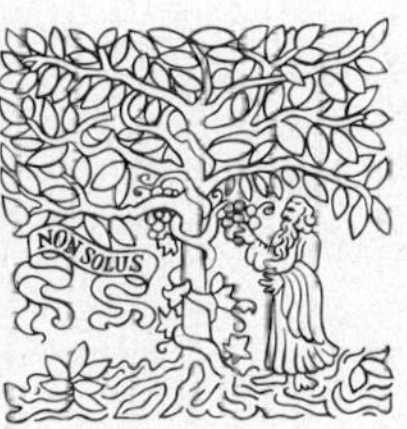

ELSEVIER
AMSTERDAM – NEW YORK – OXFORD
1986

ISBN 0-444-80762-4 (volume)
ISBN 0-444-80104-9 (series)

Published by:
Elsevier Science Publishers B.V. (Biomedical Division)
P.O. Box 211
1000 AE Amsterdam
The Netherlands

Sole distributors for the USA and Canada:
Elsevier Science Publishing Company, Inc.
52 Vanderbilt Avenue
New York, NY 10017
USA

Library of Congress Cataloging in Publication Data

Marcus Wallenberg Symposium (1985: Saltsjöbaden, Sweden)
Coexistence of neuronal messengers.

(Progress in brain research; v. 68)
Sponsored by the Wallenberg Foundation for International Cooperation in Science.
Bibliography: p.
Includes index.
1. Neurotransmitters — Congresses. 2. Neuropeptides — Congresses. 3. Neural transmission — Congresses. I. Hökfelt, Tomas. II. Fuxe, Kjell, 1938. III. Pernow, Bengt. IV. Marcus Wallenberg Foundation for International Cooperation in Science. V. Title. VI. Series.

QP376.P7 vol. 68 612′.82 s 86-16198
[QP364.7] [599′.0188]
ISBN 0-444-80762-4 (U.S.)

Printed in The Netherlands

List of Contributors

T. W. Abrams, Howard Hughes Medical Institute, Center for Neurobiology and Behavior, Department of Physiology and Psychiatry, Columbia University College of Physicians and Surgeons, 722 West 168th Street, New York, NY 10032, U.S.A.
C. Adler, Department of Psychiatry, New York University Medical Center, New York, NY 10016, U.S.A.
J. E. Adler, Cornell University Medical College, 515 East 71st Street, New York, NY 10021, U.S.A.
L. F. Agnati, Department of Human Physiology, University of Modena, Modena, Italy
H. Alho, Laboratory of Preclinical Pharmacology, National Institute of Mental Health, Saint Elizabeths Hospital, Washington, DC 20032, U.S.A.
K. Andersson, Department of Histology, Karolinska Institutet, S-10401 Stockholm, Sweden
T. Bartfai, Department of Biochemistry, Arrhenius Laboratory, University of Stockholm, S-10691 Stockholm, Sweden
L. Bassas, Diabetes Branch, National Institute of Arthritis, Diabetes and Digestive and Kidney Diseases, National Institutes of Health, Bethesda, MD 20892, U.S.A.
F. Benfenati, Department of Human Physiology, University of Modena, Via Campi 287, 41100 Modena, Italy
A. Björklund, Department of Histology, Lund University, S-22362 Lund, Sweden
H. Björklund, Department of Histology, Karolinska Institutet, S-10401 Stockholm, Sweden
I. B. Black, Cornell University Medical College, 515 East 71st Street, New York, NY 10021, U.S.A.
F. E. Bloom, Division of Preclinical Neuroscience and Endocrinology, Scripps Clinic and Research Foundation, 10666 North Torrey Pines Road, La Jolla, CA 92037, U.S.A.
W. D. Branton, Department of Physiology, School of Medicine, University of California, San Francisco and Howard Hughes Medical Institute, San Francisco, CA 94143, U.S.A.
M. J. Brownstein, Laboratory of Cell Biology, NIMH, Bethesda, MD 20205, U.S.A.
E. Brodin, Department of Pharmacology, Karolinska Institutet, S-10401 Stockholm, Sweden
G. Burnstock, Department of Anatomy and Embryology and Centre for Neuroscience, University College London, Gower Street, London WC1E 6BT, U.K.
V. F. Castellucci, Howard Hughes Medical Institute, Center for Neurobiology and Behavior, Departments of Physiology and Psychiatry, Columbia University College of Physicians and Surgeons, 722 West 168th Street, New York, NY 10032, U.S.A.
J.-P. Changeux, Institut Pasteur, Paris, France
E. Collier, Diabetes Branch, National Institute of Arthritis, Diabetes and Digestive and Kidney Diseases, National Institutes of Health, Bethesda, MD 20892, U.S.A.
E. Costa, Laboratory of Preclinical Pharmacology, National Institute of Mental Health, Saint Elizabeths Hospital, Washington, DC 20032, U.S.A.
M. Costa, Departments of Physiology and Anatomy and Histology, and the Center for Neuroscience, School of Medicine, Flinders University of South Australia, Bedford Park, SA 5042, Australia
J. N. Crawley, Electrophysiology and Behavioral Neuropharmacology Units, Clinical Neuroscience Branch, NIMH, Bethesda, MD, U.S.A.
F. dePablo, Diabetes Branch, National Institute of Arthritis, Diabetes and Digestive and Kidney Diseases, National Institutes of Health, Bethesda, MD 20892, U.S.A.
J. C. Eccles, Max-Planck-Institut für biofysikalische Chemie, Göttingen, F.R.G.
L. Edvinsson, Departments of Pharmacology, Clinical Pharmacology and Histology, University of Lund, S-22362 Lund, Sweden
E. Ekblad, Departments of Pharmacology, Clinical Pharmacology and Histology, University of Lund, S-22362 Lund, Sweden
L.-G. Elfvin, Department of Anatomy, Karolinska Institutet, S-22362 Stockholm, Sweden
B. Everitt, Department of Anatomy, Cambridge University, Cambridge, U.K.
P. Ferrero, Laboratory of Preclinical Pharmacology, National Institute of Mental Health, Saint Elizabeths Hospital, Washington, DC 20032, U.S.A.
G. A. Foster, Department of Physiology, University College, Cardiff, U.K.
J. Freedman, Department of Histology, Karolinska Institutet, S-10401 Stockholm, Sweden

J. B. Furness, Departments of Physiology and Anatomy and Histology, and the Center for Neuroscience, School of Medicine, Flinders University of South Australia, Bedford Park, SA 5042, Australia
E. J. Furshpan, Department of Neurobiology, Harvard Medical School, Boston, MA 20115, U.S.A.
K. Fuxe, Department of Histology, Karolinska Institutet, S-10401 Stockholm, Sweden
F. H. Gage, Department of Neuroscience, University of California, San Diego, La Jolla, California, U.S.A.
I. L. Gibbins, Departments of Physiology and Anatomy and Histology, and Center for Neuroscience, School of Medicine, Flinders University of South Australia, Bedford Park, SA 5042, Australia
D. L. Glanzman, Howard Hughes Medical Institute, Center for Neurobiology and Behavior, Departments of Physiology and Psychiatry, Columbia University College of Physicians and Surgeons, 722 West 168th Street, New York, NY 10032, U.S.A.
P. Goelet, Howard Hughes Medical Institute, Center for Neurobiology and Behavior, Departments of Physiology and Psychiatry, Columbia University College of Physicians and Surgeons, 722 West 168th Street, New York, NY 10032, U.S.A.
M. Goldstein, Department of Psychiatry, New York University Medical Center, New York, NY 10016, U.S.A.
A. Guidotti, Laboratory of Preclinical Pharmacology, National Institute of Mental Health, Saint Elizabeths Hospital, Washington, DC 20032, U.S.A.
R. Håkanson, Departments of Pharmacology, Clinical Pharmacology and Histology, University of Lund, S-22362 Lund, Sweden
A. Härfstrand, Department of Histology, Karolinska Institutet, S-10401 Stockholm, Sweden
R. D. Hawkins, Howard Hughes Medical Institute, Center for Neurobiology and Behavior, Departments of Physiology and Psychiatry, Columbia University College of Physicians and Surgeons, 722 West 168th Street, New York, NY 10032, U.S.A.
V. R. Holets, Department of Histology, Karolinska Institutet, S-10401 Stockholm, Sweden
T. Hökfelt, Department of Histology, Karolinska Institutet, S-10401 Stockholm, Sweden
D. W. Hommer, Electrophysiology and Behavioral Neuropharmacology Units, Clinical Neuroscience Branch, NIMH, Bethesda, MD 20205, U.S.A.
K. Iverfeldt, Department of Biochemistry, Arrhenius Laboratory, University of Stockholm, S-10691 Stockholm, Sweden
L. L. Iversen, Merck Sharp and Dohme Research Laboratories, Neuroscience Research Centre, Terlings Park, Eastwick Road, Harlow, U.K.
Y. N. Jan, Department of Physiology, School of Medicine, University of California, San Francisco and Howard Hughes Medical Institute, San Francisco, CA 94143, U.S.A.
A. M. Janson, Department of Histology, Karolinska Institutet, S-10401 Stockholm, Sweden
E. R. Kandel, Howard Hughes Medical Institute, Center for Neurobiology and Behavior, Departments of Physiology and Psychiatry, Columbia University College of Physicians and Surgeons, 722 West 168th Street, New York, NY 10032, U.S.A.
N. Kusano, Department of Psychiatry, New York University Medical Center, New York, NY 10016, U.S.A.
E. F. LaGamma, Cornell University Medical College, 515 East 71st Street, New York, NY 10021, U.S.A.
S. C. Landis, Department of Neurobiology, Harvard Medical School, Boston, MA 20115, U.S.A.
D. LeRoith, Diabetes Branch, National Institute of Arthritis, Diabetes and Digestive and Kidney Diseases, National Institutes of Health, Bethesda, MD 20892, U.S.A.
M. A. Lesniak, Diabetes Branch, National Institute of Arthritis, Diabetes and Digestive and Kidney Diseases, National Institutes of Health, Bethesda, MD 20892, U.S.A.
R. W. Lind, The Salk Institute for Biological Studies, La Jolla, CA 92307, U.S.A.
J. Å. Lindgren, Department of Biochemistry, Karolinska Institutet, S-10401 Stockholm, Sweden
B. Lindh, Department of Anatomy, Karolinska Institutet, S-10401 Stockholm, Sweden
J. M. Lundberg, Department of Pharmacology, Karolinska Institutet, S-10401 Stockholm, Sweden
S. Mackey, Howard Hughes Medical Institute, Center for Neurobiology and Behavior, Departments of Physiology and Psychiatry, Columbia University College of Physicians and Surgeons, 722 West 168th Street, New York, NY 10032, U.S.A.
S. G. Matsumoto, Department of Neurobiology, Harvard Medical School, Boston, MA 20115, U.S.A.
B. Meister, Department of Histology, Karolinska Institutet, S-10401 Stockholm, Sweden
E. Meller, Department of Psychiatry, Millhauser Laboratories, New York University Medical Center, New York, NY 10016, U.S.A.
É. Mezey, Laboratory of Cell Biology, NIMH, Bethesda, MD 20205, U.S.A.
P. G. Montarolo, Howard Hughes Medical Institute, Center for Neurobiology and Behavior, Departments of Physiology and Psychiatry, Columbia University College of Physicians and Surgeons, 722 West 168th Street, New York, NY 10032, U.S.A.

A. Neumeyer, Department of Histology, Karolinska Institutet, S-10401 Stockholm, Sweden
S.-O. Ögren, Astra Läkemedel AB, R and D Laboratories, S-15185 Södertälje, Sweden
M. Olasmaa, Department of Pharmacology, University of Uppsala, Box 591, S-75124 Uppsala, Sweden
L. Olson, Department of Histology, Karolinska Institutet, S-10401 Stockholm, Sweden
A. G. E. Pearse, Royal Postgraduate Medical School, London W12 0HS, U.K.
B. Pernow, Department of Clinical Physiology, Karolinska Hospital, S-10401 Stockholm, Sweden
H. S. Philips, Department of Physiology, School of Medicine, University of California, San Francisco and Howard Hughes Medical Institute, San Francisco, CA 94143, U.S.A.
E. M. Pich, Department of Psychiatry, New York University Medical Center, New York, NY, U.S.A.
C. Post, Astra Pharmaceuticals, S-15185 Södertälje, Sweden
D. D. Potter, Department of Neurobiology, Harvard Medical School, Boston, MA 20115, U.S.A.
J. Roth, Diabetes Branch, National Institute of Arthritis, Diabetes and Digestive and Kidney Diseases, National Institutes of Health, Bethesda, MD 20892, U.S.A.
M. Ruggeri, Department of Histology, Karolinska Institutet, S-10401 Stockholm, Sweden
D. W. Y. Sah, Department of Neurobiology, Harvard Medical School, Boston, MA 20115, U.S.A.
B. Samuelsson, Department of Biochemistry, Karolinska Institutet, S-10401 Stockholm, Sweden
M. R. Santi, Laboratory of Preclinical Pharmacology, National Institute of Mental Health, Saint Elizabeths Hospital, Washington, DC 20032, U.S.A.
P. E. Sawchenko, The Salk Institute for Biological Studies, La Jolla, CA 92307, U.S.A.
S. Schacher, Howard Hughes Medical Institute, Center for Neurobiology and Behavior, Departments of Physiology and Psychiatry, Columbia University College of Physicians and Surgeons, 722 West 168th Street, New York, NY 10032, U.S.A.
M. Schalling, Department of Histology, Karolinska Institutet, S-10401 Stockholm, Sweden
M. Schultzberg, Department of Histology, Karolinska Institutet, S-10401 Stockholm, Sweden
L. R. Skirboll, Electrophysiology and Behavioral Neuropharmacology Units, Clincal Neuroscience Branch, NIMH, Bethesda, MD 20205, U.S.A.
W. Staines, Department of Histology, Karolinska Institutet, S-10401 Stockholm, Sweden
L. Stjärne, Department of Physiology, Karolinska Institutet, S-10401 Stockholm, Sweden
F. Sundler, Departments of Pharmacology, Clinical Pharmacology and Histology, University of Lund, S-22362 Lund, Sweden
L. W. Swanson, The Salk Institute for Biological Studies, La Jolla, CA 92307, U.S.A.
L. Terenius, Department of Pharmacology, Uppsala University, S-75124 Uppsala, Sweden
C. Wahlestedt, Departments of Pharmacology, Clinical Pharmacology and Histology, University of Lund, S-22362 Lund, Sweden
I. Zini, Department of Human Physiology, University of Modena, Via Campi 287, 41100, Modena, Italy
M. Zoli, Department of Human Physiology, University of Modena, Modena, Via Campi 287, 41100, Italy

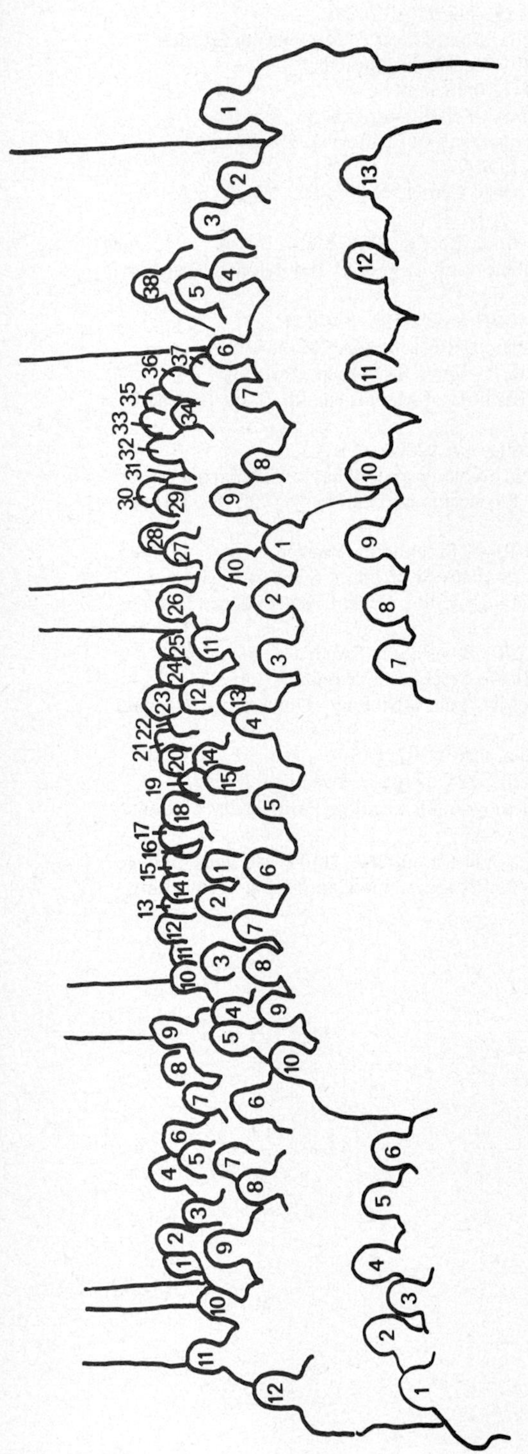

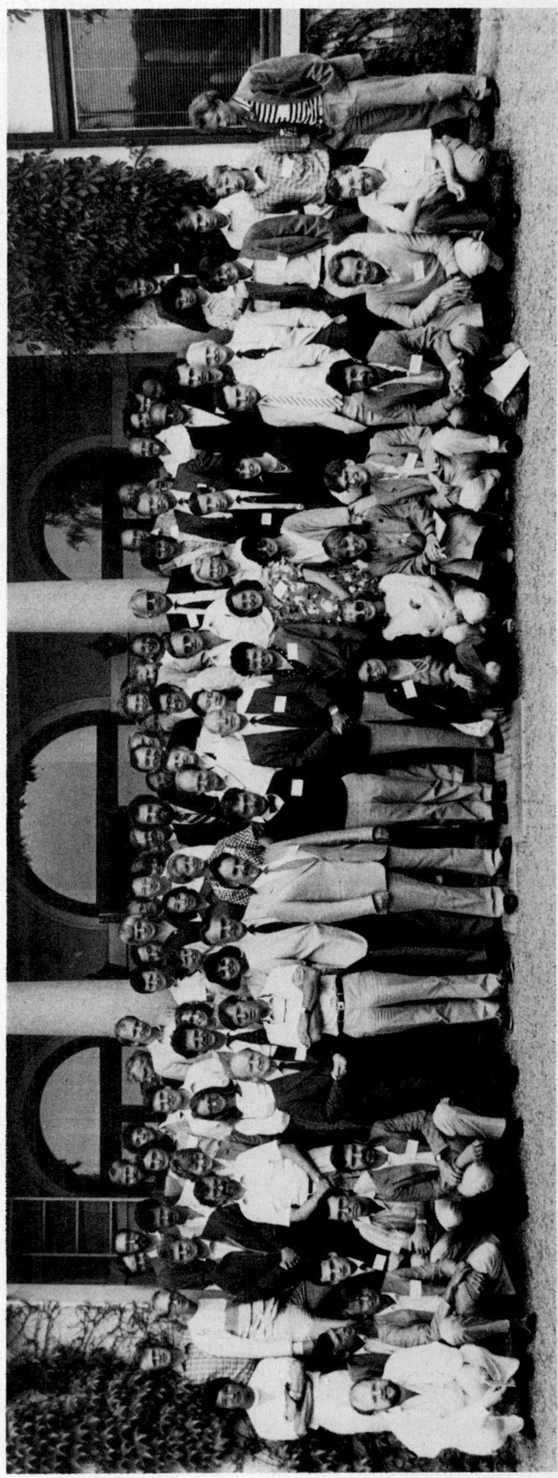

List of participants

The Marcus Wallenberg Symposium on Coexistence of Neuronal Messengers:
A New Principle in Chemical Transmission
Saltsjöbaden, Stockholm, June 26–28, 1985

Front row, sitting:
1 Håkan Hallman
2 Bertil Fredholm
3 Lars Olson
4 Anders Härfstrand
5 Michele Zoli
6 Gösta Jonsson
7 Sandra Ceccatelli
8 Marjut Olasmaa
9 Majbritt Giacobini
10 Gabriel von Euler
11 William Staines
12 Marcello Costa
13 David Potter

Center section:
1 Beatriz Bolioli
2 Vicky Holets
3 Christiane Ayer-LeLievre
4 Sir John Eccles
5 Floyd Bloom
6 Geoffrey Burnstock
7 Bengt Pernow
8 Zsuzsanna Wiesenfeld
9 Anthony Pearse
10 Viktor Mutt

Second row, left section:
1 Annica Dahlström
2 Ming-Shi Jiang
3 Edith Heilbronn
4 Lana Skirboll
5 Larry Swanson
6 Marianne Schultzberg
7 Maria Eriksdotter-Nilsson
8 Leif Bertilsson
9 Björn Lindh
10 Andreas Henschen
11 Elvar Theodorsson-Norheim
12 Matsuhiro Nagata

Second row, right section:
1 Tor Melander
2 Tomas Geijer
3 Jacob Freedman
4 Michael Broomé
5 Xia-Ying Hua
6 Knut Schmidt-Nielsen
7 Kurt Andersson
8 Ann Neumeyer
9 Björn Meister
10 Britta Werner
11 Derek LeRoith
12 O. Humberto Viveros
13 Kerstin Uvnäs-Wallensten
14 Menek Goldstein
15 Tomas Hökfelt

Back row:
1 Åke Ljungdahl
2 ?
3 Nils Lindefors
4 Johan Häggblad
5 Elisabet Björklund
6 Peter Karlsson
7 Barry Everitt
8 Manfred Karobath
9 Åke Seiger
10 Ira Black
11 Tetsuyuki Tsutsumi
12 Lars Terenius
13 David Ingvar
14 Gabriel Fried
15 Anna-Lena Hulting
16 Lars-Gösta Elfvin
17 Olle Johansson
18 Michael Brownstein
19 Nigel Newberry
20 Jean-Pierre Changeux
21 Leslie Iversen
22 Ann-Charlotte Granholm
23 Tamas Bartfai
24 Scott Whittemore
25 Eric Kandel
26 Sune Rosell
27 Anette Hemsén
28 Rolf Håkanson
29 Christer Owman
30 Jesse Roth
31 Margareta Stensdotter
32 Frank Sundler
33 Anders Franco-Cereceda
34 Mario Herrera-Marschitz
35 Jan Lundberg
36 Emanuel Nwanze
37 Antonio Cintra
38 Graham Lees

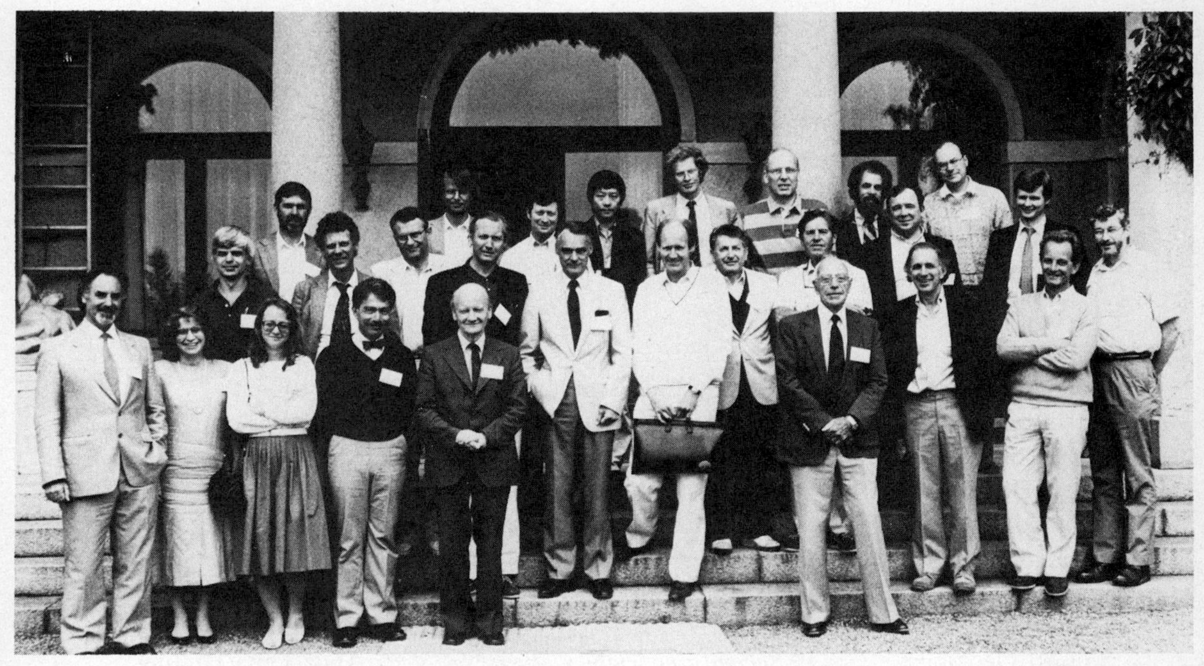

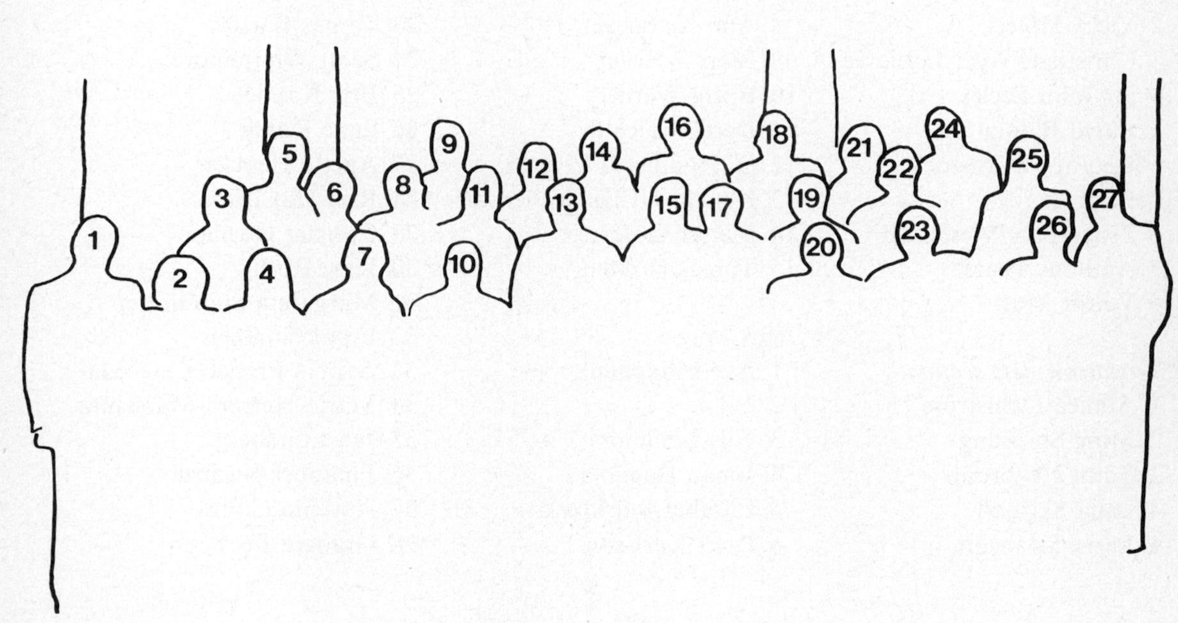
1
2
3
4
5
6
7
8
9
10
11
12
13
14
15
16
17
18
19
20
21
22
23
24
25
26
27

List of chairmen and speakers

The Marcus Wallenberg Symposium on Coexistence of Neuronal Messengers:
A New Principle in Chemical Transmission
Saltsjöbaden, Stockholm, June 26–28, 1985

1 Geoffrey Burnstock
2 Lana Skirboll
3 Lars Terenius
4 Marianne Schultzberg
5 Gösta Jonsson
6 Larry Swanson
7 Floyd Bloom
8 Lennart Stjärne
9 Lars Olson
10 Viktor Mutt
11 Kjell Fuxe
12 Ira Black
13 Bengt Pernow
14 Yuh Nung Jan
15 Tomas Hökfelt
16 Tamas Bartfai
17 Menek Goldstein
18 Jesse Roth
19 Anthony Pearse
20 Sir John Eccles
21 Michael Brownstein
22 Jean-Pierre Changeux
23 Eric Kandel
24 Rolf Håkanson
25 Jan Lundberg
26 Marcello Costa
27 David Potter

Preface

Interest in chemical transfer of information has a long tradition in Swedish biomedical research. This work started with Ulf von Euler, who discovered three compounds, which belong to distinctly separate classes of chemicals, but all of which are of importance in chemical transmission in the endocrine and in the nervous system: substance P, prostaglandins and noradrenaline. The research area outlined by von Euler was then explored by scientists all over the world and also intensely here in Sweden. Nils-Åke Hillarp, Arvid Carlsson and Bengt Falck are known as outstanding representatives of the second generation of Swedish neuroscientists involved in neurotransmitter research and they have in turn fostered a new generation of enthusiastic students carrying on the work. The three organizers of the present conference in Saltsjöbaden, outside Stockholm, in June 1985, and at the same time the editors of this volume, owe these eminent scientists gratitude for providing the basis for their scientific careers and introducing them into neuroscience research — Bengt Pernow carried out his thesis work on substance P under the guidance of Ulf von Euler, and Kjell Fuxe and Tomas Hökfelt were pupils of Nils-Åke Hillarp. It is therefore a great honor and pleasure to dedicate the present volume to the memory of the late Professors Ulf von Euler and Nils-Åke Hillarp.

The theme of the present volume of Progress in Brain Research, coexistence of multiple messengers in neurons and endocrine cells, represents a logical continuation of the work carried out by von Euler and Hillarp. The concomitant occurrence of biogenic amines and peptide hormones was first demonstrated in endocrine cells by Pearse in London and by Owman, Håkanson and their colleagues in Lund. The possibility that such coexistence could also be present in neurons was first indicated in studies on invertebrates, where biochemical studies could be used for analysis of transmitter content in single nerve cells due to their considerable size. The complexity of the mammalian neuron systems and the comparatively small size of their neurons required morphological methods for establishment of coexistence: a natural development of the techniques intiated by Hillarp and his colleagues.

Today multiple examples of different types of coexistence have been observed mainly with histochemical techniques, but our understanding of the physiological significance of this phenomenon is still unclear. It was the aim of this conference to analyze the functional aspects of coexistence, and for this purpose, leading scientists from various fields within the neurosciences were invited to Stockholm. We are grateful that they accepted and for their valuable contribution during the meeting which is now documented in the form of the chapters which make up this volume. We hope that the conference, which also was attended by many young scientists from Sweden, will stimulate further research in this area, both locally here in Sweden and in laboratories in other countries as a result of this volume of Progress in Brain Research.

The conference in Saltsjöbaden was sponsored by the Wallenberg Foundation for International Cooperation in Science. Only through their whole-hearted support and generosity was it possible to hold this conference, which took place at the Grand Hotel in Saltsjöbaden outside Stockholm in a lecture hall devoted to the memory of one of Swedens most remarkable industrialists, Dr. Marcus Wallenberg. His deep interest in research and insight that Swedish research only can survive through strong international connections have been of fundamental importance for science in Sweden and the present conference was organized and held in this spirit. We also thank Astra Pharmaceuticals and the Nobel Foundation for their support.

Stockholm, October 1985

Tomas Hökfelt
Kjell Fuxe
Bengt Pernow

Contents

List of Contributors V

List of participants (The Marcus Wallenberg Symposium) IX

List of chairmen and speakers (The Marcus Wallenberg Symposium) XI

Preface XIII

Section I — The Concept of Chemical Transmission

1. Chemical transmission and Dale's principle
John C. Eccles (Göttingen, F.R.G.) 3

2. Chemical signalling in the nervous system
Leslie L. Iversen (Harlow, U.K.) 15

Section II — Multiple Messengers — Overview and Evolution Aspects

3. The diffuse neuroendocrine system: peptides, amines, placodes and the APUD theory
A. G. E. Pearse (London, U.K.) 25

4. Coexistence of neuronal messengers — an overview
Tomas Hökfelt, Vicky R. Holets, William Staines, Björn Meister, Tor Melander, Martin Schalling, Marianne Schultzberg, Jacob Freedman, Håkan Björklund, Lars Olson, Björn Lindh, Lars-Gösta Elfvin, Jan M. Lundberg, Jan Åke Lindgren, Bengt Samuelsson, Bengt Pernow, Lars Terenius, Claes Post, Barry Everitt and Menek Goldstein (Stockholm and Uppsala, Sweden; Cambridge, U.K. and New York, NY, U.S.A.) 33

5. Molecules of intercellular communication in vertebrates, invertebrates and microbes: do they share common origins?
Jesse Roth, Derek LeRoith, Maxine A. Lesniak, Flora dePablo, Lluis Bassas and Elaine Collier (Bethesda, MD, U.S.A.) 71

Section III — Invertebrates and Developmental Aspects

6. Convergence of small molecule and peptide transmitters on a common molecular cascade
V. F. Castelluci, S. Schacher, P. G. Montarolo, S. Mackey, D. L. Glanzman, R. D. Hawkins, T. W. Abrams, P. Goelet and E. R. Kandel (New York, NY, U.S.A.) 83

7. Transmitter status in cultured sympathetic principal neurons: plasticity, graded expression and diversity
David D. Potter, Steven G. Matsumoto, Story C. Landis, Dinah W. Y. Sah and Edwin J. Furshpan (Boston, MA, U.S.A.) 103

8. Impulse activity differentially regulates co-localized transmitters by altering messenger RNA levels
I. B. Black, J. E. Adler and E. F. LaGamma (New York, NY, U.S.A.) 121

9. Coexistence during ontogeny and transplantation
M. Schultzberg, G. A. Foster, F. H. Gage, A. Björklund and T. Hökfelt (Södertälje, Lund, Stockholm, Sweden and Cardiff, U.K.) 129

Secton IV — Multiple Peptide Systems

10. Genetic background for multiple messengers
Floyd E. Bloom (La Jolla, CA, U.S.A.) 149

11. Multiple chemical messengers in hypothalamic magnocellular neurons
Michael J. Brownstein and Éva Mezey (Bethesda, MD, U.S.A.) . . . 161

12. Regulation of multiple peptides in CRF parvocellular neurosecretory neurons: implications for the stress response
L. W. Swanson, P. E. Sawchenko and R. W. Lind (La Jolla, CA, U.S.A.) 169

Section V — Peripheral Systems

13. Purines as cotransmitters in adrenergic and cholinergic neurones
G. Burnstock (London, U.K.) 193

14. The LHRH family of peptide messengers in the frog nervous system
W. D. Branton, H. S. Phillips and Y. N. Jan (San Francisco, CA, U.S.A.) 205

15. Chemical coding of enteric neurons
M. Costa, J. B. Furness and I. L. Gibbins (SA, Australia) 217

16. Multiple co-existence of peptides and classical transmitters in peripheral autonomic and sensory neurones — functional and pharmacological implications
Jan M. Lundberg and Tomas Hökfelt (Stockholm, Sweden) 241

17. On the possible roles or noradrenaline, adenosine 5′-triphosphate and neuropeptide Y as sympathetic co-transmitters in the mouse vas deferens
Lennart Stjärne and Jan M. Lundberg (Stockholm, Sweden) 263

18. Neuropeptide Y: coexistence with noradrenaline. Functional implications
R. Håkanson, C. Wahlestedt, E. Ekblad, L. Edvinsson and F. Sundler (Lund, Sweden) 279

Section VI — Central Systems

19. Aspects on the information handling by the central nervous system: focus on cotransmission in the aged rat brain
L. F. Agnati, K. Fuxe, M. Zoli, E. Merlo Pich, F. Benfenati, I. Zini and M. Goldstein (Modena, Italy, Stockholm, Sweden and New York, NY, U.S.A.) 291

20. Morphofunctional studies on the neuropeptide Y/adrenaline costoring terminal systems in the dorsal cardiovascular region of the medulla oblongata. Focus on receptor-receptor interactions in cotransmission
K. Fuxe, L. F. Agnati, A. Härfstrand, A. M. Janson, A. Neumeyer, K. Andersson, M. Ruggeri, M. Zoli and M. Goldstein (Stockholm, Sweden, Modena, Italy and New York, NY, U.S.A.) 303

21. Functional consequences of coexistence of classical and peptide neurotransmitters
Tamas Bartfai, Kerstin Iverfeldt, Ernst Brodin and Sven-Ove Ögren (Stockholm and Södertälje, Sweden) 321

22. Characterization of central neuropeptide Y receptor binding sites and possible interactions with α_2-adrenoceptors
Menek Goldstein, Norifumi Kusano, Charles Adler and Emmanuel Meller (New York, NY, U.S.A.) 331

23. Neuropeptide Y receptor interaction with beta-adrenoceptor coupling to adenylate cyclase
Marjut Olasmaa and Lars Terenius (Uppsala, Sweden) 337

24. Cotransmission at GABAergic synapses
E. Costa, H. Alho, M. R. Santi, P. Ferrero and A. Guidotti (Washington, D.C., U.S.A.) 343

25. Functional studies of cholecystokinin-dopamine co-existence: electrophysiology and behavior
L. R. Skirboll, J. N. Crawley and D. W. Hommer (Bethesda, MD, U.S.A.) 357

Section VII — Synthesis

26. Coexistence of neuronal messengers and molecular selection
Jean-Pierre Changeux (Paris, France) 373

Subject Index 405

SECTION I

The Concept of Chemical Transmission

T. Hökfelt, K. Fuxe and B. Pernow (Eds.),
Progress in Brain Research, Vol. 68

CHAPTER 1

Chemical transmission and Dale's principle

John C. Eccles*

Max-Planck-Institut für biofysikalische Chemie, Göttingen, F.R.G.

Dale's principle

Some years ago, Potter et al. (1981) published a very critical appraisal of Dale's principle as applied to the single transmitter version, which they called by the strange name "The popular Dale's principle". They concluded that this version should be relegated to history, and that the multiple transmitter version in the context of the chemical unity of the neurone seems premature.

I will be concerned in correcting some misunderstandings and re-establishing the usage of the term Dale's principle in line with Dale's pioneering thoughts (Dale, 1952). The first full statement of Dale's principle was in my Herter Lectures of 1955, published in Eccles (1957, p. 212). "According to a principle first enunciated by Dale (1935b), which may be called Dale's principle, any one class of nerve cells operates at all of its synapses by the same chemical transmission mechanism. This principle stems from the metabolic unity of a single cell, which extends to all of its branches".

It should be noted that the term "the same chemical transmission mechanism" could cover any number of chemical transmitter substances. It is also in accord with Dale's (1935a) original statement in his Nothnagel Lecture (November 12, 1934) in which he emphasized "the fact that the chemical function appeared to be a function not merely of the nerve ending, but of the whole neurone (Letter by Dale to me 1st October, 1953 quoted in Eccles, 1976).

There has been an unfortunate misunderstanding in respect of the term "principle". I was guided by the Oxford English Dictionary, where the scientific sense of "principle" is given as "A highly general or inclusive theorem", and not in the much more exalted sense quoted by Potter et al. (1981) from Webster's American Dictionary. In contrast in my review article (Eccles, 1962, p. 159), I "proposed to adopt Dale's principle as a provisional hypothesis and on this basis the problem of synaptic transmitters will be examined in relation to the known synaptic connections in the spinal cord".

There seems to be an insinuation by Potter et al. (1981) that I had done a disservice to Dale by associating his name with a Principle, whereas all he expressed was a conjecture that "would serve as a hint"; but his achievement was to propose the metabolic unity of the whole neurone — the soma and all of the axon with its branches. In 1934, this was a great theoretical advance. The first experimental evidence for this conjecture came from the demonstration that acetylcholine was the transmitter not only of the peripheral neuromuscular synapses, but also of the central synapses of motor axon collaterals on Renshaw cells (Fig. 1). This happens to be the first identification of a synaptic transmitter in the vertebrate central nervous system. Strangely, we did not mention Dale in the preliminary report (Eccles et al., 1953), but instead referred to Feldberg's (1950) review. However, I sent the manuscript to Dale, and he replied at length in a letter

* *Address for correspondence:* John C. Eccles, CH 6611 CONTRA (TI), Switzerland.

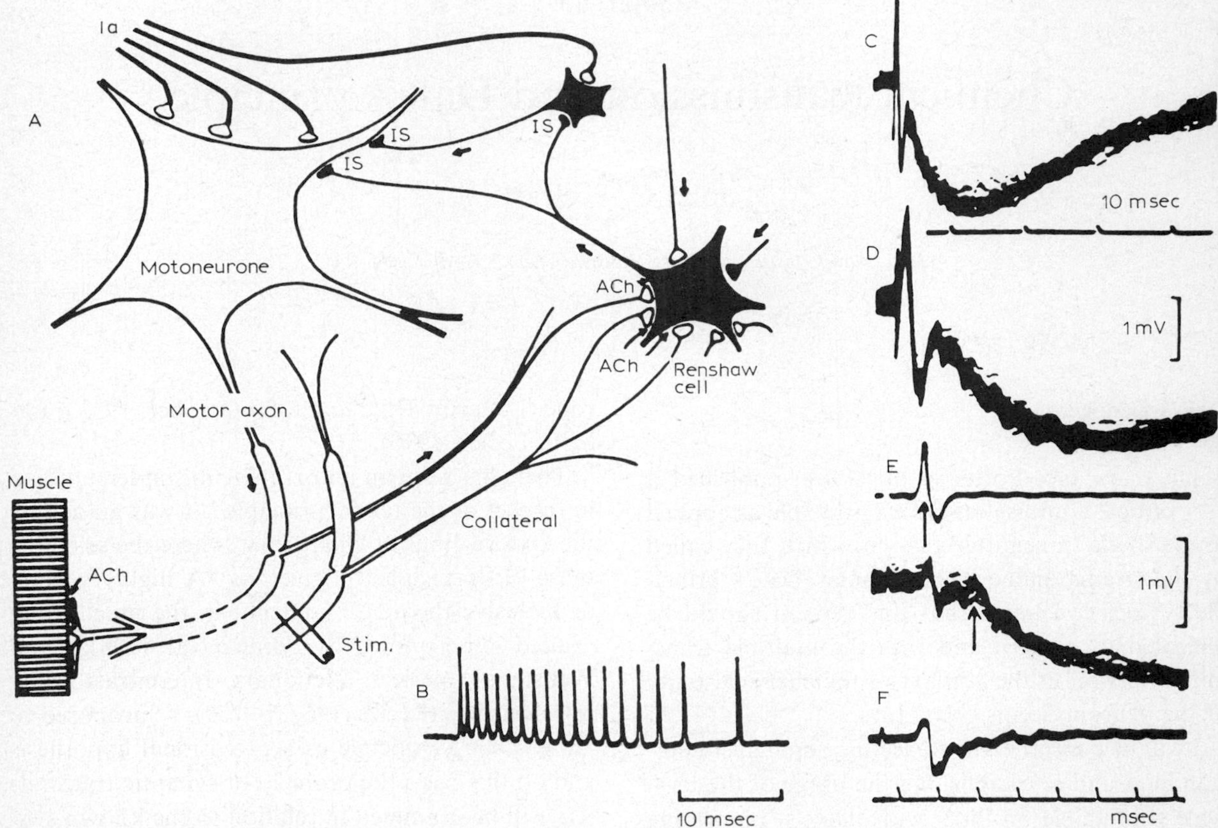

Fig. 1. Feedback inhibition via Renshaw cells. IS, signifies inhibitory synapses and, ACh, excitatory operating with acetylcholine as transmitter. Single stimulation of motor axons as indicated (STIM) evokes a repetitive discharge of a Renshaw cell (B) and IPSP of the motoneurone (recorded intracellularly) as shown at a slow sweep (C) and at faster sweeps (D, E). F is extracellular control to show onset of IPSP at arrow. (Eccles et al., 1954.)

(October 1st, 1953) quoted in Eccles (1976) mentioning that the cholinergic action of motor axon collaterals could have been predicted from his Nothnagel Lecture of 1934. In a later letter (August 25–26th, 1954) commenting on a manuscript containing a preliminary report on inhibitory neurones (Eccles et al., 1954), Dale returns to the metabolic unity of the neurone in a remarkable passage.

"I am still interested, however, in the question why the transmitter and its enzyme systems should be present, not merely at the axon ending, though there apparently in special concentration, but also all along the length of the axon, and apparently in the cell body. I suppose that, like a cytoplasmic process of any other cell, the axon and its ending must be dependent on the nucleus of the cell body for the maintenance of their integrity and special constituents. Certainly if the axon is cut, one of the earliest effects is the disappearance of the transmitter from the axon ending, and the failure of synaptic transmission, even before the conduction of the impulse as far as the ending has been noticeably affected. One must suppose, I think, that there is a constant drift of transmitter, with its associated enzymes, from the cell body down the axon, so that there is an accumulation at the ending, and ready replacement there of what is discharged by the impulse".

In 1934, he had developed his original concept on the metabolic unity of the neurone. It was on this 1934 concept and on this remarkable letter that I dared to coin the term "Dale's principle". Dale, himself, was naturally a little coy about the term,

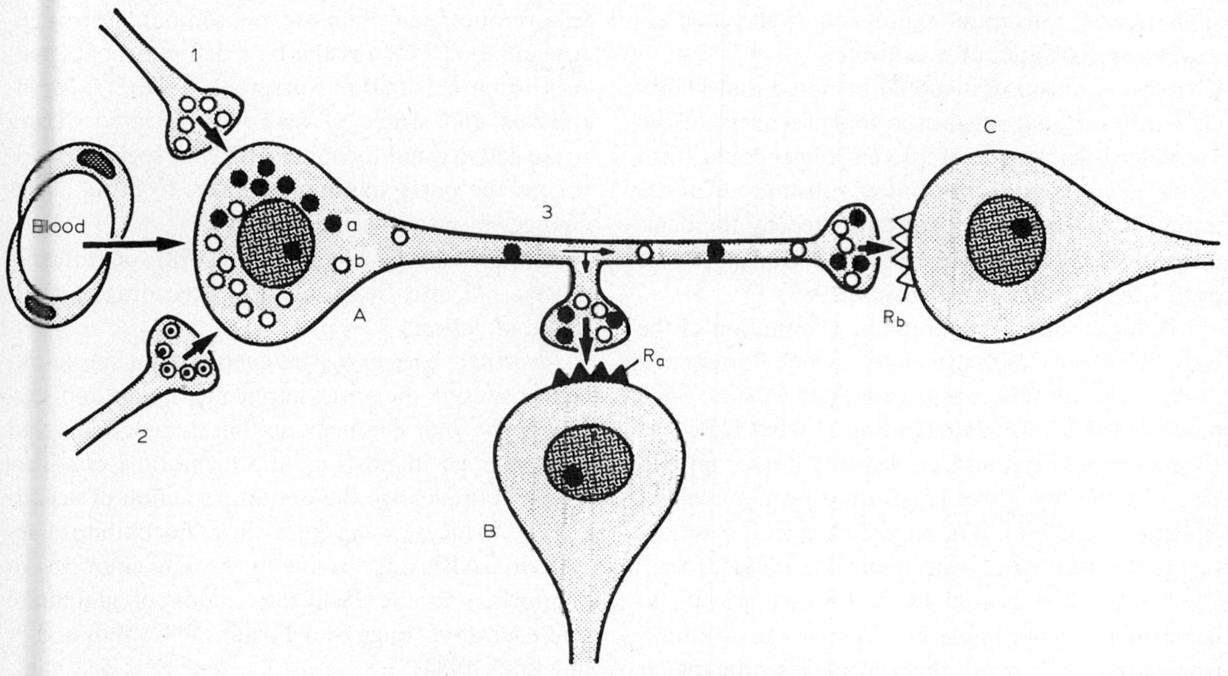

Fig. 2. A hypothetical neural system. Neuron A synthesizes two different neuroactive peptides (a and b), and innervates two neurones (B and C), one of which has receptors only for a (R_a), and the other only for b (R_b). Neurone A in turn receives two excitatory inputs (1 and 2), each mediated by a different neurotransmitter. Both of these inputs are also assumed to release a molecule that stimulates the synthesis of either peptide a or peptide b. Molecules of peptides are shown to travel down the axon and its branches in accord with Dale's principle. (Swanson, 1983.)

but he never forbade its usage. On the contrary, we were devoted friends from the 1930's onwards, as revealed by his many letters, and our friendship flourished with the years with visits to his home when I went to London every year. Moreover, he continued to propose me for scientific awards. I am embarrassed to give these personal details, but there has been an unfortunate belief that because we were for many years scientific disputants we were also personal enemies! Nothing could be further from the truth.

In retrospect, I am happy to have attached the name of Dale to a principle that he proposed and that continues to be a most valuable scientific hypothesis. As defined in 1955 (Eccles, 1957), the "metabolic unity of a neurone" can accommodate any number of transmitters. The unity comprises holistically the immense diversity of the metabolic processes in the nucleus and soma of a neurone and the flow of substances down the axon to its terminals. In Fig. 2, Swanson (1983) gives an excellent illustration for two transmitter substances showing that the two classes of vesicles generated in the soma are transported anterogradely down the axon and its collateral branch. By contrast, impulse propagation may be blocked in some collaterals because of a low safety factor (Krnjevic and Miledi, 1958, 1959; Waxman, 1972; Grossman et al., 1973). Impulse blockage is not known to affect anterograde transport, so Fig. 2 correctly depicts extension of the metabolic unity of the neurone to all of its axonal synapses. Dendro-dendritic or soma-dendritic synapses (Shepherd, 1985, p. 159) are better placed to participate in the metabolic unity of the neurone. The finding of Ochs et al. (1978) that axonal transport peripherally from the dorsal root ganglion is 3 to 5 times faster than the central transport provides no impediment to the concept of the similarity of transmitter expression at all synapses, axonal or dendritic, of a neurone.

In this connection it should be noted that Dale's (1935a,b) original suggestion that discovery of the vasodilator substance of afferent fibres could form a clue to the central transmitter substance of those fibres has recently been substantiated by the demonstration that substance P is the transmitter at both sites (Otsuka and Konishi, 1983).

In conclusion, there should be elimination of the term "Popular Dale's principle", which Potter et al. (1981) also call the single-transmitter version. Such terms reflect a misunderstanding of what Dale and I were proposing, and have led to a most confused story on the first three pages and the summary of Potter et al. (1981). (On page 2 chemical manufacturing is misquoted as mechanical manufacturing!) With that debris cleared away, it is now possible to consider the remarkable new discoveries of multitransmitters and relate them to Dale's principle as "authentically" defined on page 212 of Eccles (1957).

The multiplicity of synaptic transmitter substances

In the 1930's, there was recognition of only two transmitter substances, acetylcholine and adrenaline. For the central nervous system the most important additions have been the inhibitory transmitters, GABA and glycine, and the excitatory transmitters glutamate and aspartate. Noradrenaline, serotonin and dopamine have also been important additions with well recognized nuclei in the brain and the diffuse widely distributed fine fibre systems.

However, now the immunochemical techniques (Hökfelt et al., 1977, 1980) have demonstrated a large number of peptides that clearly are not transmitters in the classical sense, but nevertheless appear to participate in synaptic transmission. Iversen (1984) lists 32 that are constituents of neurones and nerve terminals in the mammalian central nervous system. A variety of functions have been suggested with corresponding names (Dismukes, 1979): neurohormones, neurohumors, neuromodulators, neuroregulators! Perhaps the best definition of a neurotransmitter is that of Burnstock (1976). "It is synthesized and stored in neurones, released during nerve activity and then interacts with specific receptors in the postsynaptic membrane to bring about changes in postsynaptic activity."

As stated by McGeer et al. (1978), neurotransmitters fall into two categories according to their mode of action.

Ionotropic transmitter action occurs at special receptor sites on the postsynaptic membrane and rapidly opens ionic channels, so that there is a fast and large change in postsynaptic membrane conductance. Examples are the excitatory action of acetylcholine at nicotinic receptor sites, the inhibitory action of GABA and glycine in opening chloride ion channels, and the excitatory action of glutamate and aspartate (Fagg and Foster, 1982; Wilkund et al., 1982, 1984).

In contrast, metabotropic transmitter action is effective postsynaptically by stimulating adenylate cyclase to give increased production of cyclic nucleotides with the consequent metabolic change in the postsynaptic cell by the second messenger system. This action is much slower and produces at the most a small conductance change and potential in the postsynaptic membrane. Examples are acetylcholine at muscarinic receptor sites, serotonin and the catecholamines.

In addition to these two specific categories of classical transmitter actions, there are the less well defined actions of the peptides (Hökfelt et al., 1977, 1980) which seem to qualify as neurotransmitters according to the Burnstock (1976) definition.

As stated by Hökfelt et al. (1980), several examples are known where a regulatory peptide occurs together with a classical transmitter. Using immunohistochemical methods, Johansson et al. (1981) have demonstrated the existence of three putative transmitters in many neurones, 5-HT, substance P and TRH, and have presented evidence that these neurones of the medulla oblongata project to the spinal cord. It is of particular interest that, in the nerve terminals of the adrenal medulla, peptides and catecholamines are stored in the same synaptic vesicles and are cosecreted on stimulation (Viveros et al., 1983).

The liberation of transmitter substances

There is overwhelming evidence that the emission of transmitter from the presynaptic terminals (boutons) is quantal for the classical transmitters, and that this quantal emission is due to the exocytosis of synaptic vesicles (Kelly et al., 1979). By electron microscopic studies (Gray, 1963, 1966) and the freeze fracture technique (Akert et al., 1972, 1975; Akert, 1973) it has been recognized that a highly organized structure, the presynaptic vesicular grid, plays the key role in vesicular exocytosis. As indicated in the idealized diagram of Fig. 3, there is usually only one presynaptic vesicular grid for each bouton in the central nervous system, and it has a paracrystalline structure with hexagonal arrays of synaptic vesicles separated by the presynaptic dense projections. A comparable structure has been found for the inhibitory boutons on the Mauthner cells of goldfish (Triller and Korn, 1982).

With intracellular recording from a motoneurone

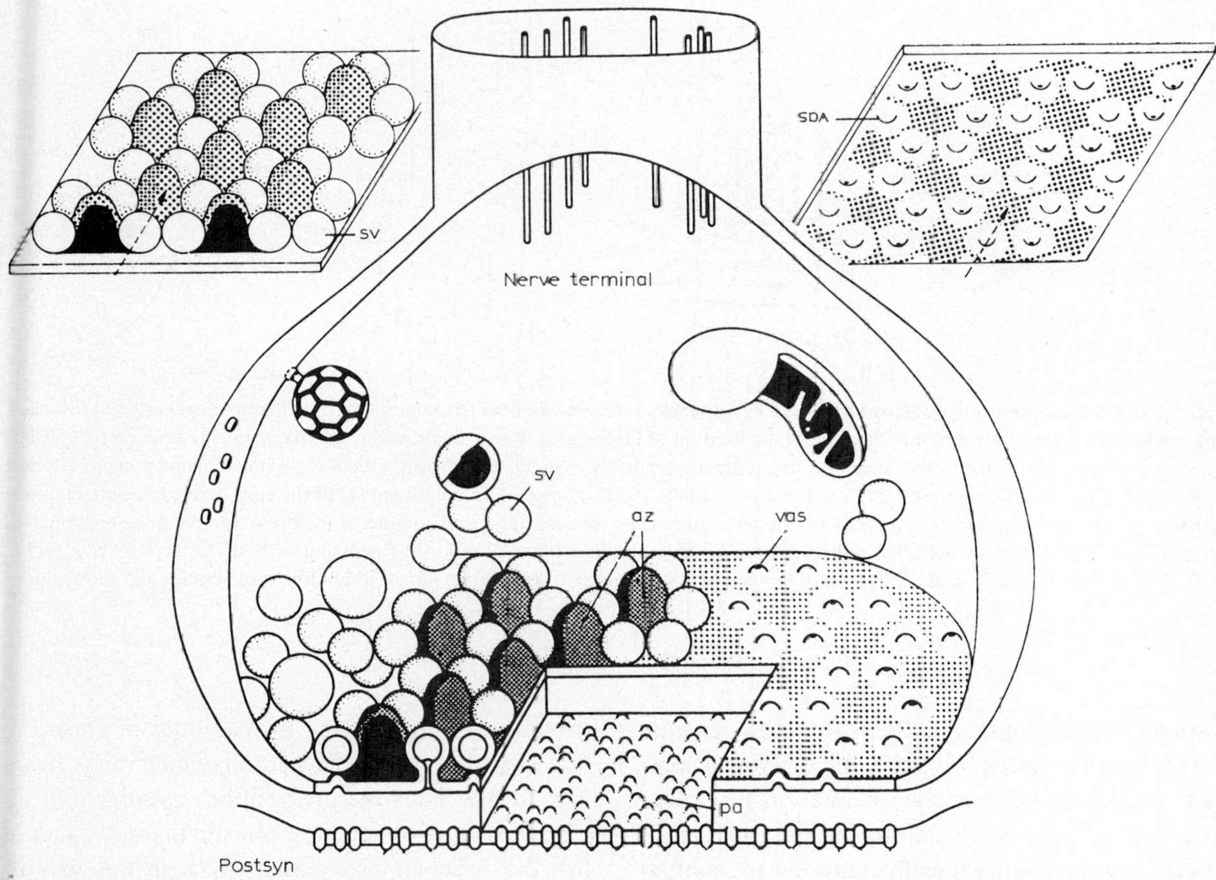

Fig. 3. Schema of mammalian central synapse. Nerve terminal finishes in the expanded bouton that is cut away to show the synaptic vesicles (SV) and the dense projections from the presynaptic membrane (AZ), that are arranged in a paracrystalline structure, the presynaptic vesicular grid, which is seen as a plate in inset above and to the left. To the right, the grid is shown cut away to reveal the attachment sites of the synaptic vesicles, vas, also shown above and to the right. The central part of the bouton is cut away to show the postsynaptic membrane (postsyn) with particle aggregations (pa). (From Akert et al., 1975.)

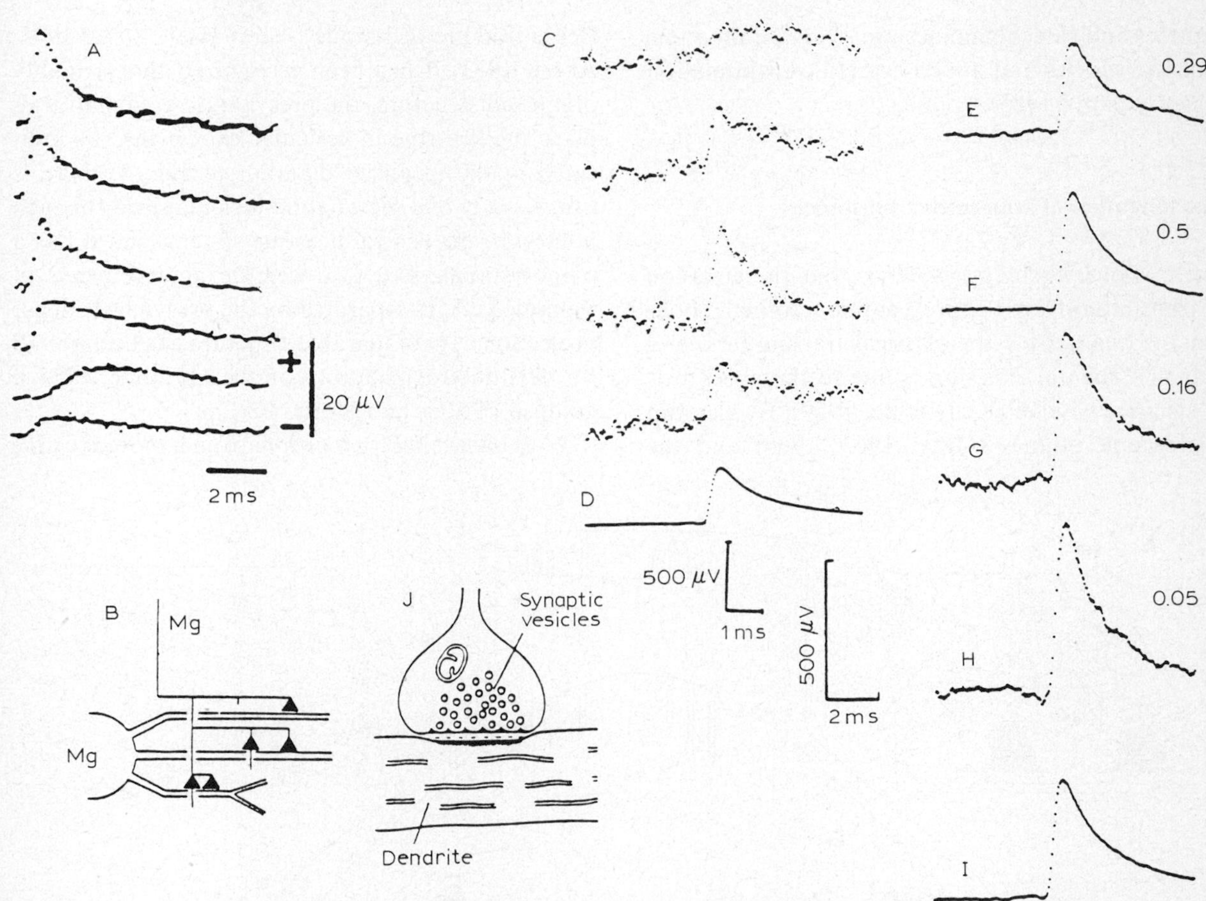

Fig. 4. (A) Averaged recordings of epsps produced by impulses in the same Ia fiber terminating on six different motoneurones (Mendell and Henneman, 1971). (B) Summary diagram of the location of Ia synapses from a single medial gastrocnemius Ia fibre on to a medial gastrocnemius motoneurone at five sites on three different dendrites as indicated (Brown, 1981). (C) Four individual epsps selected from a population of 800 responses. (D) The average of all the 800 responses. (E) Component (1) of the epsp derived from fluctuation analysis. (F, G, H) Components 2, 3 and 4 of this same fluctuation analysis. The probabilities of the occurrence of these components are indicated to the right of each. I is the reconstructed epsp obtained by adding (I) weighted sum of E, F, G, H; 0.29 E + 0.5 F + 0.16 G + 0.05 H. (Jack et al., 1981a.) (J) Drawing of a synapse on a dendrite to show the bouton with vesicles and the synaptic cleft.

a single Ia presynaptic impulse is found to generate a wide range of epsps (Fig. 4C). By applying a complex technique of fluctuation analysis to many hundreds of successive unitary epsps, Jack et al. (1981) have related these fluctuations to quantal emission from the several boutons of that fibre on that motoneurone. For example, in Fig. 4E–H there are the computed epsps for four boutons of the presynaptic fibre. The fluctuations of Fig. 4C are attributable to the varying probabilities of emission of a quantum from each bouton, which range from 0.05 to 0.5. Thus the presynaptic vesicular grid of a bouton (Fig. 3) acts in a holistic manner to control the vesicular exocytosis, which in this way is limited to less than one for a presynaptic impulse, and often to a very low probability. The mean probability is usually about 1 in 3 for a bouton.

Korn and Faber (1986) have carried out a similar

investigation on the epsps produced in a Mauthner cell of a goldfish by single presynaptic impulses. There were fluctuations similar to those of Fig. 4C, and by a different analytical procedure, binomial analysis, they also have found that the vesicular emission from a bouton by a presynaptic impulse is less than unity and with a mean probability of about 0.3.

There are comparable fluctuations in the intracellular epsps produced by single presynaptic impulses in the granule cells of the hippocampus (McNaughton et al., 1981). It can be predicted that analysis will also reveal that there is a probability of quantal emission of much the same range as those already calculated in Fig. 4E–H and by Korn and Faber (1986).

In the mammalian peripheral nervous system, a sympathetic nerve fibre to a muscle fibre of the ductus deferens, Cunnane and Stjärne (1982, 1984) have reported a precise analysis of transmitter output by a single nerve impulse from a varicosity. Intracellular recording from a muscle fibre revealed that there was a mono-quantal release of transmitter, presumably adenosine triphosphate (ATP) (Sneddon and Westfall, 1984) with the very low probability of 0.002 to 0.03. This release is believed to be vesicular and to be from a preferred site of the varicosity. Could this controlled exocytosis be from a primitive presynaptic vesicular grid?

The probabilistic factor for a bouton can be varied up or down by appropriate treatment. It is increased by increase in extracellular Ca^{2+}, by a prior presynaptic stimulation and by 4 amino-pyridine (Jack et al., 1981). It is depressed by high frequency stimulation, being halved at 30 Hz (Korn and Faber, 1985). Evidently alteration of probability of vesicle exocytosis is an important method of varying synaptic transmission.

It is not known if there is a presynaptic vesicular grid for the catecholamine and ATP boutons and varicosities. The presence of large granular vesicles (LGV) might raise a problem (Descarries et al., 1975, 1977; Chan-Palay, 1976) because they could not be accommodated in the tightly structured presynaptic vesicular grid (Fig. 3). However, LGVs may be storage and metabolic sites and not used in exocytosis. In boutons or varicosities there is always a plenitude of small clear vesicles for exocytosis. In Fig. 3, a few large vesicles are shown adjacent to the presynaptic vesicular grid, but not in it. However, most serotonin and catecholamine emission seems to occur in a non-synaptic manner from the assembled vesicles in the varicosities. Descarries et al. (1975) estimate that only 5% of serotonin varicosities make synaptic contacts, and Descarries et al. (1977) gave a similar low figure for noradrenergic varicosities. Chan-Palay (1976) found that some serotonin varicosities are placed so as to secrete into cerebrospinal fluid. They do not act synaptically. Dismukes (1979) discusses at length the possibility of non-synaptic release of transmitter from varicosities of the non-myelinated axons in the brain. There seems to be no doubt that the released transmitter has to diffuse some distance to the receptor sites on the postsynaptic membrane.

Cosecretion of ATP and noradrenaline occurs for the sympathetic nerve varicosities on the ductus

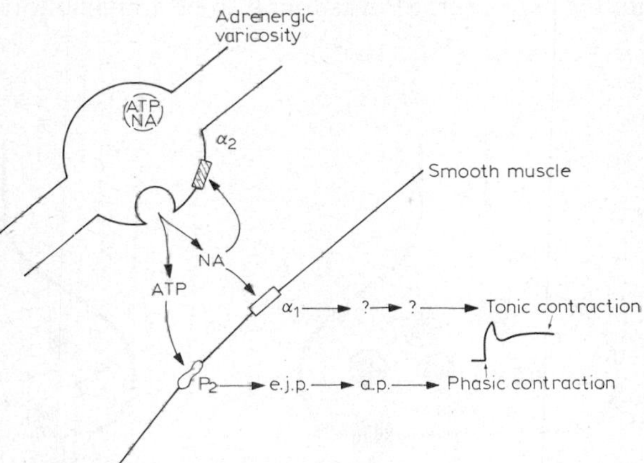

Fig. 5. Schematic representation of the co-transmitter hypothesis proposed for guinea pig vas deferens. When the nerve varicosity is depolarized, it releases ATP and NA which act on P_2 and α_1-receptors respectively of the smooth muscle cell. The first phase of the contractile response results from the action of ATP depolarizing the cell and depends on the summation of e.j.p.s to fire action potentials (a.p.). The second phase is mediated by α_1-receptors by a mechanism which is independent of action potentials. NA may also regulate release presynaptically via α_2-receptors. (Sneddon and Westfall, 1984.)

deferens. By pharmacological analysis, Sneddon and Westfall (1984) have identified the fast acting transmitter as ATP, the slow being noradrenaline. Both these transmitters appear to be contained in the same vesicles, as is illustrated in Fig. 5.

A different situation may exist for peptide transmitters (Iversen et al., 1980). In a very careful study on immunoreactive substance P (SP), di Figlia et al. (1982) have shown dense aggregations of LGVs in some boutons, and in some sections the LGVs appear to be engaged in a presynaptic vesicular grid formed by presynaptic dense projections as diagrammed in Fig. 3. There are grave technical difficulties in studying the probability of vesicular exocytosis from substance P boutons because the postsynaptic membrane reacts with the extreme slowness of a metabotropic response. Otsuka and Konishi (1983) found that the epsps of inferior mesenteric ganglion cells had a rising phase of several seconds and a total duration of about 30 sec. They even suggest that, in the dorsal horn of the spinal cord, SP may be co-released from certain primary afferent terminals together with a fast-acting transmitter. However, SP was found to be a much more effective excitant than L-glutamate by a factor of over 1000 times on a molar basis (Otsuka and Konishi, 1983). Iversen (1984) suggested that the slow SP depolarization may have a modulatory role in making the neurones more sensitive to the transmitters. A similar suggestion was made by Nicoll et al. (1980) with respect to the very slow excitatory action of SP and TRH on frog motoneurones. Koketsu (1984) describes examples of postsynaptic modulation up or down of nicotinic cholinergic excitation of frog sympathetic ganglion cells. It was up for ATP and down for 5-HT, NA, substance P and LHRH.

Possible modes of interaction of cosecreted transmitters

Figure 5 illustrates a simple presynaptic feedback, noradrenalin inhibiting vesicular emission (Sneddon and Westfall, 1984). Figure 6 (Burnstock, 1981) gives an interesting illustration of varieties of transmitter interaction. Presynaptic feedbacks are postulated to be negative controls of transmitter re-

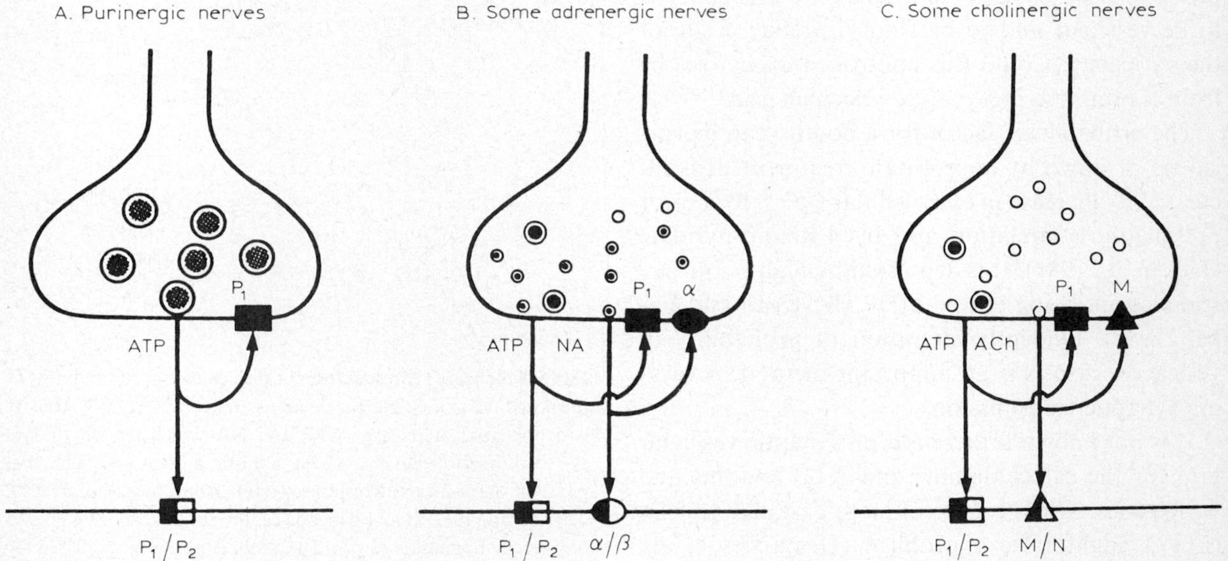

Fig. 6. Schematic representation of presynaptic neuromodulation of transmitter release. (A) Reduction of ATP release by activation of presynaptic P_1 purinoceptors. (B) Reduction of noradrenaline release by activation of presynaptic alpha-adrenoceptors and P_1 purinoceptors. (C) Reduction of ACh release by activation of presynaptic muscarinic and P_1 purinoceptors. (Burnstock, 1981.)

lease, especially the ATP control of the purinergic, noradrenergic and cholinergic nerve terminals. It is now suggested that the presynaptic feedback could be effected by a reduction in the probability of vesicular exocytosis. However, presynaptic feedback could also increase the probability of vesicular exocytosis, as has been found for 4 amino-pyridine (Jack et al., 1981).

The most important examples of cosecretion are for a classical transmitter and a peptide, almost 30 examples being listed in Table 1 of Lundberg and Hökfelt (1983). It seems likely that this cosecretion provides the opportunity for a significant interaction. In some examples the peptide may modulate the action of the classical transmitter. In other cases they may act in parallel in the transmission, the fast classical transmitter action being continued by the slow peptide action, as is illustrated by Lundberg and Hökfelt (1983, Fig. 6).

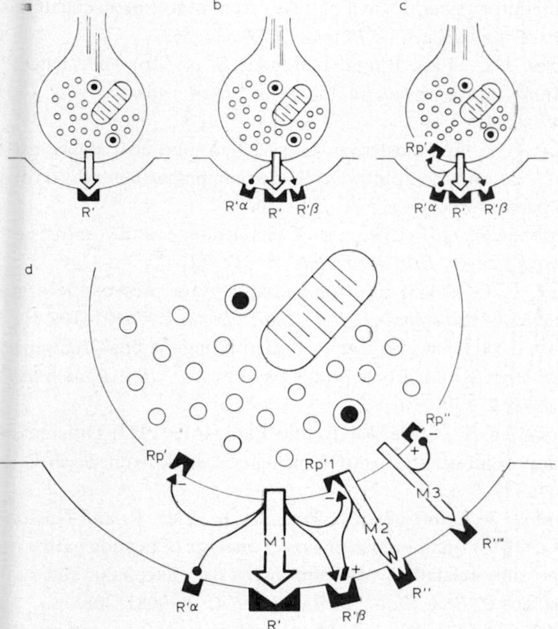

Fig. 7. Schematic illustration of the development of the concept of chemical transmission. (a) One transmitter acts on one postsynaptic receptor (R'). (b) One transmitter acts on multiple types of postsynaptic receptors (R'α R'β). (c) The transmitter acts in addition on a presynaptic receptor (Rp'). (d) Multiple compounds (M 1–3), possibly differentially stored in small vesicles (classical transmitter) and in large dense-core vesicles (classical transmitter plus peptide), are released from the same nerve ending. The main possible interactions are indicated by arrows and signs. (Lundberg and Hökfelt, 1983.)

Of particular interest is the feedback from the peptide on to the presynaptic terminal as is illustrated in Fig. 7. There would be an effective feedback action if the peptide modulator were to change the probability of exocytosis from the bouton either up or down, as described by Jack et al. (1981) and Korn and Faber (1985). It could certainly be the most direct way to modulate the synaptic transmission. If the probability of vesicle emission from boutons or varicosities could be determined as in Fig. 4E–H, the effect of the cosecreted modulator could be studied.

Conclusions

A tremendous effort has been made to establish the multiplicity of synaptic transmitter substances for a single neurone and its synaptic endings. The next stage is to elucidate the manner in which these substances are secreted by a presynaptic nerve impulse. Cosecretion raises many problems: (1) does each small clear vesicle store the cosecreted transmitters, despite their apparent absence in immunocytochemical testing? (2) Are the different transmitters stored in separate small vesicles, despite the evidence for their cosecretion in vesicular exocytosis (Cunnane and Stjärne, 1982, 1984) and as illustrated in Fig. 5? (3) Are the large granular vesicles (LGV) with their specific transmitters, ATP or peptides, also concerned in the exocytosis of their contained transmitters? (4) Are LGVs in some way attached to the presynaptic vesicular grid, perhaps on its edges in readiness for release, as seems to be indicated for the large vesicles in Fig. 3? (5) The physiological meaning of cosecretion has to be studied exhaustively to give further experimental basis for the rather speculative diagrams of Figs. 5, 6 and 7; (6) The quantal probability of exocytosis has to be investigated, but that may be beyond present techniques.

This conference has opened up immense experimental and theoretical fields, as is evidenced from the six problems listed above. The physiological significance of the multiplicity of neurotransmitters raises a tremendous challenge to both experimental and theoretical investigations.

References

Akert, K. (1973) Dynamic aspects of synaptic structure. *Brain Res.*, 49: 511–518.

Akert, K., Pfenninger, K., Sandri, C. and Moor, H. (1972) Freeze etching and cytochemistry of vesicles and membrane complexes in synapses of the central nervous system. In G. Pappas and D. F. Purpura (Eds.), *Structure and Function of Synapses,* Raven Press, New York, pp. 67–86.

Akert, K., Peper, K. and Sandri, C. (1975) Structural organization of motor end plate and central synapses. In P. G. Waser (Ed.), *Cholinergic Mechanisms,* Raven Press, New York, pp. 43–57.

Brown, A. G. (1981) *Organization in the Spinal Cord: The Anatomy and Physiology of Identified Neurones,* Springer-Verlag, Berlin–Heidelberg–New York, 238 pp.

Burnstock, G. (1976) Do some nerve cells release more than one transmitter?, *Neuroscience,* 1: 239–248.

Burnstock, G. (1981) Neurotransmitters and trophic factors in the autonomic nervous system. *J. Physiol.*, 313: 1–35.

Chan-Palay, V. (1976) Serotonin axons in the supra- and subependymal plexuses and in the leptomeninges: their roles in local alteration of cerebrospinal fluid and vasomotor activity. *Brain Res.*, 102: 103–130.

Cunnane, J. C. and Stjärne, L. (1982) Secretion of transmitter from individual varicosities of guinea-pig and mouse vas deferens: all-or-none and extremely intermittent. *Neuroscience,* 7: 2565–2576.

Cunnane, T. C. and Stjärne, L. (1984) Transmitter secretion from individual varicosities of guinea-pig and mouse vas deferens: highly intermittent and monoquantal. *Neuroscience,* 13: 1–20.

Dale, H. H. (1935a) Reizübertragung durch chemische Mittel im peripheren Nervensystem. *Sammlung von der Nothnagel-Stiftung* veranstalteten Vorträge, Heft 4, 1–23. Urban & Schwarzenberg, Berlin, Wien.

Dale, H. H. (1935b) Pharmacology and nerve endings. *Proc. Roy. Soc. Med.*, 28: 319–332.

Dale, H. H. (1952) *Transmission of Effects from Nerve Endings,* Oxford University Press, London.

Descarries, L., Beaudet, A. and Watkins, K. C. (1975) Serotonin nerve terminals in adult rat neocortex. *Brain Res.*, 100: 563–588.

Descarries, L., Watkins, K. C. and Lapierre, Yves (1977) Noradrenergic axon terminals in the cerebral cortex of rat. III. Topometric ultrastructural analysis. *Brain Res.*, 133: 197–222.

DiFiglia, M., Aronin, N. and Leeman, S. E. (1982) Light microscopic and ultrastructural localization of immunoreactive substance P in the dorsal horn of monkey spinal cord. *Neuroscience,* 7: 1127–1139.

Dismukes, R. K. (1979) New concepts of molecular communication among neurones. *Behav. Brain Sci.*, 2: 409–448.

Eccles, J. C. (1957) *The Physiology of Nerve Cells,* Johns Hopkins Press, Baltimore.

Eccles, J. C. (1962) Spinal neurones: Synaptic connexions in relation to chemical transmitters and pharmacological responses. In B. Uvnäs (Ed.), *Proc., First Inter. Pharmacol. Meeting,* 8: 157–182, Pergamon Press, Oxford.

Eccles, J. C. (1976) From electrical to chemical transmission in the central nervous system. *Notes and Records. Roy. Soc.*, 30: 219–230.

Eccles, J. C., Fatt, P. and Koketsu, K. (1953) Cholinergic and inhibitory synapses in a central nervous pathway. *Austr. J. Sci.*, 16: 50–54.

Eccles, J. C., Fatt, P. and Koketsu, K. (1954a) Cholinergic and inhibitory synapses in a pathway from motor-axon collaterals to motoneurones. *J. Physiol.*, 126: 524–562.

Eccles, J. C., Fatt, P. and Landgren, S. (1954b) The "Direct" Inhibitory pathway in the spinal cord. *Austr. J. Sci.*, 16: 130–134.

Fagg, G. E. and Foster, A. C. (1983) Amino acid neurotransmitters and their pathways in the mammalian central nervous system. *Neuroscience,* 9: 701–720.

Feldberg, W. (1950) The role of acetylcholine in the central nervous system. *Brit. Med. Bull.*, 6: 312–321.

Gray, E. G. (1963) Electron microscopy of presynaptic organelles of the spinal cord. *J. Anat. (Lond.),* 97: 101–106.

Gray, E. G. (1966) Problems of interpreting the fine structure of vertebrate and invertebrate synapses. *Int. Rev. Gen. Exper. Zool.*, 2: 139–170.

Grossman, Y., Spira, M. E. and Parnas, I. (1973) Differential flow of information into branches of a single axon. *Brain Res.*, 64: 379–386.

Hökfelt, T., Ljungdahl, A., Terenius, L., Elde, R. and Nilsson, G. (1977) Immunohistochemical analysis of peptide pathways possibly related to pain and analgesia: enkephalin and substance P. *Proc. Natl. Acad. Sci. USA,* 74: 3081–3085.

Hökfelt, T., Lundberg, J. M., Schultzberg, M., Johansson, O., Skirboll, L., Änggård, A., Fredholm, B., Hamberger, B., Pernow, B., Rehfeld, J. and Goldstein, M. (1980) Cellular localization of peptides in neural structures. *Proc. roy. Soc. (Lond.) B,* 210: 63–77.

Iversen, L. L. (1984) Amino acids and peptides: fast and slow chemical signals in the nervous system. *Proc. roy. Soc. (Lond.) B,* 221: 245–260.

Iversen, L. L., Lee, C. M., Gilbert, R. F., Hunt, S. and Emson, P. C. (1980) Regulation of neuropeptide release. *Proc. roy. Soc. (Lond.) B,* 210: 91–111.

Jack, J. J. B., Redman, S. J. and Wong, K. (1981) The components of synaptic potentials evoked in cat spinal motoneurones by impulses in single group Ia afferents. *J. Physiol.*, 321: 65–96.

Johansson, O., Hökfelt, T., Pernow, B., Jeffevate, S. L., White, N., Steinbusch, H. W. M., Verhofstad, A. A. J., Emson, P. C. and Spindel, E. (1981) Immunohistochemical support for three putative transmitters in one neurone: coexistence of 5-hydroxytryptamine, substance P and thyrotropin releasing hormone-like immunoreactivity in medullary neurons projecting to the spinal cord. *Neuroscience*, 6: 1857–1881.

Kelly, R. B., Deutsch, J. W., Carlson, S. S. and Wagner, J. A. (1979) Biochemistry of neurotransmitter release. *Ann. Rev. Neurosci.*, 2: 399–446.

Koketsu, K. (1984) Modulation of receptor sensitivity and action potentials by transmitters in vertebrate neurones. *Jap. J. Physiol.*, 34: 945–960.

Korn, H. and Faber, D. S. (1986) Regulation and significance of probabilistic release mechanisms at central synapses. In G. M. Edelman, W. E. Gall and W. M. Cowan (Eds.), *New Insights into Synaptic Function*, Neuroscience Research Foundation, Inc., J. Wiley & Sons, Inc., New York.

Krnjevic, K. and Miledi, R. (1958) Failure of neuromuscular propagation in rats. *J. Physiol.*, 140: 440–461.

Krnjevic, K. and Miledi, R. (1959) Presynaptic failure of neuromuscular propagation in rats. *J. Physiol.*, 149: 1–22.

Lundberg, J. M. and Hökfelt, T. (1983) Coexistence of peptides and classical neurotransmitters. *Trends Neurosci.*, 6: 325–333.

McGeer, P. L., Eccles, J. C. and McGeer, E. G. (1978) *Molecular Neurobiology of the Mammalian Brain*, Plenum Press, New York.

McNaughton, B. L., Barnes, C. A. and Andersen, P. (1981) Synaptic efficiency and EPSP summation in granule cells of rat fascia dentata studied in Vitro. *J. Neurophysiol.*, 46: 952–966.

Mendell, L. M. and Henneman, E. (1971) Terminals of single Ia fibers: location, density and distribution within a pool of 300 homonymous motoneurones. *J. Neurophysiol.*, 34: 171–187.

Nicoll, R. A., Alger, B. E. and Jahr, C. E. (1980) Peptides as putative excitatory neurotransmitters: carnosine, enkephalin, substance P and TRH. *Proc. roy. Soc. (Lond.) B*, 210: 133–149.

Ochs, S., Erdman, J., Jersild, R. A. and McAdoo, V. (1978) Routing of transported materials in the dorsal root and nerve fiber branches of the dorsal root ganglion. *J. Neurobiol.*, 9: 465–481.

Otsuka, M. and Konishi, S. (1983) Substance P — the first peptide neurotransmitter?, *Trends Neurosci.*, 6: 317–320.

Potter, D. D., Furshpan, E. J. and Landis, S. C. (1981) Multiple transmitter status and "Dale's Principle". *Neurosci. Commentaries*, 1: 1–9.

Shepherd, G. M. (1983) *Neurobiology*, Oxford University Press, New York and Oxford, 436 pp.

Sneddon, P. and Westfall, D. P. (1984) Pharmacological evidence that adenosine triphosphate and noradrenaline are co--transmitters in the guinea-pig vas deferens. *J. Physiol.*, 347: 561–580.

Swanson, L. W. (1983) Neuropeptides — new vistas on synaptic transmitters. *Trends Neurosci.*, 6: 294–295.

Triller, A. and Korn, H. (1982) Transmission at a central inhibitory synapse. III. Ultrastructure of physiologically identified and stained terminals. *J. Neurophysiol.*, 48: 708–736.

Viveros, O. H., Diliberto, E. J. and Daniels, A. J. (1983) Biochemical and functional evidence for the cosecretion of multiple messengers from single and multiple compartments. *Fed. Proc. Fed. Amer. Soc. exp. Biol.*, 42: 2923–2928.

Waxman, S. C. (1972) Regional differentiation of the axon. A review with special reference to the concept of the multiplex axon. *Brain Res.*, 47: 269–288.

Wilkund, L., Toggenburger, G. and Cuenod, M. (1982) Aspartate: possible neurotransmitter in cerebellar climbing fibers. *Science, N.Y.*, 216: 78–80.

Wilkund, L., Toggenburger, G. and Cuenod, M. (1984) Selective retrograde labelling of the rat olivocerebellar climbing fiber system with D-(^{3}H) Aspartate. *Neuroscience*, 13: 441–468.

T. Hökfelt, K. Fuxe and B. Pernow (Eds.),
Progress in Brain Research, Vol. 68

CHAPTER 2

Chemical signalling in the nervous system

Leslie L. Iversen

Merck Sharp and Dohme Research Laboratories, Neuroscience Research Centre, Terlings Park, Eastwick Road, Harlow, U.K.

Development of concepts of chemical transmission

Our understanding of chemical signalling in the nervous system has advanced considerably since Elliott and Dale first elaborated the concept in the early part of this century (for review see Dale, 1954). They first proposed that the actions of nerves on peripheral muscle might be mediated by the release of adrenaline and acetylcholine. Our most detailed understanding of the process of chemical transmission still comes from the many studies that have been made of the neuromuscular junction (Katz, 1969). This system has consequently dominated our thinking about neurotransmitters and the way in which they act. It may not, however, be an accurately representative model. The neuromuscular junction is adapted for fast signalling and for the amplification of digital information. It allows the relatively tiny motor nerve terminals to control the activity of large muscle fibres, and information transfer occurs between nerve and muscle by the gating of ion channels which open and close within millisecond time intervals. The system is capable of discriminating nerve firing frequencies as high as several hundred impulses per second. Information transfer depends entirely on the precise point-to-point anatomical connections made between particular motor nerves and innervated muscles, and inhibitory circuits operate, in vertebrates at least, only at the central nervous system level. We have come to realise that many other chemical signalling mechanisms in the nervous system do not have these properties.

The development of knowledge of the roles of acetylcholine and noradrenaline in the peripheral autonomic nervous system during the first half of the century revealed that the actions of these neurotransmitters on smooth muscle, glands and other peripheral organs were often more diffuse in character. There is little precise anatomical wiring and few point-to-point synaptic connections, and the actions of the transmitters on their targets are often slow in onset and prolonged in duration. It also became apparent that the same transmitter could act on different receptors in different tissues to elicit qualitatively different actions. Thus, the effects of acetylcholine on autonomic target tissues involve muscarinic receptors, mediating slow actions that do not involve the rapid gating of ion channels, in contrast to the nicotinic receptors for acetylcholine at the neuromuscular junction. It is fitting that the present Symposium is dedicated to the memories of Professors U. S. von Euler and N. A. Hillarp who contributed so importantly to our understanding of the monoamine neurotransmitters.

The concept that chemical transmission is the predominant mode of information transfer between neurones in the central nervous system was one that physiologists at first resisted strenuously (Eccles, 1964). The discovery that catecholamines exist in discrete neuronal pathways within the mammalian CNS was a major advance during the 1950's and 1960's (Vogt, 1954; Fuxe, 1965), making it difficult to contest the involvement of these substances as CNS transmitters, although we still have only an incomplete understanding of their precise roles.

With increasing knowledge of the biochemical mechanisms associated with adrenergic neurones came increasing sophistication in understanding the process of chemical neurotransmission. The work of Greengard (1978) and others pointed to the involvement of cyclic nucleotide formation and protein phosphorylation as metabolic responses often triggered by monoamine transmitters in target cells, a type of response that is quite different in character from the fast opening of an ion channel. In recent years, the role of membrane phosphoinositides, inositol phosphates and diacylglycerol in another major "second messenger" signalling system triggered by many neurotransmitters has also been recognised (Berridge, 1984).

The description of the "autoreceptor" and other presynaptic receptors which control the amount of transmitter released from presynaptic terminals in response to nerve activity introduced a novel mechanism for modulating the function of chemically transmitting junctions (Carlsson, 1975; Langer, 1977).

The discovery of the neuropeptides as a large new family of chemical messengers in the nervous system has again radically altered our thinking about the process of chemical transmission (Hökfelt et al., 1980; Bloom, 1983; Iversen, 1983). Whereas in 1970 we considered the possibility that there might be as many as 10 different neurotransmitters, in 1985 the advent of the "peptide revolution" has brought the total number close to 50. Furthermore, the discovery that peptides may co-exist with each other or with other transmitters in the same neurones has increased even further the complexity of chemical signal processes (for review see Lundberg and Hökfelt, 1983).

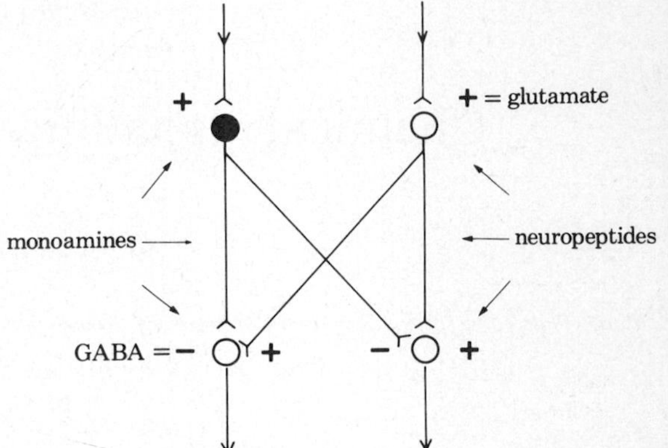

Fig. 1. Hypothetical role of GABA and glutamate as fast "ON" and "OFF" signals in anatomically addressed, point-to-point transfer of information in CNS. Monoamines and neuropeptides are postulated to act as modulators of function in the fast neural circuits. (From Iversen, 1984.)

Fast and slow chemical signalling and chemically addressed communication

Some of the differences between fast point-to-point neural circuits and slower more diffuse acting systems have been alluded to above. Figure 1 represents a simplistic view of how such systems may interact in the CNS. We now recognise that the amino acids GABA and glutamate probably represent the principal fast chemical signalling agents for OFF and ON responses respectively (Iversen, 1984). Almost all of the other brain chemical messengers may be thought of as slow-acting modulators of the mainline fast-transmitting pathways. The monoamines and neuropeptides may serve principally to modify the excitability of groups of nerve cells, operating in a slow and prolonged manner, often triggering sustained metabolic changes in the target cells (e.g. changes in the state of phosphorylation of membrane proteins). This is clearly an over-simplification: GABA and glutamate are not the only fast-acting transmitters in the mammalian CNS. Glycine may be added, at least in spinal cord, and acetylcholine acts on fast nicotinic receptors in some brain areas. Thus, the same transmitter (e.g. acetylcholine) may act both as a "fast" or as a "slow" signal depending on which receptors are concerned. The same may hold for amino acid transmitters, where multiple receptor sub-types are also emerging (Watkins and Evans, 1981; Bowery et al., 1983). However, the concept of "neuromodulation" as a common mode of chemical signalling is a useful one. It suggests, for example, that precise

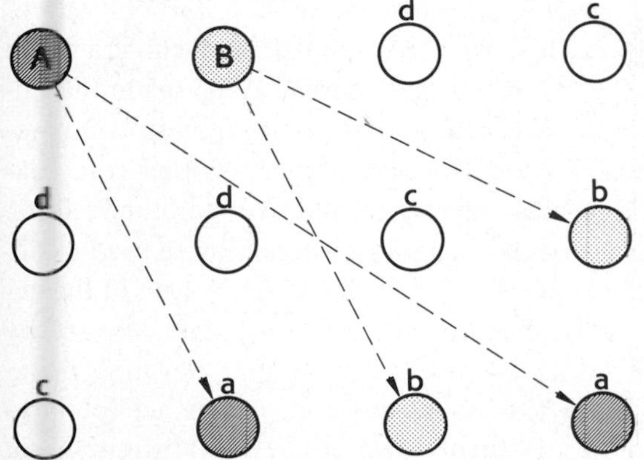

Fig. 2. The concept of "chemically addressed" transfer of information between neurones. Cells A and B release neurotransmitters A and B diffusely, but these can only be recognised by cells that possess the appropriate surface receptors (a and b).

anatomical connections between presynaptic terminals and effector cells may not always be needed or even desirable. If the function is to modify the properties of groups of neurones rather than those of individual cells, the chemical transmitter may be released in a diffuse manner, as has been suggested for catecholamines and 5-HT in brain (Descarries et al., 1975).

This concept can be taken further, as Horridge (1961) suggested. He proposed a number of hypothetical means of communication among populations of neurones. One of these he called a "chemically addressed" system, in which there was no need at all for specific anatomical connections. If different neurones release different transmitters, and if only some target cells possess receptors for these substances then a specific transfer of information is still possible (Fig. 2). This would be in contrast to the "anatomically addressed" system which corresponds to our conventional view of the nervous system. Schmitt (1984) in a valuable recent review comes to a similar conclusion, and describes what he calls the "parasynaptic" mode of communication.

In reality, many of the processes of chemical communication in the nervous system probably lie between these two extremes. In the peripheral autonomic nervous system, for example, one can discern an intermediate form — in which the neurotransmitters and neuropeptides are not released in an anatomically random manner, but there are often relatively large distances between the nerve terminals and their effector cells (Burnstock, 1981).

The recognition that the number of chemical messengers in the nervous system is large, and the further discovery that individual neurones may release mixtures of these substances makes the idea of "chemically addressed" information transfer a particularly interesting and topical one. It might even hold a key to understanding the biological significance of the phenomenon of co-existence of neuronal messengers. If one assumes that there are 50 different chemical messenger substances in the mammalian nervous system, and that all possible permutations among these are possible, then there are no less than 1,225 different permutations which neurones could contain and release, assuming they were only to contain co-existing pairs of substances. Fifty, however, is a conservative estimate of the total number of chemical messengers likely to exist in the nervous system. Furthermore, examples have already been described of neurones which contain 3, 4, 5 or even 6 different bioactive substances (see Hökfelt et al.; Costa et al., this volume). The number of chemically distinct permutations that are possible, therefore, is very large, running to many thousands. This "chemical coding" of neurones offers rich possibilities for the "chemically addressed" mode of information transfer, operating in parallel to the conventional "anatomically addressed" circuits. To understand this hypothesis we will need to know a great deal more about the mechanisms used by target cells to decipher such chemically coded information. While knowledge of the actions of neurotransmitters and neuropeptides on target cells has advanced rapidly in recent years, the great majority of studies have focussed on the actions of single substances, applied one at a time — less is known of the consequences of the exposure of cells to mixtures of agonists.

Biological effects elicited by mixtures of agonists

The concept of synergism

The actions of multiple agonists on target cells takes many forms. If one considers the interactions of two agonists, assuming that both act in similar directions, the overall effect may be simply additive or, more interestingly, there may be synergism, i.e. the combined effect is greater than the sum of the individual effects. These two phenomena are not always easily distinguished experimentally, although the above forms a useful operational definition (Gardner and Jensen, 1981).

Effects of multiple agonists on secretory cells

Some of the best studied examples of multiple agonist effects come from studies of the actions of secretagogues on glandular cells. The experiments of Gardner and Jensen (1981) on pancreatic acinar cells are particularly informative. These cells exhibit secretory responses to a number of different groups of agonists, each acting on distinct populations of cell surface receptors, these include cholinergic (muscarinic); cholecystokinin/gastrin; bombesin/litorin; tachykinin; secretin/VIP and cholera toxin (Fig. 3). Gardner and Jensen (1981) made the important observation that some agonist combinations exhibited synergism, whereas other combinations resulted merely in additive secretory effects. The nature of the agonist interaction seemed to depend on the cellular mechanism involved in the action of the secretagogue. Some agonists act by stimulating adenylate cyclase and elevating intracellular cAMP concentration; others act (perhaps through a PI breakdown mechanism) by mobilising intracellular calcium. When agonists acting by similar mechanisms were used together, the effects were additive; synergism was seen only when agonist mixtures containing compounds that act by different mechanisms were used.

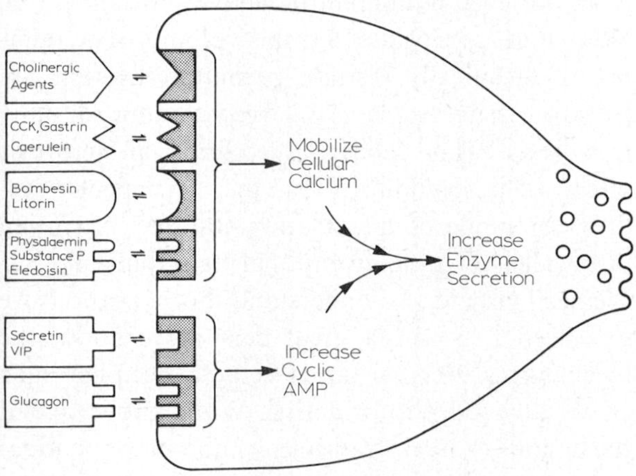

Fig. 3. Pancreatic acinar cells represent a useful model for studying agonist interactions. They respond to multiple classes of secretagogues, acting through distinct cell surface receptors; some agonists act principally by mobilising intracellular calcium, others by increasing cAMP formation. (From Gardner and Jensen, 1981.)

This observation may be of considerable relevance to understanding the biological significance of co-secretion of transmitters in the nervous system. Of the co-existing mixtures that have been described in neurones so far, it is common to find that the individual components act on different second messenger systems in target cells (Table I).

Another example of synergism has been described by Lundberg and Hökfelt (1983) in salivary gland, where they reported that acetylcholine (cal-

TABLE 1

Second messenger coupling of neuropeptide and monoamine responses

Inositol phospholipid hydrolysis activation	Adenylate cyclase
Acetycholine-muscarinic	Dopamine
Noradrenaline-α-adrenoceptors	Noradrenaline-β-adrenoceptors
Histamine-H_1 receptors	Histamine-H_2 receptors
5-Hydroxytryptamine	5-Hydroxytryptamine
Substance P	Vasoactive intestinal polypeptide
Neurotensin	Vasopressin-V_2 receptors
Cholecystokinin	
Vasopressin-V_1 receptors	

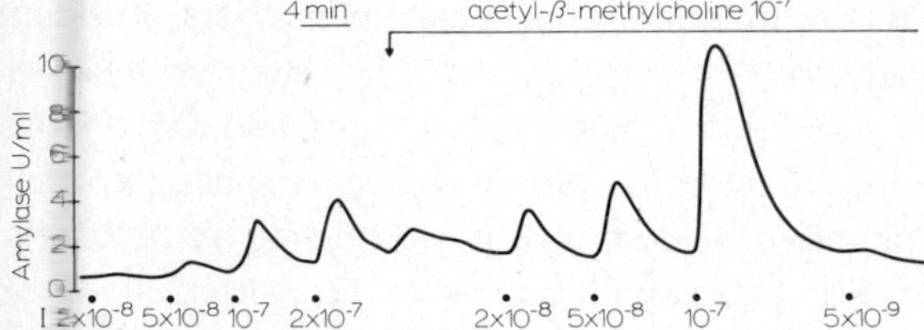

Fig. 4. Amylase release from rat parotid slices in response to isoprenaline (I) is greatly increased in presence of a muscarinic cholinergic stimulant, acetyl-β-methylcholine (10^{-7} M). Doses are given as mmol $\cdot$ l^{-1}. (From Templeton, 1980.)

cium mobilising) effects were amplified by VIP (adenylate cyclase activation). A similar amplification was observed previously between a cholinomimetic (acetyl-β-methylcholine) and an adrenoceptor stimulant (isoprenaline) in stimulating α-amylase release from rat parotid slices *in vitro* (Templeton, 1980) (Fig. 4). In recent collaborative studies

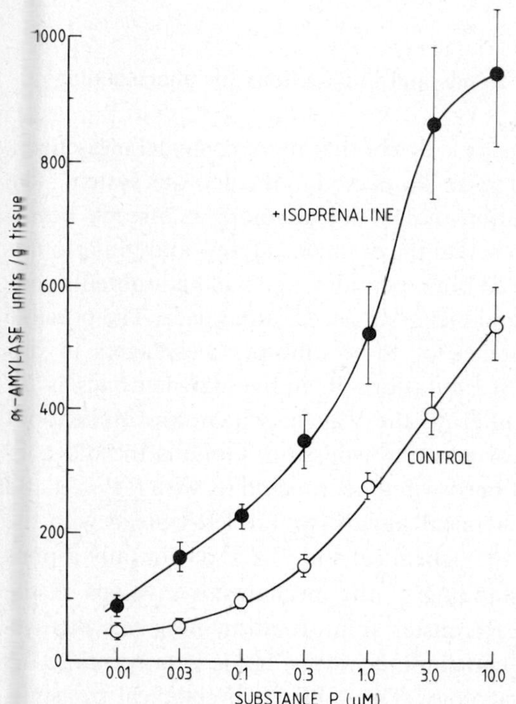

Fig. 5. Amylase release from rat parotid slices in response to substance P is enhanced by the presence of isoprenaline at a concentration (2 nM) which does not by itself cause any secretory response. (Figure redrawn from Arkle et al., 1985.)

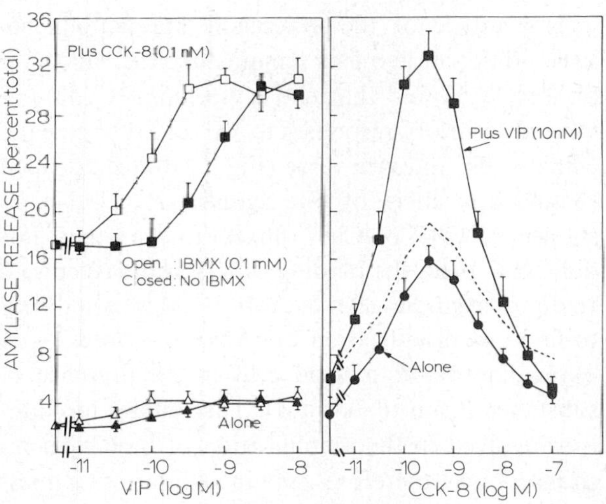

Fig. 6. Synergism between cholecystokinin C-terminal octapeptide (CCK-8) and vasoactive intestinal polypeptide (VIP) in stimulating amylase release from pancreatic acinar cells. CCK-8 greatly increases the secretory response to VIP, and the phosphodiesterase inhibitor isobutylmethylxanthine (IBMX) further enhances the VIP response. Similarly, VIP enhances the response to CCK-8 which remains biphasic in character. (From Collen et al., 1982.)

using this system, we have observed that isoprenaline considerably amplified the effects of substance P as a secretagogue (Arkle et al., 1985) (Fig. 5).

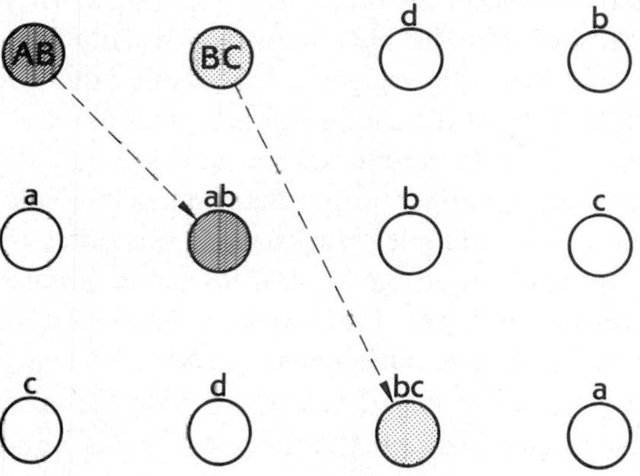

Fig. 7. Synergism between co-secreted neurotransmitters could increase the specificity of "chemically addressed" communication in the nervous system. If one assumes that transmitters A, B or C alone are unable to trigger a response in target cells but that synergistically interacting combinations are required, then only those target cells that possess the correct combination of surface receptors can respond (cf. Fig. 2).

The nature of the synergistic interactions between different agonists remains unclear. Collen et al. (1982) showed that cholecystokinin (CCK) enhanced secretory responses to VIP in rat pancreatic acinar cells, and vice versa (Fig. 6). But they failed to find any effect of one agonist on cellular responses (cAMP or Ca^{2+} fluxes) to the other, nor did CCK affect the binding of VIP to its receptors. In our own studies (Arkle et al., 1985) we also failed to find any modification of cAMP responses to isoprenaline in rat parotid cells in the presence of substance P (up to 100 μM). The cellular mechanism involved in the amplification of biological responses must, therefore, remain an interesting question for future research. The occurrence of synergism, however, raises interesting possibilities for enhancing the specificity of chemically addressed information transfer (Fig. 7).

Other agonist interactions

There are many other possible biological effects of mixtures of bioactive substances. Lundberg and Hökfelt (1983) have discussed the possible importance of co-secretion of substances with differing durations of action, so that the effects of one persist long after those of the other have diminished. They also showed that VIP may interact with cholinergic mechanisms in salivary gland by directly influencing the affinity of the cholinergic receptors for cholinergic ligands. In other cases one agonist may limit the actions of another, rather than enhancing. Substance P, for example, blocks tissue responses to nicotinic cholinergic agents, in CNS and in adrenal (for review see Ryall, 1982) without itself exerting any direct actions. One could conceive of many other possible forms of interaction: for example, one substance might protect the other by inhibiting its inactivation by metabolism or tissue uptake.

Interactions may not always take place between "slow" or "modulatory" transmitters. A number of examples are known of peptides co-existing with GABA in cortical inter-neurones, which appear to violate such a principle.

Nor is it even necessary to consider that synergistically interacting chemical messengers must always arise by co-secretion. They may be released by independent neuronal systems and act on the same target cells. Bloom and colleagues (see this volume) have described powerful synergistic effects of VIP and noradrenaline in rat cortex, both in terms of stimulating cAMP levels (Magistretti and Schorderet, 1985) and in the ability of VIP to inhibit neural firing (Ferron et al., 1985). They postulate that noradrenaline released diffusely by the tangentially arranged noradrenergic innervation to cortex may impinge on the vertically oriented VIP system to activate just those regions of cortex in which VIP neurones are active.

Receptor interactions may also take place at glial cells as well as neurones. Niehoff and Mudge (1985) have described a potentiating effect of somatostatin on cAMP responses to adrenoceptor stimulation in rat astrocytes, suggesting that both amine and peptide receptors also exist on non-neural cells.

Future trends and implications for pharmacology

There is little doubt that more chemical messengers remain to be discovered in the nervous system. The application of DNA technology is already beginning to reveal the existence of new and hitherto unsuspected brain peptides, and will undoubtedly continue to do so at an accelerating pace. The possible co-existence of these multiple messengers in different permutations in individual neurones is already altering the way in which we think about chemical neurotransmission. Gone is the old concept of hard-wired neural circuits with fast ON and OFF chemical signals, we are left instead with the era of the "chemical soup" and as yet only a poor understanding of the mechanisms involved in the chemical transfer of information in the nervous system. The future, however, holds great promise for pharmacology. The subtlety of chemical transmission is far greater than we had hitherto imagined, but the possibilities for selective pharmacological manipulation are also correspondingly larger. In the sympathetic nervous system, for example, it may be possible to alter the function of the system in particular innervated tissues without altering the properties of the whole system as with present day adrenergic drugs. In the brain, similarly, it may be possible to modify adrenergic or cholinergic function in particular brain regions without directly interfering with adrenergic or cholinergic mechanisms.

References

Arkle, S., Iversen, L. L., Michalek, R., Poat, J. A. and Templeton, D. (1985) The effect of isoprenaline on the secretory response to substance P in the rat parotid salivary gland. *Brit. J. Pharmacol.*, 86: 701.

Berridge, M. J. (1984) Inositol triphosphate and diacyclglycerol as second messengers. *Biochem. J.*, 220: 345–360.

Bloom, F. E. (1983) The endorphins: a growing family of pharmacologically pertinent peptides. *Ann. Rev. Pharmacol.*, 23: 151–170.

Bowery, N. G., Hill, D. R. and Hudson, A. L. (1983) Characteristics of $GABA_B$ receptor binding sites on rat whole brain synaptic membranes. *Brit. J. Pharmacol.*, 78: 191–206.

Burnstock, G. (1981) Neurotransmitters and trophic factors in the autonomic nervous system. *J. Physiol. (Lond.)*, 313: 1–35.

Carlsson, A. (1975) Receptor mediated control of dopamine metabolism. In E. Usdin and W. E. Bunney Jr. (Eds.), *Pre- and Postsynaptic Receptors*, Marcel Dekker, New York, pp. 49–65.

Collen, M. J., Sutliff, V. E., Pan, G. Z. and Gardner, J. D. (1982) Postreceptor modulation of action of VIP and secretin on pancreatic enzyme secretion by secretagogues that mobilize cellular calcium. *Amer. J. Physiol.*, 242: G423–428.

Dale, H. H. (1954) The beginnings and the prospects of neurohumoral transmission. *Pharmacol. Rev.*, 6: 7–13.

Descarries, L., Beaudet, A. and Watkins, K. C. (1975) Serotonin nerve terminals in adult rat neocortex. *Brain Res.*, 100: 563–588.

Eccles, J. C. (1964) *The Physiology of Synapses*, Springer-Verlag, Berlin.

Ferron, A., Siggins, G. R. and Bloom, F. E. (1985) Vasoactive intestinal polypeptide acts synergistically with norepinephrine to depress spontaneous discharge rates in cerebral cortical neurons. *Proc. nat. Acad. Sci. USA*, 82: 8810–8812.

Fuxe, K. (1965) Evidence for the existence of monoamine neurones in the central nervous system. IV. Distribution of monoamine nerve terminals in the central nervous system. *Acta physiol. Scand.*, 64, Suppl. 247: 39–85.

Gardner, J. D. and Jensen, R. T. (1981) Regulation of pancreatic exocrine secretion in vitro: the action of secretagogues. *Phil. Trans. B*, 196: 17–26.

Greengard, P. (1978) *Cyclic Nucleotides, Phosphorylated Proteins and Neuronal Function*, Raven Press, New York.

Hökfelt, T., Lundberg, J. M., Schultzberg, M., Johansson, O., Skirboll, L., Anggard, A., Fredholm, B., Hamberger, B., Pernow, B., Rehfeld, J. and Goldstein, M. (1980) Cellular localization of peptides in neural structures. *Proc. roy. Soc. B*, 210: 63–77.

Horridge, G. A. (1961) The organization of the primitive central nervous system as suggested by examples of inhibition and the structure of the neuropile. In *Nervous Inhibition*, Pergamon Press, Oxford, pp. 395–409.

Iversen, L. L. (1983) Nonopioid neuropeptides in mammalian CNS. *Ann. Rev. Pharmacol.*, 23: 1–27.

Iversen, L. L. (1984) The Ferrier Lecture, 1983: Amino acids and peptides: fast and slow chemical signals in the nervous system? *Proc. roy. Soc. B*, 221: 245–260.

Katz, B. (1969) *The Release of Neural Transmitter Substances*, Sherrington Lectures X, Liverpool University Press.

Langer, S. Z. (1977) Presynaptic receptors and their role in the regulation of transmitter release. *Brit. J. Pharmacol.*, 60: 481–497.

Lundberg, J. M. and Hökfelt, T. (1983) Coexistence of peptides and classical neurotransmitters. *Trends Neurosci.*, 6: 325–333.

Magistretti, P. J. and Schorderet, M. (1985) Norepinephrine and histamine potentiate the increase in cyclic adenosine 3′5′-monophosphate elicited by vasoactive intestinal polypeptide in mouse cerebral cortical slices: mediation by α_1-adrenergic and H_1-histaminergic receptors. *J. Neurosci.*, 5: 363–368.

Niehoff, D. L. and Mudge, A. W. (1985) Somatostatin alters β-adrenergic receptor-effector coupling in cultured rat astrocytes. *EMBO J.*, 4: 317–321.

Ryall, R. (1982) Modulation of cholinergic transmission by substance P. In R. Porter and M. O'Connor (Eds.), *Substance P in the Nervous System, CIBA Foundation Symposium 92*, Pitman, London, pp. 267–276.

Schmitt, F. O. (1984) Molecular regulators of brain function: a new view. *Neuroscience*, 4: 994–1004.

Templeton, D. (1980) Augmented amylase release from rat parotid gland slices, in vitro. *Pflügers Arch. ges. Physiol.*, 384: 287–289.

Vogt, M. (1954) The concentration of sympathin in different parts of the central nervous system under normal conditions and after the administration of drugs. *J. Physiol. (Lond.)*, 123: 451–481.

Watkins, J. C. and Evans, R. H. (1981) Excitatory amino acid transmitters. *Ann. Rev. Pharmacol.*, 21: 165–204.

SECTION II

Multiple Messengers — Overview and Evolutionary Aspects

T. Hökfelt, K. Fuxe and B. Pernow (Eds.),
Progress in Brain Research, Vol. 68

CHAPTER 3

The diffuse neuroendocrine system: peptides, amines, placodes and the APUD theory

A. G. E. Pearse

Royal Postgraduate Medical School, London W12 OHS, U.K.

Introduction

The association between amine hormone/transmitters and peptide hormone/transmitters is properly linked with the names of the two men honoured by this Symposium, Ulf von Euler and Nils-Åke Hillarp. The association now seems clear enough yet it was not always so, despite early suggestions by De Robertis (1964) and Scharrer (1969) relating to the function of neurones. For neuroendocrine cells it became evident, to me, only in 1964 when the parafollicular cells of the thyroid and ultimobranchial glands were shown to possess all the "amine-handling qualities of the other peptide-producing cells of the pre-APUD series (pituitary, gastrointestinal, pancreatic). The parafollicular cells later became the C (for calcitonin) cells when their production of this peptide was proved (Pearse, 1966a).

The co-existence of neuronal messengers of the two classes (amine and peptide), in endocrine cells widely distributed throughout the body, was laid down as the cornerstone of the original APUD concept (Pearse, 1966b,c). Their collective co-synthesis and co-secretion remains to this day the cornerstone of its successor, the APUD theory.

The APUD Theory

The original concept was based on the possession, by a series of presumptive or proven peptide hormone-producing cells, of a set of seven characteristics delineated by the acronym APUD. The term embraced the following (Pearse, 1968):

- Amine production and/or
- Amine precursor uptake
- Amino acid decarboxylase
- High esterase/cholinesterase levels
- High α-glycerophosphate dehydrogenase
- Ultrastructurally identifiable "endocrine" granules
- Specific peptide immunocytochemistry

At the outset, the last "characteristic" was almost wholly putative, since few APUD cells could be matched with a known peptide, or even with a known amine. This was due to the small number of biologically active peptides recorded at that time, and to the lack of sensitivity of existing cytochemical methods for amines.

To the first list, as set forth above, was soon added an eighth characteristic, masked metachromasia, attributed to the presence of proteins with a high cellular content of side-chain carboxyl groups (Solcia et al., 1968; Pearse, 1969). Many different suggestions were later put forward as to the nature and identity of the proteins responsible for this effect, and for the associated characteristic of argyrophilia.

New characteristics

Today, 20 years on, the total number of APUD cells exceeds 40 and a substantial proportion can be matched with known peptides and amines. Little has changed otherwise, except that almost 20 new characteristics have been described which are common to neurones in general and to the neuroendocrine cells of the APUD series. Most of them have restricted expression in cells of both classes but three are worthy of note. Two of the three have emerged as critically important indicators for neuroendocrine function while the third, the D of APUD which for many years signified the presumptive presence of the decarboxylase, is now firmly established as a true neuroendocrine function.

Neurone-specific enolase

The first of the two new indicator characteristics is known as neurone-specific enolase (NSE). This acidic soluble protein was originally extracted and purified from brain tissue by Moore and McGregor (1965), and designated by them 14.3.2. Subsequently found to be an isomer of the glycolytic enzyme 2-phospho-D-glycerate hydrolyase (enolase), the gene coding for its expression was first considered to be restricted to neurones (Marangos et al., 1978). The name NSE has been retained although it soon became clear that some APUD cells, at least, could express this neuronal isomer (Schmechel et al., 1978). NSE has now been shown to be present in all APUD cells, without exception, as well as in a high proportion of nerve cells. The main difference between the two cell types is that in the majority of neurones only specific γ-isomer is found whereas in APUD cells, and in many interneurones, both the γ- and the more universal α-isomer are co-expressed. Of particular interest, in this context, is the appearence of the γ-isomer in developing cells of the two classes. In neurones, it appears only when division has ceased and synaptic axonal contacts have been established. In the APUD endocrines, on the contrary, the γ-isomer is present at a very early stage of development. In the rat, for instance, neuronal NSE appears only at about day 9 after birth. Endocrine NSE, however, can be detected in the embryo from day E12.

Neuronal NSE is thus a marker for the late transformation of a cell committed to neural function. APUD NSE is to be interpreted rather as an indicator of the onset of neuroendocrine determination even though its role in the cell, or for that matter in the neurone, has not yet been established.

Chromogranin A

The second of the new neuroendocrine characteristics is the presence, in the storage granules, of another acidic protein, chromogranin A (CgA). This is the major soluble protein of the storage granules of the adrenomedullary cells (Smith and Winkler, 1967) in which it accounts for half the total matrix protein. It is co-secreted with the catecholamines after splanchnic stimulation (Blaschko et al., 1967). Two groups of workers, more or less simultaneously, demonstrated immunocytochemically that CgA is present in the majority of peptide-secreting neuroendocrine cells, as well as in their neoplastic counterparts (Lloyd and Wilson, 1983; O'Connor et al., 1983). It is detectable, of course, only in cells containing a sufficient number of storage granules, and with difficulty or not at all in poorly granulated examples.

The primary concern of CgA is considered to be with the binding of amine products rather than their synthesis, or the synthesis or storage of any peptide components of the granules. Human CgA contains 31.53% (g/100 g) of glutamic acid and 8.46% of aspartic acid (O'Connor et al., 1984) and Varndell et al. (1984) have surmised that this feature is responsible for the paracytochemical property of argyrophilia which is an almost invariable property of neuroendocrine granules. It is equally likely to be the protein responsible for their masked metachromasia.

Interim conclusions

It is possible to conclude, at this stage, (1) that the APUD cells constitute a diffusely distributed collection of neuroendocrine cells that may fairly be described as a system, and (2) that the manifestly neuronal properties of the cells signify only neuroendocrine function, and not a neuroectodermal origin. These two premisses provide the basis for the establishment of a Diffuse Neuroendocrine System (DNES).

So far then, the matter is a simple one. Peptides and amines are potentially co-produced and co-secreted by all neuroendocrine cells even though amine production often remains potential rather than actual. The matter becomes complicated only when one begins to ask questions, as did von Euler (1980) when he was obliged to conclude that "the full significance of the simultaneous occurrence of an amine, like 5-hydroxytryptamine, and a peptide like substance P, in the same cell has not been elucidated". Thus we are constrained to ask:

(1) Why do neuroendocrine cells express so many diverse neuronal functions.

(2) Why do both neurones and neuroendocrine cells co-produce and co-secrete so many and diverse combinations of peptides and amines.

The shortest, and most accurate answer must be "don't know" but, as a direct effect of some new cytochemical observations, it is possible to offer a revised account of the nature, and perhaps the origin, of a significant proportion of APUD cells. Exceptions, for the time being must be still the cells of the gastroenteropancreatic and genitourinary members of the series and, for oncologists, all neoplastic neuroendocrine cells wherever they may arise.

Placodal contributions to the DNES

Cells from the principal and minor placodes, local thickenings of the general head and trunk ectoderm of the embryo, provide a variety of neuroectodermal contributions to both the nervous system and the DNES. Cells from the rhombencephalic neural crest make a similar double contribution. Most of the neurones in the cranial sensory ganglia are derived from the neural crest but the trigeminal (V) has neurones of mixed placodal and crest origin. In the trunk ganglia (geniculate VII, petrosal IX, nodose X), on the contrary, all the neurones are placodal and the crest contributes only the glial satellite cells (Narayanan and Narayanan, 1980; Thiery and Le Douarin, 1981).

If, for the present purposes, we except the brain, the pineal gland and the olfactory system, all of which are indisputably placodal, the first DNES component we must consider is the anterior hypophysis. Recent cytochemical evidence supports its identity as a placode, and this accords with the long held view of at least a minority of embryologists. The endocrine cells of the hypophysis are APUD cells although, in the majority of species, overt amine-handling functions are restricted to the corticotrophs. Human and mouse prolactin cells have been shown to decarboxylate dopa (Takor-Takor and Pearse, 1973) and Iturriza et al. (1983) found that rat prolactin cells, in renal capsule transplants, could express tyrosine hydroxylase and synthesise dopamine although they do not normally do so.

The nature of the so-called folliculo-stellate cells of the hypophysis remained an enigma until recent cytochemical investigations, carried out by two separate groups of workers (Cocchia and Miani, 1980; Nakajima et al., 1980) demonstrated their possession of the glial marker protein S-100.

There are two possible explanations for the coexistence in the hypophysis of placodal endocrine cells and glial satellite cells. Both could be, as in the central nervous system, the progeny of a single neuroectodermal precursor. This cell would give rise equally to neurones and glia. Alternatively, the endocrine cells could be ectodermal, as indeed they are, and the folliculo-stellate cells a glial component of neural crest origin. Some observers specifically deny the reality of a crest contribution to the anterior hypophysis (Levy et al., 1980) but others (Rosenquist, 1981) do allow an input from this source to Rathke's pouch. Of these two premises, the second is the more attractive. If it is true, we can regard the hypophysis as the originally bilateral equivalent of a cranial or trunk sensory ganglion with placodal endocrine and crest-derived satellite cells.

The thyroid and ultimobranchial C cells need only brief consideration. They are proved derivatives of neural crest and are therefore placodal in the broad sense since the crest, derived from the junctional region between ectoderm and neural folds, can legitimately be so regarded.

Next on the list for consideration are the endocrine cells of the parathyroid gland. These founder members of the APUD series, failing to satisfy a sufficiency of the requisite criteria, were removed from the list in 1966. Sometimes temporarily reinstated, their apparent failure to express either amine-handling functions or the specific enolase (NSE) provided an absolute requirement for exclusion. Apart from their possessions of endocrine storage granules the only other APUD characteristic shown by parathyroid cells is their high content of α-glycerophosphate dehydrogenase, considered to reflect high levels of synthesis of α-phosphatidic acid and phosphoglycerides. This characteristic they share with neurones. When it became apparent that the chief cell storage granules contain the neuroendocrine marker CgA (O'Connor et al., 1983) urgent reappraisal of the status of the cells was required.

The parathyroid glands have always been regarded as derivatives of the 3rd and 4th endodermal pharyngeal pouches but Pearse and Takor-Takor (1976, 1979) provided morphological evidence that the anuran parathyroid was wholly ectodermal in origin, and hence to be regarded as a placode. For avian and mammalian species, a double origin from ectoderm and endoderm was accepted but it was concluded that "placodal ectoderm probably constitutes the major component of both avian and mammalian parathyroid glands". I see no reason to modify this conclusion, particularly in view of the latest evidence (Weber et al., 1985) that both normal and neoplastic human parathyroid tissues contain NSE levels significantly higher than those attributable to their autonomic nerve supply.

If the presence of significant NSE levels in the chief cells can be confirmed in other species, the parathyroid must be reinstated as a full member of the APUD series despite its non-expression of the amine-handling facility. This lack is the more extraordinary if one considers the significance of the presence in its granules of the amine storage protein CgA.

TABLE I

Cell type	NE cell origin	Satellite origin
Hypothalamic	N	N (glia)
Olfactory	Plac	(NC)
Pineal	N	N
Pituitary	Plac	NC
Thyroid C	NC	nil
Parathyroid	Plac	nil
Merkel	Plac	(NC)
Adrenomedullary	NC	NC
Cranial ganglion	N/Plac	NC
Trunk ganglion	Plac	NC

High levels of NSE are present in the Merkel cells of mammalian epidermis (Gu et al., 1981) but their chromogranin content is not demonstrable cytochemically since the cells are always poorly granulated. While there is some doubt as to the origin of these cutaneous mechanoreceptor cells, it is increasingly likely that they are placodal rather than neural crest derivatives. As such they are therefore recorded in Table I, below, although complete proof of this origin is not yet available.

Three possible DNES recipients of a placodal component remain for discussion. These are the carotid body and the adrenal medulla and paraganglia. A number of different origins have been proposed, in the past, for the carotid body, including the ectobranchial placodes (Murillo-Ferrol, 1967). It was conclusively demonstrated by Le Douarin et al. (1972), using the biological marker system in quail-chick chimaeras, that the type 1 cells are neural crest derivatives, and Fontaine (1973) showed that in these two species the cells are true APUD cells although they produce two different amines, 5-hydroxytryptamine in the chick and dopamine in the quail (Pearse et al., 1973). The type 2 supporting cells of the carotid body have presumably the same origin as the type 1 cells, although an ectobranchial placodal contribution to the carotid body has never been excluded.

The adrenomedullary endocrine cells, shown conclusively by Teillet and Le Douarin (1974) to be derived from the neural crest, are supported by glial type satellite cells containing the marker protein S-100 and presumably sharing the same origin. No other placodal component has been suggested as contributing to either class of cell. The constitution of the paraganglia is precisely the same as that of the adrenal medulla.

Table I summarises the established or possible origins of the neuroendocrine cells listed, and of their satellites where present. For comparison, the status of the neurones and satellites of the sensory ganglia is appended.

Concluding comments

Perusal of the facts presented generates a host of questions, of which the most outstanding fall into three distinct groups:

(1) Why do neuroendocrine APUD cells co-express such a wide variety of neuronal functions?

(2) If the parathyroid is a neuroendocrine placode, why is there no glial component, and no amine production?

(3) In the neuroendocrine APUD cells, is there a causal relationship between the production of amines and/of peptides?

The answers to all these questions are far from satisfactory but an attempt to answer them cannot be avoided.

Neuroendocrine functions in APUD cells

"Being of diverse origin they have evolved similar biochemical mechanisms for the production of ...... polypeptides" (Pearse, 1969). This was one of the original suggestions put forward to account for the common characteristics shared by all neuroendocrine cells, and particularly for their co-production of amines and peptides. Whether their origin is diverse or not, is this still a reasonable speculation? Clearly it is not for few of the functions which the cells share with neurones can be linked directly with any particular aspect of their metabolism. In particular, their early expression of NSE remains an enigma.

I have attempted here, once again, leaving aside the controversial gastrointestinal/pancreatic and genitourinary groups of APUD cells, to link the other groups together by postulating a more or less common origin from committed neuroendocrine stem cells. Inclusion of the parathyroid is still provisional but for the others existing evidence is more than sufficient to justify their revised status.

The parathyroid as a placode

Neuroendocrine and neural placodes are generally associated with a glial component of neural crest origin. Why then has the parathyroid no glial component (and no crest component except for the variable presence in the gland of calcitonin-secreting C cells). Why is CgA present in the storage granules when apparently no amine is co-stored with parathyroid hormone; and why, until now, has no other neuroendocrine peptide been shown to be co-synthesised and stored? No easy answer to the first question is to be found, but evidence has recently been provided (Weber et al., 1985) for the presence in the parathyroid of significant amounts of somatostatin. One distinct and significant difference between the parathyroid and the other neuroendocrine cells of the DNES should always be remembered. This is that the parathyroid is some 200 million years junior in evolutionary terms, to all the other members of the system.

Co-existence of amines and peptides in neuroendocrine cells

This question has been outstanding since the original formulation of the APUD theory. An attempt was made by Welsch and Pearse (1969) to elucidate the role of the amine-handling function in thyroid C cells, but no specific relationship was found between amine levels and the synthesis of the protein (cholinesterase) which was used as a marker for general protein synthesis and secretion. Modern studies, using more appropriate neuroendocrine markers, are certainly overdue. Viveros and his colleagues (Viveros et al., 1983) have proposed, for adrenomedullary cells and by inference for all neurones and neuroendocrine cells, a complex arrangement of secreting compartments for the export of multiple transmitters. While stressing the fact that co-existence cannot be construed as co-storage, they were unable to supply evidence of any causal relationship between pairs of transmitters. No significant evidence on this point appears to be available from other sources.

I am obliged, therefore, to fall back on a long-held personal view of the evolutionary sequence of events, unsubstantiated by experimental evidence and hence totally speculative. This is that a need for storage of the original amine hormone/transmitter, produced by the single cell neuroendocrine ancestor, required the synthesis of storage proteins (and other granule constituents). One of these might be the primeval CgA while others would be ancestral prepropeptides. Thus the association between amines and peptides would be fortuitous or at the least indirect, and synthesis of the one would clearly be independent of the other and independently variable. Thus cells of a single type would (do) vary their expressed peptide levels, their expressed amine levels, and the identities of both amine and peptide so as to provide an exceedingly broad spectrum of variations.

Some aspects of these hypotheses, such as the evolutionary back tracing of CgA and of amine storage in general, can be tested immediately with little difficulty, others must await the application of modern cytochemical and hybridocytochemical technology.

References

Blaschko, H., Comline, R. S., Schneider, R. H., Silver, M. and Smith, A. D. (1967) Secretion of a granule protein, chromogranin, from the adrenal gland after splanchnic stimulation. *Nature (Lond.)*, 215: 58–59.

Cocchia, D. and Miani, N. (1980) Immunocytochemical localization of the brain-specific S-100 protein in the pituitary gland of adult rat. *J. Neurocytol.*, 9: 771–782.

De Robertis, E. D. P. (1964) *Histophysiology of Synapses and Neurosecretion*, Pergamon Press, Oxford, pp. 1–24.

Fontaine, J. (1973) Contribution a l'étude du dévelopment du corps carotidien et du corps ultimobranchial des oiseaux. *Arch. Anat. Micr. Morph. Exp.*, 62: 89–100.

Gu, J., Polak, J. M., Tapia, F. J., Marangos, P. J. and Pearse, A. G. E. (1981) Neurone-specific enolase in the Merkel cell of mammalian skin. *Amer. J. Pathol.*, 104: 63–68.

Iturriza, F. C., Rubio, M. C., Gomez Dumm, C. L. A. and Zieher, L. M. (1983) Catecholamine metabolising enzymes and synthesis of dopamine in normal and grafted pituitary pars distales. *Neuroendocrinology*, 37: 371–377.

Le Douarin, N., Le Liévre, C. and Fontaine, J. (1972) Recherches expérimentale sur l'origine embryologique du corps carotidien chez les oiseaux. *C. R. Acad. Sci. (Paris)*, 275: 583–586.

Levy, N. B., Andrew, A., Rawdon, B. B. and Kramer, B. (1980) Is there a ventral neural ridge in chick embryos? Implications for the origin of adenohypophyseal and other APUD cells. *J. Embryol. exp. morphol.*, 57: 71–78.

Lloyd, R. V. and Wilson, B. S. (1983) Specific endocrine tissue marker defined by a monclonal antibody. *Science*, 222: 628–630.

Marangos, P. J., Zis, A. P., Clark, R. L. and Goodwin, F. K. (1978) Neuronal non-neuronal and hybrid forms of enolase in brain: Structural, immunological and functional comparison. *Brain Res.*, 150: 117–133.

Moore, B. W. and McGregor, D. (1965) Chromatographic and electrophoretic fractionation of soluble proteins of brain and liver. *J. Biol. Chem.*, 240: 1947–1953.

Murillo-Ferrol, N. L. (1967) The development of the carotid body in Gallus domesticus. *Acta Anat. (Basel)*, 68: 102–126.

Nakajima, T., Yamaguchi, H. and Takahashi, K. (1980) S-100 protein in folliculo-stellate cells of the rat anterior pituitary lobe. *Brain Res.*, 191: 523–531.

Narayanan, C. H. and Narayanan, Y. (1980) Neural crest and placodal contributions in the development of the glossopharyngeal complex of the chick. *Anat. Rec.*, 196: 71–82.

O'Connor, D. T., Burton, D. and Deftos, L. J. (1983) Immunoreactive human chromogranin A in diverse polypeptide hormone producing tumors and normal endocrine tissues. *J. clin. Endocr.*, 57: 1084–1086.

O'Connor, D. T., Frigon, R. P. and Sokoloff, R. L. (1984) Human chromogranin A: purification and characterization from catecholamine storage vesicles of pheochromocytoma. *Hypertension*, 6: 2–12.

Pearse, A. G. E. (1966a) The cytochemistry of the thyroid C cells and their relationship to calcitonin. *Proc. roy. Soc. B*, 164: 478–487.

Pearse, A. G. E. (1966b) 5-Hydroxytryptophan uptake by dog thyroid C cells and its possible significance in polypeptide hormone production. *Nature (Lond.)*, 211: 598–600.

Pearse, A. G. E. (1968) Common cytochemical and ultrastructural characteristics of cells producing polypeptide hormones (the APUD series) and their relevance to thyroid and ultimobranchial C cells and calcitonin. *Proc. roy. Soc. B,* 170: 71–80.

Pearse, A. G. E. (1969) Random coil conformation of polypeptide hormone precursor protein in endocrine cells. *Nature (Lond.),* 221: 1210–1211.

Pearse, A. G. E. and Takor-Takor, T. (1976) Neuroendocrine embryology and the APUD concept. *Clin. Endocr.,* 5, Suppl.: 2295–2443.

Pearse, A. G. E. and Takor-Takor, T. (1979) Embryology of the diffuse neuroendocrine system and its relationship to the common peptides. *Fed. Proc.,* 38: 2288–2294.

Pearse, A. G. E., Polak, J. M., Rost, F. W. D., Fontaine, J., Le Liévre, C. and Le Douarin, N. (1973) Demonstration of the neural crest origin of type 1 (APUD) cells in the avian carotid body, using a cytochemical marker system. *Histochemie,* 34: 191–203.

Rosenquist, G. C. (1981) Epiblast origin and early migration of neural crest cells in the chick embryo. *Dev. Biol.,* 87: 201–211.

Scharrer, B. (1969) Neurohumors and neurohormones. *J. Neurovisc. Relations,* Suppl. 9: 1–20.

Schmechel, D., Marangos, P. J. and Brightman, M. (1978) Neurone-specific enolase is a marker for peripheral and central neuroendocrine cells. *Nature (Lond.),* 276: 834–836.

Smith, A. D. and Winkler, H. (1967) Purification and properties of an acidic protein from chromaffin granules of bovine adrenal medulla. *Biochem. J.,* 103: 483–492.

Solcia, E., Vasallo, G. and Capella, C. (1968) Selective staining of endocrine cells by basic dyes after acid hydrolysis. *Stain Technol.,* 43: 257–263.

Takor-Takor, T. and Pearse, A. G. E. (1973) Cytochemical identification of human and murine corticotrophs and somatotrophs as APUD cells. *Histochemie,* 37: 207–214.

Teillet, M. A. and Le Douarin, N. M. (1974) Détermination par la méthode des greffes hétérospécifiques d'ebauches neurales de caille sur l'embryo de poulet, du niveau du névraxe dont les cellules médullosurrénaliennes. *Arch. Anat. micro. Morph. exp.,* 63: 51–61.

Thiery, J. P. and Le Douarin, N. M. (1981) Mechanisms and migration and differentiation of neural crest cells. In C. Raybaud, R. Clement, G. Lebreuil and J.-L. Bernard (Eds.), *Pediatric Ocology,* Excerpta Medica, Amsterdam, pp. 3–18.

Varndell, I. M., Bishop, A. E., Lloyd, R. V., Wilson, B. S., Grimelius, L., Pearse, A. G. E. and Polak, J. M. (1984) Chromogranin A immunocytochemistry: possible correlation with Grimelius argyrophilia. *J. Pathol.,* 143: 199A–200A.

Viveros, O. H., Diliberta, E. J. and Daniels, A. J. (1983) Biochemical and functional evidence of the co-secretion of multiple messengers from single and multiple compartments. *Fed. Proc.,* 42: 2923–2928.

Weber, C., Marangos, P., Richardson, S., LoGerfo, P., Hardy, M., Feind, C. and Reetsma, K. (1985) Presence of enolase and somatostatin in human parathyroid tissues. *Proc. Amer. Ass. Endocr. Surgeons* (Abstract), p. 15.

Welsch, U. and Pearse, A. G. E. (1969) Elecyron cytochemistry of butyryl cholinesterase and acetylcholinesterase in thyroid and parathyroid C cells under normal and experimental conditions. *Histochemie,* 7: 1–10.

T. Hökfelt, K. Fuxe and B. Pernow (Eds.),
Progress in Brain Research, Vol. 68

CHAPTER 4

Coexistence of neuronal messengers — an overview

Tomas Hökfelt[1,*], Vicky R. Holets[1], William Staines[1], Björn Meister[1], Tor Melander[1], Martin Schalling[1], Marianne Schultzberg[1], Jacob Freedman[1], Håkan Björklund[1], Lars Olson[1], Björn Lindh[2], Lars-Gösta Elfvin[2], Jan M. Lundberg[3], Jan Åke Lindgren[4], Bengt Samuelsson[4], Bengt Pernow[5], Lars Terenius[6], Claes Post[7], Barry Everitt[8] and Menek Goldstein[9]

Department of [1]Histology, [2]Anatomy, [3]Pharmacology and [4]Biochemsitry, Karolinska Institutet, Stockholm, [5]Department of Clinical Physiology, Karolinska Hospital, Stockholm, [6]Department of Pharmacology, Uppsala University, Uppsala, [7]Astra Pharmaceuticals, Södertälje, Sweden, [8]Department of Anatomy, Cambridge University, Cambridge, U.K., and [9]Department of Psychiatry, New York University Medical Center, New York, NY, U.S.A.

Introduction

Involvement of a chemical messenger in the transmission of nerve impulses between neurons and effector cells was first recognized in the peripheral nervous system (PNS) by Elliott (1905) in the beginning of this century (see Dale 1935 and book edited by Stjärne et al., 1981). Firm evidence for chemical transmission in the central nervous system (CNS) was, however, obtained considerably later (Eccles et al., 1954). Much interest has been focused on identifying potential chemicals which could be involved in transmission at synapses. For a long time the number of candidates was small and included catecholamines and acetylcholine (ACh). With regard to the CNS, ACh was the only generally accepted transmitter for quite some time (see Eccles, 1964, 1976), but the number of candidates increased fairly rapidly. Thus, in 1954 Vogt (1954) showed that noradrenaline (NA) has an uneven distribution in the brain, adding a further compound with a possible transmitter role. The histofluorescence studies of Hillarp, Falck, Carlsson, Fuxe, Dahlström and their collaborators strongly supported this view, by, for the first time demonstrating the cellular localization of a transmitter candidate (noradrenaline) in the microscope with formaldehyde-induced fluorescence (Carlsson et al., 1962; Dahlström and Fuxe, 1964, 1965; Fuxe, 1965a,b). It soon became clear that also the NA precursor dopamine (DA) may have an independent role in the CNS, possibly as a transmitter in basal ganglia (see Carlsson et al., 1958). In the 1960's the amino acids came into focus. Evidence was presented that γ-aminobutyric acid (GABA) and glycine may represent important inhibitory transmitters in the brain and that glutamate may act as an excitatory transmitter (see e.g. books edited by Roberts et al., 1976 and by Fonnum, 1978).

During the 1970's an explosive development took place in the area of peptides which today outnumber the classical transmitters in the brain and periphery (see Snyder, 1980). The rapid progress in biochemistry has turned out many new peptides and peptide families and left us in a situation, where our understanding of the possible physiological significance of peptides in neurotransmission is fragmentary. For some of these peptides a transmitter

* *Address for correspondence:* Tomas Hökfelt, Department of Histology, Karolinska Institutet, Box 60400, S-104 01 Stockholm, Sweden.

role has been suggested, for example, for substance P (Otsuka and Takahashi, 1977; Pernow, 1983). Therefore, our view on chemical transmission has become more complex and differentiated. Apparently the various types of compounds differ in parameters such as time course and mechanisms of action. For example, amino acids seem to be involved in fast transmission processes, whereas neuropeptides and monoamines often exert effects with slow onset and of a long duration (see Bloom, 1979; Iversen, 1984; Schmitt, 1984).

The huge number of transmitter candidates has raised the question whether or not there is room in the nervous system to "accommodate" each of them in individual systems, and a partial answer to this question is that in many cases more than one type of messenger molecule may be present in a neuron. Thus, as initially observed in endocrine cells (see Pearse, 1969; Owman et al., 1973) and in invertebrates (see Osborne, 1983), and as earlier discussed by Burnstock (1976) and Smith (1976), there is evidence that neurons may produce, store and perhaps release several messengers (see Hökfelt et al., 1980a,b, 1982, 1984b; Potter et al., 1981; Osborne, 1983a; and books edited by Cuello, 1982; Osborne, 1983b; Chan-Palay and Palay, 1984).

The development in the field of neurotransmitter receptors has been equally dynamic. Starting with a one transmitter — one receptor model (Fig. 1A), it was later realized that a transmitter may act at multiple postsynaptic receptor sites (e.g. α- and β-receptors) (Fig. 1B) and also that presynaptic receptors exist (Fig. 1C) (for reference see book edited by Stjärne et al., 1981). Today advanced methods are available for characterization of various transmitter receptor sites (see Snyder, 1979), and there are now data demonstrating a multiplicity of ion channels of different type, which could represent the receptive post- (or pre-) synaptic counterpart of multiple synaptic messengers (see e.g. Siegelbaum and Tsien, 1983; Hille, 1984).

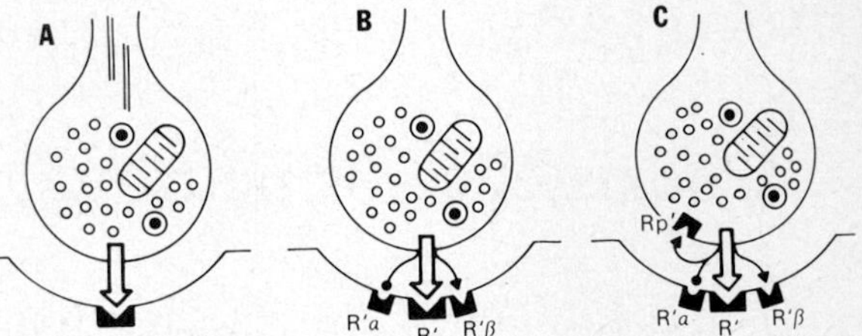

Fig. 1A–C. Schematic illustration of the development of the transmitter-receptor relation. Initially a transmitter was assumed to react with a single type of postsynaptic receptor (A). It was then recognized that the same receptor could act at different types of postsynaptic receptors (α-, β-receptors etc.) (B) More recently it has been realized that there also exist presynaptic receptors (autoreceptors) (C).

The finding of multiple messengers in a neuron raises a number of questions concerning the process of chemical transmission. In this article we would like to briefly summarize some aspects on these problems. The work on coexisting messenger molecules is up till now very much based on histochemical studies, mainly immunohistochemistry (see Coons, 1958), which permits visualization of several antigens in one cell. We would therefore first like to briefly discuss some aspects on this method, which has been the basis for much of our work.

Aspects on methodology

Multiple antigens in a neuron can be demonstrated with various approaches (Fig. 2). First, the *"adjacent section"* method can be employed (Fig. 2-I). Consecutive sections are incubated with different primary antisera. The strength of this technique is

Fig. 2. Schematic illustration of three different approaches (I–III) to visualize two antigens in the same cell. (I) Thin adjacent sections (A and B) are incubated with antiserum to substance P (SP) (B) and 5-hydroxytryptamine (5-HT), respectively. Cells I–III can be recognized in both sections, and one, no. 3 has both antigens, whereas 1 and 2 contain SP- and 5-HT-LI, respectively. Note that with this approach coexistence in nerve terminals can not be demonstrated in view of their small size. (II) With the elution/restaining technique one section (A′) is incubated with SP antiserum, the staining pattern is photographed and the section is eluted. After control incubation with FITC conjugated antibodies, which should reveal complete lack of fluorescence (B′), the same section is restained with 5-HT antiserum and the staining pattern photographed (C′) and compared with the previous one. Again, it can be established

I. ADJACENT SECTIONS

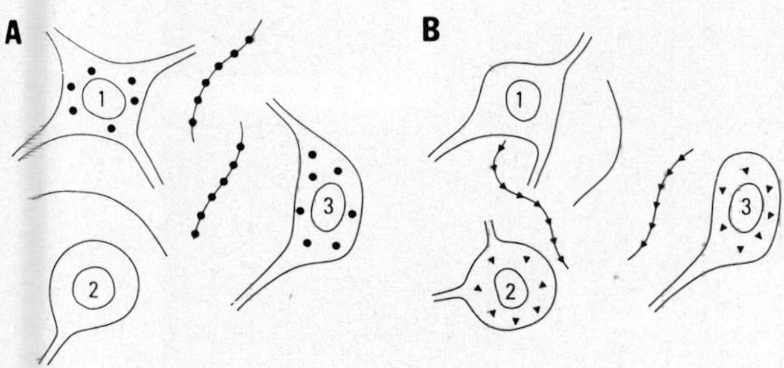

II. ELUTION/RESTAINING

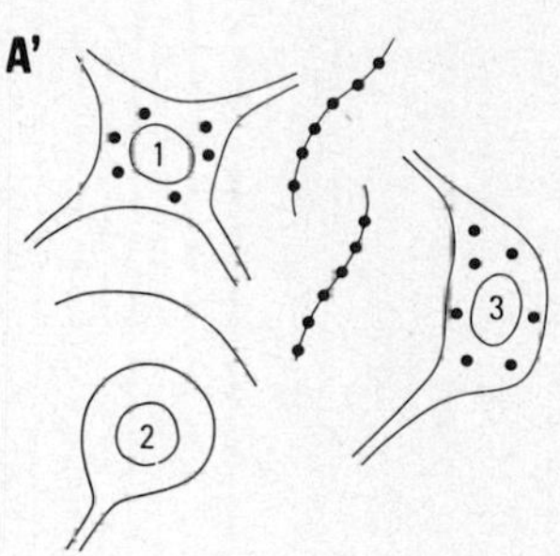

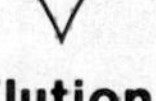

Elution

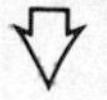

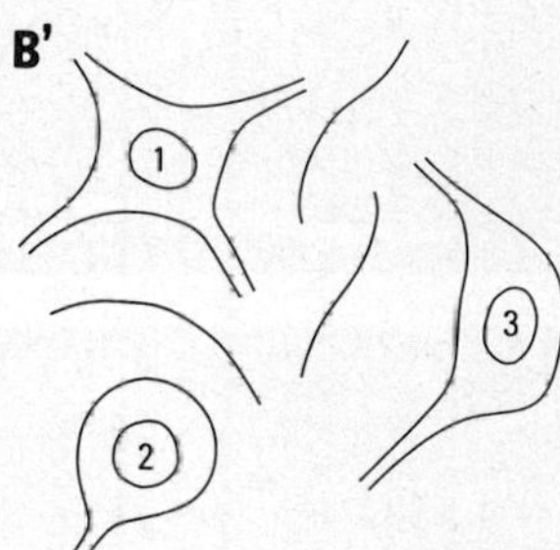

Restaining

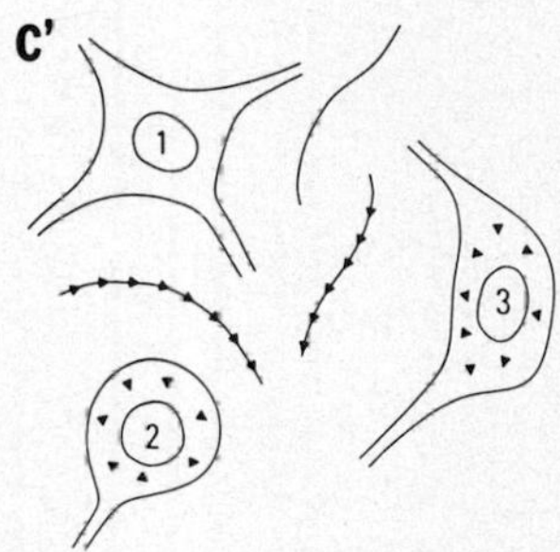

III. DOUBLE-STAINING

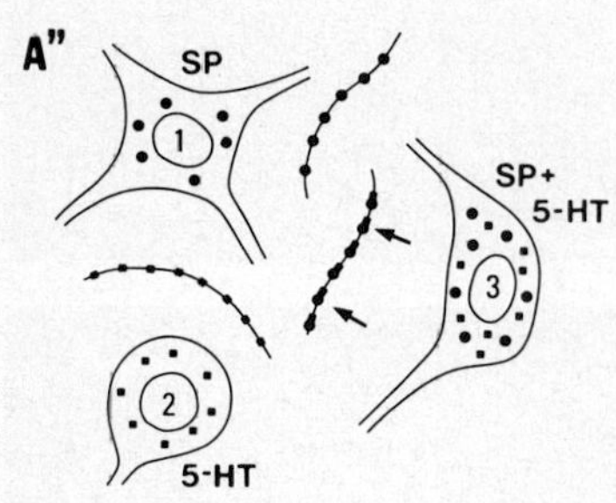

Primary antibody	Secondary antibody
Rabbit anti-SP	Swine anti-rabbit FITC ●● green
Rabbit anti-5-HT	Swine anti-rabbit FITC ▲▲ green
Guinea-pig anti-5-HT	Goat anti-guinea-pig TRITC ■■ red

that cell no. 3 contains both antigens. (III) With the double-staining technique a section (A″) is incubated with a mixture of SP antiserum raised in rabbit and 5-HT antiserum raised in guinea pig. The secondary antibodies are labeled with green fluorescent, FITC conjugated swine anti-rabbit antibodies and red fluorescent, TRITC conjugated goat anti-guinea pig antibodies. By switching between the two filters, it can be directly established that cell no. 3 contains both antigens. In addition, it can be shown that some nerve endings (arrows) contain both compounds.

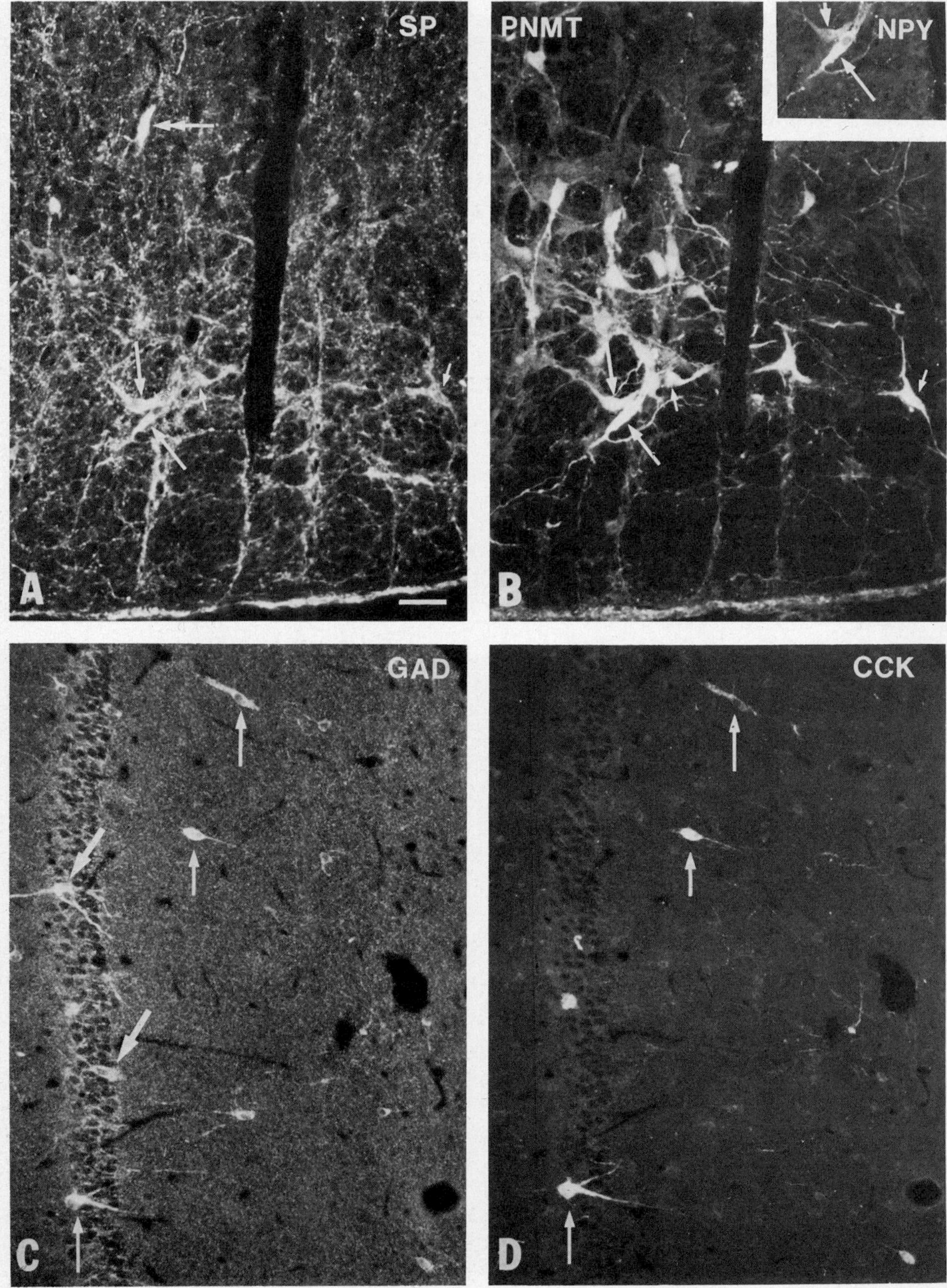
SP
PNMT
NPY
GAD
CCK
A
B
C
D

that no interference between antisera can occur, and thus no problems of specificity are encountered. The procedure is critically dependent on the relation between the size of the immunoreactive structures and the thickness of the sections. Provided that the sections are thin enough, the same cell body can often be identified in two or even more consecutive sections. The use of thick sections (50–100 μm), cut on a Vibratome or cryostat, as often used in conjunction with the peroxidase-antiperoxidase (PAP) method (Sternberger et al., 1970), precludes the use of the *"adjacent section"* method. With cryostat sections, which often are about 10–15 μm thick, proper identification is sometimes difficult to carry out. At 5 μm thickness acceptable results are mostly obtained, but the immunostaining of such thin sections may sometimes not be satisfactory. Ideally, plastic or epoxy resin embedded material should be used, allowing sections to be cut at 1 μm or even less (see e.g. Berod et al., 1984).

Secondly, *"elution-restaining"* methods can be used (Fig. 2-II). Nakane (1968) first showed that one staining pattern can be eluted and the same section then reincubated with a new antiserum and analyzed for identity of labeled cells. Using the peroxidase method, dyes with various colors can be used, and in this way double labeling can be directly seen in the same section. With fluorescence methods, the first staining pattern has to be photographed before elution (Fig. 2-II). The procedure of Tramu et al. (1978) is much used and is based on acid potassium permanganate as eluent. A disadvantage with this approach is that the elution procedure may partially or completely destroy antigens. Thus, antisera to certain antigens may not be used in this procedure. Also, negative results obtained after restaining may merely mean that the second antigen has been destroyed and should therefore be interpreted with caution. Thus, these types of studies are preferably carried out with "powerful" antisera, which give a strong immunostaining, even when part of the antigen in the section has been destroyed. It should also be emphasized that proper control incubations have to be carried out to ensure complete elution of the first antibody.

Finally, the *"direct double-staining"* method can be used, if antisera raised in different species are available. Thus, two antigens can be simultaneously visualized in the same section using secondary antibodies labeled with different dyes, for example, red fluorescent tetramethylrhodamine isothiocyanate (rhodamine; TRITC) and green fluorescent fluorescein isothiocyanate (FITC) (Fig. 2-III). Mainly because antisera usually are raised in rabbits and proper combination possibilities have been lacking, this approach has not been extensively used up till now. It will certainly be more often applied with the introduction of monoclonal antibodies as well as antisera raised in goats, guinea pigs and other species. With this technique one can directly decide whether coexistence is present or not by switching between filter combinations for red and green fluorescence (Figs. 3, 8 and 18). In Fig. 3A,B we have used this double-labeling technique to demonstrate that some adrenaline neurons of the C1 group (Hōkfelt et al., 1973, 1974, 1984c), visualized by the adrenaline-synthesizing enzyme phenylethanolamine-*N*-methyltransferase (PNMT) contain substance P-like immunoreactivity (LI), confirming recently

Fig. 3A–D. Immunofluorescence micrographs of two sections incubated according to the double-staining technique. A and B are taken from the ventrolateral medulla oblongata and C and D from the hippocampal formation. A and B show the same section incubated with a mixture of antiserum to substance P (SP) and phenylethanolamine-*N*-methyltransferase (PNMT), a marker for adrenaline neurons. The section has then in addition been eluted and restained with antiserum to neuropeptide Y (NPY) (inset). C and D show the same section which has been incubated with antiserum to the GABA synthesizing enzyme glutamic acid decarboxylase (GAD) and cholecystokinin (CCK) (D). A and C have been labeled with green fluorescent, FITC conjugated antibodies and B and D with red fluorescent, TRITC conjugated antibodies. (A,B) Some cells (arrows) contain both SP- and PNMT-LI, as well as NPY-LI. Single cells (double headed arrow) contain only SP-LI, but most cells are PNMT-positive/SP-negative. (C,D) Many cells (thin arrows) contain both GAD- and CCK-LI and other neurons (thick arrows) apparently contain only GAD-LI. Bar indicates 50 μm. All micrographs have the same magnification.

published results by Lorenz et al. (1985). Thus, substance P-LI (Fig. 3A) is demonstrated with a rat monoclonal antibody and green FITC-induced fluorescence and PNMT-LI (Fig. 3B) with a rabbit antiserum and red rhodamine-induced fluorescence. In addition, the inset to Fig. 3B shows neuropeptide (NPY)-LI in two cells which also contain substance P- and PNMT-LI. The NPY-LI was demonstrated after elution of the substance P and PNMT antisera and restaining with NPY antiserum (see Fig. 2-II). A further example of coexistence is shown with the double-staining method using a sheep antibody against glutamic acid decarboxylase (GAD) (Fig. 3C), a marker for GABA neurons, and a rabbit antibody to cholecystokinin (CCK) (Fig. 3D). Proper control experiments and selection of appropriate secondary antisera have to be carried out to avoid false positives, for example, due to the fact that the secondary antisera react with each other.

The immunohistochemical technique represents a powerful method with apparent advantages and a virtually unlimited potential, but problems with specificity and sensitivity are present. When using immunological techniques the peptide field represents a particularly difficult situation with regard to specificity, since structurally similar peptides ("peptide families") exist. Thus, the antisera raised against a certain peptide may cross-react with other members of the family and, of course, also with other peptides (proteins) containing related amino acid sequences. Expressions such as "substance P-like immunoreactivity", "substance P-immunoreactive" or "substance P-positive" are therefore often used in immunohistochemical and radioimmunological studies.

The sensitivity problem is of equal importance from many points of view, and negative immunohistochemical results should always be interpreted with caution. The intensity of the immunoreaction can vary considerably with different antisera raised against the same immunogen. Also, factors such as fixative and the immunohistochemical method may markedly influence the sensitivity. Future methodological improvements will probably allow detection of further cell bodies and fibers containing a certain antigen. This aspect should be kept in mind, especially when discussing problems related to coexistence, i.e. for example, whether or not a certain peptide occurs only in a subpopulation of neurons. In this context it may be pointed out that the occurrence of peptides in cell bodies in the CNS is almost always demonstrated after colchicine treatment, i.e. after arrest of axonal transport and accumulation of peptides synthesized in the cell body (see Dahlström, 1971). One may therefore expect that the more peptide a neuron synthesizes, the more peptide should accumulate in the cell body and the more easy it should be detectable with immunohistochemistry. Thus, the neurons with very low (undetectable) levels of peptides, may be neurons, in which the peptides are not so important.

Overview of coexistence situations

Coexistence of several potential synaptic messengers has been observed in an increasing number of neuron systems. It is important to note that different types of combinations of compounds can be recognized (Table I). Most interest has so far been focused on the occurrence of a classical transmitter, such as NA, together with one or more peptides in the same neuron in the CNS (Table II). Many cases of neurons have been observed containing more than one peptide, but so far no classical transmitter. Examples of this are hypothalamic neurosecretory cells which release their content into the blood stream, either into the hypophysial portal capillary system in the median eminence or into the systemic

TABLE I

Different types of coexistence situations

Classical transmitter + peptide(s)
Classical transmitter + classical transmitter
Classical transmitter + peptide + ATP
Peptide + peptide
Peptide + leukotriene (?)

TABLE II

Immunohistochemical evidence for coexistence of classical transmitters and peptides in the central nervous system (selected cases)

Classical transmitter	Peptide[a]	Brain region (species)	References
Dopamine	CCK	Ventral mesencephalon (rat, cat, mouse, monkey, man?)	Hökfelt et al., 1980c,d, 1985
	Neurotensin	Ventral mesencephalon (rat)	Hökfelt et al., 1984a
		Hypothalamic arcuate nucleus (rat)	Ibata et al., 1983; Hökfelt et al., 1984a
Norepinephrine	Enkephalin	Locus coeruleus (cat)	Charnay et al., 1982; Leger et al., 1983
	NPY	Medulla oblongata (man, rat)	Hökfelt et al., 1983; Everitt et al., 1984a
		Locus coeruleus (rat)	Everitt et al., 1984a
	Vasopressin	Locus coeruleus (rat)	Caffé and van Leeuwen, 1983
Epinephrine	Neurotensin	Medulla oblongata (rat)	Hökfelt et al., 1984a
	NPY	Medulla oblongata (rat)	Everitt et al., 1984a
	Substance P	Medulla oblongata (rat)	Lorenz et al., 1985
	Neurotensin	Solitary tract nucleus (rat)	Hökfelt et al., 1984a
	CCK	Solitary tract nucleus (rat)	Hökfelt et al., 1985
5-HT	Substance P	Medulla oblongata (rat, cat)	Chan-Palay et al., 1978; Hökfelt et al., 1978; Chan-Palay, 1979; Johansson et al., 1981; Lovick and Hunt, 1983
	TRH	Medulla oblongata (rat)	Johansson et al., 1981
	Substance P + TRH	Medulla oblongata (rat)	Johansson et al., 1981
	CCK	Medulla oblongata (rat)	Mantyh and Hunt, 1984
	Enkephalin	Medulla oblongata, pons (cat)	Glazer et al., 1981; Hunt and Lovick, 1982
		Area postrema (rat)	Armstrong et al., 1984
ACh	Enkephalin	Superior olive (guinea pig)	Altschuler et al., 1983
		Spinal cord (rat)	Kondo et al., 1985
	Substance P	Pons (rat)	Vincent et al., 1983
	VIP	Cortex (rat)	Eckenstein and Baughman, 1984
	Galanin	Basal forebrain (rat)	Melander et al., 1985
	CGRP	Medullary motor nuclei (rat)	Takami et al., 1985
GABA	Motilin(?)	Cerebellum (rat)	Chan-Palay et al., 1981
	Somatostatin	Thalamus (cat)	Oertel et al., 1983
		Cortex, hippocampus (rat, cat, monkey)	Hendry et al., 1984; Jirikowski et al., 1984; Schmechel et al., 1984; Somogyi et al., 1984
	CCK	Cortex (cat, monkey)	Hendry et al., 1984; Somogyi et al., 1984

TABLE II *contd.*

Classical transmitter	Peptide[a]	Brain region (species)	References
	NPY	Cortex (cat, monkey)	Hendry et al., 1984
	Galanin	Hypothalamus (rat)	Melander et al., 1986
	Enkephalin	Retina (chicken)	Watt et al., 1984
		Ventral pallidum (rat)	Zahm et al., 1985
	Opioid peptide	Basal ganglia (rat)	Oertel and Mugnaini, 1984
Glycine	Neurotensin	Retina (turtle)	Weiler and Ball, 1984

[a] This column contains the peptide against which the antiserum used for immunohistochemistry was raised. The exact structure of the peptide coexisting with the classical transmitter has mostly not been defined.

circulation in the posterior lobe of the pituitary gland (see Bargmann and Scharrer, 1951). Brownstein et al. (this volume) give an overview of such neurons in the paraventricular and supraoptic nuclei. The apparent lack of a classical transmitter in neurons may be due to the fact that for a long time there has been no good histochemical markers for several of these transmitters, such as ACh, glutamate, glycine and histamine. However, recently techniques been developed to visualize, directly or indirectly, some of them and there are thus better possibilities to demonstrate whether some neurons produce and release peptides but no classical transmitter or whether all neurons have a classical transmitter.

Many studies now suport the view that ATP may act as transmitter in several peripheral systems (see Burnstock, 1985 and this volume, and Stjärne and Lundberg, this volume). Electrical stimulation of sympathetic nerves to the vas deferens causes a biphasic response. The initial twitch contraction may be related to ATP release and the second slow concentration to NA (see Burnstock, 1985). Immunohistochemical studies have demonstrated NPY-LI in these nerves (Lundberg et al., 1982b), and this peptide has in this tissue been shown to inhibit release of NA (Allen et al., 1982; Lundberg et al., 1982b; Ohhashi and Jacobowitz, 1983; Stjärne and Lundberg, 1984). Thus, these neurons may contain three different types of messengers, NA, ATP and a peptide.

Some neurons may contain more than one classical transmitter. Thus, 5-hydroxytryptamine (5-HT) and GABA seem to be present in some pontine neurons (Belin et al., 1983). In the hypothalamic arcuate nucleus some neurons may contain both GABA and DA (Everitt et al., 1984b). In the posterior hypothalamus magnocellular neurons contain both GABA and histamine (Takeda et al., 1984).

A special case of coexistence of two classical transmitters is found in the pineal gland. Here the sympathetic nerves contain both NA and 5-HT (Owman, 1964; Jaim-Etcheverry and Zieher, 1971). It is assumed that, whereas NA is synthesized in these nerves, 5-HT is produced in the adjacent pinealocytes. It is then taken up by the membrane pump of the sympathetic neurons and is accumulated together with NA in the storage vesicles (see Smith, 1976, Jaim-Etcheverry and Zieher, 1982). These nerves may also contain octopamine (Molinoff and Axelrod, 1969; Jaim-Etcheverry and Zieher, 1975) and thus store three different biogenic amines.

In the search for novel types of messenger molecules, we have recently analyzed some compounds belonging to the arachidonic acid metabolites, the leukotrienes (see Samuelsson, 1983). Using different types of biochemical analytical techniques and bioassay, evidence has been presented that under certain conditions leukotriene C_4 (LTC_4), LTD_4 and LTE_4 can be formed in the brain (Dembinska-Kieć et al., 1984; Lindgren et al., 1984; Moskowitz et al., 1984). The exact site of formation has not been fully characterized, but there is evidence that formation does not occur in blood vessels (Moskowitz et al., 1984), and nervous tissue may therefore be responsible. Additional immunohistochemical evidence suggests that the neurosecretory luteinizing hormone releasing hormone (LHRH)-neurons involved in control of LH from the anterior pituitary gland may produce an LTC_4-like compound (Hulting et al., 1984, 1985; Lindgren et al., 1984).

Differential coexistence situations

Central nervous system

Numerous coexistence situations have been observed in the brain and spinal cord. Initially catecholamines and 5-HT were identified as classical transmitters, but more recently there are also multiple examples involving ACh and GABA (Table II). For example, many GABA neurons in cortical areas contain one or more peptides (Hendry et al., 1984; Schmechel et al., 1984; Somogyi et al., 1984). An example of coexistence of the GABA-synthesizing enzyme GAD and CCK-LI is shown in Fig. 3C,D using the double-labeling technique.

TABLE III

Summary of differential coexistence patterns of neuropeptide Y (NPY)-, neurotensin (NT)- and galanin (GAL)-like immunoreactivity in catecholamine (CA) neuron groups

Area	Catecholamine	CA/NPY Coexistence	CA/NT Coexistence	CA/GAL Coexistence
(1) Ventrolateral medulla oblongata	NA (A1 group)	Yes, major	No	Yes, single
	A (C1 group)	Yes complete	No	No
(2) Dorsal medulla oblongata (dorsal vagal complex)	NA (A2 group)	Yes, minor	No	Yes, minor
	A (C2 group)	Yes, complete	No	No
	A (C2, dorsal group)	(?)	Yes, partial	No
(3) Area postrema	NA	No	No	No
(4) Pons, locus coeruleus	NA (A6 group)	Yes, partial	No	Yes, major
(5) Pons	NA (A4 group)	Yes, major	No	Yes, major
	NA (A5 group)	No	No	No
	NA (A7 group)	No	No	No
(6) Mesencephalon, ventral tegmental area and substantia nigra	DA (A8-10 groups)	No	Yes, minor (A10)	No
(7) Hypothalamus, periventricular groups including arcuate nucleus	DA (A12 and A14 groups)	No	Yes, partial (A12)	Yes, partial
(8) Zona incerta	DA (A11 and A13 groups)	No	No	No
(9) Olfactory bulb	DA (A17)	No	No	No

For fine neuroanatomical details, particularly with regard to the nucleus of the solitary tract (A2/C2) groups), see Everitt et al. (1984), Hökfelt et al. (1984a) and Melander et al. (1986), from where the results for this table have been taken. Nomenclature is according to Dahlström and Fuxe (1964) and Hökfelt et al. (1984d). A = adrenaline; DA = dopamine; NA = noradrenaline.

A common principle often observed has been that only a subpopulation of certain systems seem to exhibit a certain combination of messengers. For example, 5-HT neurons in the lower medulla oblongata (Dahlström and Fuxe, 1964) contained substance P (Chan-Palay et al., 1978; Hökfelt et al., 1978) and also a thyrotropin-releasing hormone (TRH)-like peptide (Hökfelt et al., 1980b; Johansson et al., 1981; Gilbert et al., 1982), whereas the rostral 5-HT cell groups in the pontine and mesencephalic raphe areas seemed to lack these peptides (Hökfelt et al., 1978). Furthermore, the proportions of 5-HT neurons containing substance P- and TRH-like immunoreactivities in the medullary raphe nuclei seem to vary in relation to the subregion in this area. For example, in the arcuate nucleus of the medulla oblongata the neurons seem to have a high proportion of 5-HT-positive/peptide-negative neurons, whereas a high proportion of neurons containing all three compounds are found in the nucleus raphe pallidus (Johansson et al., 1981).

Differential colocalization of classical transmitters and peptides can also be demonstrated for catecholamine neurons. In the CNS some catecholamine neurons have been shown to contain an NPY-like peptide (Everitt et al., 1984a), others, a neurotensin (NT)-like peptide (Hökfelt et al., 1984a) or a galanin-like peptide (Rökaeus et al., 1984; Melander et al., 1986). These findings are summarized in Table III, demonstrating that many neurons in the noradrenergic A1 and adrenergic C1 cell groups in the ventrolateral medulla oblongata contain NPY-like immunoreactivity (nomenclature according to Dahlström and Fuxe, 1964; Hökfelt et al., 1984d). In the locus coeruleus 25% of all neurons contain this peptide (Holets et al., 1986), whereas no DA neurons have been shown to be NPY-immunoreactive (A8-A17). In some areas numerous NPY-immunoreactive and catecholamine cells are present, but they form distinctly separate populations. Thus, the very high numbers of NPY-positive cells in the arcuate nucleus are different from the dopaminergic A12 group (Everitt et al., 1984a, 1986). Neurotensin shows, in comparison, only a minor degree of coexistence. Thus, some cells of the small sized adrenaline cells of the so-called dorsal strip (C2 dorsal) in the nucleus tractus solitarii and a small proportion of the A10 DA cells in the ventral tegmental area are NT-immunoreactive (Hökfelt et al., 1984a). A substantial portion of the DA cells of the A12 group in the arcuate nucleus do, however, exhibit NT-LI. A third type of immunoreactivity, galanin-like immunoreactivity is found mainly in the locus coeruleus and in the arcuate nucleus (Rökaeus et al., 1984; Holets et al., 1986; Melander et al., 1986).

An example of a pronounced catecholamine-peptide coexistence is the DA/CCK neuron in the rat ventral mesencephalon, which also exhibits a marked regional variation with virtually no coexistence in cell bodies in the pars reticulata of the substantia nigra and an almost total coexistence in its pars lateralis (Hökfelt et al., 1980c,d). We are in the process of defining more exactly the distribution

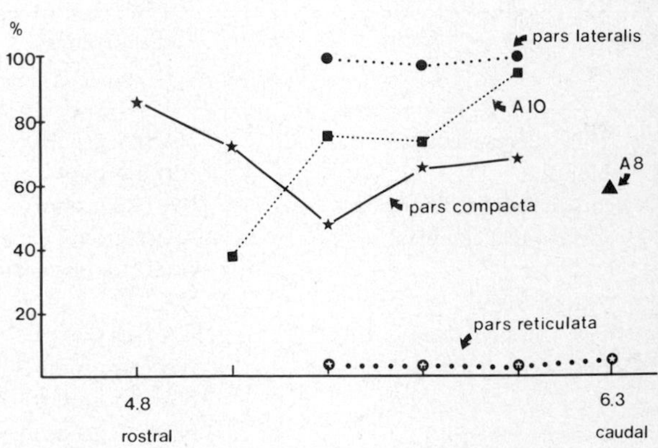

Fig. 4. Schematic illustration of the percentage of dopamine (DA) neurons containing cholecystokinin (CCK)-LI in various subregions of the ventral mesencephalon at different rostral-caudal levels (the most rostral level is approximately 4.8 mm behind Bregma, the most caudal point 6.3 mm behind the Bregma) and sections have been analyzed at 0.3 mm intervals. Areas analyzed are pars compacta, pars lateralis and pars reticulata of the substantia nigra as well as the ventral tegmental area (A10 DA cell group) and the A8 DA cell group in the mesencephalic reticular formation. Note high proportion of DA/CCK coexistence in pars lateralis and low percentage in pars reticulata. In the ventral tegmental area there is an increasing incidence of coexistence in the caudal direction. Fur further detail see text.

and percentage of DA cells containing CCK-like immunoreactivity. Figure 4 represents an attempt to schematically present preliminary results on the percentage of DA/CCK neurons in five different subregions of the ventral mesencaphalon and at six different rostrocaudal levels. It is noteworthy that the coexistence in the A10 group markedly increases in the caudal direction. In the pars compacta a reversed tendency can be observed but there is an increase in its caudal parts. In the original study, a fairly low degree of coexistence was seen in the latter region (Hökfelt et al., 1980d), but it seems as if the use of improved fixation as well as new antisera results in an increased number of CCK-immunoreactive cells. In Fig. 5, which is a low-power immunofluorescence micrograph taken from Hökfelt et al. (1984d) showing the distribution of DA (tyrosine hydroxylase (TH)-positive) cells at one particular rostro-caudal level, we have indicated the approximate percentage of DA/CCK coexistence in various subregions of the ventral mesencephalon.

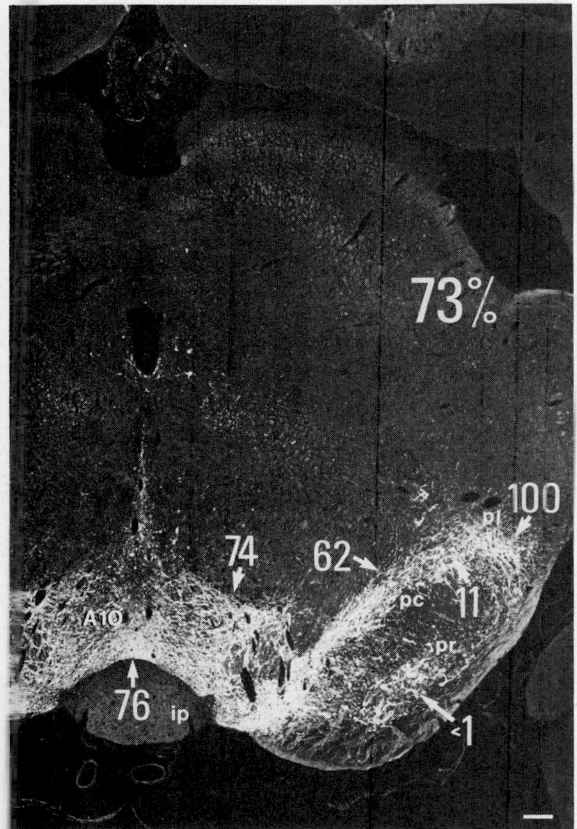

Fig. 5. Immunofluorescence micrographs of the mesencephalon after incubation with antiserum to tyrosine hydroxylase, a marker for dopamine (DA) neurons. The micrographs give an overview of the distribution of DA neurons and an approximate percentage of DA/cholecystokinin (CCK) coexistence has been indicated in various subregions of the ventral mesencephalon. At this particular level 73% of all DA cells contain CCK-LI. ip = Interpeduncular nucleus; pc = pars compacta; pl = pars lateralis; and pr = pars reticulata of the subsantia nigra. A10 = dopamine cell bodies in the ventral tegmental area. Bar indicates 200 μm.

The present findings raise an interesting question in terms of correlation between coexistence in cell bodies and terminal areas. In an early study (Hökfelt et al., 1980c) it was noted that overlapping terminal fields containing TH- and CCK-like immunoreactivity, respectively, was only observed in limited areas of the forebrain, i.e. in the medial caudal parts of nucleus accumbens and tuberculum olfatorium, in the periventricular zone of the caudate nucleus and in the tail of the caudate nucleus, as well as in the central amygdaloid nucleus. In other DA projection fields, such as a head of the caudate nucleus, the well known dense fiber network of DA fibers was seen, but no corresponding CCK fibers. This was assumed to correlate to the low percentage of DA/CCK coexistence in cell bodies observed in the main part of zona compacta. With the higher percentage observed now with improved fixation methods and antisera one should expect a more extensive CCK distribution in the forebrain. Several explanations can be forwarded such as a considerably lower content of CCK-LI in DA neurons projecting into the head of the caudate nucleus as compared to those projecting to the caudal, medial nucleus accumbens and tuberculum olfactorium. Another possibility is that the CCK precursor is differentially processed in the different systems. The antibody used by us more recently is directed towards the mid portion of CCK(1-33) and does not react with the octapeptide of CCK. It can therefore not be excluded that DA neurons process their CCK precursor in a different way, and that, therefore, the CCK-like peptide in some terminal areas, such as the head of the caudate nucleus, can not be visualized with conventional CCK antisera.

An intersting coexistence interaction involving a galanin-like peptide has been observed in the rat basal forebrain (Melander et al., 1985). Thus, galanin-LI has been found in some cholinergic neurons in the medial septal nucleus and in the vertical and horizontal limbs of the nucleus of the diagonal band with projections to cortical regions. On the other hand, no evidence was found for coexistence of galanin and ACh in the nucleus basalis of Meynert or in cortical areas (Melander et al., 1985). Thus, also this combination of classical transmitter and peptide exhibits an apparent differential distribution.

Peripheral nervous system

A further example of differential coexistence has been found in the peripheral nervous system in the coeliac-superior mesenteric ganglion complex in the guinea pig. It was earlier observed that a population of the noradrenergic neurons in this ganglion contains somatostatin-LI (Hökfelt et al., 1977a). In addition, a small population of neurons contained vasoactive intestinal polypeptide (VIP)-LI (Hökfelt et al., 1977b). Using an antiserum raised to avian pancreatic polypeptide (APP), a further noradrenergic cell population could be distinguished which appeared complementary to the somatostatin positive cell bodies (Lundberg et al., 1982c). Biochemical analysis has revealed that the compound reacting with APP antiserum in all probability represents an NPY-like peptide (Lundberg et al., 1984). In fact, using antiserum to this peptide it has been definitely demonstrated that the somatostatin and NPY-immunoreactive cell bodies occupy different territories in the ganglion (Fig. 6A,B) (Lindh et al., 1986). Only a small degree of overlap exists and a few cell bodies contain both peptides (see below).

Functional significance

The functional significance of subgrouping is still in many cases very unclear. Holets et al. (1986) have contributed some interesting information to this problem. In a detailed analysis of the locus coeruleus it was observed that about 25% of all NA neurons contained NPY-LI. Furthermore, the projections of these neurons were analyzed using retrograde tracing with a fluorescent dye, Fast Blue,

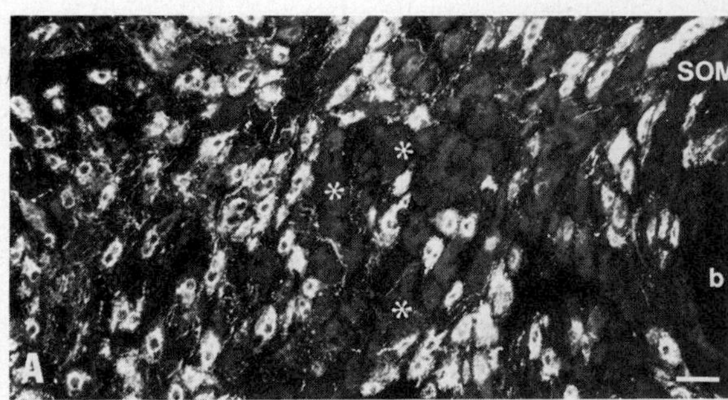

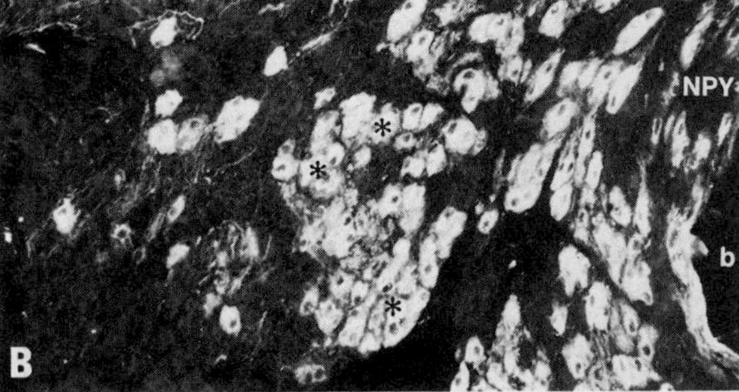

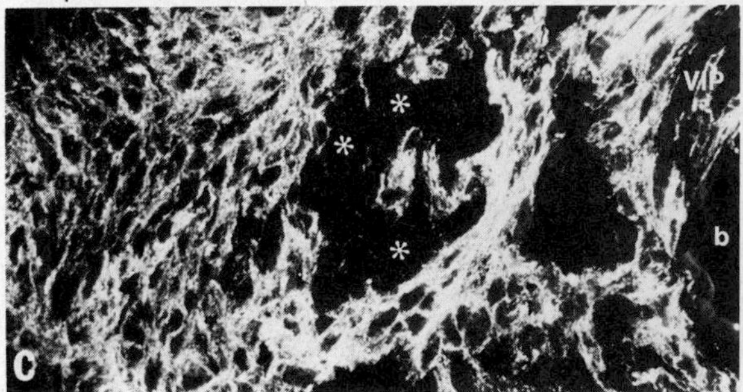

Fig. 6. Immunofluorescence micrographs of adjacent sections of the coeliac-superior mesenteric ganglion complex of the guinea pig after incubation with antiserum to somatostatin (SOM). (A), neuropeptide Y (NPY) (B) and vasoactive intestinal polypeptide (VIP) (C). Note complementary distribution of SOM- and NPY-immunoreactive principal ganglion cells and that CIP-positive fibers virtually exclusively terminate around SOM-positive cells (C). Asterisks indicate NPY-positive, SOM-negative cells, which are virtually devoid of VIP-positive fibers. b = Blood vessel. Bar indicates 50 μm.

combined with immunohistochemistry (see Hökfelt et al., 1983b; Skirboll et al., 1984). It was observed that noradrenergic neurons in the locus coeruleus containing NPY preferentially projected to the hypothalamus giving rise to bilateral projections, whereas only a smaller proportion of these neurons projected to the cerebral cortex and the spinal cord (Holets et al., 1986). The cortical projections were almost exclusively ipsilateral. These findings indicate that subdivision of transmitter specific groups of neurons by a peptide may be related to the target areas of the projections. This possibility has been further evaluated in transplantation experiments (see Schultzberg et al., this volume).

Also in the peripheral system, results indicate that neurons containing different types of coexistence combinations may project differentially. This has been observed in the analysis of the distribution of the preganglionic fibers to the coeliac-superior mesenteric ganglion complex, which, as described above, contains two main population of cells, NA/NPY- and NA/somatostatin-positive ones (Fig. 6A,B). Thus, preganglionic fibers containing, for example, the VIP/PHI (Fig. 6C)- and dynorphin-like immunoreactivities terminate virtually exclusively in those parts of the ganglion containing somatostatin-positive neurons (Lundberg et al., 1982c; Lindh et al., 1986). These fibers in all probability originate from the gastrointestinal wall, as deduced from an analysis of the inferior mesenteric ganglion (Dalsgaard et al., 1983). This would suggest that mainly the somatostatin-positive cells are involved in the reflex loop between ganglion and intestine.

Projections of somatostatin- and NPY-immunoreactive noradrenergic cell bodies from the coeliac-superior mesenteric ganglion complex have also been demonstrated by Costa, Furness and their collaborators (Furness et al., 1983; Costa and Furness, 1984). They were able to demonstrate that the major targets for the noradrenaline/NPY neurons were the intestinal blood vessels, in agreement with studies on many other peripheral tissues showing a close relation between NA/NPY neurons and the vascular system (Lundberg et al., 1980, 1982c,d). In contrast, the NA/somatostatin neurons projected to the submucous ganglia and the mucosa. A third population of noradrenergic nerves lacking the two peptides projected to the myenteric ganglia. Taken together these findings strongly suggest a distinct chemical coding of neuron populations in the prevertebral ganglia and gastrointestinal tract and that these subgroups of peripheral neurons may be involved in regulation of different peripheral functional events.

Chemical heterogeneity of brain nuclei

The immunohistochemical analysis of individual nuclei in the CNS has also demonstrated that a marked heterogeneity with regard to classical transmitters can exist, which then is enhanced when considering coexisting peptides. In this context, the locus coeruleus discussed above represents an unusual nucleus, since it almost exclusively contains noradrenergic cell bodies. So far, only two coexisting peptides have been encountered in the rat, NPY and galanin. In most other regions the heterogeneity is extensive, for example, the arcuate nucleus in the basal hypothalamus, which is involved in the gating and regulation of neuroendocrine information to the anterior and intermediate lobe of the pituitary gland. Thus, this nucleus contains somatostatin, NPY, NT, growth hormone-releasing factor (GRF), galanin, a variety of opioid peptide-immunoreactive neurons as well as neurons containing classical transmitters such as DA, GABA and in all probability ACh (Fig. 7) (for refs., see Everitt et al., 1985). Analysis of possible coexistence situations have revealed that several combinations of compounds can be observed (Everitt et al., 1986; Meister et al., 1985a,b). Thus, TH-LI coexists with GABA, NT, GRF and/or galanin. On the other hand, NPY- and somatostatin-positive neurons seem to represent essentially separate populations and so far no classical transmitters have been observed in these neurons. The neuroendocrine system may offer good possibilities to evaluate the significance of these types of coexistence.

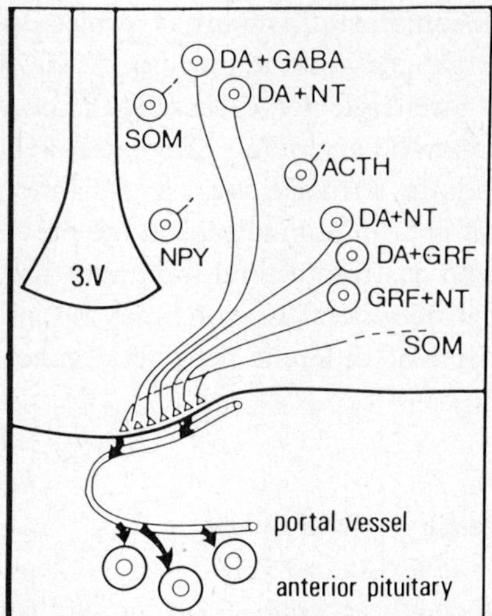

Fig. 7. Schematic illustration of the content and coexistence of various transmitters and peptides in the arcuate nucleus of the hypothalamus. The dopaminergic nature of the ventrolateral TH-positive neurons is at present under study (Meister et al., 1985).

Species variation of coexistence situations

The occurrence of coexistence combinations during phylogeny has only been studied to a limited extent. There are examples both of maintenance and variation between different species. For example, NA and somatostatin coexist in the guinea pig and rat but not in the cat (Lundberg et al., 1982c). In the CNS, DA/CCK-immunoreactive neurons in the ventral nesencephalon has been analyzed to some extent. Thus, DA neurons in this area contain CCK-LI in mouse, rat, cat, monkey and probably man (see Hökfelt et al., 1980c,d, 1985). However, certain differences can be observed (Table IV). Thus, in the cat, the zona compacta of the substantia nigra contained the highest proportions of DA/CCK coexistence. In the monkey, coexistence has so far only been observed in the midline area, i.e. the area corresponding to the A10 dopamine group. Overlapping distribution of DA and CCK fibers have been observed in, e.g. nucleus accumbens (Fig. 8A,B), but not in the nucleus caudatus putamen, suggesting nerve terminal coexistence patterns similar to the ones seen in the rat (Hökfelt, Staines, Björklund, Frey, Rehfeld and Goldstein, in preparation). In the rat, a marked regional distribution has been observed as described above. In the mouse, coexistence of this type has been observed mainly in the ventral tegmental area (A10) (Sundblad, Staines, Hökfelt, Jonsson, Frey, Reh-

TABLE IV

Dopamine-CCK coexistence in different regions of five species*

	Rat	Cat	Monkey	Mouse	Guinea pig
Substantia nigra (A9 group)			0?	0?	0
Pars compacta		+ + + +			
Rostral	+ + + +				
Mid	+ +				
Caudal	+ + +				
Pars lateralis	+ + + + +	+ + + +			
Pars reticulata	(+)	0			
Ventral tegmental area (A10 group)			+	+ + +	0
Anterior	+ + +	+ +			
Posterior	+ + + +	+			

* An estimation of the approximate percentage of DA cell bodies containing CCK-like immunoreactivity (LI) is given; CCK-LI is present in all (+ + + + +), in most (+ + + +), in moderate numbers (+ + +), in low numbers (+ +), in single (+) or in none (0) of the DA cell bodies. From Hökfelt et al. (1985).

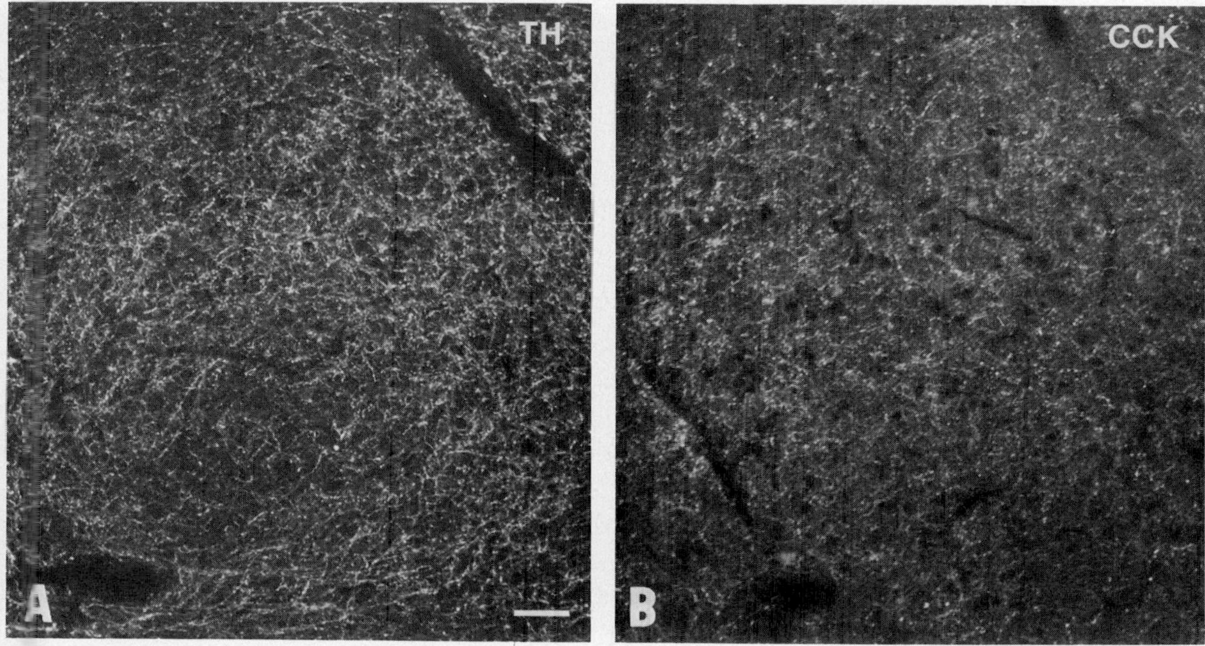

Fig. 8A,B. Immunofluorescence micrographs of the nucleus accumbens of monkey after incubation with antiserum to tyrosine hydroxylase (TH), a marker for dopamine (DA) nerve endings in this area, and cholecystokinin (CCK). The DA and CCK-positive fibers exhibit a high degree of overlap, although the TH-positive fibers are more distinct and appear somewhat more numerous. These findings suggest presence of a CCK-like peptide in DA neurons projecting to the nucleus accumbens also in the monkey. Bar indicates 50 μm.

feld and Goldstein, in preparation). No CCK-LI has been observed in the guinea pig ventral mesencephalon, where some cells instead contained an enkephalin-like peptide (unpublished observations). Further studies of other types of coexistence situations as well as studies including more diverse species are in progress.

Differential release of coexisting messenger molecules

When trying to evaluate the potential significance of coexistence of multiple messengers, a key question is if and how these compounds can produce selective and differential responses. Several possibilities to achieve this can be considered. One mechanism would be that the neuron always releases all types of messenger molecules at the same time and that, for example, selectivity and specificity is dependent on type and distribution of the receptors (see below). Another alternative is that the neuron has the capacity to release the messengers differentially. This question has been examined by studying whether the messengers are stored in the same or in different subcellular organelles within the nerve terminals.

Nerve endings in general contain at least two types of vesicles, the synaptic vesicles with a diameter of about 500 Å and a larger type of vesicle (diameter about 1000 Å), often characterized by an electron dense-core and termed large dense-core vesicles. The most simple approach to analyze this question is probably electron microscopic immunocytochemistry. Most studies with this technique have demonstrated that peptides in general are present exclusively in large dense-core vesicles (for review see Fried, 1982). However, also when anti-

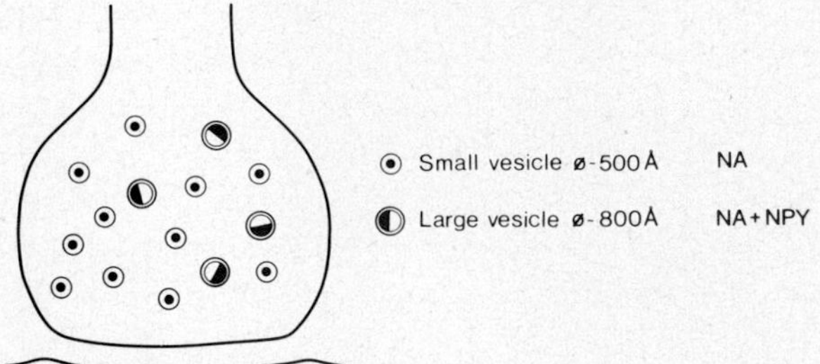

Fig. 9. Schematic illustration of our present view on the subcellular distribution of coexisting noradrenaline (NA) and neuropeptide Y (NPY) in the vas deferens of the rat. The small vesicles contain only NA, whereas both NA and NPY are present in the large vesicles.

serum to 5-HT is used, a similar distribution is seen (see e.g. Pelletier et al., 1981), in spite of the fact that it is generally accepted that 5-HT and catecholamines are stored both in small and large vesicles (see Hökfelt, 1968). In view of this possible artefact in electron microscopic immunocytochemical studies, we have employed a different approach, subcellular fractionation combined with differential centrifugation. With this method it was found that in the cat salivary gland (Lundberg et al., 1981) and in the rat vas deferens (Fried et al., 1985) classical transmitters and peptides may partially be stored in different compartments. Thus, ACh as well as NA can be found both in a light and a heavy fraction which, upon ultrastructural analysis, contains preferentially small synaptic vesicles and large dense-core vesicles, respectively. In contrast, VIP (coexisting with ACh) and NPY (coexisting with NA) principally only appear in the heavy fractions, suggesting storage exclusively in large dense-core vesicles (Fig. 9). Thus, if mechanisms exist allowing selective activation of the two types of vesicles upon arrival of nerve impulses, it should be possible to obtain differential release. We have suggested that such activation could be frequency coded — at low nerve impulse flow small vesicles release the classical transmitter, at higher frequencies large vesicles release in addition, both peptide and classical transmitter (see Lundberg and Hökfelt, 1983).

The possible differential subcellular localization of classical transmitter and peptide may be taken as basis for reflections on evolutionary aspects on the coexistence phenomenon and chemical transmission process. The possible localization of the peptides exclusively to large granular vesicles, and the presence of classical transmitters in both large and the small vesicles may be a consequence of evolutionary events. Thus it may be speculated that large vesicles may represent an older form of messenger storage. The large neuronal vesicles are similar to the vesicles found in endocrine cells, and coexistence and corelease of different types of messenger molecules may therefore represent an old phenomenon. With evolution and the demand for faster processing of information and thus faster transmission of nerve impulses, it may be speculated that small vesicles were developed in the nerve endings and that they were equipped with messenger molecules of the classical transmitter type, for example, ACh, amino acids or biogenic amines.

Coexistence and plasticity

An interesting issue is whether or not coexistence combinations represent stable situations. For example, is coexistence of a classical transmitter and a peptide always confined to the same subpopulation of neurons or do changes occur?; can the proportion of coexisting messengers change with time, for example in a daily or an annual rhythm?; can the proportion of the coexisting messengers change with function, for example, during low or high neuronal activity?, etc. Most interesting results in this respect have been obtained in ontogenetic studies, where neurons apparently can express different messenger molecules during development (see Black et al. and Potter et al., both this volume). Also after transplantation within the CNS, there is some evidence that neurons may change their phenotopy (see Schultzberg et al., this volume).

In the following, we would briefly like to discuss some experiments in adult animals, which indicate that peripheral noradrenergic neurons may change their expression of messenger molecules after experimental procedures (see Björklund et al., 1985).

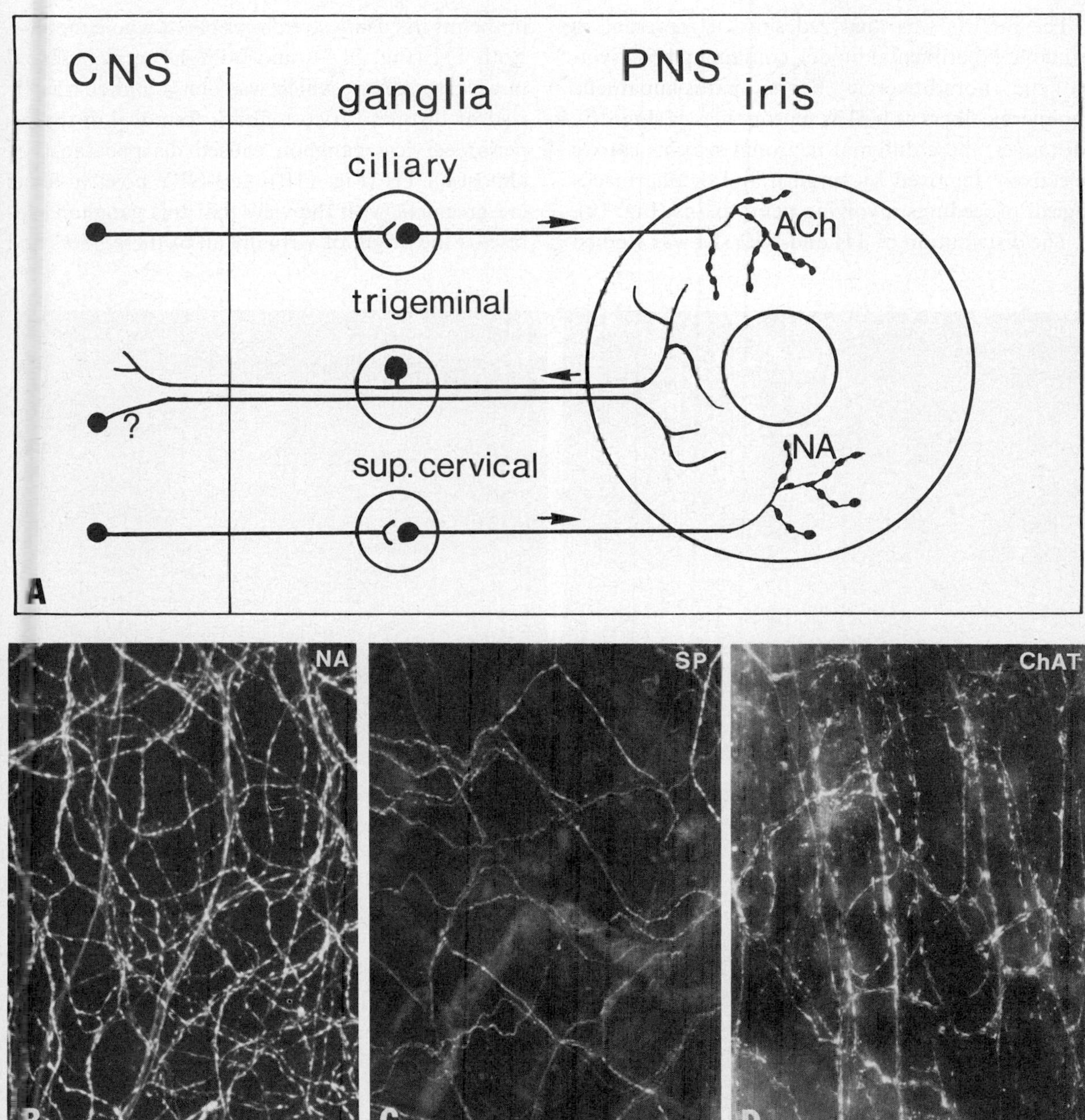

Fig. 10. Illustration of the rat iris as an experimental model. (A) Iris receives a parasympathetic, cholinergic innervation from the ciliary ganglion, the sensory innervation from the trigeminal ganglion and sympathetic, noradrenergic fibers from the superior cervical ganglion. (B–D). The three types of fibers can be visualized histochemically: noradrenaline (NA)-containing fibers form a dense plexus as shown with formaldehyde-induced fluorescence (B), whereas the sensory substance P (SP)-containing fibers are present in lower numbers (C). The parasympathetic, cholinergic fibers can be demonstrated with antibodies to cholinacetyltransferase (ChAT) (D).

The rat iris was analyzed since it represents a valuable experimental model, containing both sympathetic noradrenergic fibers, parasympathetic cholinergic fibers as well as sensory nerves (Fig. 10). Moreover, these different neuronal systems can be selectively removed by surgical and/or pharmacological procedures involving neurotoxins (Fig. 10).

The distribution of TH and NPY-LI was studied in the rat iris using stretch-prepared whole mounts. Both TH (Fig. 11A)- and NPY-LI were observed in a nerve plexus, which was dense and characterized by distinct varicose fibers. Removal of the superior cervical ganglion caused disappearance of almost all TH (Fig. 11B)- and NPY-positive fibers in agreement with the view that this ganglion represents the origin of virtually all of these fibers and

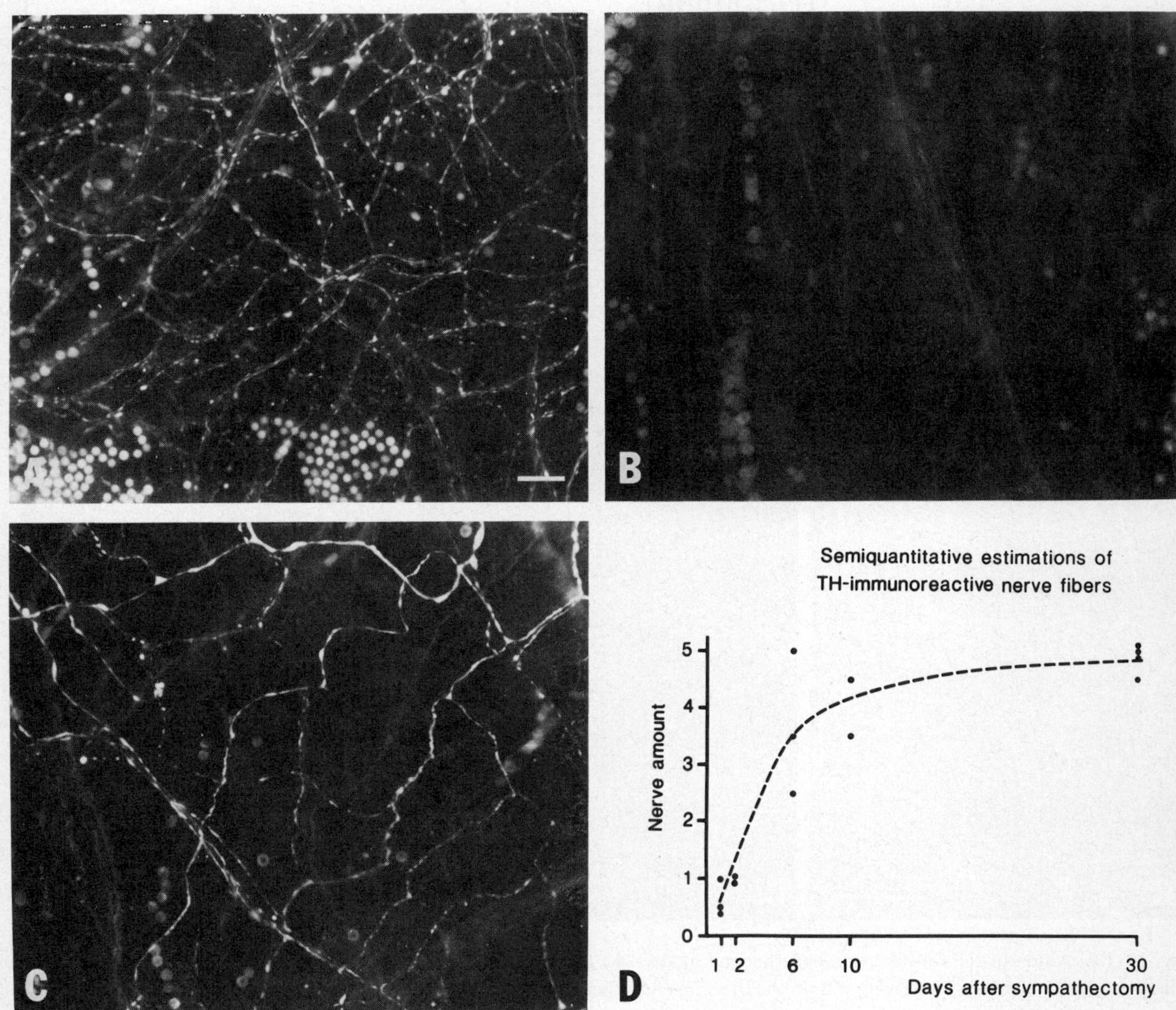

Fig. 11. Immunofluorescence micrographs (A–C) of iris of control rat (A), of rat one day after sympathectomy (B) and of rat 4 months after sympathectomy (C) after incubation with antiserum to tyrosine hydroxylase (TH). Note complete disappearance of TH-positive fibers one day after operation and reappearance of fluorescent fibers after 4 months. In D the density of TH-positive nerves has been estimated subjectively at different time intervals after sympathectomy. Bar indicates 50 μm. A–C have the same magnification. (From Björklund et al., 1985.)

thus contains NPY- and TH-positive cell bodies. In fact, it has earlier been demonstrated that NPY-LI is present in a subpopulation of the superior cervical ganglion cells (Lundberg et al., 1982c, 1983). When analyzing irides 4 weeks after sympathectomy, a substantial number of TH (Fig. 11C)- and NPY-immunoreactive fibers were observed indicating reappearance of these fiber populations. The same irides were analyzed with the formaldehyde-induced fluorescence method of Falck and Hillarp and no positive fibers could be observed in these long-term sympathectomized animals. The appearance of TH- and NPY-positive fibers in sympathetically denervated iris showed a clear time dependency (Fig. 11D). The newly appeared TH- and NPY-positive nerves were less varicose and had a lower fluorescence intensity and were not associated with blood vessels, when compared with fibers seen in untreated rats. The lack of formaldehyde-induced fluorescence indicated that the newly appeared NPY/TH-positive fibers were not regenerating sympathetic nerves. Therefore, the parasympathetic ciliary ganglion was removed bilaterally to cause degeneration of the cholinergic fibers in the rat iris (see Fig. 10A). In such rats, which had been bilaterally sympathectomized one month before, a marked decrease in the number of TH- and NPY-positive fibers was seen as compared to the iris which had been subjected to sympathectomy alone. Thus, the present experiments suggest that adult cholinergic neurons in vivo are capable of expressing adrenergic characteristics under the present experimental conditions (sympathectomy) (Björklund et al., 1985).

Interactions between peptides and classical transmitters

Interactions which may take place between a classical transmitter and a peptide, released from the same nerve endings, have been explored only to a limited extent. Perhaps the best evidence for interaction has been obtained in studies on the peripheral nervous system, especially the salivary gland of the cat and vas deferens of the rat (Lundberg et al., 1982a; see Lundberg and Hökfelt, this volume and Stjärne and Lundberg, this volume), and on autonomic ganglia of the bull frog (Jan and Jan, 1983; see Jan and Jan, this volume). Some results from studies on central nervous tissue are also available.

Interaction at the postsynaptic level

In the cat salivary gland both the sympathetic and parasympathetic nerves contain a biologically active peptide. NPY is present in a population of the sympathetic noradrenergic fibers, mainly innervating blood vessels (Lundberg et al., 1982d) and VIP occurs in the parasympathetic cholinergic fibers (Lundberg et al., 1979). As shown by Lundberg, Änggård and collaborators (see Lundberg et al., 1982a), this classical experimental model offers favorable conditions for analysis of the role of transmitters and peptides in the control of secretion and blood flow through the gland. In brief, these experiments have shown that ACh induces both secretion and increase in blood flow, effects which both are atropine-sensitive. VIP alone increases blood flow but has no apparent effect on secretion. However, VIP potentiates ACh-induced secretion and when ACh and VIP are infused together additive effects on blood flow are observed (see Lundberg et al., 1982a). In the sympathetic system, both NA and NPY cause vasoconstriction, whereby NPY exhibits a slowly developing, long-lasting effect (Lundberg and Tatemoto, 1982). Thus, both in sympathetic and parasympathetic nerves, peptides and classical transmitter may cooperate at the postsynaptic level in causing the physiological response(s).

Evidence for cooperativity at the postsynaptic level has been obtained in the CNS. In studies on the effect of intravenously administered TRH on the stretch reflex in chronically spinalized or 5-HT neurotoxin-treated rats, Barbeau and Bédard (1981) have demonstrated a marked activation of the stretch reflex. A similar effect was seen after administration of the 5-HT precursor 5-hydroxytryptophan (5-HTP) (see also Andén et al., 1964). The effect of TRH could be blocked by previous administration of a 5-HT antagonist. These findings suggested that TRH may act as a site closely associated with the 5-HT receptor (Barbeau and Bedard, 1981). In view of the similarity to the response caused by 5-HTP, it may be suggested that TRH and 5-HT cooperate at synapses in the ventral horn of the spinal cord, possibly directly or indirectly influencing motoneurons and the muscles involved in the stretch reflex.

Results from some behavioral studies also suggest interaction between 5-HT and TRH. Thus, sexual behavior in the male rat was studied after intrathecal (Yaksh and Rudy, 1976) application of 5-HT (50 μg), substance P (10 μg) or TRH (10 μg) or combinations of these compounds (Hansen et al., 1983). Several parameters such as number of mounts and intromissions, latencies (mount, intromission and ejaculation) as well as postejaculatory interval were analyzed. No significant effects of 5-HT or substance P were observed in these experiments when given alone, and the effects of TRH were very small (Hansen et al., 1983; Svensson and Hansen, unpublished results). However, when given together, 5-HT and TRH caused a marked increase in both mount and intromission latency (from about 0.2 min to more than 7 min). None of the other parameters studied were affected by the combined administration of these compounds (Hansen et al., 1983). Thus, these results are in agreement with the results of Barbeau and Bedard (1981) obtained in the spinal model described above, suggesting an interaction of 5-HT and TRH at a postsynaptic level (Fig. 12).

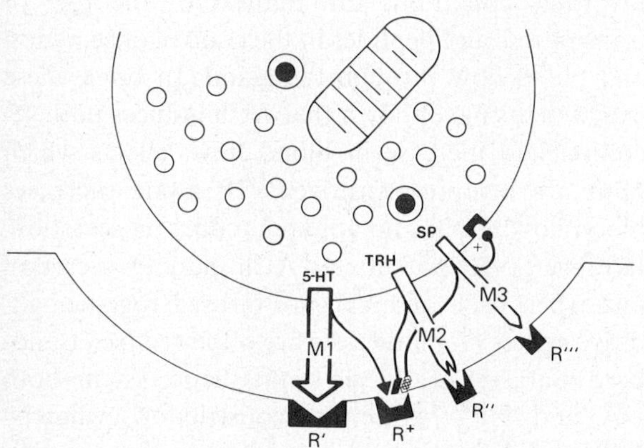

Fig. 12. Schematic illustration of a nerve ending containing three messenger molecules, 5-hydroxytryptamine (5-HT), thyrotropin--releasing hormone (TRH) and substance P (SP) and their possible interactions with receptors of different type and location. For example, TRH may act at a postsynaptic receptor closely associated with the 5-HT receptor. There is evidence that SP may act on a presynaptic, inhibitory 5-HT receptor. It may also have action at postsynaptic sites. For further details, see text.

Experimental studies on possible postsynaptic interactions

The results described above suggest that messengers released from the same nerve endings may act on closely coupled receptors and, that, perhaps a certain degree of "cross-talk" can occur between the different ligands and their receptors. Here we would like to discuss some experimental studies on spinal cord which may be related to this question (Freedman et al., 1985; Post et al., 1985).

It has been observed that substance P antagonists may cause neuronal damage (Hökfelt et al., 1981; Post and Paulsson, 1985). In the latter study, the antagonist was administered intrathecally and caused a marked necrosis of the gray matter of the spinal cord (Fig. 13A–D) (Freedman et al., 1986; Post and Paulsson, 1985; Post et al., 1985), resulting in persistent motor impairment. Furthermore, it was demonstrated that repeated treatment with the

Fig. 13. Immunofluorescence micrographs of the ventral horn of the spinal cord of untreated rat (A,B), rat treated with intrathecal injection of a substance P (SP) antagonist (C,D) and rat pretreated with thyrotropin-releasing hormone (TRH) intravenously before and after administration of the SP antagonist (E,F). Sections have been incubated with antiserum to calcitonin gene-related peptide (CGRP) as a marker for motoneurons (arrows) (A,C,E) and 5-hydroxytryptamine (5-HT) (B,D,F). Treatment with SP antagonist causes complete disappearance of motoneurons and marked changes in the 5-HT fiber plexus (C,D). These effects are completely counteracted by pretreatment with TRH (E,F). Such rats exhibit an appearance similar to the one seen in untreated rats (A,B). Bar indicates 50 μm. All micrographs have the same magnification.

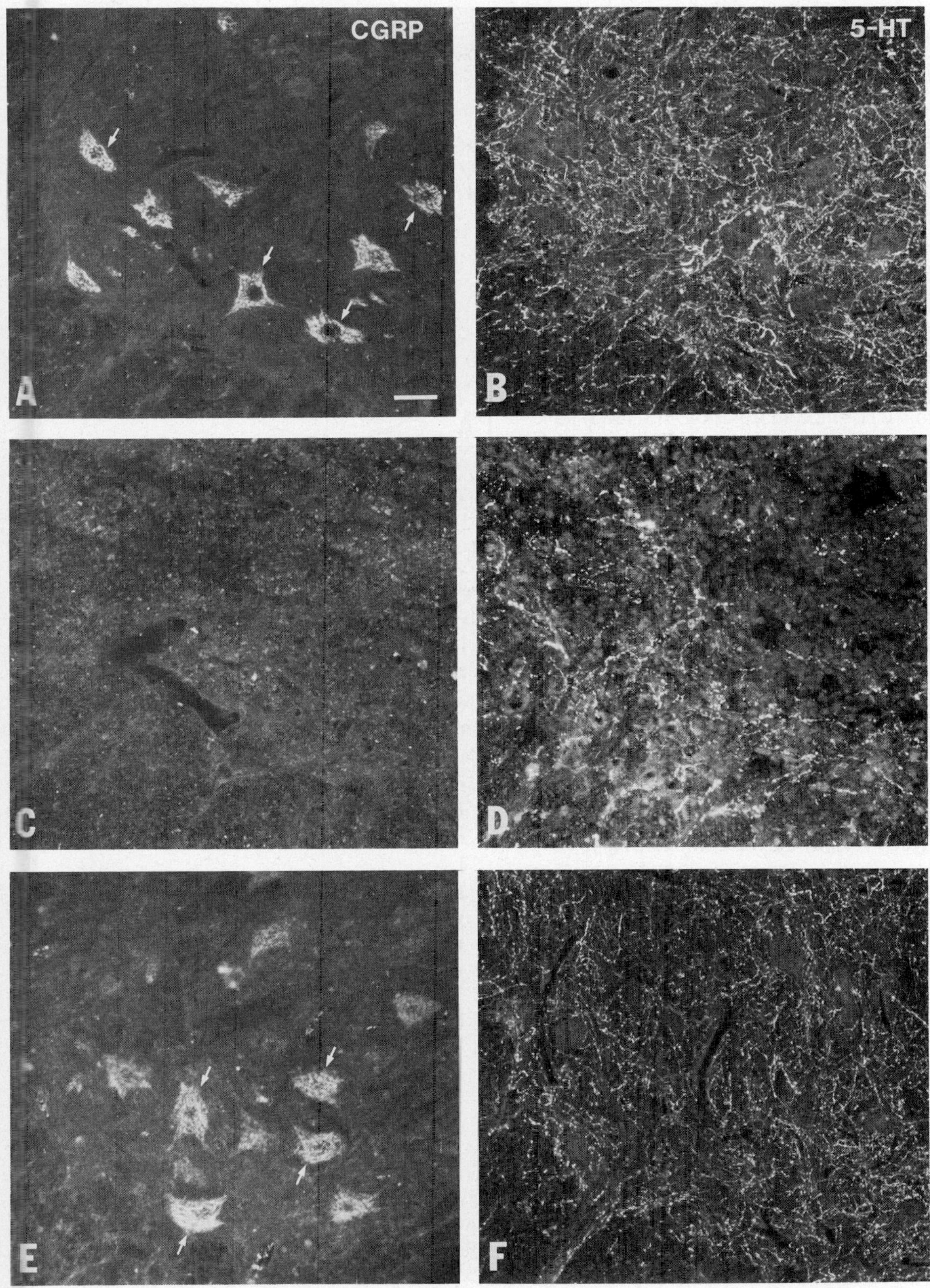
CGRP
5-HT
A
B
C
D
E
F

tripeptide TRH before and after injection of the substance P antagonist prevented the necrotic changes induced by the antagonist (Fig. 13E,F) (Freedman et al., 1985; Post et al., 1985). This is interesting also in relation to earlier results demonstrating that TRH is efficient in treating experimental (compression) spinal injury (Faden et al., 1981).

We have speculated that our findings are related to effects on blood vessels or to the coexistence of 5-HT, TRH and substance P in bulbospinal descending neurons probably innervating motoneurons. In the latter case, the necrotic effect may be due to an action of the substance P antagonist on substance P receptors. These receptors may also be sensitive to TRH, since Sharif and Burt (1983) have demonstrated that substance P and substance P analogues affects in vitro binding of TRH to spinal cord isolated membranes. Furthermore, as discussed above, interaction between 5-HT and TRH on the same or closely related receptors has been demonstrated (Barbeau and Bedard, 1981). We would therefore like to suggest that the protective effect of TRH is exerted via blockade of substance P receptors preventing access of the substance P antagonist to the receptor (see Fig. 12). If this hypothesis is correct and taken together with findings discussed above, interesting views open up on our possibilities to influence receptor function. Maybe a broader range of compounds is available to affect a certain receptor and maybe combination of several ligands can be used to more efficiently affect receptor function. This may have an impact on our future approach to drug development.

Interaction at the presynaptic level

In the rat vas deferens NA and NPY coexist in the sympathetic nerves (Lundberg et al., 1982d). Here NPY in a dose-dependent manner inhibits the electrically induced contraction of vas deferens, which seems to be due to inhibition of NA release (Allen et al., 1982; Lundberg et al., 1982d; Ohhashi and Jacobowitz, 1983; Stjärne and Lundberg, 1984; see Stjärne and Lundberg, this volume).

In the CNS evidence has been obtained for interaction of peptide and classical transmitter in the release process. Thus, in the cat a large proportion of the nigral DA neurons contain a CCK-like peptide and, correspondingly, dense networks of CCK- and tyrosine hydroxylase-immunoreactive fibers can be seen in the nucleus caudatus putamen (Hökfelt et al., 1985). Thus, in comparison to the rat (Hökfelt et al., 1980d) a fairly rich source of tissue with nerve endings presumably containing both DA

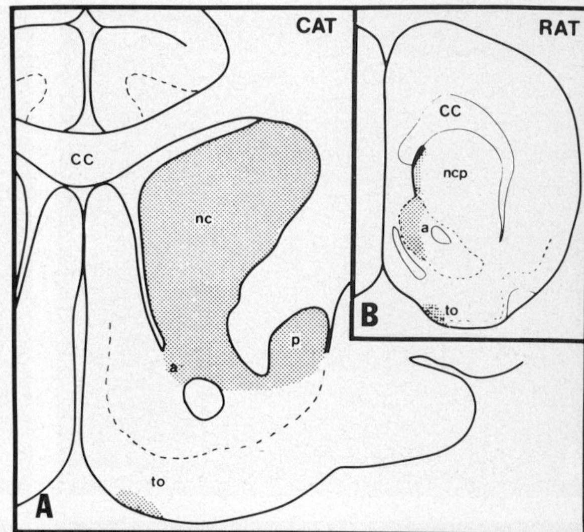

Fig. 14. Comparison of the size of the forebrain areas containing dopamine/cholecystokinin coexistence in the cat (A) and rat (B).

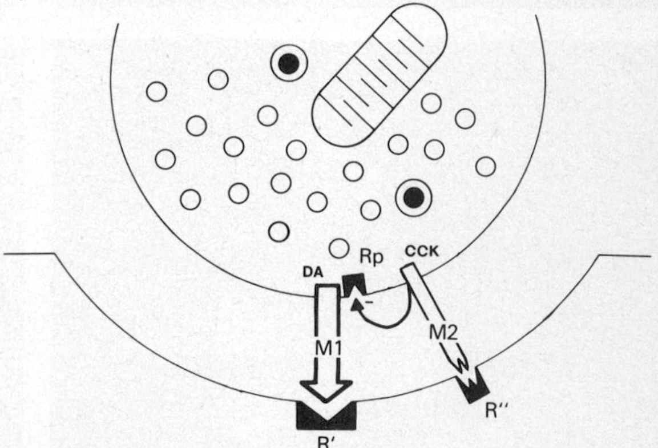

Fig. 15. Schematic illustration of a nerve ending containing dopamine (DA) and cholecystokinin (CCK). Evidence is discussed in the text, suggesting that a CCK-like peptide can inhibit release of DA by action on a presynaptic receptor.

and CCK-LI is available for in vitro release studies (Markstein and Hökfelt, 1984). This is illustrated in Fig. 14. The effects of CCK-8 were studied on basal and electrically evoked tritium outflow from slices of the nucleus caudatus putamen of cat after preincubation with tritiated DA. The tritium outflow was Ca^{2+}-dependent and abolished by tetrodotoxin. The sulphated, but not the unsulphated form of CCK-8, inhibited both basal and electrically evoked tritium outflow in concentrations down to 10^{-14} M. A CCK-like peptide released from DA nerve endings in the caudate-putamen of the cat may therefore exert an inhibitory action on DA release, perhaps as a mechanism to prevent excessive release of this catecholamine (Fig. 15).

A different type of possible presynaptic interaction in the release process has been described for substance P at the spinal cord level. There Mitchell and Fleetwood-Walker (1981) analyzed the effect of peptides on potassium-induced release of 5-HT in spinal cord slices. Neither substance P nor TRH influenced potassium-induced tritium outflow. However, after addition of cold 5-HT to the bath in a concentration known to activate the inhibitory presynaptic 5-HT receptor, substance P, but not TRH, counteracted the inhibition of tritium outflow caused by cold 5-HT. These experiments were interpreted to indicate that substance P blocks the 5-HT presynaptic receptor, and consequently 5-HT induced inhibition of release (Mitchell and Fleetwood-Walker, 1981). Thus, substance P may enhance transmission at 5-HT synapses, as does TRH (see above), but the two peptides cause this principally in different ways, TRH via a postsynaptic and substance P by a presynaptic action (Fig. 12). In Fig. 16 we have speculated how such interactions could take place in the ventral horn of the spinal cord.

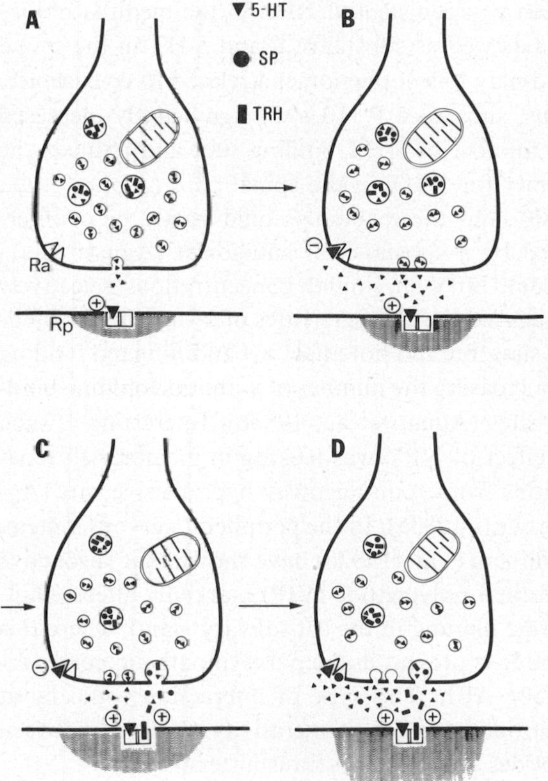

Fig. 16. Schematic illustration of a nerve ending in the ventral horn containing three messenger candidates, 5-hydroxytryptamine (5-HT), substance P (SP) and thyrotropin-releasing hormone (TRH) and the hypothetical events occurring during increasing impulse activity (A–D). At low impulse activity only 5-HT is released from small synaptic vesicles and activates a postsynaptic receptor (Rp). With increasing frequency 5-HT release increases and 5-HT also reaches presynaptic inhibitory autoreceptors (Ra), preventing further release of 5-HT and thus limiting the postsynaptic response (B). At high impulse traffic the large storage vesicles are activated, releasing not only 5-HT but also SP and TRH. Hereby TRH cooperates with 5-HT at a site closely coupled to the 5-HT receptor causing further activation of the postreceptor structure (C). Finally, SP blocks the effect of 5-HT on the inhibitory autoreceptor, allowing further 5-HT release and maximal activation of the postsynaptic membrane (D) (From Hökfelt et al., 1984b.)

Receptor-receptor interactions

Evidence has recently been presented that peptides can regulate the binding characteristics of monoamine receptors (see Agnati et al., 1984; Agnati et al. and Fuxe et al., this volume). In some cases, e.g. for DA and CCK peptides in the striatum and 5-HT and substance P in the cortex, this interaction may not be directly related to coexistence of these compounds. On the other hand, interactions between α_2-agonists and NPY in the medulla oblongata as well as substance P and 5-HT in the spinal cord may reflect phenomena related to coexistence. Thus, substance P (10 μM) significantly increased the number of 5-HT binding sites and reduced the affinity for 5-HT in the spinal cord (Agnati et al., 1980), and these actions could partly be counteracted by a substance P antagonist (Agnati et al., 1983c). NPY in similar concentrations selectively influenced the characteristics of α_2-adrenergic binding sites, but did not affect α_1- and β-ligand binding by increasing the number of *p*-aminoclonidine binding sites (Agnati et al., 1983b). Interestingly, such an effect of NPY was lacking in membrane preparations from spontaneously hypertensive rats (Agnati et al., 1983a). In the peripheral nervous system, Lundberg et al. (1982b) have shown that vasoactive intestinal polypeptide (VIP) markedly affects cholinergic binding in the cat salivary gland, where this peptide is present in the parasympathetic nerves releasing ACh. This type of interaction could be at least one basis for cooperativity observed between peptides and classical transmitters.

Distribution of receptors for coexisting messengers — autoradiographic studies

The studies related above, as well as findings described earlier in this article on, for example, the blocking effect of 5-HT antagonists on TRH-induced effects in the ventral horns of the spinal cord (Barbeau and Bedard, 1981), suggest that the receptors for coexisting classical transmitter and peptide may be closely related functionally. Only few studies have, however, dealt with the morphological, anatomical localization of such receptors. We have therefore compared the distribution of the α_2-agonist *p*-aminoclonidine and NPY. We have assumed that these two ligands may label receptors for, respectively NA/adrenaline and NPY, which are known to coexist in systems in the medulla oblongata (Everitt et al., 1984a). Using the autoradiographic technique of Young and Kuhar (1979), it was observed that both ligands exhibited distinct distribution patterns as shown in Fig. 17A,B. In fact, the two compounds exhibited very similar distribution patterns with high concentrations mainly in two areas, the superficial layers of the spinal trigeminal nucleus (ntV) and the dorsal vagal complex including nucleus commissuralis (ncom) (Fig. 17A,B). These findings confirm earlier autoradiographic demonstrations of high α_2-binding in these areas (Young and Kuhar, 1980; Palacios and Wamsley, 1984) as well as the biochemical demonstration of NPY binding sites in the rat brain (Undén et al., 1985). However, a comparison between the distribution of the presumable endogenous ligands, NA/adrenaline and NPY reveal that only in the dorsal vagal complex is there agreement with the distribution of the receptors. Thus, in the dorsal vagal complex a dense network of fibers containing both adrenaline and NPY has been demonstrated (Everitt et al., 1984), making likely that the overlap of receptor distribution corresponds to the distribution of nerve endings containing coexisting NPY and adrenaline. The spinal trigeminal nucleus contains a very dense NPY plexus in the superficial layers well overlapping with the NPY receptor distribution (Fig. 17C), but only a sparse network of NA fibers with a fairly even distribution within the nucleus (Fig. 17D) and no adrenaline fibers at all (see Moore and Card, 1984). Thus, there is an apparent mismatch problem, since the number of α_2-receptors appears much too high in the superficial layers of this nucleus, when comparing the number of noradrenergic or adrenergic fibers in this area.

Mismatch of receptors and endogenous ligands is not uncommon and has recently been discussed by Kuhar (1985), who mentioned several explanations. Here we would like to raise a further possibility. It may be speculated that the mismatch case observed in the present study may be related to coexistence. It is proposed that coupled receptors for coexisting endogenous ligands may occur, not only in areas where presynaptic elements containing the coexisting compounds occur but also in areas containing only one of the endogenous ligands. It may therefore be that the α_2- part of the α_2/NPY recep-

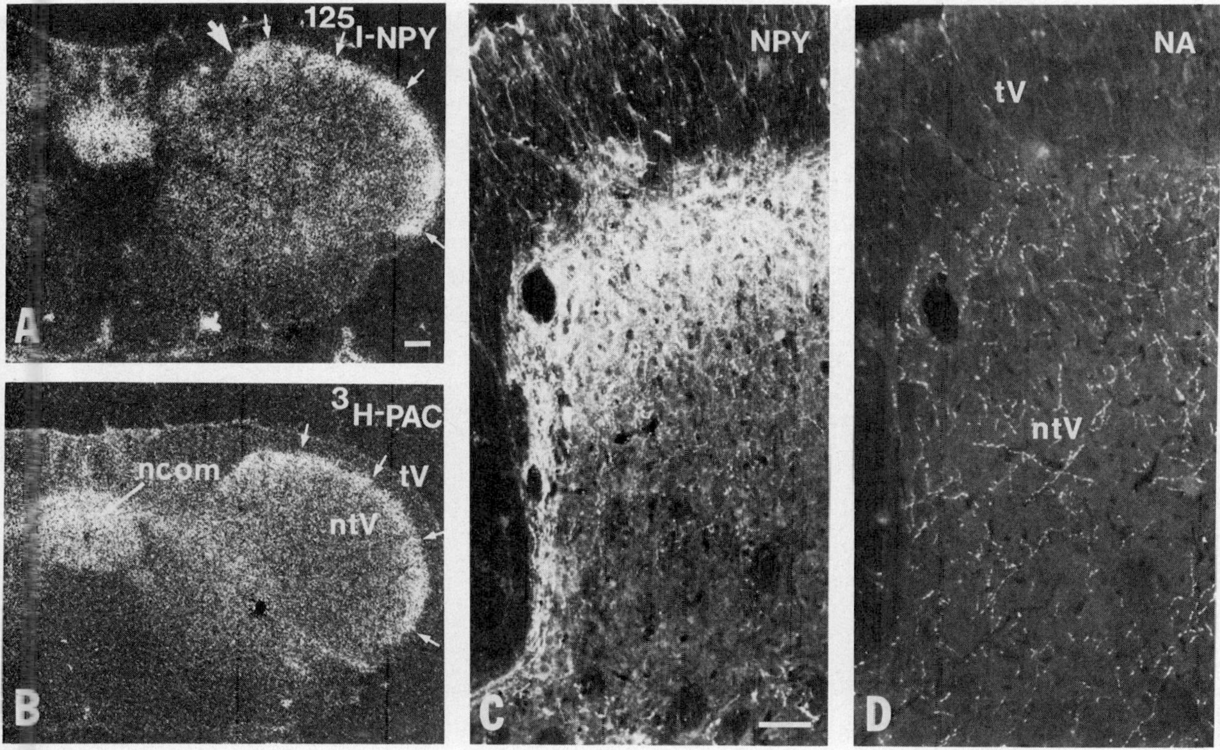

Fig. 17A–D. Autoradiographs of the lower medulla oblongata after incubation with [^{125}I]neuropeptide Y (NPY) (A) and *p*-[^{3}H]aminoclonidine (PAC) (B) and immunofluorescence micrographs of the dorsomedial part of the spinal tract nucleus of the trigeminal nerve (ntV) after incubation with antiserum to NPY and dopamine-β-hydroxylase (DBH), a marker for noradrenaline (NA) nerve fibers (D). Immunofluorescence micrographs have been taken from approximately the area indicated by arrow in A. (A,B) The two ligands show similar distribution patterns with high grain concentrations in the dorsal vagal complex, including the nucleus commissuralis (ncom) and in the superficial layers of the ntV (small arrows). (C,D) In contrast, a marked difference is seen between distribution of NPY- and DBH-immunoreactive fibers. The former show a dense network in the superficial layers of the ntV corresponding to the ligand binding (C). The NA fibers form a sparse, fairly regular plexus within the entire nucleus (D). tV = Tract of the spinal trigeminal nerve. Bar indicates 200 μm for A and B and 50 μm for C and D.

tor complex in this particular area may not be functionally important, but may only be present as a "silent" moiety. Alternatively, NA may act on the receptor after diffusion over a long distance.

Peptide-peptide interaction in the periphery and spinal cord

On the basis of recombinant DNA and molecular biological techniques a novel peptide has recently been discovered. Thus, analysis of the nucleotide sequence of the calcitonin gene provided evidence for the existence of a calcitonin gene-related peptide (CGRP) (Amara et al., 1982). From the base sequence the amino acid sequence was deduced and a synthetic peptide produced. Using antibodies to this peptide in immunohistochemical (and radioimmunological) studies, it could be demonstrated that CGRP is expressed in nervous tissues, and has a characteristic and unique distribution pattern including presence in primary sensory neurons (Rosenfeld et al., 1983). Several groups have observed that these CGRP-positive primary sensory neurons are identical to previously described substance P systems (Fig. 18A,B). (Gibson et al., 1984; Wiesen-

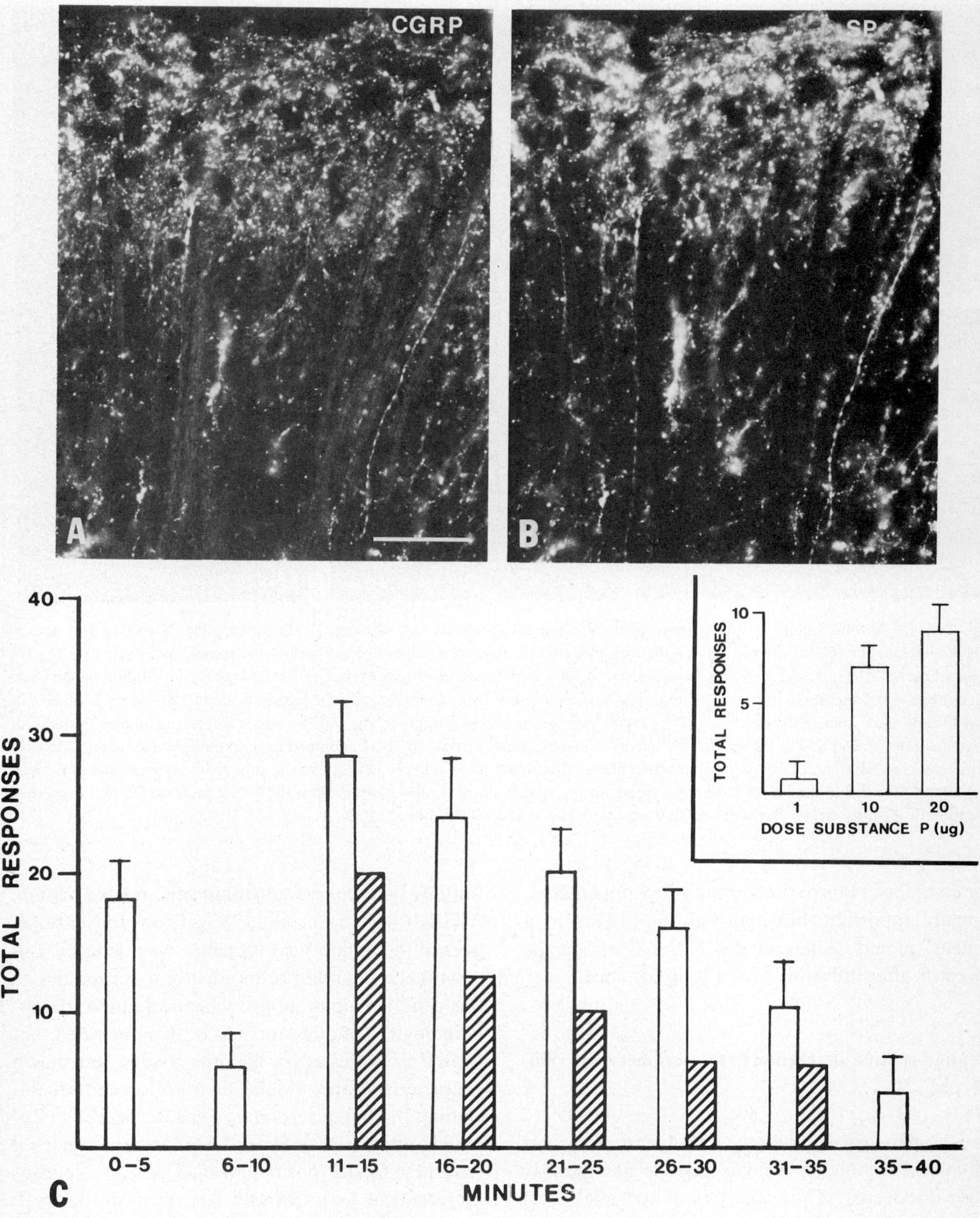
CGRP
A
SP
B
TOTAL RESPONSES
40
30
20
10
0-5
6-10
11-15
16-20
21-25
26-30
31-35
35-40
MINUTES
C
TOTAL RESPONSES
10
5
1
10
20
DOSE SUBSTANCE P (ug)

feld-Hallin et al., 1984; Gibbins et al., 1985; Lee et al., 1985; Lundberg et al., 1985; Tschopp et al., 1985). Several biological effects have been described for CGRP, for example, it exerts a vasodilatory action when administered peripherally (Rosenfeld et al., 1983; Brain et al., 1985). In view of the coexistence of substance P and CGRP in primary sensory neurons, we have attempted to analyze possible sites of interaction both in the periphery as well as in the spinal cord. These studies have revealed interesting types of interactions (Wiesenfeld-Hallin et al., 1984; Lundberg et al., 1985).

Interaction of substance P and CGRP has been analyzed at the level of the spinal cord by administration of these peptides onto the lumbar spinal cord via an intrathecal catheter according to Yaksh and Rudy (1976) (Wiesenfeld-Hallin et al., 1984). In this model, substance P has previously been shown to cause a behavior, characterized by caudally directed biting and scratching (Hylden and Wilcox, 1981; Piercey et al., 1981; Seybold et al., 1982). In our study, substance P (1, 10 and 20 μg) exhibited a dose-dependent behavior lasting for a few minutes, confirming the results mentioned above. Administration of CGRP alone in doses up to 20 μg does not induce any observable effects. However, if substance P (10 μg) and CGRP (20 μg) were injected together, a marked increase in the duration of the response to more than 30 min could be observed (Fig. 18C). The mechanism(s) underlying this dramatic effect has been analyzed by Terenius and collaborators. CGRP was found to potently inhibit a substance P endopeptidase which had been isolated from human CSF (Le Greves et al., 1985). This suggests that CGRP may enhance transmission at substance P synapses by inhibiting its degrading enzyme (Fig. 19) and may represent

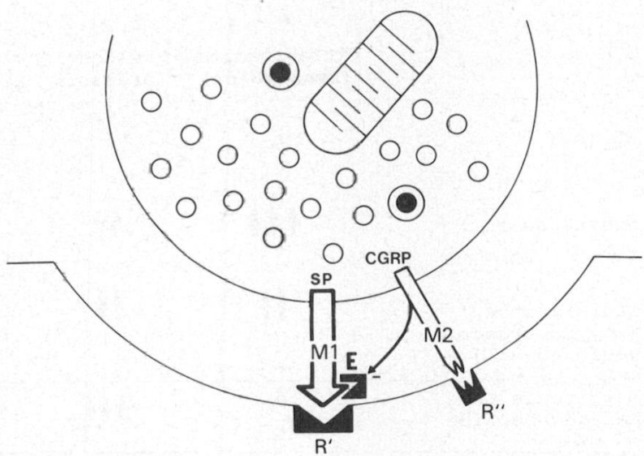

Fig. 19. Schematic illustration of a nerve ending containing substance P (SP) and calcitonin gene-related peptide (CGRP). Evidence discussed in the text supports the idea that CGRP may inhibit an endopeptidase, responsible for inactivation of SP. This could thus be the mechanism underlying the prolongation of the scratching and biting behavior induced by combined administration of SP and CGRP (see Fig. 18C).

a further type of interaction of two compounds released from the same nerve endings.

In peripheral tissues substance P and CGRP show a differential pattern of activities (Lundberg et al., 1985) (Fig. 20). Interesting similarities and differences were observed. Both compounds decreased blood pressure. However, substance P strongly increased extravasation and increased insufflation pressure in the lungs, whereas CGRP did not affect these functions. In contrast, CGRP markedly increased heart rate, ventricular rate and ventricular tension, which did not seem to be affected by substance P. These primary neurons in addition contain several other members of the tachykinin family (see Hua et al., 1985), neurokinin A (neurokinin-α, substance K, neuromidin L) (Kangawa et al., 1983; Kimura et al., 1983; Nawa et al., 1983;

Fig. 18A–C. Immunofluorescence micrographs of the dorsal horn of the spinal cord of a double stained section using goat antiserum to calcitonin gene-related peptide (CGRP) (A) and rabbit antiserum to substance P (SP) (B). C shows a drawing of the response of rats to intrathecally applied substance P (1, 10 and 20 μg) (inset) and of combined administration of CGRP (open bars, 10 μg SP + 20 μg CGRP; hatched bars 1 μg SP + 20 μg CGRP). (A,B) By switching between filters for red fluorescent CGRP (A) and green fluorescent SP (B) it can be demonstrated that most fibers in the dorsal horn contain both peptides. Bar indicates 50 μm. (C) SP alone (inset) causes a small number of caudally directed biting and scratching responses, a behavior which lasts for up to 5 min. The combined administration of the peptide markedly prolongs this behavior, which has a duration of up to 40 min. With the highest doses there is an indication of a biphasic response (open bars).

	Extravasation (Evan's Blue)	Blood pressure	Insufflation pressure	Heart rate	Ventricular rate	Ventricular tension
Saline	0	0	0	0	0	0
Substance P	↑↑↑	↓↓	↑↑	0	0	0
Neurokinin A (α, Substance K, Neuromedin L)	↑↑	↓↓	↑↑↑	↓↓	↓↓	↓↓
Calcitonin Gene Related Peptide	0	↓↓↓	0	↑↑↑	↑↑↑	↑↑
Capsacin	↑↑	↓↓	↑↑↑	↑↑	↑↑	↑
Neurokinin B (β, Neuromedin K)	↑↑	↓↓	↑↑	0	0	0

Fig. 20. Schematic illustration of peripheral effects induced by some tachykinins, calcitonin gene-related peptide (CGRP) and capsaicin. Substance P and neurokinin A as well as CGRP have been demonstrated to occur in the same primary sensory neurons. Capsaicin is a drug which acutely causes release of peptides present in fine caliber primary sensory neurons. Neurokinin B is a tachykinin, which so far has not been demonstrated in primary sensory neurons. For further details see text.

Minamino et al., 1984) and neuropeptide K (Tatemoto et al., 1985). Neurokinin A exerts some effects similar to substance P and others to CGRP and in addition some opposite to CGRP. Since little is known about actual release of these compounds or interaction at the receptor level, these results are at the moment complex and difficult to explain. Focusing on substance P/CGRP interactions, it may

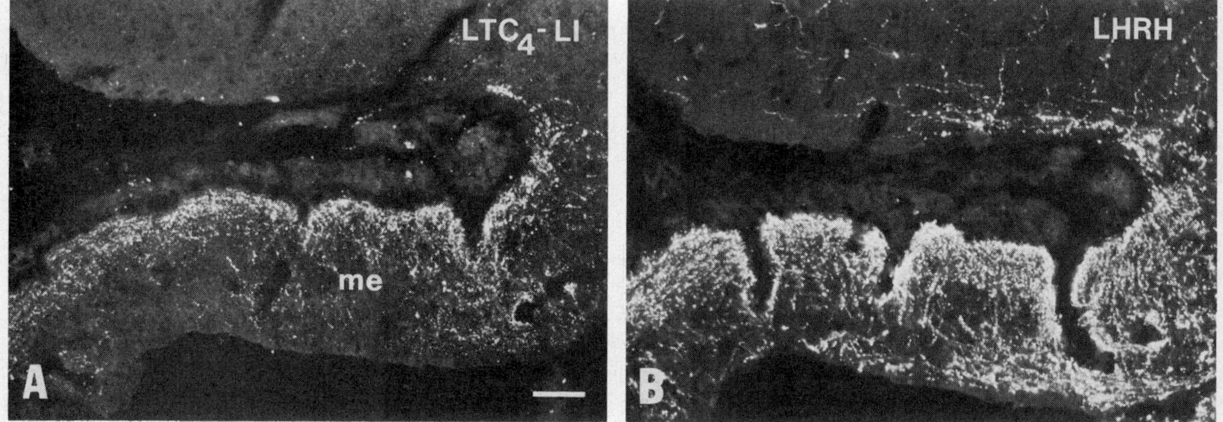

Fig. 21. Immunofluorescence micrographs of adjacent sections of the basal surface of hypothalamus and median eminence (me) of guinea pig after incubation with antiserum raised to LTC_4 conjugated with bovine serum albumin (A) and to luteinizing hormone releasing hormone (LHRH). The two antisera give a staining pattern which shows a high degree of overlap. The LHRH-positive network appears somewhat stronger and perhaps somewhat more extensive. Bar indicates 50 μm.

be speculated that different tissues and components of tissues have different receptor populations. Thus, for example, heart tissue may have CGRP receptors, whereas substance P receptors are lacking on heart muscle cells. Under such circumstances the neuron would not need to be able to differentially release CGRP and substance P, but specificity of action is achieved by absence or presence of the receptors for the respective peptide on the postsynaptic cells.

Evidence for novel types of coexisting messengers — leukotrienes

Recently evidence has been presented that various members of the leukotriene family (see Samuelsson, 1983) can be produced in the brain, possibly by nervous tissue (Dembinska-Kieć et al., 1984; Lindgren et al., 1984; Moskowitz et al., 1984). With high performance liquid chromatography (HPLC), radioimmunoassay and bioassay, formation of LTC_4, LTD_4 and LTE_4 was demonstrated in slices of brain tissue incubated with arachidonic acid and the ionophore A23187 (Lindgren et al., 1984). LTC_4 biosynthesis showed regional patterns with the lowest production in median eminence and highest in hypothalamus and cerebellum, being almost 10 times higher in the hypothalamus than in the cerebellum. Using an antiserum raised against LTC_4 conjugated to bovine serum albumin (BSA) (Aeringhaus et al., 1982), attempts were made to determine the cellular localization by immunohistochemistry. Numerous immunoreactive cell bodies were observed in many parts of the brain (Lindgren et al., 1984), but in control experiments, it was not possible to abolish the staining patterns, except for one region — the median eminence. Here a dense fiber network in the lateral part of the median eminence was seen. Comparative studies demonstrated that the LTC_4-positive fibers were identical to LHRH nerve endings, showing coexistence of the two compounds (Hulting et al., 1985).

These findings suggest involvement of a LTC_4-like compound in control of LH release from the anterior pituitary gland. In fact, in studies on rat anterior pituitary cells in vitro it was shown that LTC_4 in the picomolar range can release LH but not growth hormone (Hulting et al., 1984, 1985). In contrast, the LTC_4 precursor LTB_4 had no effect on the release of these two hormones. The stimulatory effect of LTC_4 was seen after 0.5 h incubation but not after 3 h, suggesting a fairly rapid but transient effect. In contrast, LHRH released LH with a slow onset but with a longer duration. These findings indicate that LH release from gonadotro-

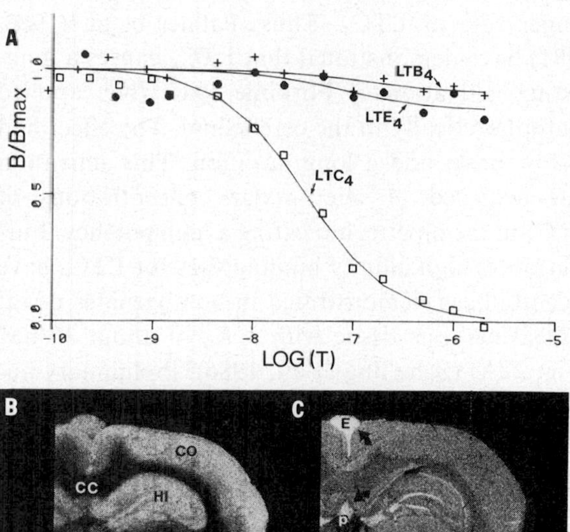

Fig. 22A–C. (A) Equilibrium binding analysis for LTC_4 (□), LTB_4 (+) and LTE_4 (●). One specific binding site with a K_D of about 31 mN and B_{max} of about 41 mol/mg of protein for the whole brain membrane preparation is demonstrated. The analysis of equilibrium binding for LTB_4 and LTE_4 suggests one weak, low capacity binding site for these ligands. (B,C) Autoradiographs of adjacent sections incubated with tritiated LTC_4 (B) and LTB_4 (C). LTC_4 binding shows high grain density in cortex (CO) and hippocampus (hi) with a variable binding in the thalamus (TH) and hypothalamus (HY). In contrast, LTB_4 binding is even in all brain areas, with higher concentrations in plexus choroideus (p) and epiphysis (E) and in ependymal cells. CC = Corpus callosum.

pins in the anterior pituitary may be under dual control, a fast acting factor related to an LTC_4-like compound in addition to the conventional LH releaser, LHRH.

Recent studies have demonstrated that LTC_4-like material can be observed in LHRH fibers in the external layer of the median eminence of several other species, including guinea pig (Fig. 21), rabbit, monkey and man but not in mouse (Hökfelt et al., 1986), suggesting that involvement of an LTC_4-like compound in the control of pituitary LH release may be common among mammals.

These findings support earlier evidence for a messenger role of LTC_4. Thus, Palmer et al. (1980, 1981) have demonstrated that LTC_4 causes a long-lasting activation of Purkinje cells when applied iontophoretically in the cerebellum. The effect had a slow onset and a long duration. This activation was achieved at micromolar concentrations of LTC_4 in the pipette, indicating a high potency. Furthermore, high affinity binding sites for LTC_4 have recently been demonstrated in homogenates of rat central nervous tissue with a K_D of about 30 nM (Fig. 22A) (Schalling et al., 1986). Preliminary autoradiographic studies have shown that $[^3H]LTC_4$ binding to sections of the brain exhibits a differential distribution pattern which is clearly different from the one seen for LTB_4 (Fig. 22B,C) (Schalling, Hökfelt, Lindgren and Samuelsson, in preparation). Thus, leukotrienes or a similar compound(s) may represent a novel type of messenger molecule(s) in the nervous system. Clearly, the results described above are very preliminary and need further substantiation.

Conclusions

The present article deals with results demonstrating that neurons often contain more than one chemical compound, and these may act as messengers. Different types of coexistence situations have been described including (1) a classical transmitter and one or more peptides, (2) more than one classical transmitter, and (3) a classical transmitter, a peptide and ATP. The functional significance of these histochemical findings are at present difficult to evaluate, but in studies on the PNS evidence has been obtained that classical transmitter and peptide are co-released and interact in a cooperative way on effector cells. In addition to enhancement, there is also evidence that other types of interaction may occur, for example, the peptide may inhibit the release of the classical transmitter. Also in the CNS indirect evidence is present for similar mechanisms, i.e. to strengthen transmission at synaptic (or non-synaptic) sites and also for peptide inhibition of release of a classical transmitter. Thus, coexistence should not be looked upon as a uniform phenomenon, but multiple types of interaction may provide a mechanism for obtaining differential responses and for conveying an increased number of messages.

It is important to note that the different types of compounds discussed here not necessarily have to be involved in the process of transmission at synapses but could also participate in other events, for example, to have trophic effects or induce other types of long-term events in neurons and effector cells. It has, for example, been shown that substance P exerts growth stimulatory effects on smooth muscle cells (Nilsson et al., 1985). It may

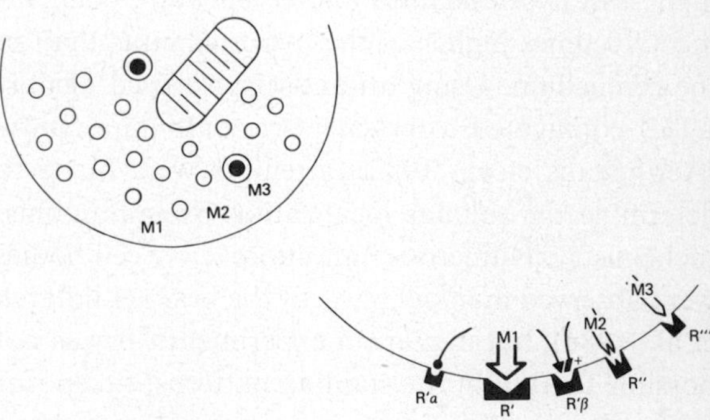

Fig. 23. Schematic illustration of our "view" on the present situation for the functional analysis of the significance of coexisting messengers. In a few years knowledge has accumulated on coexistence situations in the presynaptic nerve endings as well as possible postsynaptic interactions and mechanisms, but much work remains to tie this information together into a meaningful picture of the events going on at synapses involving multiple messengers.

be argued that the fact that the coexistence phenomenon indeed occurs, provides a basis that peptides may well be involved in other functions, since they are present in neurons which already have a transmitter at their disposal, the classical transmitter.

Multiple messengers may provide the means for increasing the capacity for information transfer in the nervous system. Considering the large number of neurons and the even larger number of nerve endings, one may wonder why it should not be sufficient with one transmitter at each synapse. However, although redundancy is an important feature of the CNS, one should bear in mind the enormous operational capacity of our brain and, it may, in fact, be necessary to use the huge but still finite number of neurons in the most efficient way. Transmission via multiple messengers may be a way to achieve the outstanding performance of our neuronal machinery.

It is, however, at this point also necessary to look upon the coexistence phenomenon with critical eyes in view of the discrepancy between the extensive immunohistochemical findings and the meager physiological evidence. It can, in fact, not be excluded that coexistence of multiple messengers is a paraphenomenon, which could represent a consequence of evolution. Perhaps peptides have been important messengers early in evolution, but have later on been replaced by more efficient, small-molecule transmitters and the peptides could very well be carried along more or less as "silent passengers".

We have tried to illustrate the present situation, as we see it (see Fig. 23). Thus, a wide range of data are available with regard to coexistence in the presynaptic part of the neuron and interesting information has been collected with regard to interaction at the receptor level, but much work needs to be done to establish if and how these results fit into physiological events in the nervous system.

Acknowledgements

This research was supported by grants from the Swedish Medical Research Council (04X-2887; 12X-5189), Knut and Alice Wallenbergs Stiftelse, Petrus och Augusta Hedlunds Stiftelse and Magnus Bergvalls Stiftelse. We thank Ms. W. Hiort, Ms. S. Nilsson and Ms. A. Peters for excellent technical assistance and Ms. E. Björklund for skilful help in preparing the manuscript. We thank Ragnar Mårtensson for supplying the fluorescence micrograph used in Fig. 5.

Some results in this review article are taken from ongoing collaborative research with colleagues as indicated by the papers referred to (see reference list). We thank in particular Professor Claudio Cuello, Department of Pharmacology and Therapeutics, McGill University, Montreal, Canada for substance P antiserum, Dr. Robert Elde, Department of Anatomy, University of Minnesota, Minneapolis, Minn., U.S.A. for somatostatin antiserum, Professor Jan Fahrenkrug, Department of Clinical Chemistry, Bispbjerg Hospital, Copenhagen, Denmark for VIP and PHI antisera, Professor Jan Fischer, Orthophädische Universitätsklinik Balgrist, Zürich, Switzerland for CGRP antiserum, Professor Carlo Patrono, Department of Pharmacology, Universita Cattolica, Rome, Italy for LTC_4 antiserum, Professor Jens Rehfeld, Department of Clinical Chemistry, Rigshospitalet, Copenhagen, Denmark, Dr. Paul Salvaterra, Division of Neuroscience, Beckman Research Institute, City of Hope, Duarte, Calif., U.S.A. for ChAT antiserum and Dr. Albert Verhofstad, Department of Anatomy and Embryology, Katholieke Universiteit Nijmegen, The Netherlands for 5-HT antiserum.

References

Aehringhaus, U., Wölbling, R. H., König, W., Patrono, C., Peskar, B. M. and Peskar, B. A. (1982) Release of leukotriene C_4 from human polymorphonuclear leucocytes as determined by radioimmunoassay. *FEBS Lett.*, 146: 111–114.

Agnati, L. F., Fuxe, K., Zini, I., Lenzi, P. and Hökfelt, T. (1980) Aspects on receptor regulation and isoreceptor identification. *Med. Biol.*, 58: 182–187.

Agnati, L. F., Fuxe, K., Benfenati, F., Battistini, Härfstrand, A., Hökfelt, T, Cavicchioli, L., Tatemoto, K. and Mutt, V.

(1983a) Failure of neuropeptide Y in vitro to increase the number of α_2-binding sites in membranes of medulla oblongata of the spontaneous hypertensive rat. *Acta physiol. Scand.*, 119: 309–312.

Agnati, L. F., Fuxe, K., Benfenati, F., Battistini, Härfstrand, A., Hökfelt, T., Tatemoto, K. and Mutt, V. (1983b) Neuropeptide Y in vitro selectively increases the number of α_2-adrenergic binding sites in membranes of the medulla oblongata of the rat. *Acta physiol. Scand.*, 118: 293–295.

Agnati, L. F., Fuxe, K., Benfenati, F., Zini, I. and Hökfelt, T. (1983c) On the functional role of coexistence of 5-HT and substance P in bulbospinal 5-HT neurons. Substance P reduces affinity and increases density of ^{3}H-5-HT binding sites. *Acta physiol. Scand.*, 117: 299–301.

Agnati, L. F., Fuxe, K., Benfenati, F., Battistini, N., Zini, I., Camurri, M. and Hökfelt, T. (1984) Postsynaptic effects of neuropeptide comodulators at central monoamine synapses. In E. Usdin, A. Carlsson, A. Dahlström and J. Engel (Eds.), *Neurology and Neurobiology, Vol. 8B: Catecholamines, Part B: Neuropharmacology and Central Nervous System — Theoretical Aspects,* Alan R. Liss, Inc., New York, pp. 191–198.

Allen, J. M., Tatemoto, K., Polak, J. M., Hughes, J. and Bloom, S. R. (1982) Two novel related peptides, neuropeptide Y (NPY) and peptide YY (PYY) inhibit the contraction of the electrically stimulated mouse vas deferens. *Neuropeptides,* 3: 71–77.

Altschuler, R. A., Parakkal, M. H. and Fex, J. (1983) Localization of enkephalin-like immunoreactivity in acetylcholinesterase-positive cells in the guinea-pig lateral superior olivary complex that project to the cochlea. *Neuroscience,* 9: 621–630.

Amara, S. G., Jonas, V., Rosenfeld, M. G., Ong, E. S. and Evans, R. M. (1982) Alternative RNA-processing in calcitonin gene expression generates mRNAs encoding different polypeptide products. *Nature (Lond.)*, 298: 240–244.

Andén, N.-E., Jukes, M. and Lundberg, A. (1964) Spinal reflexes and monoamine liberation. *Nature (Lond.)*, 202: 1222–1223.

Armstrong, D. M., Miller, R. J., Beaudet, A. and Pickel, V. M. (1984) Enkephalin-like immunoreactivity in rat area postrema: Ultrastructural localization and coexistence with serotonin. *Brain Res.*, 310: 269–278.

Barbeau, H. and Bédard, P. (1981) Similar motor effects of 5-HT and TRH in rats following chronical spinal transection and 5,7-dihydroxytryptamine injection. *Neuropharmacology,* 20: 477–481.

Bargmann, W. and Scharrer, B. (1951) The site of origin of the hormones of the posterior pituitary. *Amer.Sci.*, 39: 255–259.

Belin, M. F., Nanopoulos, D., Didier, M., Aguera, M., Steinbusch, H., Verhofstad, A., Maitre, M. and Pujol, J. F. (1983) Immunohistochemical evidence for the presence of γ-aminobutyric acid and serotonin in one nerve cell. A study on the raphe nuclei of the rat using antibodies to glutamate decarboxylase and serotonin. *Brain Res.*, 275: 329–339.

Berod, A., Chat, M., Paut, L. and Tappaz, M. (1984) Catecholaminergic and GABAergic anatomical relationship in the rat substantia nigra, locus coeruleus, and hypothalamic median eminence: Immunocytochemical visualization of biosynthetic enzymes on serial semithin plastic-embedded sections. *J. Histochem. Cytochem.*, 32: 1331–1338.

Björklund, H.,Hökfelt, T., Goldstein, M., Terenius, L. and Olson, L. (1985) Appearance of the noradrenergic markers tyrosine hydroxylase and neuropeptide Y in cholinergic nerves of the iris following sympathectomy. *J. Neurosci.*, 5: 1633–1643.

Bloom, F. E. (1979) Contrasting principles of synaptic physiology: peptidergic and non-peptidergic neurons. In K. Fuxe, T. Hökfelt and R. Luft (Eds.), *Central Regulation of the Endocrine System,* Novel Foundation Symposium 42, Plenum Press, New York, pp. 173–187.

Brain, S. D., Williams, T. J. Tippins, J. R. Morris, H. R. and MacIntyre, I. (1985) Calcitonin gene-related peptide is a potent vasodilator. *Nature (Lond.)*, 313: 54–56.

Burnstock, G. (1976) Do some nerve cells release more than one transmitter. *Neuroscience,* 1: 239–248.

Burnstock, G. (1985) Purinergic mechanisms broaden their sphere of influence. *Trends Neurosci.*, 8: 5–6.

Caffé, A. R. and van Leeuwen, F. W. (1983) Vasopressin-immunoreactive cells in the dorsomedial hypothalamic region, medial amygdaloid nucleus and locus coeruleus of the rat. *Cell Tissue Res.*, 233: 23–33.

Carlsson, A., Lindqvist, M., Magnusson, T. and Waldeck, B. (1958) On the presence of 3-hydroxytryptamine in brain. *Science,* 127: 471.

Carlsson, A., Falck, B. and Hillarp, N.-Å. (1962) Demonstration of catecholamines with a histochemical fluorescence method. *Acta physiol. Scand.*, 56, Suppl. 56: 1–28.

Chan-Palay, V. (1979) Combined immunocytochemistry and autoradiography after in vivo injection of monoclonal antibody to substance P and ^{3}H-serotonin: Coexistence of two putative transmitters in single raphe cells and fiber plexuses. *Anat. Embryol.*, 156: 241–254.

Chan-Palay, V. and Palay, S. L. (Eds.) (1984) *Coexistence of Neuroactive Substances in Neurons,* John Wiley & Sons, New York.

Chan-Palay, V., Jonsson, G. and Palay, S. L. (1978) Serotonin and substance P coexist in neurons of the rat's central nervous system, *Proc. nat. Acad. Sci. USA,* 75: 1582–1586.

Chan-Palay, V., Nilaver, G., Palay, S. L., Beinfeld, M. C., Zimmerman, E. A., Wu, J.-Y. and O'Donohue, T. L. (1981) Chemical heterogeneity in cerebellar Purkinje cells: evidence and coexistence of glutamic acid decarboxylase-like and motilin-like immunoreactivities. *Proc. nat. Acad. Sci. USA,* 78: 7787–7791.

Charnay, Y., Léger, L., Dray, F., Bérod, A., Jouvet, M., Pujol, J. F. and Dubois, P. M. (1982) Evidence for the presence of enkephalin in catecholaminergic neurons of cat locus coeruleus. *Neurosci. Lett.*, 30: 147–151.

Coons, A. H. (1958) Fluorescent antibody methods. In J. F. Danielli (Ed.), *General Cytochemical Methods,* Academic Press, New York, pp. 399–422.

Costa, M. and Furness, J. B. (1984) Somatostatin is present in subpopulation of noradrenergic nerve fibres supplying the intestine. *Neuroscience,* 13: 911–919.

Cuello, A. C. (Ed.) (1982) *Co-transmission,* MacMillan, London and Basingstoke.

Dahlström, A. (1971) Effects of vinblastine and colchicine on monoamine containing neurons of the rat with special regard to the axoplasmic transport of amine granules. *Acta Neuropathol.,* Suppl. 5: 226–237.

Dahlström, A. and Fuxe, K. (1964) Evidence of the existence of monoamine-containing neurons in the central nervous system. I. Demonstration of monoamines in the cell bodies of brain stem neurons. *Acta physiol. Scand.,* 62, Suppl. 232: 1–55.

Dahlström, A. and Fuxe, K. (1965) Evidence for the existence of monoamine containing neurons in the central nervous system. II. Experimentally induced changes in the intraneuronal levels of bulbospinal neuron system. *Acta physiol. Scand.,* 64, Suppl. 247: 5–36.

Dale, H. (1934) Pharmacology and nerve-endings. *Proc. roy. Soc. Med.,* 28: 319–332.

Dalsgaard, C.-J., Hökfelt, T., Schultzberg, M., Lundberg, J. M., Terenius, L., Dockray, G. J. and Goldstein, M. (1983) Origin of peptide-containing fibers in the inferior mesenteric ganglion of the guinea pig: Immunohistochemical studies with antisera to substance P, enkephalin, vasoactive intestinal polypeptide, cholecystokinin and bombesin. *Neuroscience,* 9: 191–211.

Dembinska-Kieć, A., Simmet, T. and Peskar, B. A. (1984) Formation of leukotriene C_4-like material by rat brain tissue. *Eur. J. Pharmacol.,* 99: 57–62.

Eccles, J. C. (1964) *The Physiology of Synapses,* Springer-Verlag, Berlin.

Eccles, J. C. (1976) From electrical to chemical transmission in the central nervous system. *Notes and Records of the Royal Society of London,* 30: 219–230.

Eccles, J. C., Fatt, P. and Koketsu, K. (1954) Cholinergic and inhibitory synapses in a pathway from motor axon collaterals to motoneurones. *J. Physiol. (Lond.),* 126: 524–562.

Eckenstein, F. and Baughman, R. W. (1984) Two types of cholinergic innervation in cortex, one co-localized with vasoactive intestinal polypeptide. *Nature (Lond.),* 309: 153–155.

Elliott, T. R. (1905) The action of adrenalin. *J. Physiol. (Lond.),* 32: 401–407.

Everitt, B. J., Hökfelt, T., Terenius, L., Tatemoto, K., Mutt, V. and Goldstein, M. (1984a) Differential co-existence of neuropeptide Y (NPY)-like immunoreactivity with catecholamines in the central nervous system of the rat. *Neuroscience,* 11: 443–462.

Everitt, J. E., Hökfelt, T., Wu, J.-Y. and Goldstein, M. (1984b) Coexistence of tyrosine hydroxylase-like and gamma-aminobutyric acid-like immunoreactivities in neurons of the arcuate nucleus. *Neuroendocrinology,* 39: 189–191.

Everitt, B. J., Meister, B., Hökfelt, T., Melander, T., Terenius, L., Rökaeus, Å., Theodorsson-Norheim, Dockray, G.,Edwardson, J., Cuello, A.C., Elde, R., Goldstein, M., Hemmings, H., Ouimet, C., Walaas, I., Greengard, P., Vale, W., Weber, E. and Wu, J.-Y. (1986) The hypothalamic arcuate nucleus — median eminence complex: Immunohistochemistry of transmitters, peptides and DARPP-32 with special reference to coexistence in dopamine neurons. *Brain Res. Rev.* (in press).

Faden, A. I., Jacobs, T. P. and Holaday, J. W. (1981) Thyrotrophin-releasing hormone improves neurologic recovery after spinal trauma in cats. *New Engl. J. Med.,* 305: 1063–1067.

Fonnum, F. (Ed.) (1978) *Amino Acids as Chemical Transmitters,* NATO Advanced Study Institutes Series. Series A: Life Sciences, Plenum Press, New York.

Freedman, J., Hökfelt, T., Jonsson, G. and Post, C. (1986) Thyrotropin-releasing hormone (TRH) counteracts neuronal damage induced by a substance P-antagonist. *Exp. Brain Res.,* 62: 175–178.

Fried, G. (1982) Neuropeptide storage in vesicles. In R. L. Klein, H. Lagercrantz and H. Zimmerman (Eds.), *Neurotransmitter Vesicles,* Academic Press, Inc., London, pp. 361–374.

Fried, G., Terenius, L., Hökfelt, T. and Goldstein, M. (1985) Evidence for differential localization of noradrenaline and neuropeptide Y (NPY) in neuronal storage vesicles isolated from vas deferens. *J. Neurosci.,* 5: 450–458.

Furness, J. B., Costa, M., Emson, P. C., Håkanson, R., Moghimzadeh, E., Sundler, F., Taylor, J. L. and Chance, R. E. (1983) Distribution, pathways and reactions to drug treatment of nerves with neuropeptide Y- and pancreatic polypeptide-like immunoreactivity in the guinea pig digestive tract. *Cell Tissue Res.,* 234: 71–92.

Fuxe, K. (1965a) Evidence for the existence of monoamine neurons in the central nervous system. III. The monoamine nerve terminal. *Z. Zellforsch. Mikrosk. Anat.,* 65: 573–596.

Fuxe, K. (1965b) Evidence for the existence of monoamine neurons in the central nervous system. IV. The distribution of monoamine nerve terminals in the central nervous system. *Acta physiol. Scand.,* 64, Suppl. 247: 39–85.

Gibbins, I. L., Furness, J. B., Costa, M., MacIntyre, I., Hillyard, C. J. and Girgis, S. (1985) Co-localization of calcitonin gene-related peptide-like immunoreactivity with substance P in cutaneous, vascular and visceral sensory neurons of guinea pigs. *Neurosci. Lett.,* 57: 125–130.

Gibson, S. J., Polak, J. M., Bloom, S. R., Sabate, I. M., Mulderry, P. M., Ghatei, M. A., McGregor, G. P., Morrison, J. F. B., Kelly, J. S., Evans, R. M. and Rosenfeld, M. G. (1984) Calcitonin gene-related peptide immunoreactivity in the spinal cord of man and of eight other species. *J. Neurosci.,* 4: 3101–3111.

Gilbert, R. F. T., Emson, P. C., Hunt, S. P., Bennett, G. W.,

Marsden, C. A., Sandberg, B. E. B., Steinbusch, H. and Verhofstad, A. A. J. (1982) The effects of monoamine neurotoxins on peptides in the rat spinal cord. *Neuroscience,* 7: 69–88.

Glazer, E. J., Steinbusch, H., Verhofstad, A. and Basbaum, A. I. (1981) Serotonin neurons in nucleus raphe dorsalis and paragigantocellularis of the cat contain enkephalin, *J. Physiol. (Paris),* 77: 241–245.

Hansen, S., Svensson, L., Hökfelt, T. and Everitt, B. J. (1983) 5-Hydroxytryptamine-thyrotropin releasing hormone interactions in the spinal cord: effects on parameters of sexual behaviour in the male rat. *Neurosci. Lett.,* 42: 299–304.

Hendry, S. H. C., Jones, E. G., DeFelipe, J., Schmechel, D., Brandon, C. and Emson, P. C. (1984) Neuropeptide-containing neurons of the cerebral cortex are also GABAergic. *Proc. nat. Acad. Sci. USA,* 81: 6526–6530.

Hille, B. (1984) *Ionic Channels of Exitable Membranes,* Sinauer Ass. Inc., Sunderland, MS.

Hökfelt, T. (1968) In vitro studies on central and peripheral monoamine neurons at the ultrastructural level. *Z. Zellforsch.,* 91: 1–74.

Hökfelt, T., Fuxe, K., Goldstein, M. and Johansson, O. (1973) Evidence for adrenaline neurons in the rat brain. *Acta physiol. Scand.,* 89: 286–288.

Hökfelt, T., Fuxe, K., Goldstein, M. and Johansson, O. (1974) Immunohistochemical evidence for the existence of adrenaline neurons in the rat brain. *Brain Res.,* 66: 235–251.

Hökfelt, T., Elfvin, L.-G., Elde, R., Schultzberg, M., Goldstein, M. and Luft, R. (1977a) Occurrence of somatostatin-like immunoreactivity in some peripheral sympathetic noradrenergic neurons. *Proc. nat. Acad. Sci. USA,* 74: 3587–3591.

Hökfelt, T., Elfvin, L.-G., Schultzberg, M., Fuxe, K., Said, S. J., Mutt, V. and Goldstein, M. (1977b) Immunohistochemical evidence of vasoactive intestinal polypeptide-containing neurons and nerve fibers in sympathetic ganglia. *Neuroscience,* 2: 885–896.

Hökfelt, T., Ljungdahl, A., Steinbusch, H., Verhofstad, A., Nilsson, G., Brodin, E., Pernow, B. and Goldstein, M. (1978) Immunohistochemical evidence of substance P-like immunoreactivity in some 5-hydroxytryptamine-containing neurons in the rat central nervous system, *Neuroscience,* 3: 517–538.

Hökfelt, T., Johansson, O., Ljungdahl, Å., Lundberg, J. M. and Schultzberg, M. (1980a) Peptidergic neurons. *Nature (Lond.),* 284: 515–521.

Hökfelt, T., Lundberg, J. M., Schultzberg, M., Johansson, O., Ljungdahl, Å. and Rehfeld, J. (1980b) Coexistence of peptides and putative transmitters in neurons. In E. Costa and M. Trabucchi (Eds.), *Neural Peptides and Neuronal Communication,* Raven Press, New York, pp. 1–23.

Hökfelt, T., Rehfeld, J. F., Skirboll, L., Ivemark, B., Goldstein, M. and Markey, K. (1980c) Evidence for coexistence of dopamine and CCK in mesolimbic neurones. *Nature (Lond.),* 285: 476–478.

Hökfelt, T., Skirboll, L., Rehfeld, J. F., Goldstein, M., Markey, K. and Dann, O. (1980d) A subpopulation of mesencephalic dopamine neurons projecting to limbic areas contains a cholecystokinin-like peptide: evidence from immunohistochemistry combined with retrograde tracing, *Neuroscience,* 5: 2093–2124.

Hökfelt, T., Vincent, S., Hellsten, L., Rosell, S., Folkers, K., Markey, K., Goldstein, M. and Cuello, C. (1981) Immunohistochemical evidence for a "neurotoxic" action of (D-Pro^2, D-Trp^{7,9})-substance P, an analogue with substance P antagonistic activity. *Acta physiol. Scand.,* 113: 571–573.

Hökfelt, T., Lundberg, J. M., Skirboll, L., Johansson, O., Schultzberg, M. and Vincent, S. R. (1982) Coexistence of classical transmitters and peptides in neurons. In A. C. Cuello (Ed.), *Co-transmission,* MacMillan, London and Basingtoke, pp. 77–126.

Hökfelt, T., Lundberg, J. M., Lagercrantz, H., Tatemoto, K., Mutt, V., Lundberg, J. M., Terenius, L., Everitt, B. J., Fuxe, K., Agnati, L. F. and Goldstein, M. (1983a) Occurrence of neuropeptide Y (NPY)-like immunoreactivity in catecholamine neurons in the human medulla oblongata. *Neurosci. Lett.,* 36: 217–222.

Hökfelt, T., Skagerberg, G., Skirboll, L. and Björklund, A. (1983b) Combination of retrograde tracing and neurotransmitter histochemistry. In A. Björklund and T. Hökfelt (Eds.), *Handbook of Chemical Neuroanatomy, Vol. 1: Methods in Chemical Neuroanatomy,* Elsevier, Amsterdam, pp. 228–285.

Hökfelt, T., Everitt, B. J., Theodorsson-Norheim, E. and Goldstein, M. (1984a) Occurrence of neurotensinlike immunoreactivity in subpopulations of hypothalamic, mesencephalic, and medullary catecholamine neurons. *J. comp. Neurol.,* 222: 543–559.

Hökfelt, T., Johansson, O. and Goldstein, M. (1984b) Chemical anatomy of the brain. *Science,* 225: 1326–1334.

Hökfelt, T., Johansson, O. and Goldstein, M. (1984c) In A. Björklund and T. Hökfelt (Eds.), *Handbook of Chemical Neuroanatomy, Vol. 2: Classical Transmitters in the CNS, Part I,* Elsevier, Amsterdam, pp. 157–276.

Hökfelt, T., Mårtensson, R., Björklund, A., Kleinau, S. and Goldstein, M. (1984d) Distributional maps of tyrosine hydroxylase immunoreactive neurons in the rat brain. In A. Björklund and T. Hökfelt (Eds.), *Handbook of Chemical Neuroanatomy, Vol. 2: Classical Transmitters in the CNS, Part I,* Elsevier, Amsterdam, pp. 277–379.

Hökfelt, T., Skirboll, L., Everitt, B. J., Meister, B., Brownstein, M., Jacobs, T., Faden, A., Kuga, S., Goldstein, M., Markstein, R., Dockray, G. and Rehfeld, J. (1985) Distribution of cholecystokinin-like immunoreactivity in the nervous system with special reference to coexistence with classical neurotransmitters and other neuropeptides. In J. J. Vanderhaeghen and J. Crawley (Eds.), *Neuronal Cholecystokinin,* Ann. N.Y. Acad. Sci., New York.

Hökfelt, T., Schalling, M., Meister, B., Lindgren, J.-Å., Samuelsson, B. and Patrono, C. (1986) Occurrence and distribution of LTC_4-like immunoreactivity in different species including man (in preparation).

Holets, V., Hökfelt, T., Rökaeus, Å., Terenius, L. and Goldstein, M. (1986) Differential projections of locus coeruleus neurons containing tyrosine hydroxylase and neuropeptide Y and/or galanin: Innervation of the rat cerebral cortex, hypothalamus and spinal cord. *Neuroscience* (submitted).

Hua, X., Theodorsson-Norheim, E., Brodin, E., Lundberg, J. M. and Hökfelt, T. (1985) Multiple tachykinins (neurokinin A, neuropeptide K and substance P) in capsaicin-sensitive sensory neurons in the guinea-pig. *Regul. Peptides,* 13: 1–19.

Hulting, A.-L., Lindgren, J.-Å., Hökfelt, T., Heidvall, K., Eneroth, P., Werner, S., Patrono, C. and Samuelsson, B. (1984) Leukotriene C_4 stimulates LH secretion from rat pituitary cells in vitro. *Europ. J. Pharmacol.,* 106: 459–460.

Hulting, A.-L., Lindgren, J.-Å., Hökfelt, T., Eneroth, P., Werner, S., Patrono, C. and Samuelsson, B. (1985) Leukotriene C_4 as a mediator of LH release from rat anterior pituitary cells. *Proc. nat. Acad. Sci. USA,* 52: 3834–3838.

Hunt, S. P. and Lovick, T. A. (1982) The distribution of serotonin, met-enkephalin and β-lipotropin-like immunoreactivity in neuronal perikarya of the cat brain stem. *Neurosci. Lett.,* 30: 139–145.

Hylden, J. L. K. and Wilcox, G. L. (1981) Intrathecal substance P elicits a caudally-directed biting and scratching behavior in mice. *Brain Res.,* 217: 212–215.

Ibata, Y., Fukui, K., Okamura, H., Kawakami, T., Tanaka, M., Obata, H. L., Isuto, T., Terubayashi, H., Yanaihara, C. and Yanaihara, N. (1983) Coexistence of dopamine and neurotensin in the hypothalamic arcuate and periventricular nucleus. *Brain Res.,* 269: 177–179.

Iversen, L. L. (1984) Amino acids and peptides: fast and slow chemical signals in the nervous system. *Proc. roy. Soc. Lond., B,* 221: 245–260.

Jaim-Etcheverry, G. and Zieher, L. M. (1971) Ultrastructural cytochemistry and pharmacology of 5-hydroxytryptamine in adrenergic nerve endings. III. Selective increase of norepinephrine in the rat pineal gland consecutive to depletion of neuronal 5-hydroxytryptamine. *J. Pharmacol. exp. Ther.,* 178: 42–48.

Jaim-Etcheverry, G. and Zieher, L. M. (1975) Octopamine probably coexists with noradrenaline and serotonin in vesicles of pineal adrenergic nerves. *J. Neurochem.,* 25: 915–917.

Jaim-Etcheverry, G. and Zieher, L. M. (1982) Coexistence of monoamines in peripheral adrenergic neurons. In A. C. Cuello (Ed.), *Co-transmission,* McMillan Press Ltd., London and Basingtoke.

Jan, Y. N. and Jan, L. Y. (1983) A LHRH-like peptidergic transmitter capable of "action at a distance" in autonomic ganglia. *Trends Neurosci.,* 6: 320–325.

Jirikowski, G., Reisert, I., Pilgrim, Ch. and Oertel, W. H. (1984) Coexistence of glutamate decarboxylase and somatostatin immunoreactivity in cultured hippocampal neurons of the rat. *Neurosci. Lett.,* 46: 35–39.

Johansson, O., Hökfelt, T., Pernow, B., Jeffcoate, S. L., White, N., Steinbusch, H. W. M., Verhofstad, A. A. J., Emson, P.C. and Spindel, E. (1981) Immunohistochemical support for three putative transmitters in one neuron: coexistence of 5-hydroxytryptamine-, substance P-, and thyrotropin releasing hormone-like immunoreactivity in medullary neurons projecting to the spinal cord. *Neuroscience,* 6: 1857–1881.

Kangawa, K., Minamino, N., Fukuda, A. and Matsuo, H. (1983) Neuromedin K: A novel mammalian tachykinin identified in porcine spinal cord. *Biochem. Biophys. Res. Commun.,* 114: 533–540.

Kimura, S., Okada, M., Sugita, Y., Kanazawa, I. and Munekata, E. (1983) Novel neuropeptides, neurokinin α and β isolated from porcine spinal cord. *Proc. Jap. Acad.,* 59B: 101–104.

Kondo, H., Kuramoto, H., Wainer, B. H. and Yanaihara, N. (1985) Evidence for the coexistence of acetylcholine and enkephalin in the sympathetic preganglionic neurons of rats. *Brain Res.,* 335: 309–314.

Kuhar, M. J. (1985) The mismatch problem in receptor mapping studies. *Trends Neurosci.,* 5: 190–191.

Lee, Y., Kawai, Y., Shiosaka, S., Takami, K., Kiyama, H., Hillyard, C. J., Girgis, S., MacIntyre, I., Emson, P. C. and Tohyama, M. (1985) Coexistence of calcitonin gene-related peptide and substance P-like peptide in single cells of the trigeminal ganglion of the rat: immunohistochemical analysis. *Brain Res.,* 330: 194–196.

Léger, L., Charnay, Y., Chayvialle, J. A., Bérod, A., Dray, F., Pujol, J. F., Jouvet, M. and Dubois, P. M. (1983) Localization of substance P- and enkephalin-like immunoreactivity in relation to catecholamine-containing cell bodies in the cat dorsolateral pontine tegmentum: an immunofluorescence study. *Neuroscience,* 8: 525–546.

Le Grevés, P., Nyberg, F., Terenius, L. and Kökfelt, T. (1985) Calcitonin gene-related peptide is a potent inhibitor of substance P degradation. *Europ. J. Pharmacol.* (in press).

Lindgren, J. Å., Hökfelt, T., Dahlén, S. E., Patrono, C. and Samuelsson, B. (1984) leukotrienes in the rat central nervous system. *Proc. nat. Acad. Sci. USA,* 81: 6212–6216.

Lindh, B., Hökfelt, T., Elfvin, L.-G., Terenius, L., Elde, R. and Goldstein, M. (1986) Topography of NPY-, somatostatin and VIP-immunorective neuronal subpopulations in the guinea-pig celiac-superior mesenteric ganglion and their projection to the pylorus. *Cell Tiss. Res.* (submitted).

Lorenz, R. G., Saper, C. B., Wong, D. L., Ciaranello, R. D. and Loewy, A. D. (1985) Co-localization of substance P- and phenylethanolamine-N-methyltransferase-like immunoreactivity in neurons of ventrolateral medulla that project to the spinal cord: Potential role in control of vasomotor tone. *Neurosci. Lett.,* 55: 255–260.

Lovick, T. A. and Hunt, S. P. (1983) Substance P-immunoreactive and serotonin-containing neurones in the ventral brainstem of the cat, *Neurosci. Lett.,* 36: 223–228.

Lundberg, J. M. and Hökfelt, T. (1983) Coexistence of peptides and classical neurotransmitters. *Trends Neurosci.,* 6: 325–333.

Lundberg, J. M. and Tatemoto, K. (1982) Pancreatic polypeptide family (APP, BPP, NPY and PYY) in relation to sympathetic vasoconstriction resistant to α-adrenoceptor blockade. *Acta physiol. Scand.*, 116: 393–402.

Lundberg, J. M., Hökfelt, T., Schultzberg, M., Uvnäs-Wallensten, K., Köhler, C. and Said, S. (1979) Occurrence of vasoactive intestinal polypeptide (VIP)-like imunoreactivity in certain cholinergic neurons of the cat: evidence from combined immunohistochemistry and acetylcholine esterase staining. *Neuroscience*, 4: 1539–1559.

Lundberg, J. M., Hökfelt, T., Änggård, A., Kimmel, J., Goldstein, M. and Markey, K. (1980) Coexistence of an avian pancreatic polypeptide (APP) immunoreactive substance and catecholamines in some peripheral and central neurons. *Acta physiol. Scand.*, 110: 107–109.

Lundberg, J. M., Fried, G., Fahrenkrug, J., Holmstedt, B., Hökfelt, T., Lagercrantz, H., Lundgren, G. and Änggård, A. (1981) Subcellular fractionation of cat submandibular gland: comparative studies on the distribution of acetylcholine and vasoactive intestinal polypeptide (VIP). *Neuroscience*, 6: 1001–1010.

Lundberg, J. M., Hedlund, B., Änggård, A., Fahrenkrug, J., Hökfelt, T., Tatemoto, K. and Bartfai, T. (1982a) Costorage of peptides and classical transmitters in neurons. In S. R. Bloom, J. M. Polak and E. Lindenlaub (Eds.), *Systemic Role of Regulatory Peptides*, Schattauer, Stuttgart and New York, pp. 93–119.

Lundberg, J. M., Hedlund, B. and Bartfai, T. (1982b) Vasoactive intestinal polypeptide enhances muscarinic ligand binding in cat submandibular salivary gland. *Nature (Lond.)*, 295: 147–149.

Lundberg, J. M., Hökfelt, T., Änggård, A., Terenius, L., Elde, R., Markey, K. and Goldstein, M. (1982c) Organization principles in the peripheral sympathetic nervous system: Subdivision by coexisting peptides (somatostatin, avian pancreatic polypeptide and vasoactive intestinal polypeptide-like immunoreactive materials). *Proc. nat. Acad. Sci. USA*, 79: 1303–1307.

Lundberg, J. M., Terenius, L., Hökfelt, T., Martling, C. R., Tatemoto, K., Mutt, V., Polak, J., Bloom, S. and Goldstein, M. (1982d) Neuropeptide Y (NPY)-like immunoreactivity in peripheral noradrenergic neurons and effects of NPY on sympathetic function. *Acta physiol. Scand.*, 116: 477–480.

Lundberg, J. M., Terenius, L., Hökfelt, T. and Goldstein, M. (1983) High levels of neuropeptide Y in peripheral noradrenergic neurons in various mammals including man. *Neurosci. Lett.*, 42: 167–172.

Lundberg, J. M., Terenius, L., Hökfelt, T. and Tatemoto, K. (1984) Comparative immunohistochemical and biochemical analysis of pancreatic polypeptide Y in central and peripheral neurons. *J. Neurosci.*, 4: 2376–2386.

Lundberg, J. M., Franco-Cereceda, A., Hua, X., Hökfelt, T. and Fischer, J. A. (1985) Co-existence of substance P and calcitonin gene-related peptide-like immunoreactivities in sensory nerves in relation to cardiovascular and bronchoconstrictor effects of capsaicin. *Europ. J. Pharmacol.*, 108: 315–319.

Mantyh, P. W. and Hunt, S. P. (1984) Evidence for cholecystokinin-like immunoreactive neurons in the rat medulla oblongata which project to the spinal cord. *Brain Res.*, 291: 49–54.

Markstein, R. and Hökfelt, T. (1984) Effect of cholecystokinin-octa-peptide on dopamine release from slices of cat caudate nucleus. *J. Neurosci.*, 4: 570–575.

Meister, B., Hökfelt, T., Vale, W. W. and Goldstein, M. (1985a) Growth hormone releasing factor (GRF) and dopamine coexist in hypothalamic arcuate neurons. *Acta physiol. Scand.*, 124: 133–136.

Meister, B., Hökfelt, T., Vale, W. W., Sawchenko, P. E., Swanson, L. and Goldstein, M. (1985b) Coexistence of dopamine and growth hormone releasing factor (GRF) in a subpopulation of tuberoinfundibular neurons of the rat. *Neuroendocrinology*, 42: 237–247.

Melander, T., Staines, W. A., Hökfelt, T., Rökaeus, Å., Eckenstein, F., Salvaterra, P. M. and Wainer, B. H. (1985) Galanin-like immuno-reactivity in cholinergic neurons of the septum-basal forebrain complex projecting to the hippocampus of the rat. *Brain Res.*, 360: 130–138.

Melander, T., Hökfelt, T. and Rökaeus, Å. (1986) Distribution of galanin-like immunoreactivity in the rat central nervous system. *J. comp. Neurol.* (in press).

Minamino, N., Kangawa, K., Fukuda, A. and Matsuo, H. (1984) A novel mammalian tachykinin identified in porcine spinal cord. *Neuropeptides*, 4: 157–166.

Mitchell, R. and Fleetwood-Walker, S. (1981) Substance P, but not TRH, modulates the 5-HT autoreceptor in ventral lumbar spinal cord. *Europ. J. Pharmacol.*, 76: 119–120.

Molinoff, P. B. and Axelrod, J. (1969) Octopamine: normal occurrence in sympathetic nerves of rats. *Science*, 164: 428–429.

Moore, R. Y. and Card, J. P. (1984) Noradrenaline-containing neuron systems. In A. Björklund and T. Hökfelt (Eds.), *Handbook of Chemical Neuroanatomy, Vol. 2: Chemical Transmitters in the CNS, Part I*. Elsevier, Amsterdam, pp. 123–156.

Moskowitz, M. A., Kiwak, K. J., Hekimian, K. and Levine, L. (1984) Synthesis of compounds with properties of leukotrienes C_4 and D_4 in gerbil brains after ischemia and reperfusion. *Science*, 224: 886–889.

Nakane, P. K. (1968) Simultaneous localization of multiple tissue antigens using the peroxidase-labeled antibody method: a study in pituitary glands of the rat. *J. Histochem. Cytochem.*, 16: 557–560.

Nawa, H., Hirose, T., Takashima, H., Inayama, S. and Nakanishi, S. (1983) Nucleotide sequences of cloned cDNAs for two types of bovine brain substance P precursor. *Nature (Lond.)*, 306: 32–36.

Nilsson, J., von Euler, A. M. and Dalsgaard, C.-J. (1985) Stimulation of connective tissue cell growth by substance P and substance K. *Nature (Lond.)*, 315: 61–63.

Oertel, W. H. and Mugnaini, E. (1984) Immunocytochemical

studies of GABAergic neurons in rat basal ganglia and their relations to other neuronal systems. *Neurosci. Lett.*, 47: 223–238.

Oertel, W. H., Graybiel, A. M., Mungnaini, E., Elde, R. P., Schmechel, D. E. and Kopin, E. J. (1983) Coexistence of glutamic acid decarboxylate- and somatostatin-like immunoreactivity in neurons of the feline nucleus reticularis thalami. *J. Neurosci.*, 3: 1322–1332.

Ohhashi, T. and Jacobowitz, D. M. (1983) The effects of pancreatic polypeptides and neuropeptide Y on the rat vas deferens. *Peptides*, 4: 381–386.

Osborne, N. N. (1983a) Do some nerves use more than one neurotransmitter? A look at the evidence. In N. N. Osborne (Ed.), *Dale's Principle and Communication between Neurones*, Pergamon Press, Oxford and New York, pp. 83–94.

Osborne, N. N. (Ed.) (1983b) *Dale's Principle and Communication between Neurones*, Pergamon Press, Oxford and New York.

Otsuka, M. and Takahashi, T. (1977) Putative peptide neurotransmitters. *Ann. Rev. Pharmacol. Toxicol.*, 17: 425–439.

Owman, Ch. (1964) Sympathetic nerves probably storing two types of monoamines in the rat pineal gland. *Int. J. Neuropharmacol.*, 2: 97–127.

Owman, Ch., Håkanson, R. and Sundler, F. (1973) Occurrence and function of amines in polypeptide hormone producing cells. *Fed. Proc. Fed. Amer. Soc. exp. Biol.*, 32: 1785–1791.

Palacios, J. M. and Wamsley, J. K. (1984) Catecholamine receptors. In A. Björklund and T. Hökfelt (Eds.), *Handbook of Chemical Neuroanatomy, Vol. 3: Classical Transmitters and Transmitter Receptors in the CNS, Part II*, Elsevier, Amsterdam, pp. 325–351.

Palmer, M. R., Mathews, R., Murphy, R. C. and Hoffer, B. J. (1980) Leukotriene C elicits a prolonged excitation of cerebellar Purkinje neurons. *Neurosci. Lett.*, 18: 173–180.

Palmer, M. R., Mathews, W. R., Hoffer, B. J. and Murphy, R. C. (1981) Electrophysiological response of cerebellar Purkinje neurons to leukotriene C_4 and B_4. *J. Pharmacol. exp. Ther.*, 219: 91–96.

Pearse, A. G. E. (1969) The cytochemistry and ultrastructure of polypeptide hormone producing cells of the APUD series and the embryologic physiologic and pathologic implications of the concept. *J. Histochem. Cytochem.*, 17: 303–313.

Pelletier, G., Steinbusch, H. W. and Verhofstad, A. (1981) Immunoreactive substance P and serotonin present in the same dense core vesicles. *Nature (Lond.)*, 293: 71–72.

Pernow, B. (1983) Substance P. *Pharmacol. Rev.*, 35: 85–141.

Piercey, M. F., Dobry, P. J. K., Schroeder, L. A. and Einspahr, F. J. (1981) Behavioral evidence that substance P may be a spinal cord sensory neurotransmitter. *Brain Res.*, 210: 407–412.

Post, C. and Paulsson, I. (1985) Antinociceptive and neurotoxic actions of substance P analogues in the rat's spinal cord after intrathecal administration. *Neurosci. Lett.*, 57: 159–164.

Post, C., Freedman, J., Hökfelt, T., Jonsson, G., Paulsson, I., Arwesträm, E., Leander, S., Fischer, J. A. and Verhofstad, A. (1985) Neuronal damage induced by a substance P-antagonist is counteracted by thyrotropin releasing hormone. In R. Håkanson and F. Sundler (Eds.), *Tachykinin Substance P Antagonists*, Elsevier, Amsterdam, pp. 383–391.

Potter, D. D. Furshpan, E. J. and Landis, S. C. (1981) Multiple-transmitter status and "Dale's Principle". *Neurosci. Commun.*, 1: 1–9.

Roberts, E., Chase, T. N. and Tower, D. B. (1976) *GABA in Nervous System Function*, Kroc Foundation Series, Vol. 5, Raven Press, New York.

Rökaeus, Å., Melander, T., Hökfelt, T., Lundberg, J. M., Tatemoto, K., Carlquist, M. and Mutt, V. (1984) A galanin-like peptide in the central nervous system and intestine of the rat. *Neurosci. Lett.*, 47: 161–166.

Rosenfeld, M. G., Mermod, J.-J., Amara, S. G., Swanson, L. W., Sawchenko, P. E., Rivier, J., Vale, W. W. and Evans, R. M. (1983) Production of a novel neuropeptide encoded by the calcitonin gene via tissue-specific RNA processing. *Nature (Lond.)*, 304: 129–135.

Samuelsson, B. (1983) Leukotrienes: mediators of immediate hypersensitivity reactions and inflammation. *Science*, 220: 568–575.

Schalling, M., Neil, A., Terenius, L., Hökfelt, T., Lindgren, J.-Å. and Samuelsson, B. (1985) Leukotriene C_4 binding sites in the rat central nervous system. *Europ. J. Pharmacol.*, 122: 251–257.

Schimchowitsch, S., Stoeckel, M. E., Vigny, A. and Porte, A. (1983) Oxytocinergic neurons with tyrosine hydroxylase-like immunoreactivity in the paraventricular nucleus of the rabbit hypothalamus. *Neurosci. Lett.*, 43: 55–59.

Schmechel, D. E., Vickrey, B. G., Fitzpatrick, D. and Elde, R. P. (1984) GABAergic neurons of mammalian cerebral cortex: widespread subclass defined by somatostatin content. *Neurosci. Lett.*, 47: 227–232.

Schmitt, F. O. (1984) Molecular regulators of brain function: A new view. *Neuroscience*, 13: 99–100.

Schultzberg, M., Dunett, S. B., Björklund, A., Stenevi, U., Hökfelt, T., Dockray, G. J. and Goldstein, M.(1984) Dopamine and cholecystokinin immunoreactive neurones in mesencephalic grafts reinnervating the neostriatum: evidence for selective growth regulations. *Neuroscience*, 12: 17–32.

Seybold, V. S., Hylden, J. L. K. and Wilcox, G. L. (1982) Intrathecal substance P and somatostatin in rats: behaviors indicative of sensation. *Peptides*, 3: 49–54.

Sharif, N. A. and Burt, D. R. (1983) Micromolar substance P reduces spinal receptor binding for thyrotrophin-releasing hormone — possible relevance to neuropeptide coexistence? *Neurosci. Lett.*, 43: 245–261.

Siegelbaum, S. A. and Tsien, R. W. (1983) Modulation of gated ion channels as a mode of transmitter action. *Trends Neurosci.*, 6: 307–313.

Skirboll, L., Hökfelt, T., Norell, G., Philipson, O., Kuypers, J. G. J. M., Bentivoglio, M., Catsman-Berrevoets, C. E., Visser,

T. J., Steinbusch, H., Verhofstad, A., Cuello, A. C., Goldstein, M. and Brownstein, M. (1984) A method for specific transmitter identification of retrogradely labeled neurons: immunofluorescence combined with fluorescence tracing. *Brain Res. Rev.*, 8: 99–127.

Smith, A. D. (1976) Dale's principle today: Adrenergic tissues. In J. Szentágothai, J. Hámori and E. S. Vizi (Eds.), *Neuron Concept Today,* Symposium, Tihany, Akadémiai Kiado, Budapest.

Snyder, S. H. (1979) Receptors, neurotransmitters and drug responses. *New Engl. J. Med.*, 300: 465–472.

Snyder, S. H. (1980) Brain peptides as neurotransmitters. *Science,* 209: 976–983.

Somogyi, P., Hodgson, A. J., Smith, A. D., Nunzi, M. G., Gorio,A. and Wu, J.-Y. (1984) Different populations of GABAergic neurons in the visual cortex and hippocampus of cat contain somatostatin- or cholecystokinin-immunoreactive material. *Neuroscience,* 14: 2590–2603.

Sternberger, L. A., Hardy, Jr., P. H., Cuculis, J. J. and Meyer, H. G. (1970) The unlabeled antibody enzyme method of immunohistochemistry. Preparations and properties of soluble antigen-antibody complex (horseradish peroxidase-antihorseradish peroxidase) and its use in identifications of spirochetes. *J. Histochem. Cytochem.*, 18: 315–324.

Stjärne, L. and Lundberg, J. M. (1984) Neuropeptide Y (NPY) depresses the secretion of ^{3}H-noradrenaline and the contractile response evoked by field stimulation in rat vas deferens. *Acta physiol. Scand.*, 120: 477–479.

Stjärne, L., Hedqvist, P., Lagercrantz, H. and Wennmalm, Å. (Eds.) (1981) *Chemical Neurotransmission,* Academic Press, London.

Takami, K., Kawai, Y., Shiosaka, S., Lee, Y., Girgis, S., Hillyard, C. J., MacIntyre, I., Emson, P. C. and Tohyama, M. (1985) Immunohistochemical evidence for the coexistence of calcitonin gene-related peptide- and choline acetyltransferase--like immunoreactivity in neurons of the rat hypoglossal, facial and ambiguus nuclei. *Brain Res.*, 328: 386–389.

Takeda, N., Inagaki, S., Shiosaka, S., Taguchi, Y., Oertel, W. H., Tohyama, M., Watanabe, T. and Wada, H. (1984) Immunohistochemical evidence for the coexistence of histidine decarboxylase-like and glutamate decarboxylase-like immunoreactivities in nerve cells of the magnocellular nucleus of the posterior hypothalamus of rats. *Proc. nat. Acad. Sci. USA,* 81: 7647–7650.

Tramu, G., Pillez, A. and Leonardelli, J. (1978) An efficient method of antibody elution for the successive or simultaneous location of two antigens by immunocytochemistry. *J. Histochem. Cytochem.*, 26: 322–324.

Tschopp, F. A., Henke, H., Petermann, J. B., Tobler, P. H., Janzer, R., Hökfelt, T., Lundberg, J. M., Cuello, C. and Fischer, J. A. (1984) Calcitonin gene-related peptide and its binding sites in the human nervous system and pituitary. *Proc. nat. Acad. Sci. USA,* 82: 248–252.

Vincent, S. R., Satoh, K., Armstrong, D. M. and Fibiger, H. C. (1983) Substance P in the ascending cholinergic reticular system. *Nature (Lond.),* 306: 688–691.

Vogt, M. (1954) The concentration of sympathin in different parts of the central nervous system and normal conditions and after the administration of drugs. *J. Physiol. (Lond.),* 123: 451–481.

Watt, C. B., Su, Y. T. and Lam, D. M.-K. (1984) Interactions between enkephalin and GABA in avian retina. *Nature (Lond.),* 311: 761–763.

Weiler, R. and Ball, A. K. (1984) Co-localization of neurotensin-like immunoreactivity and ^{3}H-glycine uptake system in sustained amacrine cells of turtle retina. *Nature (Lond.),* 311: 759–761.

Wiesenfeld-Hallin, Z., Hökfelt, T., Lundberg, J. M., Forssmann, W. G., Reinecke, M., Tschopp, F. A. and Fischer, J. A. (1984) Immunoreactive calcitonin gene-related peptide and substance P coexist in sensory neurons to the spinal cord and interact in spinal behavioural responses of the rat. *Neurosci. Lett.*, 52: 199–204.

Yaksh, T. L. and Rudy, T. A. (1976) Chronic catheterization of the spinal subarachnoid space. *Physiol. Behav.*, 17: 1031–1036.

Zahm, D. S., Zaboszky, L., Alones, V. E. and Heimer, L. (1985) Evidence for the coexistence of glutamate decarboxylase and met-enkephalin immunoreactivities in axon terminals of rat ventral pallidum. *Brain Res.*, 325: 317–321.

Young, W. S. III and Kuhar, M. J. (1979) A new method for receptor autoradiography: (^{3}H)opioid receptors in rat brain. *Brain Res.*, 179: 255–270.

Young, W. S. III and Kuhar, M. J. (1980) Noradrenergic alpha-1 and alpha-2-receptors: light microscopic autoradiographic localization. *Proc. nat. Acad. Sci. USA,* 77: 1696–1700.

T. Hökfelt, K. Fuxe and B. Pernow (Eds.),
Progress in Brain Research, Vol. 68

CHAPTER 5

Molecules of intercellular communication in vertebrates, invertebrates and microbes: do they share common origins?

Jesse Roth, Derek LeRoith, Maxine A. Lesniak, Flora de Pablo, Lluis Bassas and Elaine Collier

Diabetes Branch, National Institute of Arthritis, Diabetes and Digestive and Kidney Diseases, National Institutes of Health, Bethesda, MD 20892, U.S.A.

Newly characterized messenger molecules as well as messengers of the traditional communication systems, the nervous and endocrine systems, are a major focus of investigation. By examining the phylogenetic origins of these messengers, as well as the emergence of ideas on the subject, we suggest a greater unity than heretofore suspected (Roth et al., 1982, 1983). With this perspective, we now review (1) materials in microbes that resemble vertebrate receptors for hormones and other intercellular messengers; (2) intercellular communication in microbes; (3) materials that resemble vertebrate hormones in microbes, higher plants, amphibian skin, and very young avian embryos.

Glandulocentric approach

We introduce here the term "glandulocentric" to indicate a traditional approach whereby each hormone was thought to be a unique product of one endocrine gland. Because the typical vertebrate endocrine gland (e.g. pituitary, adrenal, thyroid) is limited to vertebrates, its hormonal product had been thought to be similarly restricted in distribution. The one-to-one relationship between hormone and gland was similarly applied conceptually to the endocrine system in insects and in molluscs (Fig. 1).

Neuronocentric approach

We introduce here the term "neuronocentric" to indicate that subsequently, with improvements in techniques, materials similar to or identical with the peptide hormones of vertebrates were detected in vertebrate extraglandular tissues especially tumors of non-endocrine origin and neurons. Since neurons were known to occur very widely in multicellular animals, it was logical to expand the phyletic range of these peptides to coincide with that of neurons.

To explain the overlap between the vertebrate and invertebrate nervous systems and the vertebrate endocrine system, Pearse and Polak postulated that the nervous system (or some branch of it) gave rise to the vertebrate endocrine system both evolutionarily and embryologically (Pearse et al., 1980). An alternative formulation by Fujita and co-workers introduced the concept of the paraneuron and included under this rubric many cell types that secrete intercellular messenger molecules (Fujita, 1976).

Paleocentric approach

We introduce here the term "paleocentric" to indicate a proposed new approach. Recently, we and

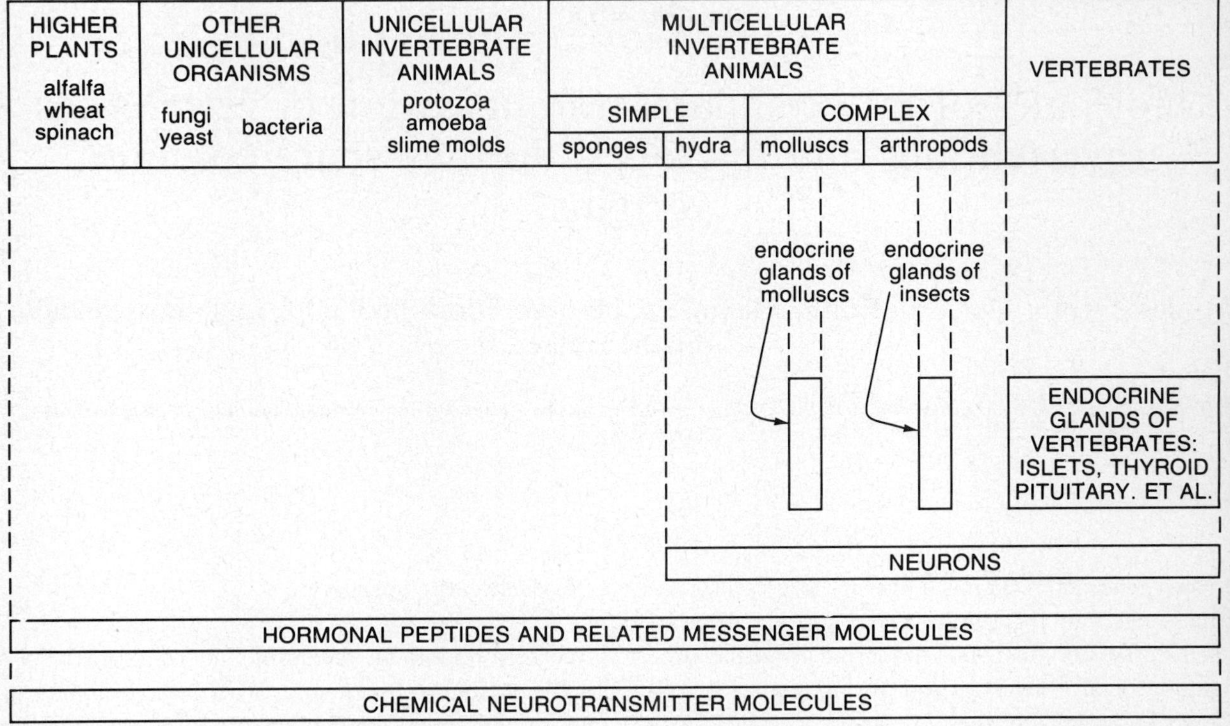

Fig. 1. Evolutionary origins of the biochemical elements of the endocrine gland and nervous systems. (Adapted from LeRoith et al., 1982b).

others have detected materials in unicellular organisms that closely resemble messenger peptides of vertebrates (Table I). On that basis we have suggested that many of the messenger peptides arose evolutionarily in microbes and were carried to the multicellular animals in typical Darwinian fashion. Rather than postulating that the nervous system was the evolutionary source for peptide messengers of vertebrates (Fig. 2B), we raise the possibility that for many peptide messengers the microbes may play that role (Fig. 2C).

Potential value of the paleocentric approach

A hypothesis such as this cannot be proven but its usefulness can be tested. First, it may unite in a rational way data that were previously fragmented (see below). Second, it provides a basis for novel predictions of experimental results.

Receptors in microbes

The presence of vertebrate-type messenger peptides in microbes leaves us with our paleocentric approach to search for evidence of receptors for vertebrate-type messengers. (Current concepts of ligand-receptor interactions at the target cell strengthen that expectation. In vertebrates, hormones and most other messenger peptides have no known function except as messengers. Further, to function as the messengers they bind to receptors and activate them. The activated receptors provide the proximate signal to the target cell.) Table II lists some well studied examples of binding substances in microbes that bear some resemblance to vertebrate-type receptors for messenger molecules. It should be noted that the TSH receptor-like material in gram-negative bacteria not only binds TSH and related vertebrate hormones but is also recognized

TABLE I

Materials in microbes that resemble messenger peptides of vertebrates

Hormone-related materials	Microbe	References
TSH	*Clostridium perfringens*	Macchia et al., 1967
hCG	Many bacteria	Acevedo et al., 1978, Maruo et al., 1979
Neurotensin	*Escherichia coli, Caulaobacter crescentus Rhodopseudomonas palustris*	Bhatnagar and Carraway, 1981
Insulin	*Escherichia coli, Tetrahymena pyriformis Neurospora crassa, Aspergillus fumigatus; Halobacterium solinarium, Bordetella pertussis*	LeRoith et al., 1980, 1981; Rubinovitz and Shiloach, 1985
ACTH; β-endorphin	*Tetrahymena pyriformis*	LeRoith et al., 1982a
Somatostatin	*Escherichia coli, Tetrahymena pyriformis, Bacillus subtilis*	Berelowitz et al., 1982; LeRoith et al., 1985a LeRoith et al., 1985b
Relaxin	*Tetrahymena pyriformis*	Schwabe et al., 1983
Calcitonin human-type	*Candida albicans, Escherichia coli*	Perez Cano et al., 1982
salmon-type	*Tetrahymena pyriformis*	Deftos et al., 1985
Arginine vasotocin	*Tetrahymena pyriformis*	Glick et al., unpublished

Non-peptide materials similar to vertebrate messenger molecules are also present in microbes. Our discussion has been restricted to peptides because with peptides, existence per se has important implications, i.e. existence of genes, conservation of DNA, natural selection. (With the non-peptides, it might be argued that the resemblance to vertebrate messengers is a coincidence, a metabolic "accident", e.g. catecholamines are only a couple of simple enzymatic steps away from tyrosine.) Until the structure of the microbial peptides is determined (or the structure of the corresponding DNA or mRNA), it is impossible to state how closely any of these microbial components resemble their vertebrate counterparts, However, since many are similar in overall size and shape, are recognized by one or more specific antibodies against the vertebrate peptides, and are recognized by receptors on vertebrate target cells, at least several regions on the surfaces of the microbial peptide must resemble their counterparts on the vertebrate peptide. Another unresolved more general problem is the relationship between proteins in prokaryotes and their counterparts in eukaryotes. When the eukaryotic peptide is a glycoprotein, what is the bacterial equivalent since prokaryotes lack typical glycoprotein structures? When the eukaryotic peptide undergoes a trypsin-like change to achieve conversion from a precursor protein to a mature protein, what is the bacterial equivalent? A third general unresolved problem is represented by the introns. Most eukaryotic genes have introns; how did the intron-less prokaryotic gene transform into the intron-containing eukaryotic gene?

by human auto-antibodies (from serum of patients with Graves' disease) directed against the TSH receptor of the human thyroid gland (Heyma et al., 1986). As a result, the microbial "receptor" has also been considered as a possible candidate for the primary immunogen in humans with Graves' disease.

The estrogen-related receptor and estrogen-mediated inhibitory effect observed in the yeast, *Paracoccidioides brasiliensis,* has been considered as a possible basis for the heavy predominance in males for serious forms of this endemic disease (non-apparent infections are equally prevalent in both sexes) (Loose et al., 1983). Finally, the pioneer work of Csaba and his colleagues on the effect of hormones on protozoa should be noted (Csaba, 1984).

Intercellular communication in microbes

Intercellular communication is widespread in microbes. An outline is provided in Table III. Thus far, none of the vertebrate-type peptide messengers has been implicated in a microbe's own communication system. However, two examples of similarity deserve special mention. In *Saccharomyces cerevi-*

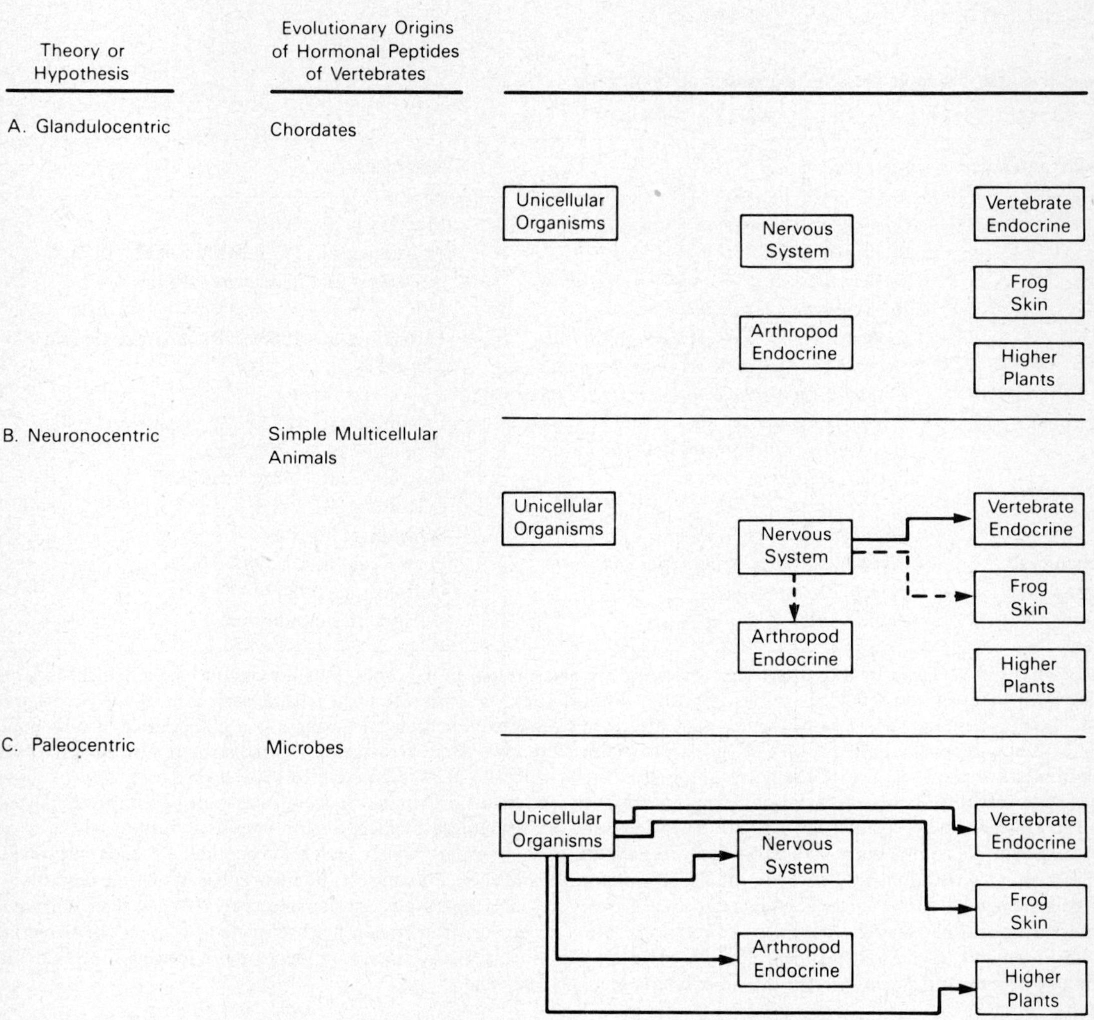

Fig. 2. This figure summarizes the successive stages in our understanding of the evolutionary origins of hormonal peptides of vertebrates.

siae, the common yeast, there are two sex types, α and A, which communicate one with the other via peptide mesengers, designated α factor and A factor (Stotzler and Duntze, 1976). Interestingly, α factor (a) structurally resembles mammalian GnRH; (b) binds to GnRH receptors, albeit with a reduced affinity; and (c) at high concentrations can act via the GnRH receptor to stimulate release of gonadotropins from the rat pituitary (Loumaye et al., 1982).

In *Achlya ambisexualis,* a unicellular water mold, "male" and "female" sex types communicate via specific steroid-like molecules, designated "oogoniol" and "antheridiol". The receptor for antheridiol (a) shows high specificity and affinity, (b) is present only in the male, and (c) is a soluble "cytoplasmic" protein that has the physical and chemical characteristics that are typical of all of the steroid receptors of vertebrates (Riehl and Toft, 1984).

Material in plants that resemble vertebrate peptide messengers

Materials that resemble vertebrate-type messenger peptides are present in plants (Table IV). The pa-

TABLE II

Hormone-binding materials in microbes that resemble vertebrate-type receptors

Hormone-like material bound	Microbe containing receptor-like binding substance	References
(1) Chorionic gonadotropin (hCG)	*Pseudomonas maltophilia*	Richert and Ryan, 1977
(2) Opioid peptides	*Amoeba proteus*	Josefsson and Johansson, 1979
(3) Thyrotropin (TSH)	*Escherichia coli, Yersinia enterocolitica*	Weiss et al., 1983; Heyma et al., 1986
(4) Corticosterone	*Candida albicans*	Loose and Feldman, 1982
(5) Estrogen	*Saccharomyces cerevisiae*	Burshell et al., 1984
	Paracoccidioides brasiliensis	Loose et al., 1983
(6) Antheridiol	*Achlya ambisexualis*	Riehl and Toft, 1984

TABLE III

Intercellular communication in unicellular organisms

(1) Phyletic range	— prokaryotes and eukaryotes
(2) Topics of discussion	— food and sex
(3) Chemical nature of messenger molecules	— peptides; nucleotides; sterols; lipids et al.
(4) Examples of elements present typical of vertebrate post-receptor systems	— cAMP; G-proteins; (cAMP) protein kinases; calmodulin et al.

TABLE IV

Materials in higher plants that resemble messenger peptides of vertebrates

Hormone-related material	Plant	References
Chorionic gonadotropin (hCG)	Alfalfa	Shomer-Ilan et al., 1973
Gonadotropin-releasing hormone (GnRH)	Oak leaves	Fukushima et al., 1976
Thyrotropin-releasing hormone (TRH)	Alfalfa	Jackson, 1981; Morley et al., 1980
Opioid ("exorphin")	Wheat	Zioudrov et al., 1979
Interferon	Tobacco	Sela, 1981
Insulin	Spinach, Lemna	Collier et al., 1986
Somatostatins-14 and -28	Spinach, Lemna*, Tobacco*	LeRoith et al., 1985c; Werner et al., 1986

* Partial characterization.

TABLE V

Multiple tissue sites of possible production of canonical hormones in vertebrates

ACTH/β-endorphin	*hCG (Braunstein et al., 1979)*
(1) Pituitary	(1) Placenta
(2) Brain (Civelli et al., 1982)	(2) Pituitary
(3) Tumors (Ratcliffe et al., 1972)	(3) Kidney
(4) Placenta (Liotta et al., 1977)	(4) Liver
(5) Lung	(5) Tumors (Odell and Wolfsen, 1980)
(6) Spleen	(6) Fetus (McGregor et al., 1984)
(7) Adrenal (Evans et al., 1983)	(7) Testes
(8) Gonads (Pintar et al., 1984)	
(9) Pancreas (Sanchez-Franco et al., 1981)	
Insulin	*Vasopressin*
(1) Pancreas	(1) Hypothalamus
(2) Central and peripheral nerves (Hendricks et al., 1983)	(2) Brain
(3) Salivary gland	(3) Adrenal
(4) Embryo	(4) Gonads (Lim et al., 1985)
(5) Placenta	

TABLE VI

Evidence that endogenous insulin functions in embryos before emergence of pancreatic insulin production

(1) Insulin is present in unfertilized eggs and in chick embryos at days 2–3 although pancreatic islets, and pancreatic production of insulin do not develop until later (dePablo et al., 1982)
(2) Receptors that prefer IGFs to insulin as well as receptors that prefer insulin to IGFs are present in chick embryos; at early times (1–2 days of embryogenesis) the former dominate (Bassas et al., 1985)
(3) Insulin at low doses (ng/embryo) accelerates growth as well as morphological and biochemical development by receptor-mediated pathways, whereas insulin at high doses (μg/embryo) causes a high ratio of death and developmental abnormalities which are unaffected by co-administration of glucose (dePablo et al., 1985a)
(4) Anti-insulin antibodies administered to embryos at day 2 cause a high incidence of death; in survivors by days 3 and 4, growth as well as morphological and biochemical development are retarded. Since those antibodies are not reactive with insulin-like growth factors, it is the neutralization of insulin or a very closely related molecule which is interfering with normal embryogenesis (dePablo et al., 1985b)

leocentric approach, which suggests that these messengers originated early in evolution before the divergence of life forms into separate kingdoms, easily accommodates these observations. A highly speculative extrapolation would lead to a search for corresponding receptors, based on the reasoning expressed earlier with regard to receptors in microbes.

Peptides in frog skin and other related observations

In our opinion, the paleocentric approach provides a logical pathway for the evolution of the frog skin as a repository of biologically active messenger-like peptides. The paleocentric approach also provides a rational understanding of several features of the nervous system that were not fully integrated into alternative theories: (a) the very large vocabulary used by the nervous system, seemingly excessive if the vocabulary had been created expressly for it; (b) the co-existence of multiple messenger molecules in individual neurons; (c) the existence of at least five and possibly more vertebrate-type neuropeptides in

TABLE VII

Biology of insulin-related materials in multicellular invertebrates

(1) Insulin immunoactive (by RIA and immunocytochemistry) and bioactive materials are widespread in insect tissues including neurons, neurosecretory organs and body fluids (Duve et al., 1979)
(2) Vertebrate insulin has typical effects on insects: adults, larvae and cells in culture (Duve et al., 1979)
(3) Insulin-binding substance with binding properties very similar to insulin receptors typical of vertebrates and receptor-linked insulin-stimulated protein kinase, an activity closely related to insulin activation of its receptor in target cells, are both present in *Drosophila* (Petruzzelli et al., 1985)
(4) The lower molecular weight form of prothoracicotrophic hormone of silkworm (4K-PTTH-II), the brain hormone which drives metamorphosis, has a 50% amino acid sequence homology with the A-chain of mammalian insulin and with the equivalent region of IGF-I. This material appears to be unreactive with typical anti-insulin sera and therefore not likely to account for the insulin RIA activity present in insects (Nagasawa et al., 1984)
(5) Insulin bioactivity and immunoactivity are present in other multicellular invertebrates. In several bivalve molluscs, the insulin was localized to the GI tract. From the effects produced by administering either glucose, insulin or insulin anti--sera, it was concluded that the endogenous insulin plays a role in normal carbohydrate metabolism (Plisetskaya et al., 1978)

the nerve net of the hydra, which is thought to be representative of the evolutionarily earliest nervous systems and composed of neurons of a single type (Grimmelikhuijzen, 1983, 1984).

The paleocentric approach is also compatible with the finding that in mammals a large number of normal (non-tumor) tissues including those not included under anyone's definition of neural tissue appear to make measurable (albeit modest) amounts of hormonal peptides (Table V). Similarly, the paleocentric approach is compatible with recent studies which show that insulin is present and functions in early embryos even before development of their pancreas or pancreatic β-cells (Table VI) (DePablo et al., 1982; Bassas et al., 1985). Similarly, the findings of insulin-related materials in multicellular invertebrates (Table VII) provides a bridge from the microbes to the vertebrates.

We conclude that many of the messenger peptides (and probably non-peptide messengers) of vertebrate as well as their receptors and many of their post-receptor components have their evolutionary origins among the microbes and appear to be distributed among a very wide range of forms of life. It is not yet known which, if any, of these ancestral molecules perform messenger functions in the microbes themselves. However, among the intercellular communication systems of microbes, several tantalizing overlaps have emerged. This approach also seems to be useful as a way of bringing together a wide range of heretofore diverse phenomena related to communication in both invertebrates, and higher plants.

Note added in proof

In recent studies messenger RNA for insulin has been identified in pituitary gland (Budd et al., 1986) and brain (Young, 1986).

References

Acevedo, M. F., Slifkin, M., Pouchet, G. R. and Pardo, M. (1978) Immunocytochemical localization of a choriogonadotropin-like protein in bacteria isolated from cancer patients. *Cancer,* 41: 1217.

Bassas, L., de Pablo, F., Lesniak, M. A. and Roth, J. (1985) Ontogeny of receptors for insulin-like peptides in chick embryo tissues: early dominance of insulin-like growth factor over insulin receptors in brain. *Endocrinology,* 117: 2321.

Berelowitz, M., LeRoith, D., von Schenk, H., Newgard, C., Szabo, M., Frohman, L. A., Shiloach, J. and Roth, J. (1982) Somatostatin-like immunoactivity and biological activity is present in T. pyriformis, a ciliated Protozoan. *Endocrinology,* 110: 1939.

Bhatnagar, Y. M. and Carraway, R. (1981) Bacterial peptides with C-terminal similarities to bovine neurotensin. *Peptides,* 2: 51.

Braunstein, G. D., Kandar, V., Rasor, J., Swaminathan, N. and Wade, M. E. (1979) Widespread distribution of chorionic gonadotropin-like substance in normal tissues. *J. clin. Endocrinol.,* 49: 917.

Budd, G.C., Pansky, B. and Cordell, B. (1986) Detection of insulin synthesis in mammalian anterior pituitary cells by immunochemistry and demonstration by in situ RNA-DNA hybridization. *J. Histochem. Cytochem.*, 34: 673.

Burshell, A., Stathis, P. A., Do, Y., Miller, S. T. and Feldman, D. (1984) Characterization of an estrogen-binding protein in the yeast Saccharomyces cerevisiae. *J. biol. Chem.*, 259: 3450.

Civelli, O., Birnberg, N. and Herbert, E. (1982) Detection and quantitation of pro-opiomelanocortin mRNA in pituitary and brain tissues from different species. *J. biol. Chem.*, 257: 6783.

Collier, E., Watkinson, A., Roth, J. and Cleland, C. F. (1986) *Endocrinology*, 118: 40 (Abstr.).

Csaba, G. (1984) The present state in the phylogeny and ontogeny of hormone receptors. *Horm. Metab. Res.*, 16: 329.

Deftos, L., LeRoith, D., Shiloach, J. and Roth, J. (1985) Salmon calcitonin-like immunoactivity in extracts of Tetrahymena pyriformis. *Horm. Metab. Res.*, 17: 82.

DePablo, F., Hernandez, E., Collia, F. and Gomez, J. A. (1985a) Untoward effects of pharmacological doses of insulin in early chick embryos: through which receptors are they mediated? *Diabetologia*, 18: 308.

DePablo, F., Girbau, M., Gomez, J. A., Hernandez, E. and Roth, J. (1985b) Insulin antibodies retard and insulin accelerates growth and differentiation in early embryos. *Diabetes*, 34: 1063.

DePablo, F., Roth, J., Hernandez, E. and Pruss, R. M. (1982) Insulin is present in chicken eggs and early chick embryos. *Endocrinology*, 111: 1909.

Duve, H, Thorpe, A. and Lazarus, N. R. (1979) Isolation of material displaying insulin-like immunological and biological activity from the brain of the blowfly. Calliphora vomitoria. *Biochem. J.*, 184: 221.

Erspamer, V. and Melchiorri, P. (1980) Correlations between active peptides of the amphibian skin and peptides of the avian and mammalian gut and brain. The gut-brain-skin triangle. *Trend. Pharmacol. Sci.*, 1: 391.

Evans, C. J., Erdelyi, E., Weber, E. and Barachas, J. D. (1983) Identification of pro-opiomelanocortin-derived peptides in the human adrenal medulla. *Science*, 221: 957.

Fujita, T. (1976) The gastro-enteric endocrine cell and its paraneuronic nature. In R. E. Coupland and T. Fujita (Eds.), *Chromafin, Enterochromafin and Related Cells*, Elsevier, Amsterdam p. 191.

Fukushima, J., Watanabe, S. and Kushima, K. (1976) Extraction and purification of substance with luteinizing hormone releasing activity from the leaves of avenasativa. *Tohoku J. exp. Med.*, 119: 115.

Grimmelikhuijzen, C. J. P. (1983) Coexistence of neuropeptides in hydra. *Neuroscience*, 4: 837.

Grimmelikhuijzen, C. J. P. (1984) Peptides in the nervous system of coelenterates. In S. Falkmer, R. Hakanson and F. Sundler (Eds.), *Evoluton and Tumour Pathology of the Neuroendocrine System*, Elsevier, Amsterdam, p. 39.

Hendricks, S. A., Roth, J., Rishi, S. and Becker, K. L. (1983) Insulin in the nervous system. In D. T. Krieger, M. Brownstein and J. B. Martin (Eds.), *Brain Peptides*, p. 903.

Heyma, P., Harrison, L. and Robins-Browne, R. (1986) (submitted).

Jackson, I. M. D. (1981) Abundance of immunoreactive thyrotropin-releasing hormone-like material in the alfalfa plant. *Endocrinology*, 108: 344.

Josefsson, J.-O. and Johansson, P. (1979) Naloxone-reversible effect of opioids on pinocytosis in Amoeba proteus. *Nature (Lond.)*, 282: 78.

LeRoith, D., Shiloach, J., Roth, J. and Lesniak, M. A. (1980) Evolutionary origins of vertebrate hormones: substances similar to mammalian insulins are native to unicellular organisms. *Proc. nat. Acad. Sci. USA*, 77: 6184.

LeRoith, D., Shiloach, J. Roth, M. and Lesniak, M. A. (1981) Insulin or a closely related molecule is native to Escherichia coli. *J. biol. Chem.*, 256: 6533.

LeRoith, D., Liotta, A. S., Roth, J., Shiloach, J., Lewis, M. E., Pert, C. B. and Krieger, D. T. (1982a) Corticotropin and β-endorphin-like materials are native to unicellular organisms. *Proc. nat. Acad. Sci. USA*, 79: 2086.

LeRoith, D., Shiloach, J. and Roth, J. (1982b) Is there an earlier phylogenetic precursor that is common to both the nervous and endocrine systems? *Peptides*, 3: 211.

LeRoith, D., Berelowitz, M., Pickens, W., Crosby, L. K. and Shiloach, J. (1985a) Somatostatin-related material in E. coli: Evidence for two molecular forms. *Biochim. biophys. Acta*, 838: 335.

LeRoith, D., Pickens, W., Vinik, A. I. and Shiloach, J. (1985b) Bacillus subtilis contains multiple forms of somatostatin-like material. *Biochem. biophys. Res. Commun.*, 127: 713.

LeRoith, D., Pickens, W., Wilson, G. L., Miller, B., Berelowitz, M., Vinik, A. I., Collier, E. and Cleland, C. F. (1985c) Somtostatin-like material is native to flowering plants. *Endocrinology*, 117: 2093.

Lim, A. T. W., Lolait, S. J., Barlow, J. W., Autelitano, D. J., Toh, B. H., Boublik, J., Abrahams, J., Johnston, C. I. and Funder, J. W. (1985) Immunoreactive arginine-vasopressin in Brattleboro rat ovary. *Nature (Lond.)*, 310: 61.

Liotta, A. S., Osathawordh, R., Ryan, D. J. and Krieger, D. T. (1977) Presence of corticotropin in human placenta demonstration of in vitro synthesis. *Endocrinology*, 101: 1552.

Loose, D. S. and Feldman, D. (1982) Characterization of a unique corticosterone-binding protein in Candida albicans. *J. biol. Chem.*, 259: 3450.

Loose, D. S., Stover, E. P., Restrepo, A., Stevens, D. A. and Feldman, D. (1983) Estradiol binds to a receptor-like cytosol binding protein and initiates a biological response in Paracoccidioides brasiliensis. *Proc. nat. Acad. Sci. USA*, 80: 7659.

Loumaye, E., Thorner, J. and Catt, K. J. (1982) Yeast mating pheromone activates mammalian gonadotrophs: Evolutionary conservation of a reproductive hormone. *Science*, 218: 1324.

Macchia, V., Bates, R. W. and Pastan, I. (1967) Purification and properties of thyroid stimulating factor isolated from Clostridium perfringens. *J. biol. Chem.*, 242: 3726.

Maruo, T., Cohen, H., Segal, S. J. and Koide, S. S. (1979) Production of choriogonadotropin-like factor by a microorganism. *Proc. nat. Acad. Sci. USA*, 76: 6622.

McGregor, N., Kuhn, R. W. and Jaffe, R. B. (1984) Biologically active choronic gonadotropin: Synthesis by human fetus. *Science*, 220: 306.

Morley, J. E., Meyer, N., Pekary, A. E., Melmed, S., Carlson, H. E., Briggs, J. E. and Hershman, J. M. (1980) A prolactin inhibitory factor with immunocharacteristics similar to thyrotropin releasing factor (TRH) is present in rat pituitary tumors (GH3&W5) testicular tissue and a plant material, Alfalfa. *Biochem. biophys. Res. Commun.*, 96: 47.

Nagasawa, H., Kataoka, H., Isogai, A., Tamura, S., Suzuki, A., Ishizaki, H., Mizoguchi, A., Fujiwara, Y. and Suzuki, A. (1984) Amino-terminal amino acid sequence of the silkworm prothoracicotropic hormone: Homology with insulin. *Science*, 226: 1344.

Odell, W. D. and Wolfsen, A. R. (1980) Hormones from tumors. Are they ubiquitous? *Amer. J. Med.*, 68: 317.

Pearse, A. G. E., Polak, J. M. and Facer, P. (1980) Neuron specific enolase in gastric and related endocrine cells. The facts and their significance. *Hepatogastroenterology*, 27: 78.

Perez-Cano, R., Murphy, P. K., Girgis, S. I., Arnett, T. R., Blankharn, I. and MacIntyre, I. (1982) Unicellular organisms contain a molecule resembling human calcitonin. *Endocrinology*, (abstract), 110: 673.

Petruzzelli, L., Herrera, R., Garcia, R. and Rosen, O. M. (1985) The insulin receptor of Drosophila melanogaster. *Cold Spring Harbor Symp.*, 3: 115.

Pintar, J. E., Schacter, B. S., Herman, A. B., Durgerian, S. and Krieger, D. T. (1984) Characterization and localization of pro-opiomelanocortin mRNA in the adult rat testis. *Science*, 225: 632.

Plisetskaya, E., Kazakow, V. K., Solititskaya, L. and Leibson, L. G. (1978) Insulin producing cells in the gut of freshwater bivalve molluscs Anodonta cygnea and Unio pictorum and the role of insulin in the regulation of their carbohydrate metabolism. *Gen. comp. Endocr.*, 35: 133.

Ratcliffe, J. G., Knight, R. A., Besser, G. M., Landon, J. and Stansfeld, A. G. (1972) Tumor and plasma ACTH concentrations of patients with and without the ectopic ACTH syndrome. *Clin. Endocr.*, 1: 27.

Richert, N. D. and Ryan, R. J. (1977) Specific gonadotropin binding to Pseudomonas maltophilia. *Proc. nat. Acad. Sci. USA*, 74: 878.

Riehl, R. M. and Toft, D. O. (1984) Analysis of the steroid receptor of Achlya ambisexualis. *J. biol. Chem.*, 259: 15324.

Roth, J., LeRoith, D., Shiloach, J., Rosenzweig, J. L., Lesniak, M. A. and Havrankova, J. (1982) The evolutionary origins of hormones, neurotransmitters, and other extracellular chemical messengers. *New Engl. J. Med.*, 306: 523.

Roth, J., LeRoith, D., Shiloach, J. and Rubinovitz, C. (1983) Intercellular communication: an attempt at a unifying hypothesis. *Clin. Res.*, 31: 354.

Rubinovitz, C. and Shiloach, J. (1985) Insulin-related material in prokaryotes. *FEMS Microbiol. Lett.* (in press).

Sanchez-Franco, F., Patel, Y. C. and Reichlin, S. (1981) Immunoreactive ACTH in the gastrointestinal tract and pancreatic islets of the rat. *Endocrinology*, 108: 2235.

Schwabe, C., LeRoith, D., Thompson, R. P., Shiloach, J. and Roth, J. (1983) Relaxin extracted from protozoa (Tetrahymena pyriformis). *J. biol. Chem.*, 258: 2778.

Sela, I. (1981) Plant-virus interaction related to resistance and localization of viral infections. *Advanc. Virus Res.*, 26: 201.

Shomer-Ilan, A., Avtalion, R. R. and Leshem, Y. (1973) Further evidence for the presence of an endogenous gonadotrophin-like plant factor, "Phytotrophin": Isolation and mechanism of action of the active principle. *Aust. J. biol. Sci.*, 26: 105.

Stotzler, D. and Duntze, W. (1976) Isolation and characterization of four related peptides exhibiting α factor activity from Saccharomyces cerevisiae. *Europ. J. Biochem.*, 65: 257.

Weiss, M., Ingbar, S. H., Winblad, S. and Kasper, D. L. (1983) Demonstration of a saturable binding site for thyrotropin in Yersinia enterocolitica. *Science*, 219: 1331.

Werner, H., Fridkin, M. and Koch, Y. (1985) Immunoreactive and bioactive somatostatin-like material is present in tobacco (*Nicotiana tabacum*). *Peptides*, 6: 797.

Young, III, W. S. (1986) Periventricular hypothalamic cells in the rat brain contain insulin mRNA neuropeptides (in press).

Zioudrov, C., Streaty, R. A. and Klee, W. A. (1979) Opioid peptides derived from food proteins. The exorphins. *J. biol. Chem.*, 254: 2446.

SECTION III

Invertebrates and Developmental Aspects

T. Hökfelt, K. Fuxe and B. Pernow (Eds.),
Progress in Brain Research, Vol. 68

CHAPTER 6

Convergence of small molecule and peptide transmitters on a common molecular cascade

V. F. Castellucci, S. Schacher, P. G. Montarolo, S. Mackey, D. L. Glanzman, R. D. Hawkins, T. W. Abrams, P. Goelet and E. R. Kandel

Howard Hughes Medical Institute, Center for Neurobiology and Behavior, Departments of Physiology and Psychiatry, Columbia University College of Physicians and Surgeons, 722 West 168th Street, New York, NY 10032, U.S.A.

Introduction

The ion channel gated by transmitters consists of at least three functional components: (1) a receptor or recognition site, (2) a channel, and (3) a gate. The receptor recognizes the transmitter and instructs the gate to open or close the channel. The channel conducts ions only when it is gated open (Fig. 1A; for discussion see Hille, 1984). In the most extensively studied class of transmitter-gated channels, the nicotinic acetylcholine (ACh) channels at the neuromuscular junction, the channel and the receptor site coexist in a single macromolecule (see Changeux et al., 1983; Karlin et al., 1983; Numa et al., 1983). A similar situation is thought to exist for glutamate, glycine, and GABA-regulated channels in the central nervous system (Sakmann et al., 1983). But, in addition to the well-studied channels that use *intrinsic receptors,* a second class of channels has now been found that is governed by *remote receptor* sites. Remote receptors communicate with their channel by means of a second messenger system, such as cAMP and the cAMP-dependent protein kinase (Fig. 1B).

Although direct evidence that ion channels in nerve cells can be controlled by remote receptors has been obtained only recently (Klein and Kandel, 1978; Castellucci et al., 1980; Kaczmarek et al., 1980; Klein et al., 1980; Levitan and Adams, 1981; Bernier et al., 1982; Siegelbaum et al., 1982), these second-messenger-mediated actions have immediately proven interesting because they differ markedly in functional character from the common *mediating* synapses that make up the basic neural circuitry for behavior. Rather than producing fast synaptic actions that *control* behavior, second mes-

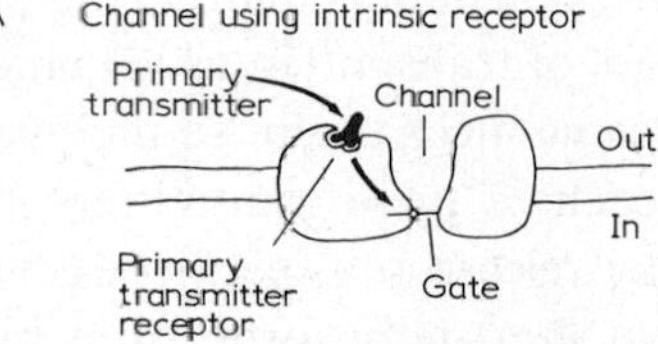

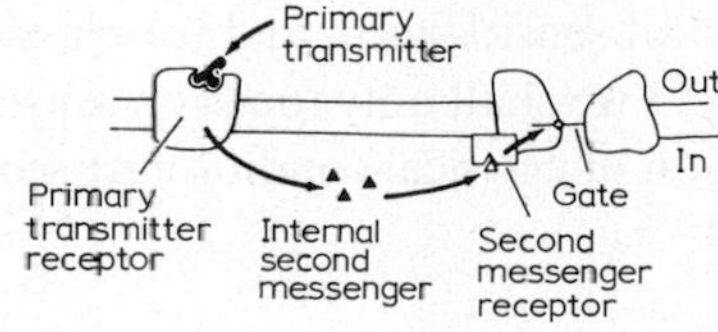

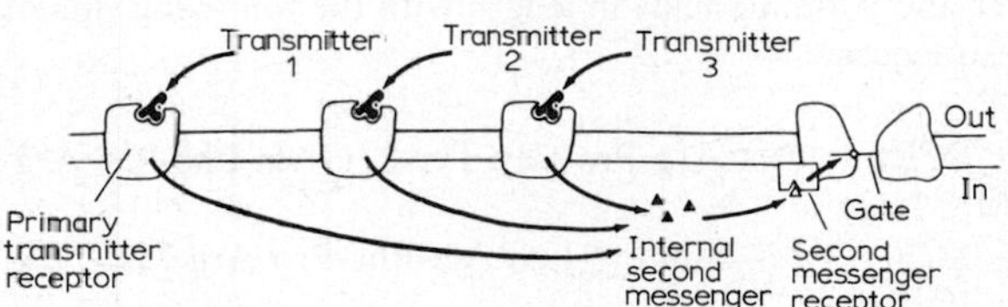

Fig. 1. Schematic diagrams illustrating the various families of ionic channels in cell membranes. (A) Channel using intrinsic receptor. (B) Channel using a single remote receptor. (C) Channel using several remote receptors. (Parts A and B are modified from Hille, 1984.)

sengers produce slow actions that *modulate* the basic neural circuitry mediating behavior. In *Aplysia,* neuronal modulation by second messengers is of further interest because it is important for two simple forms of learning: sensitization and classical conditioning.

The finding that the receptor for the action of some transmitters is at a distance from the channel and that the receptor activates the channel by means of an internal second messenger, opens up the possibility that a single species of channels can be activated by a small family of transmitters, each acting through its own remote receptors (Fig. 1C). These transmitter receptors could then instruct the channels by means of the same or different internal second messengers. We have recently encountered such a situation in *Aplysia.*

In this paper we summarize the evidence that a conventional transmitter, serotonin, and the peptides SCP_A and SCP_B* can modulate a specific K^+ channel by means of cAMP. Although the information is still fragmentary, there is the possibility that a third class of transmitter, as yet unidentified, works by the same mechanism. In modulating this K^+ channel, each of these transmitters also regulates transmitter release at a specific set of synapses involved in two short-term forms of memory each lasting minutes to hours: the memory for short-term behavioral sensitization and for classical conditioning. Here we shall only focus on sensitization. (For discussion of classical conditioning see Kandel et al., 1983.)

* The Small Cardioactive Peptides (SCPs) of *Aplysia* consist of two closely related peptides SCP_A and SCP_B, 11 and 9 amino acids in length with the following similar sequences:

SCP_A: Ala-Arg-Pro-Gly-Tyr-Leu-Ala-Phe-Pro-Arg-Met-NH_2

SCP_B: Met-Asn-Tyr-Leu-Ala-Phe-Pro-Arg-Met-NH_2 (Lloyd et al., 1984).

They are derived from a common precursor (Mahon et al., 1985). Both have identical actions in all systems so far examined, and in this chapter we shall consider them as representing one class of chemical messenger.

The specific set of connections modulated during short-term sensitization also undergoes a prolonged modulation lasting days and weeks which contributes to long-term memory for sensitization. Since several transmitters can play a similar role during short-term sensitization, we have asked: Is a single transmitter sufficient to produce the long-term changes in synaptic transmission? To what degree does this long-lasting change in the synaptic connection between the sensory and motor cells require the *cooperative* participation of several transmitters? To examine long-term sensitization, we have used dissociated cell culture and explored first the effects of a single transmitter in isolation.

Before considering these experiments, we shall briefly review some of the basic features of the gill- and siphon-withdrawal reflex, the behavioral system that we have used to study learning.

Short-term sensitization of gill- and siphon-withdrawal reflex in *Aplysia*

The defensive reflex withdrawal of the gill and siphon can be elicited by weak stimuli applied to the siphon (Fig. 2). This elementary reflex is modified by four forms of learning: habituation, sensitization, classical conditioning, and operant conditioning (Pinsker et al., 1970, 1973; Carew et al., 1981, 1983; Hawkins et al., 1985).

Sensitization is a nonassociative form of learning in which an animal learns about the properties of a single stimulus, usually a noxious one. As a result of a noxious stimulus to its tail or head, the animal learns about the presence of a dangerous stimulus and remembers to enhance its defensive responses for a varying period of time. Following a *single* noxious stimulus, an animal may show short-term memory lasting minutes to hours (Fig. 3A). But following sensitization stimuli that are repeated four or more times, an animal will remember to enhance these defensive reflexes for days or weeks (Fig. 3B; Pinsker et al., 1973; Frost et al., 1985.)

The basic reflex is controlled by a fairly simple neuronal circuit. The siphon is innervated by a clus-

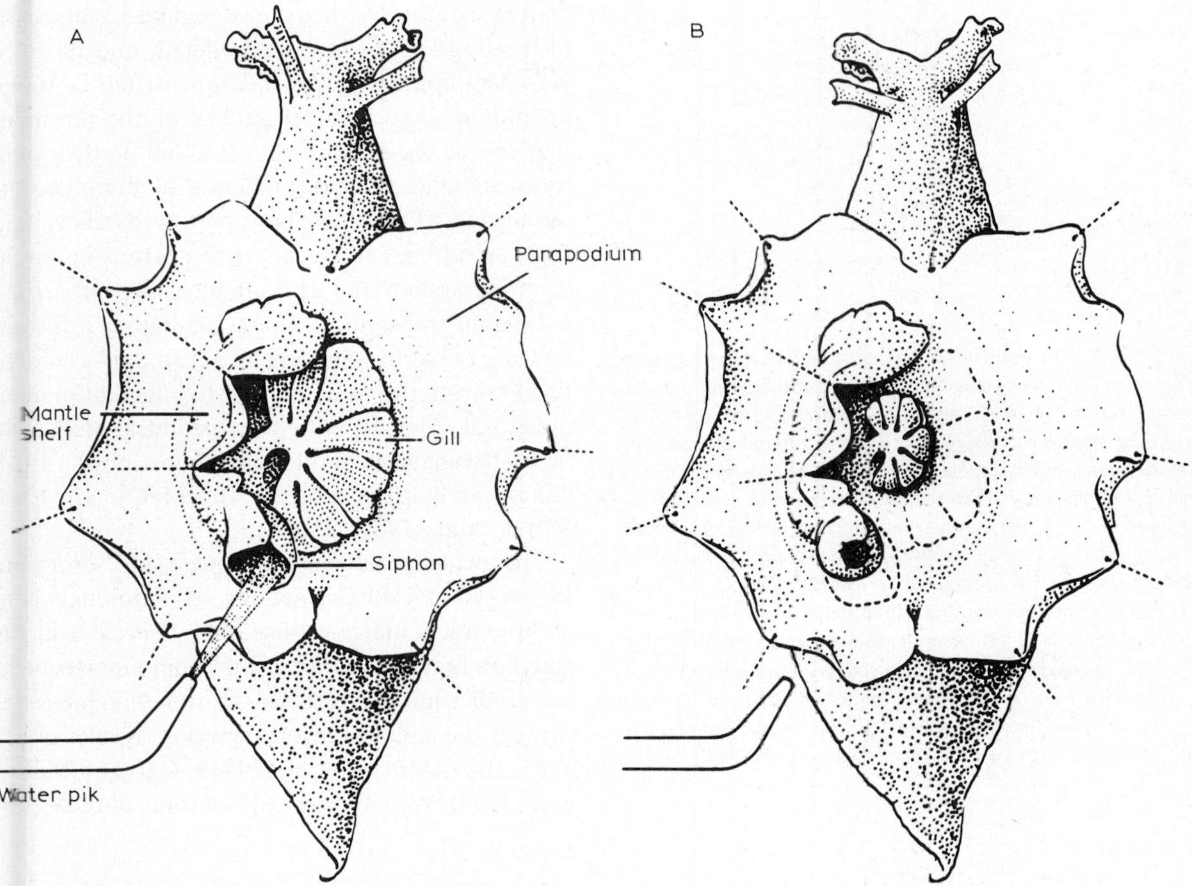

Fig. 2. Gill- and siphon-withdrawal reflex in *Aplysia*: Top view of *Aplysia* with the parapodia retracted to expose the gill and the mantle shelf. (A) Before the tactile stimulation (brief jet of water) to the siphon skin, the gill and the siphon are relaxed. (B) After the stimulation, there is a brisk contraction of the gill and the siphon. ----, Relaxed position of the two organs.

ter of about 24 sensory cells, located on the left side of the abdominal ganglion called the siphon or LE sensory neurons (Byrne et al., 1974). These sensory neurons make excitatory monosynaptic connections with interneurons and motor neurons that produce the withdrawal reflex. We will focus here only on the *monosynaptic component* of the reflex circuit which consists of the sensory neurons, the motor neurons, and the connections between them (Fig. 4; for discussion of interneurons see Byrne et al., 1978; Hawkins et al., 1981; Frost and Kandel, 1984).

How does sensitization work? A single sensitizing stimulus applied to the tail (or the neck) activates a modulatory system that consists of several sets of facilitating neurons that produce a slow modulatory excitatory synaptic potential in the sensory neurons (Klein and Kandel, 1978, 1980). This slow synaptic action lasts many minutes and has the time course of the memory for short-term sensitization. It leads, in turn, by a series of steps we shall later consider, to a process called *presynaptic facilitation*, the enhancement of transmitter release from the presynaptic terminals of the sensory neurons (Kandel and Tauc, 1965a,b; Castellucci and Kandel, 1976).

What neurons contribute to the facilitating system, and how do these neurons produce their mod-

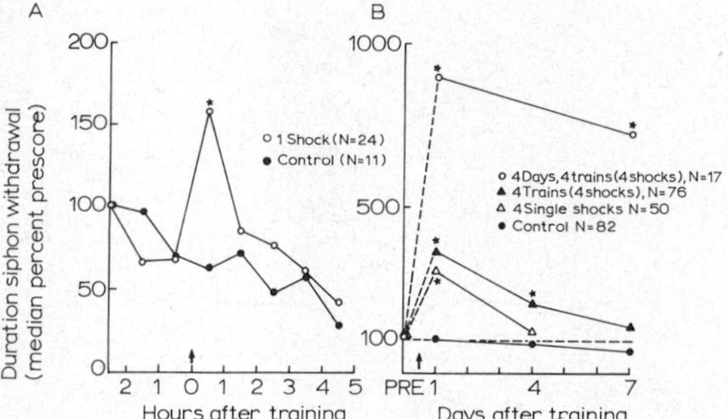

Fig. 3. Short-term and long-term sensitization of the withdrawal reflex in *Aplysia.* (A) Time course of sensitization after a single strong electrical shock to the tail or the neck of the subject (arrow). The siphon was tested once every 0.5 h and the mean of each two consecutive responses is shown. The experimental animals had significantly longer withdrawal responses than controls for more than 1 h. (B) Summary of different groups of animals receiving various amounts of stimulation. There is a gradual increase in the duration of long-term sensitization which is a function of the amount of training administered. Animals receiving four single shocks (0.5 h intervals) showed a smaller effect than animals receiving four trains of four shocks. A much larger effect is observed if four trains of four shocks are repeated for four consecutive days. Asterisks indicate points that are significantly different from control points. (From Frost et al., 1985.)

ulatory actions? We have only begun to analyze the facilitating system in cellular detail, and have, as yet, identified only a few neurons within it. Based on immunocytochemical studies of the terminals that end on the sensory neurons, and on their ability to simulate the natural action of stimuli to the tail or neck (Fig. 5), we have reason to believe that there are at least three classes of neurons in the facilitating system and each of these appears to use a different transmitter. These facilitatory transmitters are: (1) serotonin (5-HT), (2) an as yet unidentified transmitter used by the L_{29} facilitator neurons, and (3) the two related peptides, SCP_A and SCP_B (Brunelli et al., 1976; Abrams et al., 1984; Glanzman et al., 1984; Ono and McCaman, 1984; Kistler et al., 1985) (Fig. 4).

The evidence is most complete for serotonin. Bioassays of HPLC fractions of abdominal ganglion extracts indicate that 5-HT is present in the ganglion in large quantities and immunocytochemical studies have shown that serotonergic processes contact the siphon sensory neurons (Kistler et al., 1983, 1985; Abrams et al., 1984b; Ono and McCaman, 1984). We have now traced some of these pro-

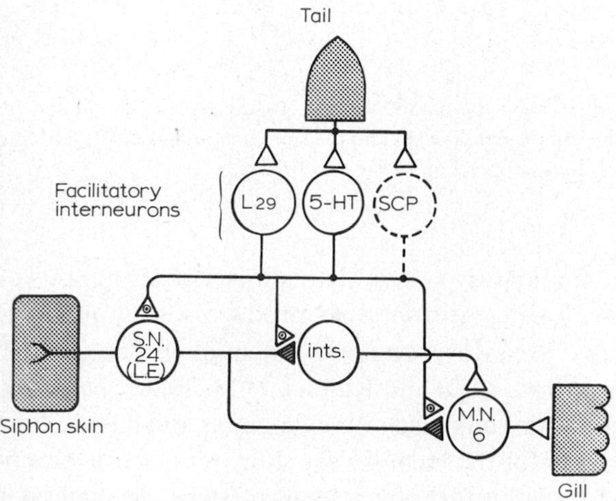

Fig. 4. Simplified diagram of the gill-withdrawal reflex in *Aplysia.* The mechanoreceptor neurons (24) carry the information from the siphon skin to interneurons and gill motor neurons (6). Stimulation of the tail (or the neck region) excites subsets of facilitator neurons which increase the synaptic transmission between the sensory neurons and their follower cells (shaded terminals). Some facilitators may be serotonergic or peptidergic (SCP). The transmitter of one identified facilitator group of interneurons (L_{29} cluster) is not yet known.

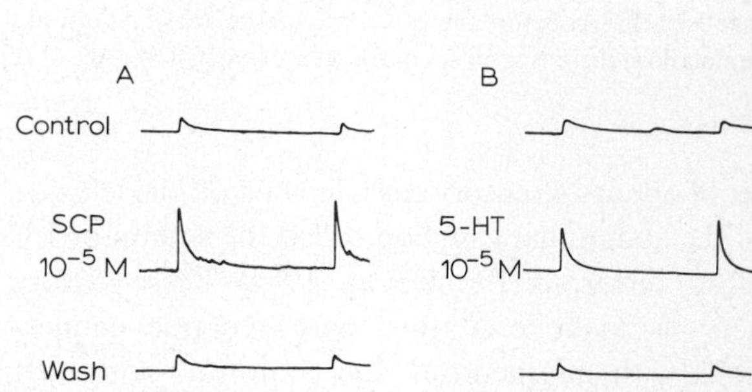

Fig. 5. Effects of 10^{-5} M SCP (A) and 10^{-5} M serotonin (B) on the gill-withdrawal reflex to siphon stimulation. The reflex was stimulated with an electrical stimulus to the siphon skin. The traces are the voltage output of a photocell located beneath the gill. Upper traces: withdrawal response immediately prior to perfusion of the transmitter onto the abdominal ganglion. Middle traces: response at the end of 3–4 min of exposure to the transmitter. Lower traces: response several minutes after the transmitter had been washed out. (From Abrams et al., 1984.)

cesses to identifiable facilitating cells in the cerebral ganglia that use 5-HT (Mackey, Glanzman, Hawkins and Kandel, unpublished data).

A second group of facilitator neurons (the L_{29} cells) uses an unidentified transmitter that may be related to 5-HT because these neurons have a high affinity uptake system for 5-HT (Bailey et al., 1983; Glanzman et al., 1984). A third group of cells, whose location has not yet been identified, are thought to use the peptides SCP_A and SCP_B. The two peptides are present in the abdominal ganglion, as indicated by bioassay of HPLC fractions of extracts from the ganglion, and by immunocytochemical studies which indicate that processes containing the SCPs come in close contact with sensory neurons (Abrams et al., 1984b; Lloyd et al., 1985).

Binding of the modulatory transmitters 5-HT and the SCPs to their receptors leads to an increase in cAMP and produces presynaptic facilitation

The binding of 5-HT or of the SCPs to their receptors on the sensory neuron leads to an increase in the intracellular level of cAMP (Bernier et al., 1982; Abrams et al., 1984b). This increase resembles that produced in these cells by stimulating the connectives, the nerves that activate the facilitating cells (Fig. 6).

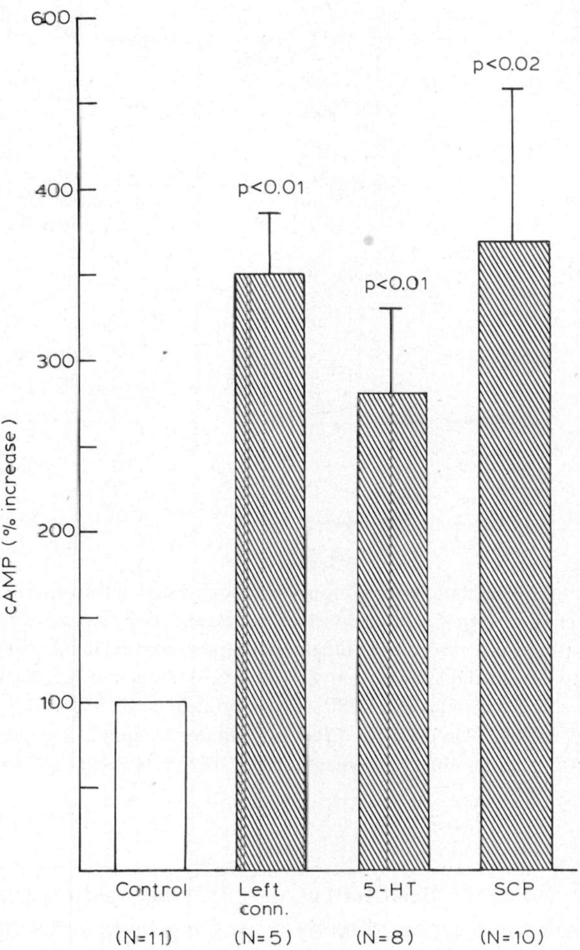

Fig. 6. Effect of facilitator cells activity, serotonin and SCP on the synthesis of cAMP in sensory cells of the abdominal ganglion. The left connective was stimulated to excite the facilitating neurons; 30 sec after the stimulation, the ganglia were frozen quickly and the sensory cells were analyzed for cAMP content. In the case of serotonin, the ganglia were exposed to the drug (2×10^{-4} M) for 5 min, then they were frozen and processed. For SCP (10^{-4} M), a 60-sec exposure to the drug was used. (Adapted from Bernier et al., 1982, and Abrams et al., 1984.)

How does the increase in cAMP participate in neuronal modulation? Stimulation of the connective that carries information from the tail or the neck to the abdominal ganglion, or intracellular stimulation of the L_{29} facilitator cells, or application of serotonin or of the SCPs, all increase synaptic transmission from siphon sensory neurons and enhance the defensive withdrawal reflex (Fig. 7). This synaptic facilitation can also be produced by injecting cAMP or the cAMP-dependent protein kinase into the sensory neuron (Figs. 7B and 8B).

In turn, nerve stimulation which excites facilitator cells in the central nervous system (Fig. $8A_1$), intracellular stimulation of L_{29} cells (Fig. $8B_2$), and application of the SCPs or 5-HT (Fig. $8A_{2,3}$), all increase the duration of each individual action potential in the cell body of the sensory neurons (Klein and Kandel, 1978; Castellucci et al., 1980). This increase in turn allows the Ca^{2+} current to stay on for a longer period of time and thereby enhances Ca^{2+} influx into the sensory neurons. A similar increase is produced by cAMP and the cAMP-dependent protein kinase (Fig. $8A_4$, B_4).

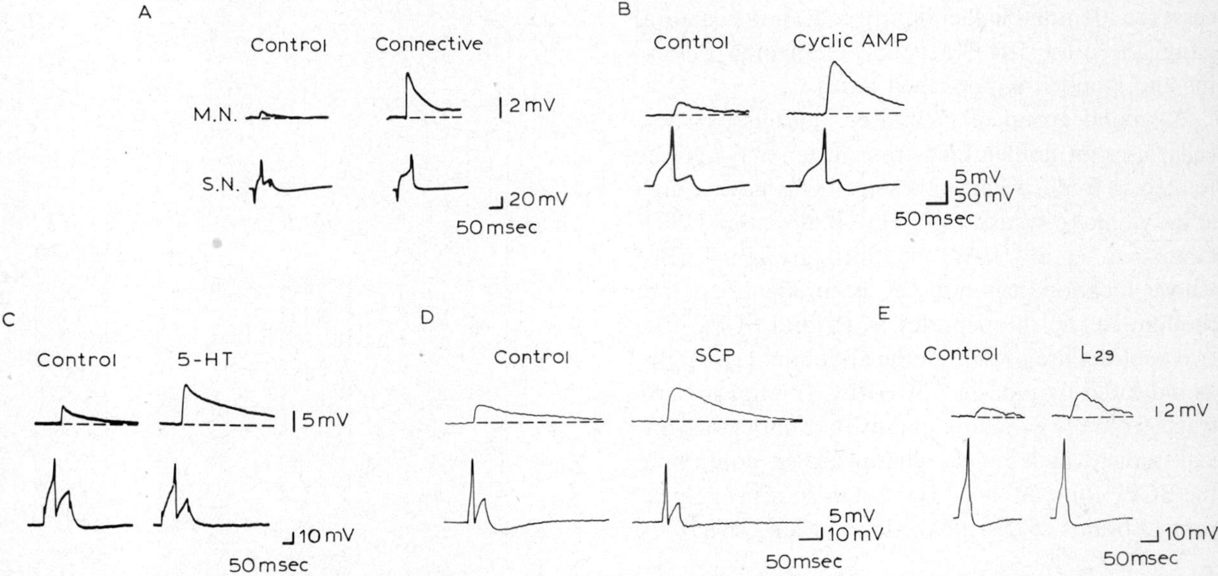

Fig. 7. Facilitation of the monosynaptic connection between the sensory neurons and motor neurons of the gill- and siphon-withdrawal reflex in *Aplysia*. In each set of traces, the lower ones are recordings from the presynaptic sensory neuron. The upper ones are intracellular recordings of the postsynaptic potential in the motor neuron. (A) The facilitator neurons were excited by a train of stimuli applied to the left connective. (From Castellucci and Kandel, 1976.) (B) Intracellular injection of cAMP in the presynaptic sensory neuron facilitates the EPSP. (From Brunelli et al., 1976.) (C) The EPSP is facilitated by application of 5-HT. (From Rayport and Schacher, 1986.) (D) The EPSP is facilitated by application of SCP. (From Abrams et al., 1984.) (E) Intracellular firing of a single L_{29} can facilitate the monosynaptic EPSP. (From Hawkins, 1981.)

Recently, Belardetti et al. (1985) have used tissue culture to record directly from the growth cones of sensory neurons, the likely precursors of the synaptic terminals, and have observed a similar broadening of the action potential. Thus, the slow modulatory synaptic actions in *Aplysia* that contribute to sensitization and act on the cell body may also be exerted on the presynaptic terminals where the broadening of the action potential can increase Ca^{2+} influx, which in turn can enhance transmitter release.

The recognition site (the receptor) for the transmitter and the ionic channel are separate protein molecules

Detailed voltage clamp studies indicate that the broadening of the sensory neuron action potential is produced by the depression of a specific K^+ current (Camardo et al., 1982; Klein et al., 1982). This finding has allowed us to ask: How is the serotonin-sensitive K^+ current modulated? Using the patch clamp technique that allowed study of the properties of individual ion channels, Siegelbaum et al. (1982) searched for and characterized a new class of K^+ channels and found it to have properties consistent with the macroscopic serotonin-sensitive K^+ current. We have therefore called this channel the *serotonin-sensitive K^+ channel* or *S channel* (Fig. 9).

How does protein phosphorylation alter channel gating? How is the K^+ current that flows through the S channel reduced by cAMP-dependent protein phosphorylation? In principle, current flow through the K^+ channel could be reduced in one of these ways: (1) by decreasing the conductance of the channel; (2) by decreasing the probability of channel opening or by increasing the probability of closing; and/or (3) by reducing the number of channels that are open in the membrane (Fig. 10). Siegelbaum et al. (1982), Abrams et al. (1984), and Shuster et al. (1985) examined this question in both cell-attached and cell-free patches and have found that serotonin, the SCPs, and cAMP act in a common manner: they reduce, in an all-or-none fashion, the number of channels that are open (Fig. 11A, B, C). Moreover, the channel can be shown to be structurally independent of the receptor. When 5-HT or either of the SCPs is applied to the cell membrane *outside* the area of the patch electrode, the ion channels *under* the patch electrode are closed even though they are not directly accessible to the transmitter. These experiments provided compelling evidence in nerve cells that a channel can be structurally independent of the receptor that regulates it.

These findings now raised the question: Is the critical substrate protein that is acted on by the protein kinase cytoplasmic, or is it membrane-associated? To address this point, Shuster et al. (1985) applied the purified catalytic subunit of cAMP-dependent protein kinase to cell-free, inside-out patches of membrane and found that the protein kinase is capable of closing the S channels (Fig. 11D). Thus, the critical substrate protein appears membrane-associated; it might be either the channel itself or a regulatory protein closely linked to the channel in the membrane.

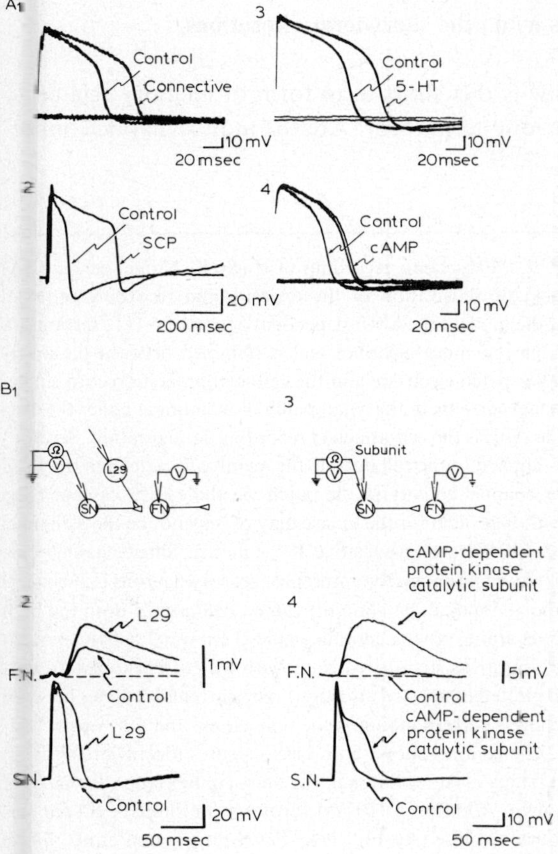

Fig. 8. (A) Increase in the duration of the sensory neuron action potential in artificial sea water containing 0.1 M tetraethylammonium. (A_1) After stimulation of the connective (the nerve pathway that mediates sensitization); (A_2) application of 1 μM SCP; (A_3) application of 0.2 mM 5-HT; and (A_4) intracellular injection of cAMP. Each trace represents superimposition of two or three action potentials evoked by a 2- to 5-msec depolarizing pulse applied intracellularly. (A_1, A_3 and A_4, from Klein and Kandel, 1978; A_2, from Abrams et al., 1984.) (B) Effects of stimulating a single facilitator neuron and of injecting the catalytic subunit of the cAMP-dependent protein kinase on the duration of the sensory neuron action potential and EPSP amplitude. (B_1) Diagram of the simplified neuronal circuit of the gill-withdrawal reflex, illustrating the experimental procedure involving stimulation of a single facilitator neuron (L_{29}) and simultaneous recording from a sensory neuron (SN) and a motor neuron (FN). (B_2) Superimposed traces of action potentials of the sensory cell and evoked EPSPs before and after intracellular stimulation of a single facilitator neuron (an L_{29} cell). (B_3) Diagram of the simplified neuronal circuit of the gill-withdrawal reflex, illustrating the experimental procedure involving the injection of the catalytic subunit into the sensory neuron. (B_4) Superimposed traces of action potentials of the sensory cell and evoked EPSP recorded in the motor neuron (FN) before and after intracellular injection of the catalytic subunit into the sensory neuron body. Injection of the catalytic subunit increased the duration of the action potential of the sensory neuron and the EPSP amplitude, simulating the action of the facilitator neuron. (B_1 and B_2, from Hawkins, 1981; B_3 and B_4, from Castellucci et al., 1980.)

The several modulatory transmitters converge on a common cascade

Based on our voltage-clamp, patch-clamp, and biochemical studies of the sensory neuron and its growth cone, we have proposed a molecular model for presynaptic facilitation (Fig. 12; for review see Kandel and Schwartz, 1982). According to this model, the transmitter released by the facilitating neurons (serotonin, the SCPs, and perhaps the transmitter of the L_{29} neurons) activate a transmitter-sensitive adenylate cyclase in the membrane of the presynaptic terminals of the sensory neurons that increases the level of cAMP within these terminals. Cyclic AMP then activates a protein kinase that phosphorylates the K^+ channel protein or a protein that is associated with it. This K^+ current normally contributes significantly to the repolarization of the action potentials and phosphorylation reduces this current. Reduction of the current prolongs the action potentials in the sensory neurons and allows more Ca^{2+} to flow into their terminals. In addition, serotonin and cAMP also act to modulate the handling of Ca^{2+} within the sensory cells (Boyle et al., 1984; Klein et al., unpublished; Hochner et al., 1985). We think this second process may allow for more effective mobilization of transmitter to release sites, a process that becomes particularly important when transmitter release is depressed (Hochner et al., 1985).

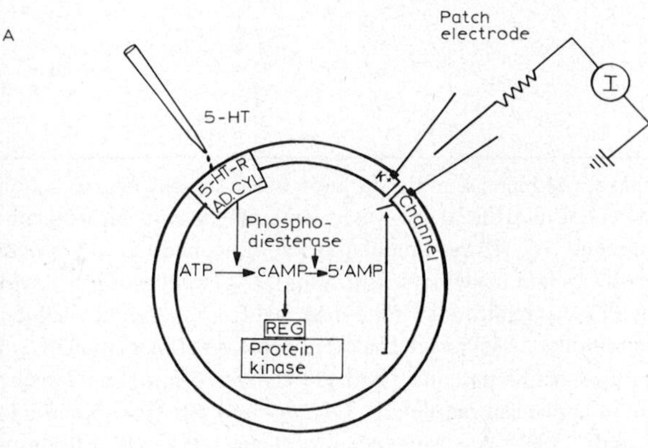

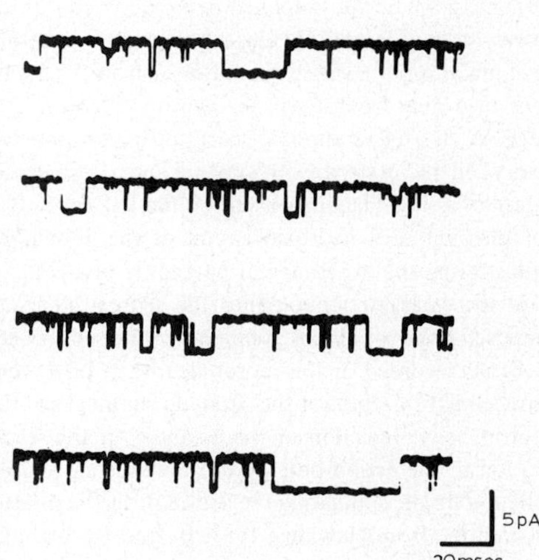

Fig. 9. Patch-clamp recording of single S channel current. (A) Schematic illustration of the experimental recording protocol and the model for cAMP-dependent action of 5-HT (serotonin). A high-resistance gigaohm seal is obtained between the extracellular patch electrode and the cell membrane to record single-channel currents in the small patch of membrane under the electrode. This is the cell-attached recording configuration. Serotonin is applied to the cell outside the membrane patch but may still alter channel activity in the patch via the cAMP cascade. The substrate protein for the kinase may or may not be the S channel itself. (B) Serotonin-sensitive K^+ channel. Single-channel current records from mechanoreceptor sensory neurons (LE cluster) in the abdominal ganglion of *Aplysia californica.* Both the bath and recording pipette contain artificial sea water. Channel openings appear as step increases in outward current (outward current plotted in upward direction). The current fluctuates between two levels corresponding to the fully closed and fully open channel. The channel shows both brief closures (downward flickers) and longer closures but is in the open configuration for most of the time. Addition of 10 μM serotonin in the bath caused this channel to close (see Fig. 11). (From Siegelbaum et al., 1982.)

Long-term synaptic alterations occur at the same locus as do the short-term alterations

How is this short-term form of memory related to the long-term form? Are the monosynaptic connec-

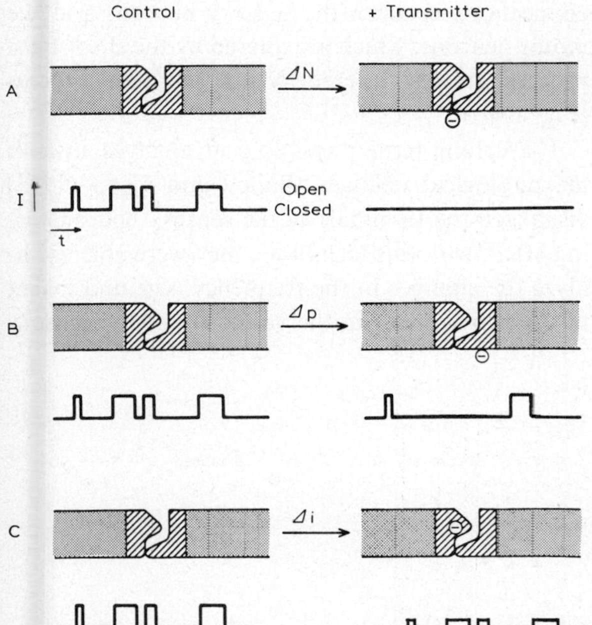

Fig. 10. Three possible mechanisms of channel modulation by neurotransmitter. Transmitter is assumed to decrease macroscopic ion conductance. Channel openings are displayed as upward going step changes in current. Three possible outcomes that could lead to a decrease in ionic current. (A) The baseline current trace shows no channel openings, corresponding to a decrease in the number (ΔN) of active channels. (B) The probability (ΔP) of channel opening is reduced. (C) The single-channel conductance is reduced, so less current flows through the channel (Δi). I = Current; t = time.

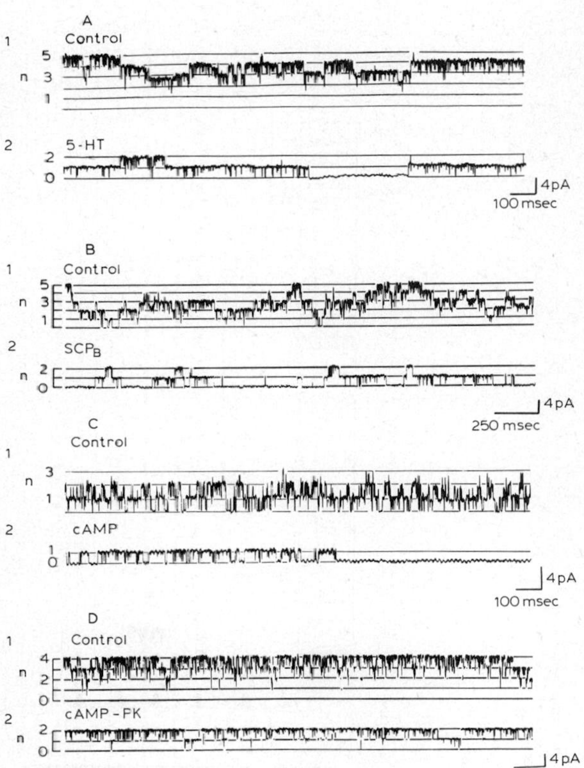

Fig. 11. Action of serotonin, SCP, cAMP and the catalytic unit of cAMP-protein kinase on single-channel current recorded from sensory neurons in the abdominal ganglion of *Aplysia californica*. (A_1) Current in the absence of serotonin. Left-hand ordinate shows the number of open channels. The current record was well fitted by a binomial distribution assuming that five channels are active in the patch and that each channel opens with a probability of 0.84. (A_2) Current obtained 2 min after addition of 30 μM serotonin to the bath. The single channel currents were recorded in response to steady depolarization of the patch membrane to 0 mV (defined as patch pipette minus cell resting potential) produced by changing the potential inside the patch pipette. The use of steady-state recording conditions minimizes interferences from other channels since steady-state depolarization inactivates much of the K^+, Na^+ and Ca^{2+} current. In contrast, serotonin-sensitive K^+ current is active during steady-state depolarizations. Note that the number of active channels is reduced from five to two. (From Siegelbaum et al., 1982.) (B_1) Current in the absence of peptide. (B_2) Current 4 min after addition of 10 μM SCP$_B$; note that the number of active channels is reduced from five to two. All records are representative samples of several minutes of recording. (From Abrams et al., 1984.) (C) Effect of intracellular injection of cAMP on single-channel current. Following establishment of the seal between patch electrode and membrane, the cell was impaled with a microelectrode filled with 1 M cAMP and cAMP was injected into cells by hyperpolarizing current pulses. (C_1) Current obtained soon after impalement of the cell with the cAMP electrode. (C_2) Current records after subsequent injection. Note that only one active channel is open and after a while this last channel is closed. (From Siegelbaum et al., 1982.) (D) Effect of cAMP-kinase on S channels in inside-out membrane patches from sensory neurons. (D_1) Before the addition of the kinase, the patch contained four active channels open for a large fraction of the time. (D_2) Three minutes after addition of cAMP-PK (0.1 μM final concentration) plus 1 mM Mg-ATP, the current level fluctuates from zero to two channels open. (From Shuster et al., 1985.)

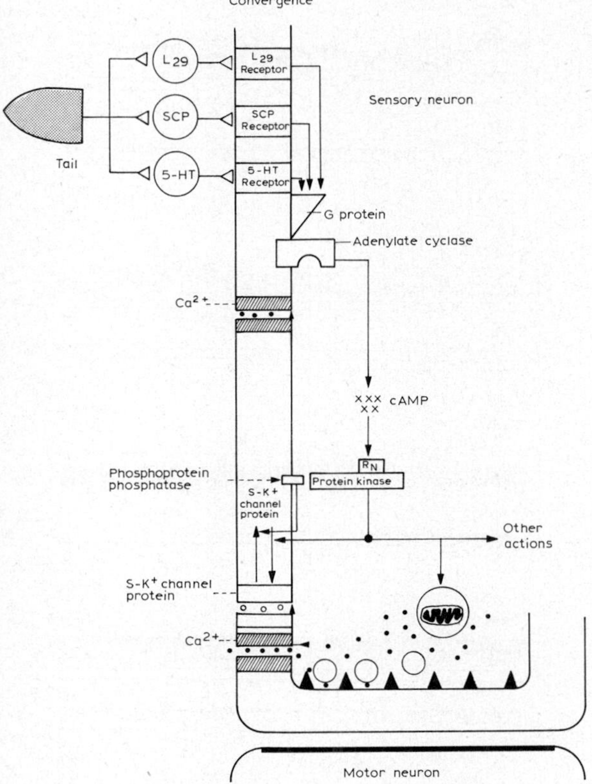

Fig. 12. Molecular model of presynaptic facilitation underlying sensitization. When excited, the various groups of facilitator neurons activate a sequence of events which lead to a cAMP-dependent phosphorylation of substrate proteins which results in the closure of a special K^+ channel and in a change in the Ca^{2+} buffering in the presynaptic terminals of the sensory neuron. The resulting increase in the duration of the sensory neuron action potential leads to an increase of Ca^{2+} current. This effect together with the increase in the free Ca^{2+} in the terminals results in an enhanced synaptic transmission.

tions which are modulated during short-term sensitization also modulated during long-term sensitization? A first step in the analysis was recently achieved by William Frost and his colleagues (1985). They measured the amplitude of the monosynaptic connections between sensory neurons and the gill motor neuron L_7 in a group of long-term sensitized animals and compared that to a control group. They found that the monosynaptic connections between the sensory neurons and the motor neurons, which are altered by the short-term process, are also altered by the long-term process (Fig. 13).

These long-term physiological changes involve morphological changes. Bailey and Chen (1983) visualized the terminals of the sensory neurons using HRP; with this technique, they were able to analyze the changes in the frequency, size and extent of the active zones in the varicosity of the sensory

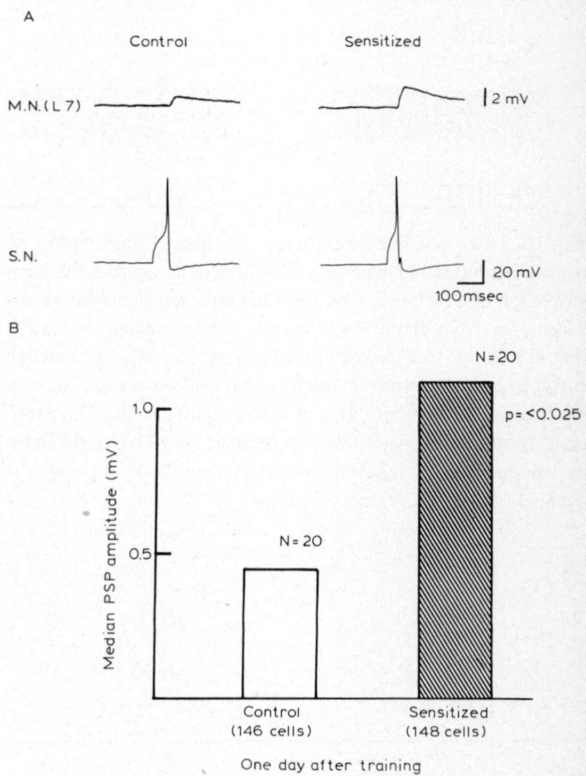

Fig. 13. EPSP data from control and long-term sensitized animals. (A) Representative monosynaptic EPSPs from siphon sensory neurons to gill motor neuron L_1. The synaptic connection on the left is from a control animal. The connection on the right is from a long-term sensitized animal examined one day after the end of training. (B) Comparison of median EPSP values from control and long-term sensitized animals examined one day after the end of training. The median value from the sensitized population is significantly larger than the median value from the control population. (Mann-Whitney *U* Test, *p* 0.025). (From Frost et al., 1985.)

neurons as well as changes in the number and distribution of the synaptic vesicles. They found that in sensitized animals a larger percentage of varicosities had an active zone than in control animals. The mean ratio of active zones to varicosities increased from 41% in control animals to 65% in long-term sensitized animals. Bailey and Chen also found that the total surface membrane area of sensory neuron active zones and the total number of vesicles associated with each release site were increased in sensitized animals. Their results suggest that active zones are plastic structures and that learning may modulate these sites to alter synaptic effectiveness. Since the observations have been made on animals that have received long-term behavioral training, the possibility exists that these morphological changes could represent an anatomical substrate for memory consolidation.

To relate these physiological and morphological changes to their molecular mechanisms, we attempted to simplify the system further. Toward this end, we carried out two sets of experiments. First, we reconstituted the monosynaptic component of the reflex system in dissociated cell culture. Second, we attempted to simulate the training using repeated applications of only one of the candidate facilitating transmitters, serotonin.

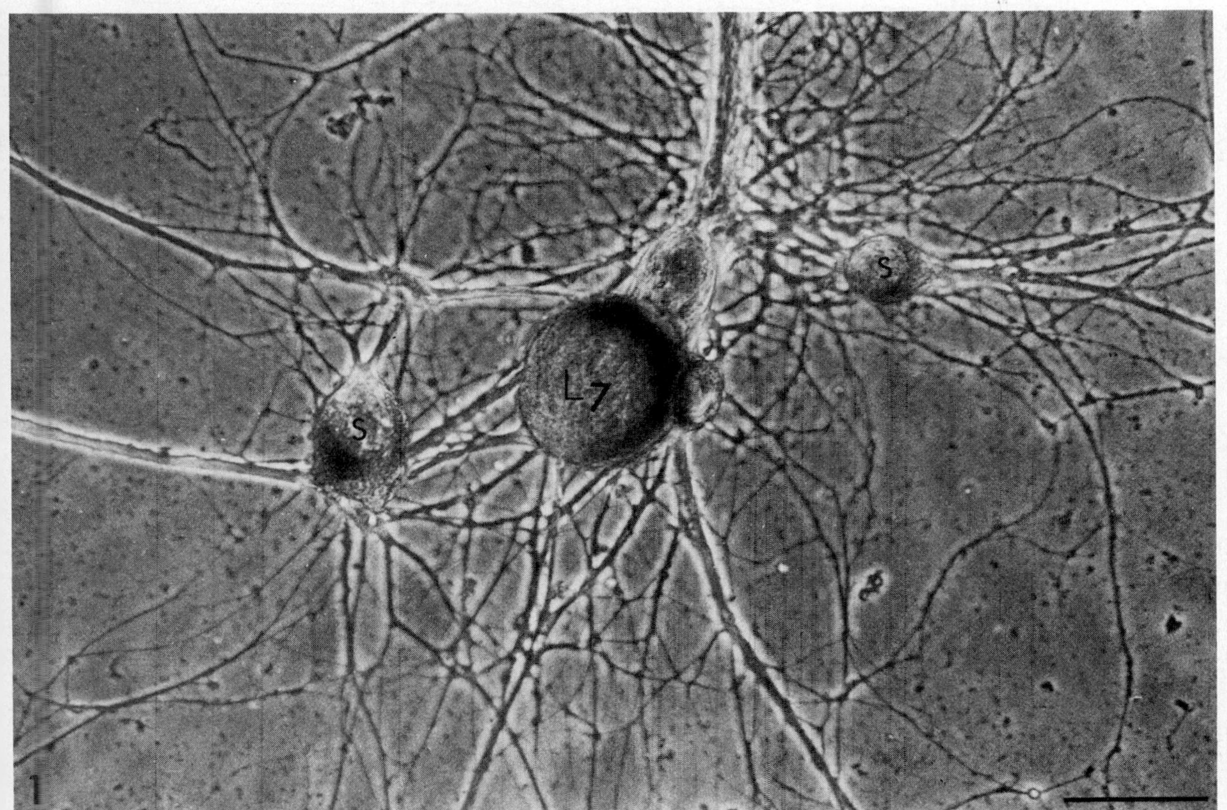

Fig. 14. Reconstitution of the monosynaptic component of the reflex mediating gill-withdrawal. The circuit consists of two LE sensory neurons and one gill motor cell L_7 after 5 days in dissociated cell culture. S = LE sensory cell; L_1 = motor cell; calibration = 100 μm. (From Rayport and Schacher, 1986.)

Reconstitution of long-term synaptic plasticity in dissociated cell culture

The monosynaptic component of the learning system for sensitization comprises three critical components: (1) sensory neurons; (2) motor neurons; and (3) facilitating neurons. We have succeeded in reconstituting this system in dissociated cell culture (Fig. 14; Rayport and Schacher, 1986). Figure 15 illustrates that sensory neurons can form chemical synapses with the identified motor cell L_7 in tissue culture. Repeated stimulation of the sensory neuron

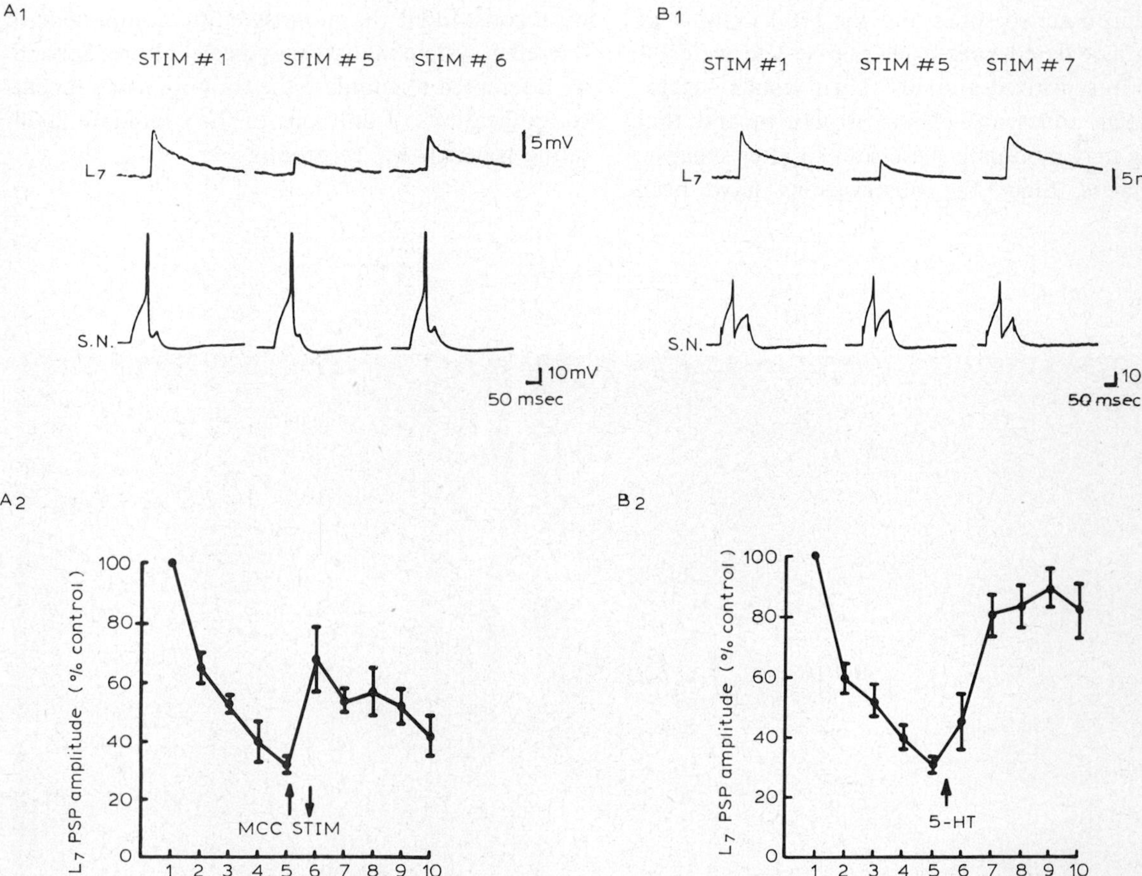

Fig. 15. Neurons of the gill-withdrawal reflex in dissociated cell culture show homosynaptic depression and heterosynaptic facilitation produced by firing of a single serotonergic cell (MCC) or 5-HT. (A_1) Sensory, motor and metacerebral (MCC) cells were simultaneously impaled with single-barreled electrodes. The motor cell was hyperpolarized 50 mV below rest. The sensory neuron was then fired with a brief intracellular depolarizing current pulse once every 20 sec. Between the fifth and sixth stimuli, the MCC was fired with a long depolarizing current step causing it to fire 3 to 5 spikes per second for 15 sec. The records show first the initial EPSP, then the fifth EPSP showing the magnitude of homosynaptic depression followed by the EPSP after MCC firing showing facilitation. (A_2) The graph summarizes the results of five experiments, normalized by adjusting the initial EPSP of each LE-L_7 connection to unity. Points are mean and standard error of the mean. (B_1) Record of the evoked EPSP in L_7 for the first, fifth and seventh intracellular stimulation of the sensory neuron. At the fifth stimulus, the EPSP is depressed. After the fifth stimulus, 5-HT was applied (2×10^{-6} M). This leads to a large facilitation of the evoked EPSP. (B_2) Summary of homosynaptic depression and 5-HT facilitation from five experiments. The LE-L_7 EPSPs were normalized relative to the initial EPSP in each experiment. Points are mean and standard error of the mean. (From Rayport and Schacher, 1986.)

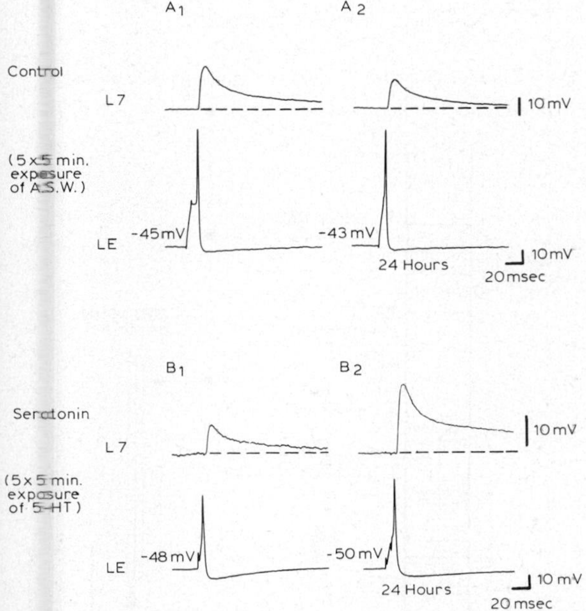

Fig. 16. Long-term facilitation in dissociated cell culture. Top trace of each pair is the intracellular recording from gill motor neuron L_7. Bottom trace is from the presynaptic sensory neuron. (A_1) Records from a control culture. On day 5, the EPSP amplitude evoked by a single sensory cell was sampled. Then a sham training with artificial seawater was carried out (5 exposures of 5 min at 15-min intervals). (A_2) The same pair of neurons were recorded from 24 h later. There was a small decrease in the EPSP amplitude. (B_1) Records from a treated culture. The protocol is identical to the one described in (A) except that the culture cells were exposed to serotonin (1×10^{-6} M). (B_2) Twenty-four hours later, the evoked EPSP is greatly facilitated.

in such a system leads to synaptic depression as in the intact ganglion, which underlies habituation. Stimulating a serotonergic neuron leads to synaptic facilitation. This facilitation is simulated by simply exposing the culture to 5-HT (Fig. 15).

Since in the intact animal, long-term sensitization lasting days can be produced by presenting four or more facilitating stimuli at regular intervals, we adapted an analogous protocol in the dissociated culture using five brief exposures to 5-HT, each separated by 15 min. During each exposure, 5-HT was applied at a concentration of 1μM for 5 min. When retested 24 h later, the change in EPSP amplitude in the 5-HT treated cultures was significantly greater than the change in EPSP amplitude in control untreated cultures (Fig. 16).

A large number of studies in intact animals have suggested that short-term memory is independent of new protein synthesis, whereas long-term memory is not (Davis and Squire, 1985). To bring this problem to the cellular level and determine whether long-lasting facilitation of this monosynaptic connection is dependent on new protein synthesis, we studied the effects of inhibitors of protein synthesis and of RNA synthesis. As a first step, we used anisomycin. This antibiotic blocks protein synthesis in culture and in the intact ganglion by more than 90% and has no detrimental effects on the direct sensory neuron-to-motoneuron connection. When anisomycin was added to cultures 60 min before starting the 5-HT protocol and kept in the cultures until one hour following the last 5-HT application, it blocked the 5-HT-induced long-term increase of EPSP amplitudes. By contrast, the exposure to anisomycin did not interfere with short-term facilitation, indicating that long- and short-term facilitation can be dissociated pharmacologically (Montarolo et al., 1985). We have now obtained similar results with emetine, and with actinomycin and α-amanitin, two inhibitors of RNA transcription.

These results suggest that learning initiates two memory traces acting on a common locus which appear to use two different mechanisms: a short-term memory which results from post-translational covalent modification, and a long-term memory that seems to result from an alteration in protein synthesis. It now remains to be determined whether the long-term process is initiated by a cAMP cascade, and therefore is in series with the short-term process, or whether a facilitatory transmitter like serotonin, acting on a separate receptor, initiates a second molecular cascade for the long-term process (Fig. 17).

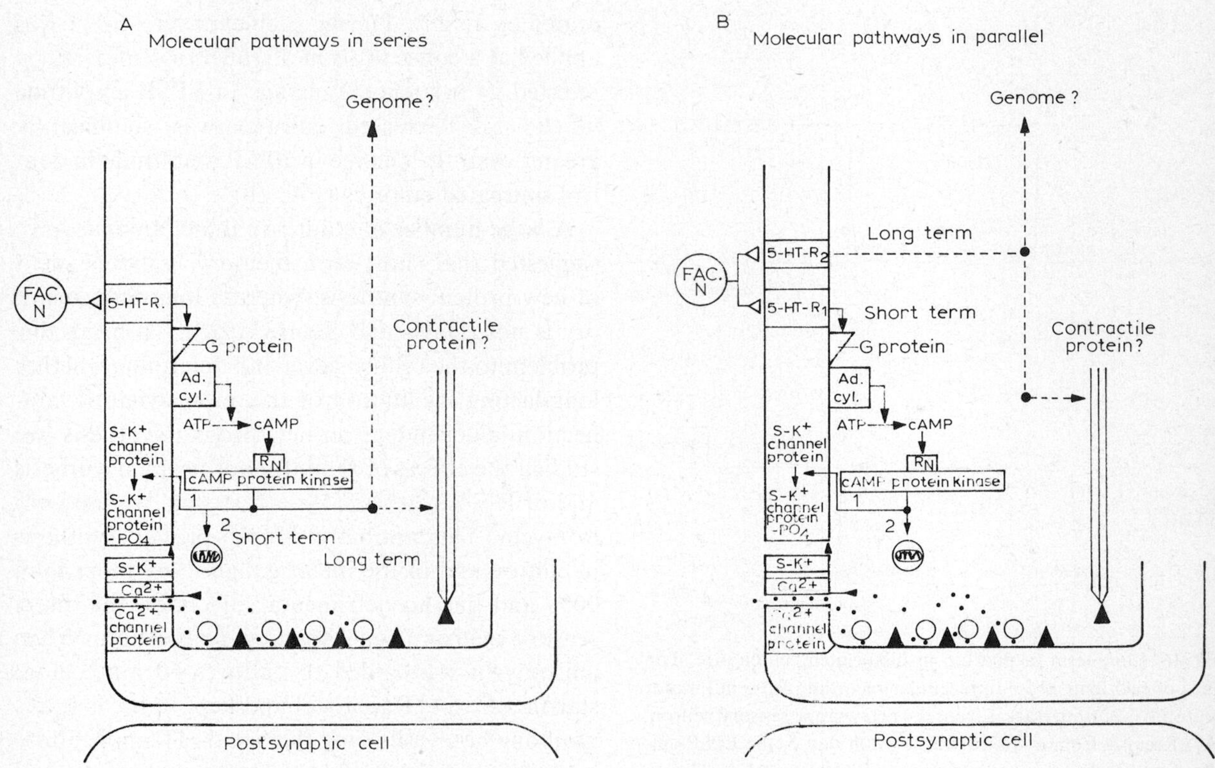

Fig. 17. Alternate models of mechanisms involved in the transition from short-term to long-term memory. The long-term memory is depicted as involving among other steps, the insertion of new active zone protein. (A) The mechanisms for short-term and long-term memory are in series. The cascade of events which arises during short-term memory triggers or signals one or more cascades that produce long-term memory. (B) The mechanisms for short-term and long-term memory are in parallel. The cascade of events which arises during short-term memory is independent from the cascade of events that will produce long-term memory. For example, one receptor (R_1) will be dedicated to the short-term process, a second receptor (R_2) will be involved in the long-term one.

An overall view

Why multiple facilitating transmitters?

The observation that there is a small family of transmitters used by the facilitation system raises the question of why there should be multiple transmitters with the same action. Whereas serotonin, the SCPs and the L_{29} transmitter all have roughly similar facilitatory effects on the sensory neurons, it is possible that there are differences in the detail of their actions.

For example, the several facilitatory transmitters may exist to mediate behavioral sensitization of differing time courses. Indeed, we have found to our surprise that the response of the sensory neurons to the peptides SCP_A and SCP_B desensitizes rapidly and tends to give rise to relatively brief short-term facilitation, whereas the response to the small molecule transmitter, 5-HT, does not desensitize readily and produces more persistent effects (Fig. 18). Thus, it is conceivable that some transmitters might support only very short-term memory for sensitization (lasting seconds to one or more minutes) and other transmitters more sustained short-term memory (lasting several minutes to one or more hours). Similarly, we know from the tissue culture experiments that 5-HT alone can signal the long-term forms of this memory. But we do not yet know whether any of the other facilitatory transmitters

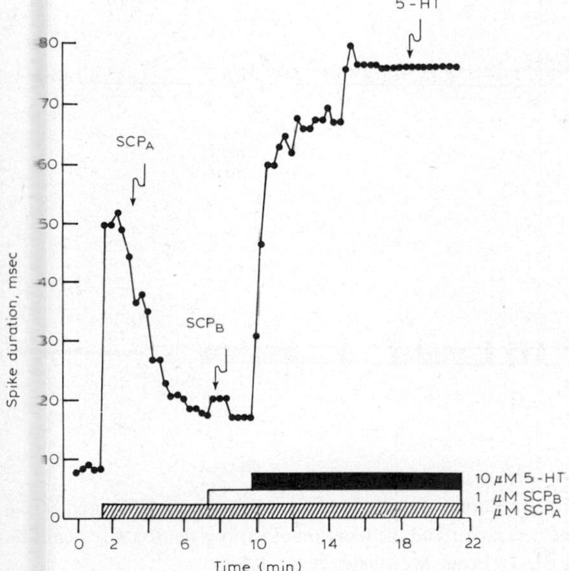

Fig. 18. Effect of desensitization to SCP on the response to serotonin. The action potential in a sensory neuron was recorded at 20-sec intervals in high-Ca^{2+}/Mg^{2+} saline with 50 mM tetraethylammonium. The responsiveness of serotonin (5-HT) was first tested with a brief exposure to 10 μM 5-HT. After washout and recovery of the action potential, the preparation was perfused with 1 μM SCP_A for the remainder of the experiment. Once the spike-broadening response to SCP_A had almost completely desensitized, 1 μM SCP_B and then 10 μM 5-HT were added to the perfusion. Note that, although the response to SCP_B was almost entirely eliminated, the response to 5-HT remained comparable with the 5-HT response at the outset of the experiment. (From Abrams et al., 1984.)

can initiate long-term sensitization by themselves.

In addition, the different facilitatory transmitters may be specific for different sensitizing stimuli. For example, L_{29} cells are activated by stimuli to the *Aplysia*'s tail but not to its head (Hawkins, unpublished results), whereas some serotonergic facilitator neurons may respond to noxious stimulation of *Aplysia*'s head as well as its tail. We will be in a better position to address this question once we have characterized the receptive fields for the various facilitatory neurons.

Finally, the different facilitatory transmitters may differ in their ability to support associative learning. As we mentioned in the beginning of this paper, *Aplysia*'s defensive withdrawal can be classically conditioned (Carew et al., 1981, 1983). The cellular basis of classical conditioning of this reflex involves a mechanism whereby activity in the sensory neurons amplifies the effects of presynaptic facilitation (Hawkins et al., 1983; Walters and Byrne, 1983). This activity-dependent amplification of presynaptic facilitation which occurs during conditioning can be mimicked by pairing sensory neuron activity with exposure to 5-HT (Abrams et al., 1983; Ocorr et al., 1985). Our preliminary evidence suggests that the Ca^{2+} influx resulting from activity in the sensory neurons interacts with the elevation of cAMP levels to potentiate transmitter release from the sensory neuron terminals (see Abrams et al., 1984a; Abrams and Kandel, 1985; Ocorr et al., 1985). 5-HT has been shown to be capable of supporting activity-dependent enhancement of presynaptic facilitation. We have yet to test the other facilitatory transmitters to see if they, too, have this capability.

Whether or not the several facilitatory transmitters differ in their precise actions, they may have synergistic effects. Thus, while release of a single transmitter may produce presynaptic facilitation of synaptic transmission from the siphon sensory neurons, release of several modulatory transmitters may greatly potentiate this presynaptic facilitation, either increasing it quantitatively or greatly prolonging it.

Following up on the results of Abrams et al. (1984b), we have begun to fractionate *Aplysia* abdominal ganglia using HPLC with the aim of isolating and characterizing other facilitatory substances. We hope in this way to be able to eventually discover the facilitatory transmitter used by the L_{29} cells and to use this additional information to distinguish among these several possibilities.

Co-reception, co-existence, co-release, and the mechanisms of learning

Recent work on learning in *Aplysia* has so far focused primarily on attempts to define some of the key elements in the facilitating system and to de-

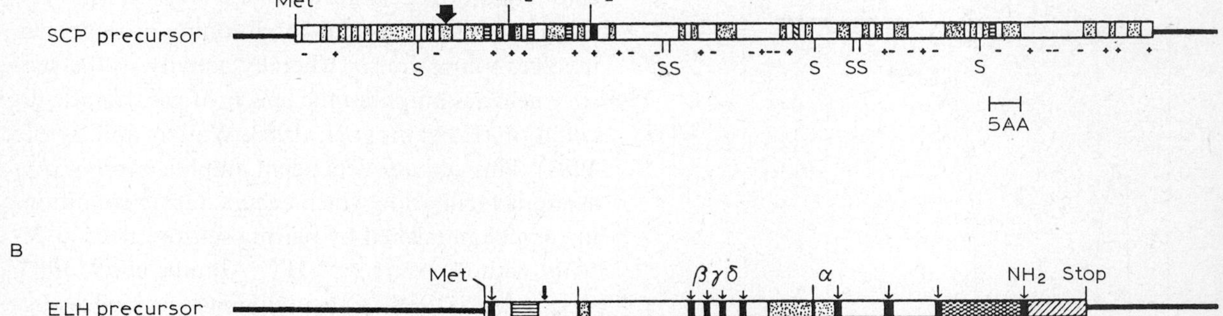

Fig. 19. Structure of two protein precursors in *Aplysia*. (A) Structure of the precursor giving rise to the two peptides SCP_A and SCP_B. (From Mahon et al., 1985.) (B) Structure of the ELH (egg-laying hormone) precursor and the location of various neuroactive peptides, such as the alpha, beta, gamma peptides, the acidic peptides, as well as ELH. (From McAllister et al., 1983.)

scribe the nature of the major transmitters involved. We are only beginning to understand the underlying cellular architecture of the facilitating system. Only once that is understood will we be in a position to see to what degree co-reception, co-existence, and co-release are likely to play a role in these forms of learning.

Co-reception refers to the fact that a single transmitter released from a single neuron can act on more than one receptor of a single target cell. First demonstrated in *Aplysia* and other invertebrates co-reception involves multiple responses of a neuron to the same transmitter (Wachtel and Kandel, 1967; Gardner and Kandel, 1972; Kehoe, 1969, 1972; for review see Kandel, 1976). The responses differ in time courses and often involve a fast synaptic action combined with a slow one. Sometimes the responses also differ in their sign, as in the case of combined excitation and inhibition. Whether co-reception occurs in the sensory neuron in response to the action of the modulatory system is not known. But it is possible, as we have argued above, that 5-HT might produce its short- and long-term actions by means of two independent receptors in parallel, one coupled to an adenylate cyclase and the other to another molecular cascade.

Co-existence and *co-release* refer to a set of processes that parallel co-reception but, instead of involving the postsynaptic side, they involve the presynaptic side. Here one or more transmitters exist in the same presynaptic neuron and are released to act on the same or different postsynaptic cells. We know equally little of the importance of co-existence and co-release for learning.

However, some understanding of the basis of transmitter co-existence comes from molecular studies of neurons that contain multiple peptide transmitters and include those that contain the SCPs. For example, Lloyd et al. (1985b) found that all neurons that contain one of the SCPs also contain the other. The co-existance of the two peptides is explained by the finding of Mahon et al. (1985) that the two peptides are encoded by a single gene. The corresponding mRNA is translated into a polyprotein that contains the sequence for both SCP_A and SCP_B (see footnote, p. 84). The polyprotein is then processed into the two active peptides which then are co-released (Fig. 19A and Lloyd et al., 1985b).

The polyprotein for the SCPs is relatively simple. Other polyproteins in *Aplysia* are considerably more complex. For example, studies of the bag cells in *Aplysia* indicate that there are five to nine genes for the egg-laying hormone (ELH). Each gene of the family encodes for a polyprotein, and each of these proteins encodes for *several different* peptides (Scheller et al., 1982, 1983a,b; Fig. 19B). Several of the peptides have been shown to have different actions on different identified cells (Scheller et al., 1983a,b). This suggested the possibility that the various peptides of a polyprotein may encode the several components that make up the fixed action pattern behavior of egg laying (McAllister et al., 1983; Scheller et al., 1983).

Although co-existence and co-release have only recently begun to be studied in *Aplysia* in relation to behavior and learning, historically *Aplysia* and other invertebrates have played an important role in the initial elucidation of this idea. (See the early studies by Brownstein et al., 1974, and Hanley et al., 1974.) Thus, there is now persuasive evidence for co-existence in *Helix* (Osborne et al., 1982; Osborne, 1984), *Aplysia* (Brown et al., 1984; Ambron et al., 1985; Lloyd et al., 1985a,b), *Tritonia* (Lloyd et al., 1981), cockroach (Adams and O'Shea, 1983), lobster (Siwicki and Kravitz, 1983), and crayfish (Bishop et al., 1984). As antibodies to more transmitter substances (particularly peptides) become available, we can expect to see more examples of co-localization and co-release within invertebrate neurons.

As yet, the functional significance of co-release is only beginning to be understood (see Lundberg, Hökfelt, this volume). Traditionally, invertebrates have provided powerful model systems for the analysis of basic principles of membrane and synaptic function and for relating these functions to behavior. Thus, it seems likely that studies of co-transmitters in invertebrates will allow detailed analyses of the behavioral significance of co-release. An important beginning was made by Adams and O'Shea (1983) who found that stimulation of an identified excitatory skeletal motoneuron in the cockroach has two effects on the target muscle: (1) it produces a fast contraction of the muscle which is associated one-to-one with transient EJPs in the muscle, and (2) a delayed slow increase in muscle tension which is not associated with depolarization of the muscle membrane. The fast contraction (and EJPs) are, presumably, due to L-glutamate, the classically-recognized transmitter at the insect neuromuscular junction. The delayed slow tension is due to release of the peptide, proctolin.

Comparable demonstrations of functional roles for co-localized transmitters within the invertebrate central nervous systems related to learning are not yet available. However, as the previous discussion indicates the study of learning in the gill- and siphon-withdrawal system of *Aplysia* provides an interesting opportunity for understanding the functional roles of different modulatory transmitters within the central nervous system.

Acknowledgements

We are grateful for the support of the European Molecular Biology Organization (P.M.), the McKnight Foundation, and the System Development Foundation.

References

Abrams, T. W. and Kandel, E. R. (1985) Roles of calcium and adenylate cyclase in activity-dependent facilitation, a cellular mechanism for classical conditioning in *Aplysia*. *J. Neurosci.*, 44: S12.

Abrams, T. W., Carew, T. J., Hawkins, R. D. and Kandel, E. R. (1983) Aspects of the cellular mechanisms of temporal specificity in conditioning in *Aplysia*: Preliminary evidence for Ca^{2+} influx as a signal of activity. *Soc. Neurosci. Abstr.*, 9: 168.

Abrams, T. W., Bernier, L., Hawkins, R. D. and Kandel, E. R. (1984a) Possible roles of Ca^{2+} and cAMP in activity-dependent facilitation, a mechanism for associative learning in *Aplysia*. *Soc. Neurosci. Abstr.*, 10: 269.

Abrams, T. W., Castellucci, V. F., Camardo, J. S., Kandel, E. R. and Lloyd, P. E. (1984b) Two endogenous neuropeptides modulate the gill and siphon withdrawal reflex in *Aplysia* by means of presynaptic facilitation involving cyclic AMP-dependent closure of a serotonin-sensitive potassium channel. *Proc. nat. Acad. Sci. USA*, 81: 7956–7960.

Adams, M. E. and O'Shea, M. (1983) Peptide co-transmitter at a neuromsucular junction. *Science*, 221: 286–289.

Ambron, R. T., Lloyd, P., Flaster, M. S. and Schacher, S. (1985) FMRFamide in neuron R2 of *Aplysia*: Evidence for a role as a second transmitter. *Soc. Neurosci. Abstr.*, 11: 483.

Bailey, C. H. and Chen, M. (1983) Morphological basis of long-term habitutation and sensitization in *Aplysia*. *Science*, 220: 91–93.

Bailey, C. H., Hawkins, R. D. and Chen, M. (1983) Uptake of (^{3}H) serotonin in the abdominal ganglion of *Aplysia californica*: Further studies on the morphological and biochemical basis of presynaptic facilitation. *Brain Res.*, 272: 71–78.

Belardetti, F., Schacher, S., Kandel, E. R. and Siegelbaum, S. A. (1985) Serotonin produces a decreased conductance EPSP and broadening of the action potential in growth cones of *Aplysia* sensory neurons. *Soc. Neurosci. Abstr.*, 11: 28.

Bernier, L., Castellucci, V. F., Kandel, E. R. and Schwartz, J. H. (1982) Facilitatory transmitter causes a selective and prolonged increase in adenosine 3′:5′-monophosphate in sensory neurons mediating the gill and siphon withdrawal reflex in *Aplysia*. *J. Neurosci.*, 2: 1682–1691.

Bishop, C. A., Wine, J. J. and O'Shea, M. (1984) Neuropeptide proctolin in postural motoneurons of the crayfish. *J. Neurosci.*, 4: 2001–2009.

Boyle, M. B., Klein, M. Smith, S. J. and Kandel, E. R. (1984) Serotonin increases intracellular Ca^{2+} transients in voltage-clamped sensory neurons of *Aplysia californica*. *Proc. nat. Acad. Sci. USA*, 81: 7642–7646.

Brown, R. O., Basbaum, A. I. and Mayeri, E. (1984) Identification of FMRF-amide immunoreactive neurons in the abdominal ganglion of *Aplysia*. *Soc. Neurosci. Abstr.*, 10: 691.

Brownstein, M. J., Saavedra, J. M., Axelrod, J., Zeman, G. H. and Carpenter, D. O. (1974) Coexistence of several putative neurotransmitters in single identified neurons of *Aplysia*. *Proc. nat. Acad. Sci. USA*, 71: 4662–4665.

Brunelli, M., Castellucci, V. F. and Kandel, E. R. (1976) Synaptic facilitation and behavioral sensitization in *Aplysia*: Possible role of serotonin and cyclic AMP. *Science*, 194: 1178–1181.

Byrne, J. H., Castellucci, V. F. and Kandel, E. R. (1974) Receptive fields and response properties of mechanoreceptor neurons innervating siphon skin and mantle shelf in *Aplysia*. *J. Neurophysiol.*, 37: 1041–1064.

Byrne, J. H., Castellucci, V. F. and Kandel, E. R. (1978) Contribution of individual mechanoreceptor sensory neurons to defensive gill-withdrawal reflex in *Aplysia*. *J. Neurophysiol.*, 41: 418–430.

Carew, T. J., Walters, E. T. and Kandel, E. R. (1981) Classical conditioning in a simple withdrawal reflex in *Aplysia californica*. *J. Neurosci.*, 1: 1426–1437.

Carew, T. J., Hawkins, R. D. and Kandel, E. R. (1983) Differential classical conditioning of a defensive withdrawal reflex in *Aplysia californica*. *Science*, 219: 397–400.

Castellucci, V. F. and Kandel, E. R. (1976) Presynaptic facilitation as a mechanism for behavioral sensitization in *Aplysia*. *Science*, 194: 1176–1178.

Castellucci, V. F., Kandel, E. R., Schwartz, J. H., Wilson, F. D., Nairn, A. C. and Greengard, P. (1980) Intracellular injection of the catalytic subunit of cyclic AMP-dependent protein kinase simulates facilitation of transmitter release underlying behavioral sensitization in *Aplysia*. *Proc. nat. Acad. Sci. USA*, 77: 7492–7496.

Changeux, J.-P., Bon, F., Cartaud, J., Devillers-Thiery, A., Giraudat, J., Heidmann, T., Holton, B., Nghiem, H. O., Popot, J. L., Van Rapenbusch, R. and Tzartos, S. (1983) Allosteric properties of the acetylcholine receptor protein from *Torpedo marmorata*. In *Molecular Biology, Cold Spring Harbor Symp. Quant. Biol.*, 48: 35–52.

Davis, H. P. and Squire, L. R. (1984) Protein synthesis and memory: A review. *Psychol. Bull.*, 96: 518–559.

Frost, W. N. and Kandel, E. R. (1984) Sensitizing stimuli reduce the effectiveness of the L_{30} inhibitory interneurons in the siphon withdrawal reflex circuit of *Aplysia*. *Soc. Neurosci. Abstr.*, 10: 510.

Frost, W. N., Castellucci, V. F., Hawkins, R. D. and Kandel, E. R. (1985) The monosynaptic connections from the sensory neurones participate in the storage of long-term memory for sensitization of the gill- and siphon-withdrawal reflex in *Aplysia*. *Proc. nat. Acad. Sci. USA*, 82: 8266–8269.

Gardner, D. and Kandel, E. R. (1972) Diphasic postsynaptic potential: A chemical synapse capable of mediating conjoint excitation and inhibition. *Science*, 176: 675–678.

Glanzman, D. L., Abrams, T. W., Hawkins, R. S. and Kandel, E. R. (1984) Extracts of L_{29} interneurones produce spike-broadening in sensory neurones of *Aplysia*. *Soc. Neurosci. Abstr.*, 10: 510.

Hanley, M. R., Cottrell, G. A., Emson, P. C. and Fonnum, F. (1974) Enzymatic synthesis of acetylcholine by a serotonin-containing neuron from *Helix*. *Nature (Lond.)*, 251: 631–633.

Hawkins, R. D. (1981) Interneurons involved in mediation and modulation of gill-withdrawal reflex in *Aplysia*. III. Identified facilitating neurons increase Ca^{2+} current in sensory neurons. *J. Neurophysiol*, 45: 327–339.

Hawkins, R. D., Castellucci, V. F. and Kandel, E. R. (1981) Interneurons involved in mediation and modulation of gill-withdrawal reflex in *Aplysia*. I. Identification and characterization. *J. Neurophysiol.*, 45: 304–314.

Hawkins, R. D., Abrams, T. W., Carew, T. J. and Kandel, E. R. (1983) A cellular mechanism of classical conditioning in *Aplysia*: Activity-dependent amplification of presynaptic facilitation. *Science*, 219: 400–415.

Hawkins, R. D., Clark, G. A. and Kandel, E. R. (1985) Operant conditioning and differential classical conditioning of gill withdrawal in *Aplysia*. *Soc. Neurosci. Abstr.*, 11: 796.

Hille, B. (1984) *Ionic Channels of Excitable Membranes*, Sinauer, Sunderland, Mass., 426 pp.

Hochner, B., Schacher, S., Klein, M. and Kandel, E. R. (1985) Presynaptic facilitation in *Aplysia* sensory neurons: A process independent of K^+ current modulation becomes important when transmitter release is depressed. *Soc. Neurosci. Abstr.*, 11: 29.

Kaczmarek, L. K., Jennings, K. R., Strumwasser, F., Nairn, A. C., Walter, V., Wilson, F. P. and Greengard, P. (1980) Microinjection of catalytic subunit of cyclic AMP-dependent protein kinase enhances calcium action potentials of bag cell neurons in cell culture. *Proc. Nat. Acad. Sci. USA,* 77: 7487–7491.

Kandel, E. R. (1976) *Cellular Basis of Behavior,* Freeman, San Francisco, pp. 281–344.

Kandel, E. R. and Schwartz, J. H. (1982) Molecular biology of an elementary form of learning: Modulation of transmitter release by cyclic AMP. *Science,* 218: 433–443.

Kandel, E. R. and Tauc, L. (1965a) Heterosynaptic facilitation in neurones of the abdominal ganglion of *Aplysia depilans. J. Physiol. (Lond.),* 181: 1–27.

Kandel, E. R. and Tauc, L. (1965b) Mechanism of heterosynaptic facilitation in the giant cell of the abdominal ganglion of *Aplysia depilans. J. Physiol. (Lond.),* 181: 28–47.

Kandel, E. R., Abrams, T. W., Bernier, L., Carew, T. J., Hawkins, R. D. and Schwartz, J. H. (1983) Classical conditioning and sensitization share aspects of the same molecular cascade in *Aplysia. Cold Spring Harbor Symp. Quant. Biol.,* 48: 821–830.

Karlin, A., Cox, R., Kaldany, R. R., Lobel, P. and Holtzman, E. (1983) The arrangement and functions of the chains of the acetylcholine receptor of *Torpedo* electric tissue. In *Molecular Biology, Cold Spring Harbor Symp. Quant. Biol.,* 48: 1–8.

Kehoe, J. S. (1969) Single presynaptic neurone mediates a two component postsynaptic inhibition. *Nature (Lond.),* 221: 866–868.

Kehoe, J. S. (1972) Ionic mechanisms of a two-component cholinergic inhibition in *Aplysia* neurons. *J. Physiol. (Lond.),* 225: 85–114.

Kistler, H. B., Hawkins, R. D., Koester, J., Steinbusch, W. M., Kandel, E. R. and Schwartz, J. H. (1985) Distribution of serotonin-immunoreactive cell bodies and processes in the abdominal ganglion of mature *Aplysia. J. Neurosci.,* 5: 72–80.

Klein, M. and Kandel, E. R. (1978) Presynaptic modulation of voltage-dependent Ca^{2+} current: Mechanism for behavioral sensitization in *Aplysia californica. Proc. nat. Acad. Sci. USA,* 75: 3512–3516.

Klein, M. and Kandel, E. R. (1980) Mechanism of calcium current modulation underlying presynaptic facilitation and behavioral sensitization in *Aplysia. Proc. nat. Acad. Sci. USA,* 77: 6912–6916.

Klein, M., Shapiro, E. and Kandel, E. R. (1980) Synaptic plasticity and the modulation of the Ca^{2+} current. *J. exp. Biol.,* 89: 117–157.

Klein, M., Camardo, J. and Kandel, E. R. (1982) Serotonin modulates a specific potassium current in the sensory neurons that show presynaptic facilitation in *Aplysia. Proc. nat. Acad. Sci. USA,* 79: 5713–5717.

Levitan, I. B. and Adams, W. B. (1981) Cyclic AMP modulation of a specific ion channel in an identified nerve cell: Possible role for protein phosphorylation. *Advanc. Cyc. Nuc. Res.,* 14: 647–653.

Lloyd, P. E., Masinovsky, B., McCaman, R. E. and Willows, A. O. D. (1981) Coexistence of a neuropeptide and acetylcholine in an identified molluskan neuron. *Soc. Neurosci. Abstr.,* 7: 637.

Lloyd, P. E., Kupfermann, I. and Weiss, K. R. (1984) Sequence and neuronal localization of a newly characterized neuropeptide in *Aplysia. Soc. Neurosci. Abstr.,* 10: 153.

Lloyd, P. E., Frankfurt, M., Kupfermann, I. and Kandel, E.R. (1985a) Colocalization of the SCPs and FMRFamide to motor neurons innervating *Aplysia* buccal muscle. *Soc. Neurosci. Abstr.,* 11: 482.

Lloyd, P. E., Mahon, A. C., Kupferman, I., Cohen, L., Scheller, R. H. and Weiss, K. R. (1985b) Biochemical and immunocytochemical localization of molluscan small cardioactive peptides in the nervous system of *Aplysia californica. J. Neurosci.,* 5: 1851–1861.

Mahon, A. C., Lloyd, P. E., Weiss, K. R., Kupfermann, I. and Scheller, R. H. (1985) The small cardioactive peptides A and B of *Aplysia* are derived from a common precursor molecule. *Proc. nat. Acad. Sci. USA,* 82: 3925–3929.

McAllister, L. B., Scheller, R. H., Kandel, E. R. and Axel, R. (1983) In situ hybridization to study the origin and fate of identified neurons. *Science,* 222: 800–808.

Montarolo, P. G., Castellucci, V. F., Goelet, P., Kandel, E. R. and Schacher, S. (1985) Long-term facilitation of the monosynaptic connection between sensory neurons and motor neurons of the gill-withdrawal reflex in *Aplysia* in dissociated cell culture. *Soc. Neurosci. Abstr.,* 11: 795.

Numa, S., Noda, M., Takahashi, H., Tanabe, T., Toyosato, M., Furutani, Y. and Kikyotani, S. (1983) Molecular structure of the nicotinic acetylcholine receptor. In *Molecular Biology, Cold Spring Harbor Symp. Quant. Biol.,* 48: 57–70.

Ocorr, K. A., Walters, E. T. and Byrne, J. H. (1985) Associative conditioning analog selectively increases cAMP levels of tail sensory neurons in *Aplysia. Proc. nat. Acad. Sci. USA,* 82: 2548–2552.

Ono, J. and McCaman, R. E. (1984) Immunocytochemical localization and direct assays of serotonin-containing neurons in *Aplysia. Neuroscience,* 11: 549–560.

Osborne, N. N. (1984) Putative neurotransmitters and their coexistence in gastropod mollusks. In V. Chan-Palay and S. L. Palay (Eds.), *Coexistence of Neuroactive Substances in Neurons,* John Wiley & Sons, New York, pp. 395–409.

Osborne, N. N., Cuello, A. C. and Dockray, G. J. (1982) Substance P and cholecystokinin-like peptides in *Helix* neruons and cholecystokinin and serotonin in a giant neurons. *Science,* 216: 409–411.

Pinsker, H. M., Kupfermann, I., Castellucci, V. F. and Kandel, E. R. (1970) Habituation and dishabituation of the gill-withdrawal reflex in *Aplysia. Science,* 167: 1740–1742.

Pinsker, H. M., Hening, W. A., Carew, T. J. and Kandel, E. R.

(1973) Long-term sensitization of a defensive withdrawal reflex in *Aplysia*. *Science,* 182: 1039–1042.

Rayport, S. G. and Schacher, S. (1986) Synaptic plasticity *in vitro:* Cell culture of identified *Aplysia* neurons mediating short-term habituation and sensitization. *J. Neurosci.,* 6: 759–763.

Sakmann, B., Bormann, J. and Hamill, O. P. (1983) Ion transport by single receptor channels. In *Molecular Biology, Cold Spring Harbor Symp. Quant. Biol.,* 48: 247–257.

Scheller, R. H., Jackson, J. R., McAllister, L. B., Schwartz, J. H., Kandel, E. R. and Axel, R. (1982) A family of genes that codes for ELH, a neuropeptide eliciting a sterotyped pattern of behavior in *Aplysia*. *Cell,* 28: 707–719.

Scheller, R. H., Jackson, J. F., McAllister, L. B., Rothman, B. S., Mayeri, E. and Axel, R. (1983a) A single gene encodes multiple neuropeptides mediating a stereotyped behavior. *Cell,* 35: 7–22.

Scheller, R. H., Rothman, B. S. and Mayeri, E. (1983b) A single gene encodes multiple peptide transmitter candidates involved in a stereotyped behavior. *Trends Neurosci.,* 6: 340–345.

Shuster, M. J., Camardo, J. S., Siegelbaum, S. A. and Kandel, E. R. (1985) Cyclic AMP-dependent protein kinase closes the serotonin-sensitive K^+ channels of *Aplysia* sensory neurones in cell-free membrane patches. *Nature (Lond.),* 313:392–395.

Siegelbaum, S. A., Camardo, J. S. and Kandel, E. R. (1982) Serotonin and cyclic AMP close single K^+ channels in *Aplysia* sensory neurones. *Nature (Lond.),* 299: 413–417.

Siwicki, K. K. and Kravitz, E. A. (1983) Proctolin in lobster: General distribution and co-localization with serotonin. *Soc. Neurosci. Abstr.,* 9: 313.

Taldany, R. G., Nambu, G. R. and Scheller, R. H. (1985) Neuropeptides in identified *Aplysia* neurones. *Ann. Rev. Neurosci.,* 8: 431–455.

Wachtel, S. S. and Kandel, E. R. (1967) A direct synaptic connection mediating both excitation and inhibition. *Science,* 158: 1206–1208.

Walters, E. T. and Byrne, J. H. (1983) Associative conditioning of single sensory neurons suggests a cellular mechanism for learning. *Science,* 219: 405–408.

T. Hökfelt, K. Fuxe and B. Pernow (Eds.),
Progress in Brain Research, Vol. 68

CHAPTER 7

Transmitter status in cultured sympathetic principal neurons: plasticity, graded expression and diversity

David D. Potter, Steven G. Matsumoto, Story C. Landis, Dinah W. Y. Sah and Edwin J. Furshpan

Department of Neurobiology, Harvard Medical School, Boston, MA 02115, U.S.A.

Introduction

This chapter summarizes recent investigations of the transmitter status of sympathetic principal neurons derived from neonatal or adult rats and grown singly in "microcultures" with cardiac cells. The work began out of an interest in the status of individual neonatal sympathetic neurons during a transition from an initial (at least) adrenergic state to a predominantly cholinergic state, under the influence of non-neuronal cells (for reviews of this phenomenon in "mass" cultures that contain several thousand neurons, see Bunge et al., 1978; O'Lague et al., 1978; Patterson, 1978; for evidence that the transition is apparently graded in rate, depending on how "cholinergic" the culture conditions are, see Landis, 1980; for evidence that under highly "cholinergic" conditions expression of adrenergic properties declines, see Patterson and Chun, 1977, and Wolinsky and Patterson, 1985; for evidence that a similar transition occurs during normal development of certain sympathetic neurons in vivo, see Landis, 1983; Landis and Keefe, 1983). One of the questions of interest was: Do the neurons phase out adrenergic properties before adopting cholinergic function (transition via a null state), or does the transition occur via a state in which both transmitters are simultaneously secreted (dual function)? This and other questions can be answered if the neurons are grown, one or a few at a time, in tiny cultures on cells such as cardiac myocytes that are sensitive to both norepinephrine (NE) and acetylcholine (ACh). These considerations led to development of the microculture procedure described below (Furshpan et al., 1976). Evidence was obtained that most (but probably not all) microcultured neurons undergo the transition and that most (perhaps all) that change transmitters do so via dual function and fine structure (see below and Furshpan et al., 1976, 1982; Landis, 1976, 1980; Potter et al., 1983, 1986; see also Johnson et al., 1976, 1980; Higgins et al., 1981; Iacovitti et al., 1981). It was also found that several other active substances are secreted by microcultured principal neurons: at least one purine (the agent that acts on the myocytes appears to be adenosine), serotonin (5-HT) and an as-yet-unidentified agent or agents called "X" (Furshpan et al., 1981, 1985b; Matsumoto et al., 1986; Sah and Matsumoto, 1986). Secretion of the five (or more) agents in various combinations and in different relative strengths creates a diversity of transmitter functions in these microcultured neurons greater than that previously reported for any type of vertebrate or invertebrate neuron; however, cytochemical evidence reported elsewhere in this volume indicates that other types of neurons are likely also to prove highly complex and diverse in function. The diversity and plasticity of the microcultured neurons are illustrated briefly in this chapter.

Methods

Our current methods for making and maintaining microcultures and for studying them electrophysiologically or with the electron microscope are described by Furshpan et al., (1986a). The major points are briefly as follows. Small domains, about 0.5 mm in diameter, to which cells can adhere on an otherwise non-wetting surface are formed by drying droplets of dissolved collagen. Dissociated

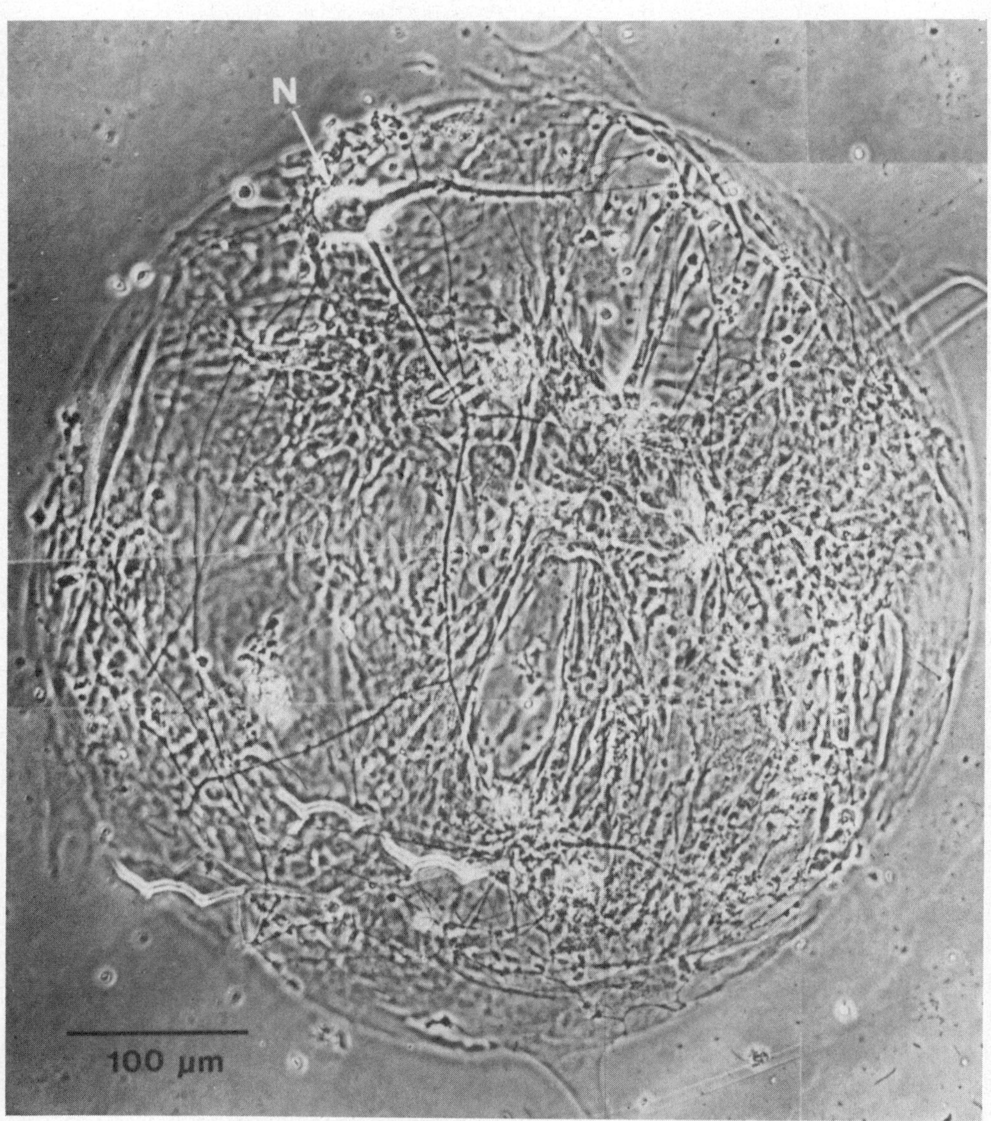

Fig. 1. A microculture containing a solitary neonate-derived principal neuron (N indicates the cell body with its eccentric nucleus) growing on cardiac cells (myocytes, fibroblasts and perhaps other types of cells) that cannot be individually resolved in this phase contrast picture. By virtue of their electrical coupling, the myocytes generally beat synchronously throughout such microcultures. In the electron microscope, a large neurite like that emerging at 3 o'clock from the cell body, has the fine structure of a dendrite, while the slender neurites have the fine structure of axons; the latter make numerous varicosities near the myocytes and often make synapses (autapses) on the cell body and dendrites (cf. Fig. 4; Furshpan et al., 1986a).

cardiac cells, usually from both atria and ventricles, are allowed to flatten on the collagen dots; they can be washed away from the untreated surface. Then dissociated principal neurons, from superior cervical ganglia of neonatal or adult rats, are added to the dish at a density so low that some microcultures receive no neurons, others only one or a few. Some neurons were grown in a medium that contained 20 mMK^+ instead of the normal 5.4 mMK^+ to enhance the probability that the neuron would display purely adrenergic status at first assay (see Walicke et al., 1977).

Under the influence of nerve growth factor, neurites grow progressively over the microculture, but not beyond its borders. The appearance in phase contrast of a microculture after 19 days is shown in Fig. 1. Many microcultures survive for 1–3 months; after such periods the density of neurites over the myocytes is often greater than that of the normal innervation of sympathetic target tissues in vivo (compare Fig. 1 of this chapter, or Fig. 1A of Furshpan et al., 1986a, with Fig. 2 of Malmfors and Sachs, 1965, or with Fig. 1a of Björklund et al., 1985).

For physiological assay the dish was perfused continuously with a warmed solution with a raised calcium concentration (2.93 mM) and reduced magnesium concentration (0.18 mM). Microelectrodes were filled with 3 M KCl. Blocking drugs were added to the perfusion fluid; agonists were often applied in brief "puffs" to the microculture from a local micropipette (method of Choi and Fischbach, 1981). For fine structural analysis of a physiologically characterized neuron, the address of the microculture in the dish was noted, the culture was fixed in glutaraldehyde (followed by OsO_4 and uranyl acetate) or in potassium permanganate and prepared for electron microscopy as described in Furshpan et al. (1985a).

A useful property of the microcultures was the high sensitivity of the physiological assay. Recordings made from widely separated myocytes in a microculture were generally similar in size and time course because the electrical coupling of the cardiac cells often made the myocyte layer effectively a single large target cell with regard to electrical activity (Furshpan et al., 1986a). The network of progressively growing neurites was confined to this target, and the numerous varicosities acted in parallel when the neuron was stimulated; consequently, the

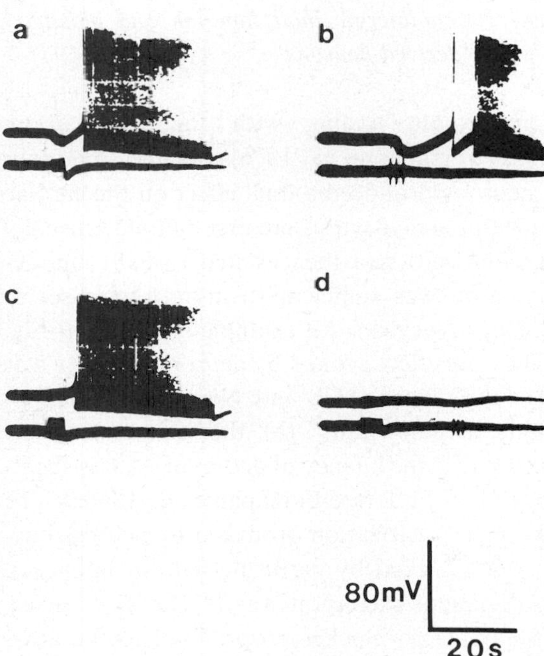

Fig. 2. Adrenergic/cholinergic dual function mimicked by applying ACh and NE from a micropipette. The solitary neonate-derived neuron was grown in high-K^+ medium for 21 days. In (a), as in most subsequent physiological records, the upper trace is an electrical recording by intracellular microelectrode from the cardiac myocytes (each myocyte impulse was accompanied by a visible beat), and the lower trace is an intracellular recording from the neuron at a gain so low that a train of neuronal impulses appears simply as a thickening or deflection of the trace. In (a), a train of neuronal impulses (50 Hz for about 2.5 sec) evoked first a hyperpolarization of the previously quiescent myocytes and then a train of myocyte impulses that lasted about 30 sec. In (b), three "puffs" of a mixture of ACh (5 μM) and NE (100 μM), each puff marked by a deflection of the lower trace, produced somewhat more intense effects than those in (a); the train of impulses lasted for 13 sec on the next sweep (not shown). When atropine sulfate (0.2 μM) was added to the perfusion fluid, the neuronally-evoked inhibition was eliminated (c); further addition of 2 μM propranolol (d) eliminated the neuronally-evoked excitation, and the more intense effects of the puffed ACh and NE (at three deflections of the lower beam) were also largely blocked. The vertical scale refers to the myocyte recordings only.

probability of detecting a weak transmitter function was increased.

Results and discussion

Adrenergic/cholinergic dual function and plasticity in neonate-derived neurons

An immediate finding with the microculture method (Furshpan et al., 1976) was that some solitary neurons produced a dual effect on the cardiac myocytes; the myocytes were first inhibited (usually hyperpolarized) and then excited (usually the depolarization was sufficient to initiate impulses in quiescent myocytes). An example is shown in Fig. 2a. The dual effect evoked by neuronal activity was also evoked when ACh and NE were applied simultaneously in "puffs" (b); the sequential effects arose because the latency of action of ACh is shorter than that of NE (see Furshpan et al., 1986a). The initial hyperpolarization produced by neuronal activity was blocked by perfusing with atropine (c); the subsequent excitation was blocked by adding the β-adrenergic blocker propranolol to the atropine solution; now activity in the neuron had no detectable effect on the myocytes, and the strong actions of the puffed ACh and NE were also largely blocked. The effects of the blockers were reversible (not shown). The similarity of action of the puffed mixture of ACh and NE to the neuronal actions and the block of both by conventional concentrations of atropine and propranolol provide strong evidence that this solitary neuron secreted both transmitters. That such neurons also synthesized both transmitters (as opposed to taking one up from the medium) was confirmed in cases where a dual-function neuron was the only neuron in the dish.

The existence of neurons that secrete both ACh and NE is consistent with other evidence that the neurons are plastic with respect to these transmitters and can change in culture from an initial (at least) adrenergic state to a (predominantly) cholinergic state; it also suggests that during the transition cholinergic function is expressed before adrenergic function is lost. This interpretation is also consistent with the finding that the relative strengths of the two functions vary, among neurons picked at random, from mainly adrenergic (like the neuron of Fig. 2) to roughly balanced (see Potter

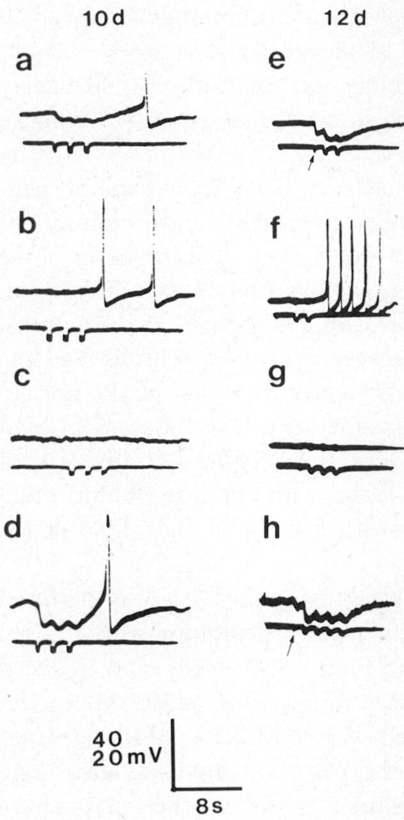

Fig. 3. Two dual-function, solitary, neonate-derived neurons grown for 10 and 12 days in microcultures. Brief trains of neuronal impulses (deflections of the lower traces in (a) and (e)), hyperpolarized the myocytes (upper traces), followed by a cardiac impulse in (a) (stimulation of the neuron at 20 Hz in (a), 40 Hz in (e); in (e), the first stimulus produced a single neuronal impulse at the arrow). When atropine sulfate was added to the perfusion fluid (0.5 μM in (b), 0.1 μM in (f), the hyperpolarization of the myocytes was blocked, the neuronally evoked effects were now purely excitatory. The excitatory effects were blocked by further addition of propranolol (0.5 μM in (c), 1 μM in (g)). After washout of the blocking drugs, the original effects were restored (d, h; the first stimulus in (h) again produced a single neuronal impulse at the arrow). Scales: 20 mV for (a–d); 40 mV for e–h myocyte traces only. The cardiac impulses in (f) were retouched for clarity.

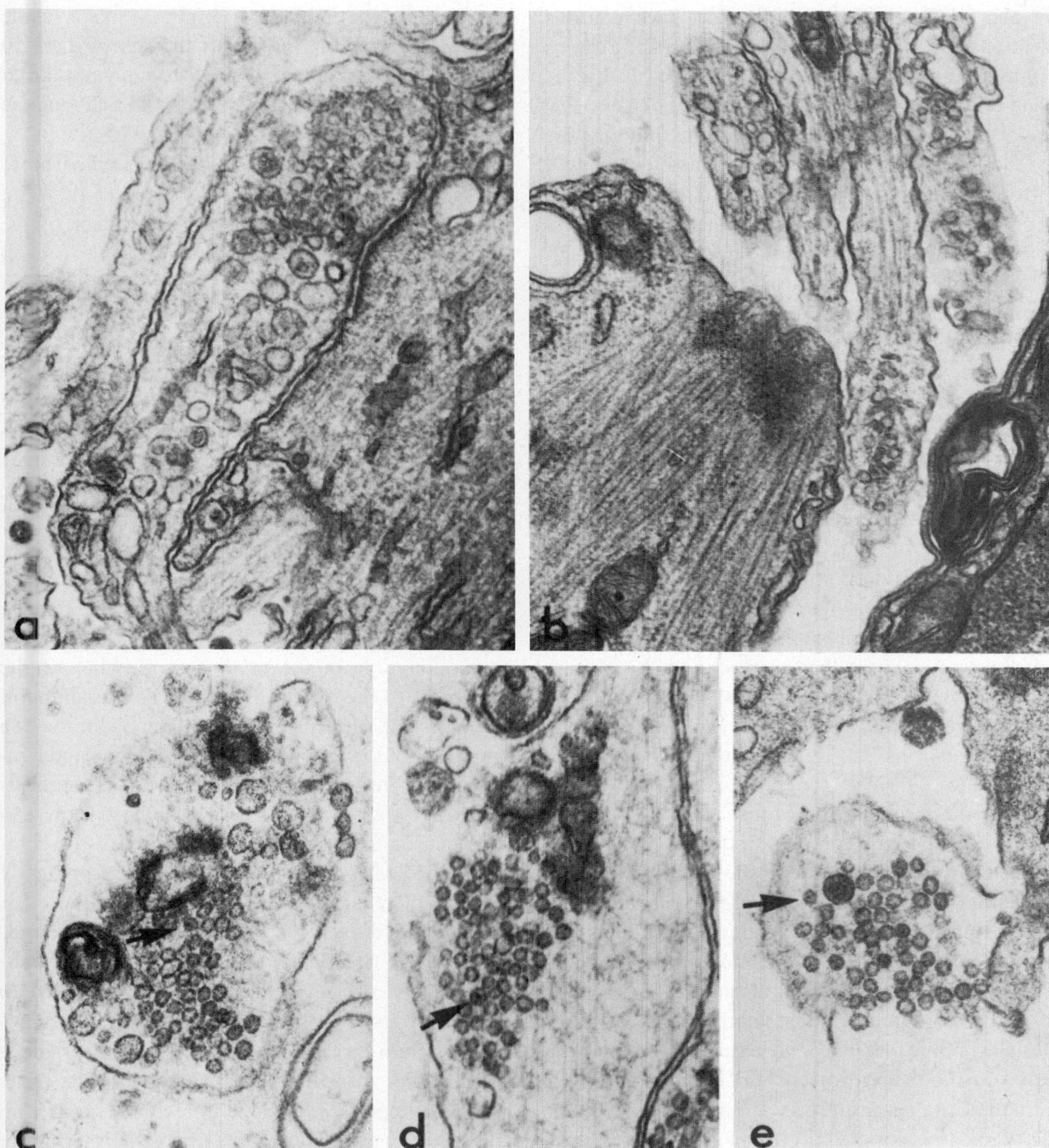

Fig. 4. The fine structure of terminals made by the 10- and 12-day solitary, neonate-derived neurons of Fig. 3. The micrograph in (a) shows an autapse on a dendrite of the 12-day neuron, fixed in 3% glutaraldehyde (note pre- and post-synaptic densities at upper right); (b) shows a grazing section through four of the neurites that grew extensively over the microculture (at the lower left and right are myocytes). Both pictures show a mixed content of synaptic vesicles, larger ones (some with stained cores) and small pleiomorphic ones. After glutaraldehyde fixation, vesicles that contain NE cannot be distinguished. The 10-day neuron was fixed in 4% potassium permanganate, to stain the cores of small NE-containing vesicles. Three varicosities of this neuron are shown in (c), (d) and (e); most of the small vesicles are empty, as is characteristic of cholinergic vesicles in vivo; a few have dense cores (arrows) and presumably contained NE. This vesicular fine structure is consistent with the relatively strong cholinergic function of this neuron, illustrated in Fig. 3 a–d. Magnification: 40,000.

et al., 1986) to mainly cholinergic. Two neurons that exerted mainly cholinergic effects as nearly as 10 and 12 days in culture are illustrated in Fig. 3. The 10-day neuron consistently evoked one or a few myocyte impulses in control solution and after the pronounced cholinergic response was blocked with atropine (b); in the 12-day neuron cholinergic function was relatively so strong that in control solution the neuron appeared purely inhibitory (e,h) although a clear weak excitatory effect was unmasked by atropine (f). Another neuron that exerted a possibly adrenergic effect so weak as to be at the limit of detection is shown in Fig. 5 (neuron N_1) discussed below.

The microculture procedure permits the fine structure and function of a particular neuron to be compared, a difficult matter in mammalian neurons in vivo (but see McGuire et al., 1984). It was found that the synapses and varicosities of dual-function neurons had a mixed content of small synaptic vesicles after permanganate fixation: small granular vesicles (SGV), the presumed site of storage of NE, interspersed with small clear vesicles (SCV), at least some of which were the presumed site of storage of ACh. Figure 4 shows terminals and varcosities of the two neurons of Fig. 3. Figure 4a, b show the appearance of small synaptic vesicles and larger ones (some with dense cores, structures currently of interest for storage of peptides) after glutaraldehyde fixation. Figure 4 c–e show the mixture of SGV and SCV characteristic of dual-function neurons, after permanganate fixation. In 10 microcultures, the pecentage of SGV among the small vesicles was counted in sections of synapses or varicosities that contained a substantial number of small vesicles. While for each neuron there was some variation in the proportion of SGV from terminal to terminal, the variation was around a single mean, as would be expected if the neuron possessed a single class of terminals of mixed fine structure, rather than two classes, one adrenergic in appearance, the other cholinergic (Potter et al., 1986). This, too, is consistent with the idea that during the transition, cholinergic properties (vesicles, synthetic mechanism and so on) are added to existing adrenergic ones; i.e. individual terminals, like a whole neuron, can be dual in status. In each of these 10 neurons, the percentage of SGV roughly paralleled the relative strengths of adrenergic and cholinergic functions.

Dual function and fine structure seemed more exotic when first discovered (Furshpan et al., 1976; Landis, 1976) amid widespread acceptance of the popular form of "Dale's Principle" (a neuron secretes only one transmitter), than they now seem given the abundant evidence for multiple-transmitter status summarized in this volume. While dual-function neurons violate the popular version of "Dale's principle", the rather uniform fine structure of their terminals is consistent with the original version of Dale's principle (a neuron secretes the same transmitter(s) from all its terminals; see Eccles, 1976; Potter et al., 1981).

We assume that the graded differences between the microcultured neurons in their effects on the myocytes, were due to differences in the relative amounts of ACh and NE secreted by the neurons, not differences in the relative sensitivities of the myocytes to the two transmitters. This assumption is consistent with the graded differences in the fine structure of the terminals described above and consistent with observations on two-neuron microcultures like that of Fig. 5 in which the response to one neuron established the sensitivity of the common pool of myocytes to a transmitter apparently lacking or relatively weakly expressed in the other neuron. Moreover, whenever moderate concentrations of ACh and NE were puffed onto a microculture, as in Fig. 2, the myocytes responded to both agents.

To obtain direct evidence for the adrenergic-to-cholinergic transition and investigate its time course, attempts were made to record serially from the same neuron. During the first assay, steps were taken to reduce contamination of the culture by microorganisms; after the assay the dish was returned to the incubator for a period of 4 to 42 days pending re-assay of the same neuron. Most such attempts ended when the dish became contaminated with microorganisms, but in 27 cases at least two assays were performed on neonate-derived neurons; these cases are illustrated and discussed in Potter et al. (1986). In 12 cases no clear change from an initial dual status occurred (five of these cases were re-assayed in less than one week). One further neuron had no effect on the myocytes at either assay (interval: 10 days). In 14 cases there was a clear change in status, always in the relatively-more-cholinergic direction. There were four neurons that acquired dual status from apparently purely adrenergic function, four that acquired apparently purely cholinergic status from dual function, five that changed from dual function to relatively-more-cholinergic dual function, and one that appeared to undergo the full adrenergic-to-cholinergic transition via dual function. These serial assays provide a particularly direct confirmation of earlier evidence for an adrenergic-to-cholinergic transition in mass cultures of neonate-derived neurons.

In the current climate, one's doubt is focussed not on the dual-function neurons but on the neurons that apparently lacked cholinergic or adrenergic function at the beginning and end of the developmental transition: perhaps such neurons are really multi-functional. Because of hyperinnervation of the myocytes, the microculture method has high sensitivity in the detection of physiological responses to released transmitters. These experiments thus also provide direct evidence that a neuron can make a qualitative change in its functionally significant transmitter status (e.g. the reduction of adrenergic function to physiologically undetectable levels). A reservation, however, about the apparent absence of cholinergic or adrenergic function at the outset or end of the transition is the possibility of transmitter actions that do not change the membrane potential or beating rate of the myocytes.

It is likely that at least some of the neurons that appeared to be purely cholinergic in the myocyte assay retained adrenergic properties — release of catecholamines below the detection sensitivity of the assay or other adrenergic attributes. One approach was to look for uptake and storage of 5-hydroxydopamine (an analogue of NE) in SGV (method of Tranzer et al., 1969). With this procedure, the serially-assayed neuron that appeared to undergo the full transition was found after the last assay to contain about 1% SGV in the sectioned varicosities (Potter et al., 1986). This residual adrenergic property is also displayed by the cholinergic sympathetic innervation of sweat glands in adult rats (Landis, 1983). In addition, there are several reports of immunoreactivity for enzymes of catecholamine metabolism in adult neurons that apparently lack adrenergic function (e.g. parasympathetic neurons: Grzanna and Coyle, 1978; Landis et al., 1983; Björklund et al., 1985; and brain neurons: Hökfelt et al., 1984; Jaeger et al., 1984; Ross et al., 1984). These observations raise the possibility of gratuitous expression of transmitter properties (i.e. expression without functional significance), and emphasize the need for both cytochemical evidence and functional assays.

With the possibility of false negatives and electrically-silent effects in mind, what proportions of neonate-derived neurons appeared to lack cholinergic or adrenergic functions? Of the 221 assays of neonate-derived neurons summarized in Fig. 7, about 29% lacked detectable cholinergic function. These neurons either never detectably entered the transition or relapsed to a state that did not include this function (apparently purely adrenergic neurons are illustrated in Furshpan et al., 1986a; see also neuron N_2 of Fig. 5 in this chapter). Of the 221 assays, 30% apparently lacked adrenergic function; these neurons either completed the transition or lacked detectable adrenergic function at the outset (apparently purely cholinergic neurons are illustrated by Furshpan et al., 1986a; Potter et al., 1986). These proportions are strongly influenced by the growth conditions and should be taken to indicate only that such neurons were not rare.

The proportion of neurons that simultaneously expressed adrenergic and cholinergic functions was substantial (94 of the 221 neonate-derived neurons of Fig. 7). Apparently the neurons express this presumed transition state for periods of several to many weeks (heterogeneity in the rate of transition is discussed in the next section). For example, 17 of the serially-assayed neurons displayed adrenergic/

cholinergic dual function at both initial and final assays; in six cases, these assays spanned intervals of 11–16 days, indicating that the whole transition would have taken about 2 weeks or longer. Landis and Keefe (1983) report that in the developing sympathetic innervation of the plantar sweat glands of rats the adrenergic-to-cholinergic transition takes about 2 weeks.

Evidence for heterogeneity in the rate of the adrenergic-to-cholinergic transition

Our observations were consistent with the idea that the rate of transition in the microculture environment was variable and also consistent with the idea that some neurons never entered the transition (i.e. their rate of transition was zero). Apparently purely adrenergic neurons were observed as late as the 12th week, apparently purely cholinergic neurons as early as the 2nd week and adrenergic/cholinergic function as late as the 16th week (Potter et al., 1986; Matsumoto et al., 1986; compare the two neurons of Fig. 3 that were predominantly cholinenergic on culture days 10 and 12). An example of this heterogeneity is the two-neuron microculture of Fig. 5. Neuron N_1 was strongly cholinergic; it drove N_2 1:1 via cholinergic synapses and exerted a strong autaptic effect on itself (not shown). To eliminate

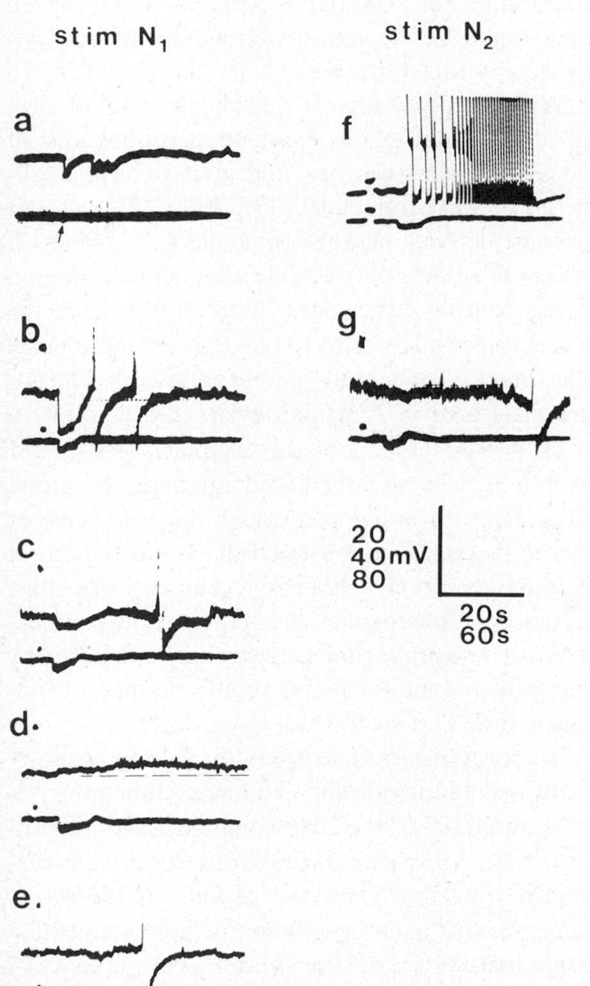

Fig. 5. Contrasting transmitter repertoires in two neonate-derived neurons grown in the same microculture for 80 days. The neurons were assayed on days 76 and 80. As no differences in status were observed, records from the two assays were pooled: (a–b) were recorded on day 76, the other records on day 80. Neuron N_1 drove neuron N_2 and itself, 1:1, via cholinergic synapses; N_2 had no detectable synaptic effect on N_1 or itself (not shown). A concentration of hexamethonium (1 mM) sufficient to eliminate the effect of N_1 on N_2 was present in all the records of this figure. The first deflections of the traces in (b–g) are calibrating steps of 10 mV. The effect of N_2 on the myocytes (f) was strongly excitatory; as this effect was blocked by 30 μM atenolol and 0.1 μM phenolamine without revealing a consistent second effect on the myocytes (g), the status of N_2 was apparently purely adrenergic. In contrast, the status of N_1 was considerably more complicated. Even single impulses produced a marked hyperpolarization of the myocytes (a) followed by a small depolarization; a train of impulses at 20 Hz in (b) produced a larger hyperpolarization followed by two myocyte impulses, even in the presence of 30 μM atenolol and 0.1 μM phentolamine. Addition of a high concentration of atropine (10 μM) in (c) only partly blocked the hyperpolarization; the atropine-resistant component was shown to be purinergic in origin by block with 8-phenyltheophylline (8-PT, nominally 3 μM) in (d). In the presence of the high concentrations of hexamethonium, atropine, atenolol, phentolamine and 8-PT, a non-adrenergic excitation remained (the NAE effect); on 1 of 5 trials a myocyte impulse was evoked (not shown). If only the adrenergic blockers were removed, an increased proportion of trials (4 of 5) evoked a myocyte impulse (e) consistent with a weak adrenergic effect. Thus, N_1 appeared to be strongly cholinergic/moderately purinergic/NAE/possibly weakly adrenergic. Vertical scale: 20 mV for (b–e, g); 40 mV for (a); 80 mV for (f). Horizontal scale: 20 sec for (a, f); 60 sec for all other traces.

synaptic interaction between N_1 and N_2 and permit their effects in the myocytes to be observed independently, a blocking concentration of hexamethonium (1 mM) was present during all the records of Fig. 5. The strong initial inhibitory effect of N_1 on the myocytes (a,b) had a double source; after a cholinergic component was blocked (compare b and c), a hyperpolarization of the myocytes persisted in the presence of 100 times the normal blocking concentration of atropine. The purinergic origin of this effect was shown by adding 8-phenyltheophylline (8-PT) to the perfusion fluid (see below). Even in the presence of adrenergic, cholinergic and purinergic blockers, a slow depolarization persisted, the NAE-effect described below; in 1 of 5 trials like that of d, this led to a myocyte impulse (not shown). When the adrenergic blockers were withdrawn (e), on 4 of 5 trials a myocyte impulse occurred; this is consistent with a very weak adrenergic effect. Thus, on day 80, N_1 was (in relative strengths) strongly cholinergic/moderately purinergic/moderately NAE/possibly very weakly adrenergic. In contrast, N_2 was strongly excitatory to the myocytes (f). As this effect was eliminated by adrenergic blockers without unmasking another consistent effect (g), on day 80, N_2 was apparently purely adrenergic.

It is noteworthy that this microculture was capable of inducing cholinergic function in N_1 (and at least permitting purinergic and NAE functions); yet after 80 days on the same pool of cardiac cells and exposed to the same medium, N_2 did not display these functions detectably. Evidently, N_2, unlike N_1, was insensitive to (stable) cholinergic induction by the cardiac cells; among the conceivable explanations for this heterogeneity is the idea that restrictions on the permitted transmitter repertoire of the neurons of the superior cervical ganglion are imposed by the day of birth, when these neurons were placed in culture, in accordance with the various target tissues that the neurons are to innervate (e.g. the heart, dilator of the iris, pineal gland, cerebral vessels, salivary glands, brown fat). Heterogeneity in the apparent rate of the adrenergic-to-cholinergic transition was only one of the ways that the microcultured neurons differed (see below).

Evidence for transmitter plasticity during development in vivo

Landis and colleagues (Landis, 1983; Landis and Keefe, 1983; Yodlowski et al., 1984; Leblanc and Landis, 1985) have provided strong evidence that the sympathetic innervation of plantar sweat glands of the rat undergoes a similar adrenergic-to-cholinergic transition, via dual status, during normal postnatal development. The elegant chick-quail transplant experiments of LeDouarin and colleagues (for a review, see LeDouarin, 1980) have shown that populations of neural crest cells destined normally to produce adrenergic cells can give rise to cholinergic cells and vice versa; in these cases it is not clear whether individual precursor cells are plastic or whether there is selection between two populations each capable of only one of these statuses. Other reports of plasticity of transmitter status during development are reviewed by Black et al. (1984; and Chapter 8, in this volume).

Adrenergic/cholinergic dual function and plasticity in adult-derived neurons

The persistence of adrenergic/cholinergic dual function in some neonate-derived neurons in microculture up to culture ages of 6 weeks or longer (Potter et al., 1986) raised the question whether neurons derived from adult ganglia could display this status. A method for isolating principal neurons from ganglia of adult rats was reported by Johnson (1978); Wakshull et al. (1979) reported that some such neurons form effective cholinergic junctions with each other or with skeletal myotubes. To discover if adult-derived neurons can display adrenergic/cholinergic status, we have placed them in microcultures with cardiac cells from hearts of newborn rats (Potter et al., 1981, 1986). A smaller proportion of adult-derived than neonate-derived neurons exerted (at least) cholinergic effects on the myocytes in the first 2 months in microculture (Potter et al., 1986); among the 83 such neurons of Fig. 7, from rats 8 weeks to about one year old, 22 displayed (at least) adrenergic/cholinergic status and only one displayed apparently purely cholinergic status. For reasons that are not understood, a smaller proportion of the at-least-cholinergic adult-derived neurons formed cholinergic synapses on themselves or a neighboring neuron than did neonate-derived neurons (Furshpan et al., 1986a).

To investigate whether adult-derived neurons acquire cholinergic function in culture (plasticity) or simply enter culture in dual status, we have made 10 preliminary serial assays of adult neurons (Potter et al., 1986). None of the 10 neurons was detectably cholinergic at first assay. Two of the 10 had cholinergic status at a later assay; one of these cases is shown in Fig. 6. On day 28 this neuron was relatively strongly adrenergic (a) and weakly purinergic (b), but when the adrenergic and purinergic effects were blocked (c), no cholinergic response to a prolonged train of neuronal impulses (20 Hz for about 14 sec) was visible. Nevertheless, the myocytes were responsive to a puff of 10 μM ACh (not shown); a significant secretion of ACh would presumably have been detected. After a further 16 days in medium equivalent to that conditioned by cardiac cells for 3 days (100% CM) the neuron displayed a pronounced cholinergic effect on the myocytes (compare d and e, before and after application of atropine) and a cholinergic autaptic effect (not shown). Thus, at first assay on day 28, the neuron had formed a sufficient number of varicosities on the myocytes to exert a pronounced adrenergic effect, but lacked a detectable cholinergic effect; exposure to CM was accompanied by acquisition of a pronounced cholinergic effect, as is characteristic of neonate-derived neurons. There seems little reason to doubt that this adult-derived neuron was plastic. It is not known whether this plasticity is a feature of the normal transmitter controls in adults or a feature induced by the process of dissociation from the ganglion; either way, the plasticity was latent for the first 4 weeks in microculture. If it is assumed that adult sympathetic principal neurons do not express adrenergic/cholinergic status in vivo (the conventional view, but see below), then the 21 other cases of this status in the 83 assays of microcultured neurons are further evidence for adrenergic-to-cholinergic plasticity in adult neurons; a demonstration of cholinergic function by itself is not clear evidence for plasticity, as it has been known for many years that some adult sympathetic principal neurons are cholinergic.

There have been reports of large changes in transmitter status in adult mammalian neurons, especially in the reproductive and digestive systems (e.g. Adham and Schenk, 1969; Sjöstrand and Swedin, 1976; Tuĉek et al., 1976; Sjöberg et al., 1977; Alm et al., 1979; Thorbert et al., 1979). A

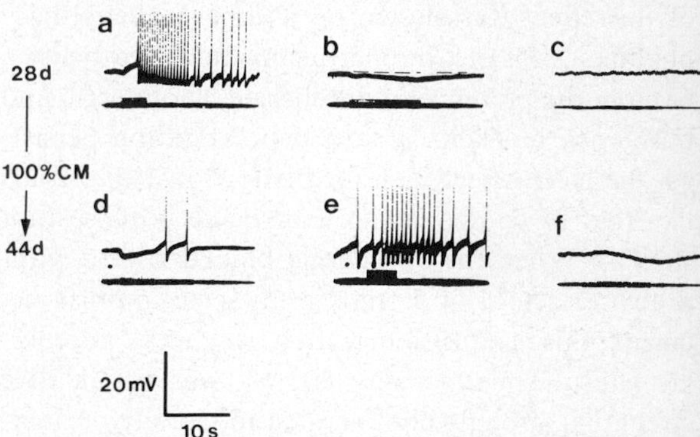

Fig. 6. Serial assay of a solitary neuron obtained from an adult (350 g) rat; the neuron was assayed on day 28 (a–c), returned to the incubator and fed thereafter with medium that contained a high concentration of the conditioned medium factor (equivalent to 100% CM); the neuron was re-assayed on day 44 (d–f). As with most adult-derived neurons, there was no autaptic effect on day 28 (not shown). The neuron had a pronounced excitatory effect on the myocytes (stimulation at 20 Hz as in the other records); this was blocked (b) by perfusion with atenolol (10 μM; a β-blocker), phentolamine (0.1 μM; an α-blocker) and atropine (0.5 μM); a small atropine-resistant hyperpolarization remained. Block of this hyperpolarization in (c), in the absence of atropine and presence of 8-phenyltheophylline (nominally 10 μM; 8-PT) established that the neuron secreted a purine (see text). As no cholinergic effect was unmasked in (c), although the myocytes were responsive to a puff of 10 μM ACh (not shown), it was concluded that the neuron was adrenergic/purinergic but not cholinergic on day 28. In contrast, at re-assay after 16 days in CM, a pronounced autaptic effect was present (not shown), and a train of neuronal impulses evoked a hyperpolarization of the myocytes (d) that was apparently eliminated by atropine (0.5 μM; e). The excitation in (e) was blocked (f) by 10 μM atenolol and 0.1 μM phentolamine. Before the responsiveness of the remaining atropine-resistant hyperpolarization to 8-PT could be checked, the cell was accidentally destroyed by the microelectrode. Thus, on day 44 this neuron was adrenergic/cholinergic and probably purinergic (see b, c). The scales apply to the myocyte traces only.

marked loss of tyrosine-hydroxylase activity and immunoreactivity was reported after axotomy of sensory neurons of the petrosal ganglion by Katz et al. (1983); it is not known whether this was the result of a change in enzyme metabolism or a change in transport (cf. Härkönen, 1964; Eränkö and Härkönen, 1965) or both. A marked increase in the substance P content of cultured explants of the superior cervical ganglion of the adult rat was reported by Adler and Black (1984). Björklund et al. (1985) report that in the sympathetically-denervated rat iris, parasympathetic axons of the ciliary ganglion acquire marked immunoreactivity for tyrosine hydroxylase and neuropeptide Y; it is possible that this is a sharp upward modulation of existing properties (Landis et al., 1983; Björklund et al., 1985). Additional descriptions of plasticity in adult neurons are given in Chapter 8 by Black and Chapter 12 by Swanson.

Is adrenergic/cholinergic dual status a transmitter option of adult sympathetic neurons in vivo?

While there is strong evidence that this status is part of the developmental program of certain rat sympathetic neurons (Landis, 1983; Landis and Keefe, 1983), there is uncertainty in adults, in spite of much work triggered by the proposal by Burn and Rand (e.g. Burn and Rand, 1959, 1960, 1965) that adult sympathetic neurons secrete both NE and ACh, and that the secretion of ACh, acting via nicotinic receptors at the terminals, causes the subsequent release of NE (the "cholinergic-link" hypothesis). Experimental evidence inconsistent with the cholinergic-link hypothesis was produced (see review by Ferry, 1966), and microculture experiments like that of Fig. 5 appear to eliminate the hypothesis in its simplest form: Neuron N_2 secreted NE (f) onto cardiac myocytes sensitive to ACh (a, b) without any sign of co-secretion of ACh (g) and in the presence of a concentration of hexamethonium sufficient to block, completely, powerful nicotinic cholinergic synapses elsewhere on N_2. Figure 7 summarizes numerous observations on microcultured neurons that displayed adrenergic function in the absence of cholinergic function (A, A/P, A/X, etc.).

However, in retrospect some other tests of the Burn and Rand idea do not seem conclusive. Tranzer et al. (1969) reported that "virtually all" small synaptic vesicles in certain sympathetic target tissues (the dilator of the iris was studied carefully) are SGV if the tissues are incubated in 5-hydroxydopamine prior to fixation; such vesicles were deemed to be adrenergic. Unfortunately, no one appears to have made a similar study of vesicles in the nictitating membrane of the cat, a tissue that has been much studied pharmacologically since the claim of Burn and Rand (1960) that the sympathetic innervation exerts a significant cholinergic effect. Investigation of this tissue has been hampered by the fact that whole nerves (not single axons) have been stimulated, and the common adrenergic and cholinergic blocking agents are not completely effective or specific, at high concentrations; a cholinergic effect has been sought against a background of an incompletely blocked excitatory effect of uncertain origin (for a recent investigation of this long-standing puzzle, see Duval et al., 1984).

Evidence consistent with weak adrenergic function in the cholinergic sympathetic innervation of the plantar sweat glands of adult rats has been obtained by Landis and colleagues: as indicated above some synaptic vesicles can store catecholamine (dense cores after incubation of the tissue in exogenous catecholamines; Landis and Keefe, 1983) and at least some of the neurons are immunoreactive for both tyrosine hydroxylase and dopamine-β-hydroxylase (Siegel et al., 1982). Given these observations and the rapidly growing evidence for unconventional transmitter statuses in peripheral neurons (see other chapters in this volume), we urge caution in interpreting earlier evidence that adult sympathetic neurons in vivo secrete NE or ACh but never both.

Purinergic status

Figures 5, 6 and 8 show atropine-resistant hyperpolarizations of the cardiac myocytes that were

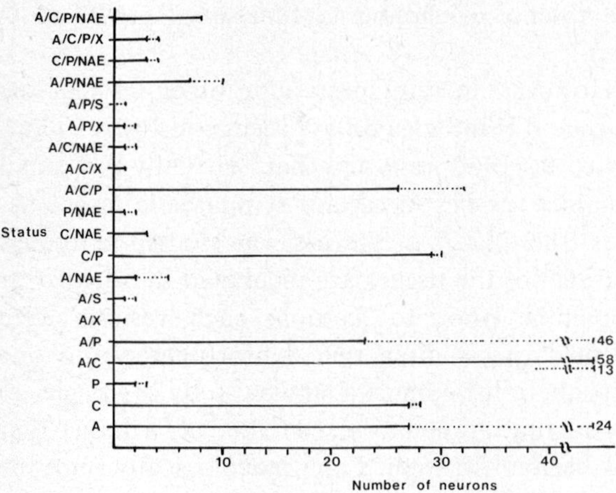

Fig. 7. The transmitter statuses of 304 reasonably well-characterized sympathetic neurons in microculture for periods of 10 days to 18 weeks; a neuron was included if the sensitivity of the assay was sufficient to determine that no substantial transmitter effect of another kind was present. A = adrenergic; C = cholinergic; P = purinergic (effect presumably exerted mainly by adenosine); S = serotonergic; X = a non-adrenergic excitatory effect insensitive to serotonergic blockers of reserpine; NAE = a non-adrenergic excitatory effect not distinguished pharmacologically as S or X; such cases would plausibly have been assignable to an S- or X-category by further analysis. The horizontal axis shows the number of neurons assigned to each status. The solid lines represent neonate-derived neurons; the dotted lines, adult-derived neurons. Numbers to the right of a line indicate the number of assays represented by the broken line segment. For reasons discussed in the text, the numbers are not a reliable measure of the incidence of each status among the microcultured neurons.

blockable with a moderate concentration of 8-PT, an agent known to block adenosine receptors (e.g. Brun, 1981). This form of transmission is described in detail in Furshpan et al. (1982, 1986b). Not only is this effect almost always blocked by adenosine receptor blockers, it is almost always diminished or eliminated by perfusing the culture with adenosine deaminase (Sigma, Type III), an enzyme reported by Sigma to be 5×10^{-5} times more active against adenosine than against AMP. While the available evidence (Furshpan et al., 1986b) does not clarify the nature of the *secreted* agent (which might be adenosine or a phosphorylated derivative or both), adenosine is plausibly the agent primarily responsible for the effect on the myocytes. In the exceptional cases of insensitivity to 8-PT or adenosine deaminase, action by ATP is a possibility.

The storage site for the secreted purine(s) has not yet been identified; the large, opaque vesicles considered of interest in purinergic transmission in vivo have not been observed in microcultured neurons that exerted pronounced purinergic effects (Furshpan et al., 1986b). Given evidence for costorage of purines with NE or ACh in small synaptic vesicles in several types of neurons, these vesicles are clearly of interest in this respect. However, it is notable that purinergic function is expressed in various strengths relative to the other two transmitters (e.g. Figs. 5, 6, 8) and that each of the three transmitters can be expressed in apparent isolation (A, C, P in Fig. 7). This clearly is inconsistent with the hypothesis that these transmitters must be secreted in a stoichiometric relation to each other and raises the possibility of independent, graded control (plasticity) of purinergic function. Figure 7 shows that purinergic function was common in neonate- and adult-derived neurons. A few microcultured neurons that exhibited apparently purely purinergic function (illustrated in Furshpan et al., 1986b) appear to be the first neurons of this status to be reported.

Non-adrenergic excitation: "X-ergic" and serotonergic functions

Many neurons exerted an excitatory effect on the myocytes (cf. Fig. 5d) that was evoked by rather prolonged trains of neuronal impulses at rather high frequency, usually had a slow onset and offset, often could not be consistently reproduced after intervals shorter than 15–30 min, sometimes fatigued irreversibly and was insensitive to high concentrations of cholinergic, adrenergic and purinergic blockers (Matsumoto et al., 1986). In some experiments, this non-adrenergic excitatory effect (NAE effect) was apparently produced by secretion of serotonin (5-HT), as it was sensitive to moderate concentrations of the 5-HT blockers methysergide or gramine, or eliminated by incubation in reserpine

(Matsumoto et al., 1986). So far, no case of serotonergic function has been seen in the absence of detectable adrenergic function, nor has it been possible to impose serotonergic function on a non-adrenergic neuron by pre-incubation in 5-HT (Sah and Matsumoto, 1986). It has been demonstrated repeatedly that adult adrenergic sympathetic neurons can take up and release exogenous 5-HT (e.g. Gershon and Ross, 1966; Thoa et al., 1969; Jaim-Etcheverry and Zieher, 1980; Koevary et al., 1983; Verbeuren et al., 1983; Kawaski and Takasaki, 1984), and this phenomenon may have physiological significance (Cohen, 1984). Sah and Matsumoto (1986) have shown that the cultured (at-least-adrenergic) neurons can take up 5-HT from the serum in the growth medium, and are now investigating whether the cultured neurons also synthesize 5-HT. While sympathetic ganglia contain 5-HT in vivo, it is not clear whether principal neurons synthesize it (see Verhofstad et al., 1981; Dun et al., 1984 for discussion).

In certain microcultures, the NAE effect was insensitive to 5-HT blockers or reserpine; this indicates that a fifth transmitter "X" is present (Matsumoto et al., 1986). We have been unable to block or mimic the X-effect with a variety of familiar agents (including the peptides VIP, somatostatin, substance P, neurotensin, NPY or PYY at concentrations between 10^{-9} and 10^{-6} M).

We place no emphasis, as noted earlier, on the relative frequencies of the statuses shown in Fig. 7. There is an under-representation of neurons of more complex statuses, as many assays of such neurons ended for various reasons before the status was fully determined. It should be emphasized that if the neurons of Fig. 7 had been assayed against a different type of target cell, many of the neurons might have been categorized differently with respect to these states; for example, cultured smooth muscle cells of the vas deferens are much less sensitive to adenosine and more sensitive to 5-HT than the cultured cardiac myocytes (Sah and Matsumoto, 1986). It should also be emphasized that if the neurons of Fig. 7 had been assayed against the full range of sympathetic target cells and their receptors, new and more complicated statuses would probably have been seen. The number of transmitter candidates under consideration in sympathetic neurons in vivo is rising rapidly. With varying degrees of confidence, the following are currently of interest: NE, ACh, dopamine, epinephrine, 5-HT, ATP, adenosine, VIP, PHI, somatostatin, substance P, the enkephalins, NPY, CGRP and a vasopressin-like substance (Hökfelt et al., 1977, 1980).

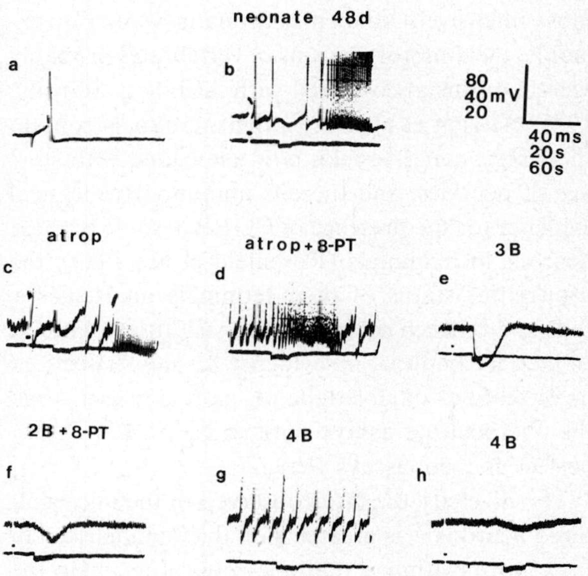

Fig. 8. A solitary, neonate-derived neuron that exhibited (at least) adrenergic/cholinergic/purinergic function after 48 days in microculture. The neuron produced no detectable autaptic effect (a). In (b, c, e, f) and (h) the first deflection on each trace is a calibrating step of 10 mV. A dual effect on the myocytes was observed (b) in the absence of drugs; the hyperpolarization was only partially blocked by atropine (1 μM) in (c), indicating the presence of a purinergic inhibition. The adrenergic effect is seen in isolation in (d), in the presence of atropine (1 μM) and 8-PT (nominally 3 μM); the purinergic effect is seen in isolation in (e), in the presence of atropine, atenolol (30 μM) and phentolamine (0.2 μM); the cholinergic effect is seen in isolation in (f), in the presence of the two adrenergic blockers (2B) and 8-PT. When all four blockers were present (g; 4B) stimulation at 10 Hz for about 16 sec had little effect on the spontaneously beating myocytes, but later (h) stimulation at 20 Hz evoked a small hyperpolarization, perhaps due to an unblocked effect of ACh or a purine. Vertical scale: 80 mV for (a), 40 mV for (b), 20 mV for other myocyte traces. Horizontal scale: 40 msec for (a), 20 sec for (b), 60 sec for other traces.

Much remains to be learned about the patterns of co-expression of these candidates.

In the context of the subject of this volume the apparently monofunctional neurons, A, C and P, are of special interest. Given the possibility that assays against other target cells would have revealed additional transmitters to which the cardiac myocytes were insensitive, coupled with concern about electrically-silent effects, it is far from certain that the neurons categorized as A, C or P were actually monofunctional. Similar concerns apply even to the most intensively studied neurons in vivo. For example, the α-motor neurons of vertebrates probably secrete purine(s) co-stored with ACh (e.g. Silinsky, 1975; Carlson et al., 1978); their terminals contain the larger, cored vesicles now associated with storage of peptides, and there is immunocytochemical evidence for the presence of CGRP in some of these neurons in mammals (Rosenfeld et al., 1983); the transmitter status of their terminals on Renshaw cells and on each other has received little attention. In fact, we know of no evidence for monofunction, in vertebrates or invertebates, more stringent than the microculture assays summarized in Fig. 7, imperfect as these assays were.

The diversity of status observed in the microcultured neurons was greater than that summarized in Fig. 7, for within a multiple-transmitter state the relative intensities of the individual effects varied in an apparently graded way. Figure 8 is included as a further illustration of the apparently graded and independent expression of purinergic with adrenergic and cholinergic functions already illustrated in Figs. 5 and 6. The solitary neuron of Fig. 8 might be characterized (relative strengths) as moderately adrenergic/weakly cholinergic/rather strongly purinergic (the three effects are seen in isolation in d, f and e). In contrast, N_1 in Fig. 5 was possibly-very-weakly adrenergic/strongly cholinergic/moderately purinergic, and the neuron of Fig. 6 was apparently moderately adrenergic/moderately cholinergic/weakly purinergic on day 44. Further examples of graded expression of the transmitter states are given in Furshpan et al. (1986b) and Matsumoto et al. (1986).

This variation in the relative strengths of adrenergic and cholinergic functions in neonate-derived neurons is comfortably accommodated in connection with a developmental transition, as discussed above. The variation in neuronal cytochemical reactivity previously reported in vivo, for a variety of synaptic functions (e.g., enzymes, transmitter candidates; e.g. Holmstedt and Sjöqvist, 1959; Härkönen, 1964; Lundberg et al., 1979) is potentially of interest in the context of transmitter plasticity. Intermediate states of transmitter expression are clearly of physiological interest, aside from serving as evidence of plasticity, as in the case described by Sawchenko and Swanson (1985).

Is the diversity of transmitter states shown in Fig. 7 an artifact of culture? Part of the diversity was apparently due to addition of cholinergic status to neurons in culture that did not express it in vivo; however, the adrenergic-to-cholinergic transition is part of the normal developmental repertoire in at least one group of sympathetic neurons. As noted above, we urge caution in assuming that co-expression of adrenergic and cholinergic function never occurs in adults in vivo. Adrenergic/ATP-ergic and cholinergic/adenosinergic neurons have been reported in vivo (see Chapter 13 by Burnstock for discussion). The ability of adrenergic neurons to take up and release 5-HT has ample precedent in vivo. If X proves to be a peptide or peptides, release with the amines or purine will be no great surprise. Much further work is required to clarify the range and incidence of transmitter states in culture and in vivo; it is possible that each of the states shown in Fig. 7, and many more, will be discovered in vivo.

Among the more exotic neurons of Fig. 7 are those with triple or quadruple function. Do neurons with such complex statuses have plausible roles in vivo? Some of the demonstrated and possible roles for multiple-function neurons have been described by Lundberg and Hökfelt (1983). It will not now be surprising if each neuron in vivo is found to secrete as many transmitters or modulators as there are cell properties, electrogenic and electrically silent, in the vicinity of the endings that require coordinated control on several time scales. This conceivably could require transmitter statuses considerably more complicated than quadruple function. There are precedents in cell biology for high orders of multiple secretory function, for example, endocrine cells that synthesize pro-opiomelanocortin or the adrenal medullary cells that collectively are reported to contain or secrete NE, epinephrine, ATP, GABA, substance P, enkephalins, dynorphin, neurotensin, NPY, VIP, somatostatin and ascorbate; textbooks assume that numerous serum enzymes and proteins are secreted by each liver cell, numerous digestive enzymes by each pancreatic acinar cell, and numerous enzymes and proteins by each prostatic gland cell.

Given the growing evidence for overlap in the secretory repertoires of neurons and endocrine cells, it is natural to wonder whether other classes of molecules are employed as transmitters or modulators. There is precedent for secretion of an enzyme (e.g. dopamine-β-hydroxylase by adrenergic cells); secretion of various other enzymes would obviously be of interest (e.g. secretion of a specific protease (see Pittman, 1983) or a specific protein kinase with ATP). Secretion of steroids would also clearly be of interest.

Summary

The classical view of transmitter status in adult mammalian sympathetic principal neurons is that two transmitters, NE and ACh, are expressed; each neuron secretes only one (monofunction), and that transmitter is expressed approximately full-on (flip-flop control with modulation around the full-on state); once the appropriate transmitter is adopted, the neuron does not change status (no plasticity). Recent work in culture and in vivo has called each of these views into question; transmitter status in these neurons is clearly considerably more complicated than was formerly thought, but we are far from a satisfactory understanding. Similar considerations apply to other types of neurons discussed in this volume. It is possible that plasticity of transmitter status, and its association with a widely graded expression of a status, will prove a widespread phenomenon in chemical transmission, like co-existence. The microculture procedure offers certain advantages in displaying and investigating the new complexities.

Acknowledgements

We are indebted to many colleagues for discussion, especially Drs. Linda Chun, Patrick Hogan, Peter MacLeish, Rae Nishi, Paul O'Lague, Paul Patterson, and Alan Willard. Expert assistance was provided by Robert Bosler, Wendy Brooks, Delores Cox, Karen Fischer, Joseph Gagliardi, Nona Hayes, Ibrahim Houri, James and Michael LaFratta, Shirley Wilson and Vivienne Yee. Conditioned medium was kindly provided by Drs. Linda Chun, Allison Doupe, Keiko Fukada and Eve Wolinsky. This work was supported by NIH grants NS11576, NS18316, NS03273 and NS02253, a Grant-in-Aid from the American Heart Association (78-964) and an AHA Established Investigator Award to SCL.

References

Adham, N. and Schenk, E. A. (1969) Automatic innervation of the rat vagina, cervix and uterus and its cyclic variation. *Amer. J. Obstet. Gynec.*, 104: 508–516.

Adler, J. E. and Black, I. B. (1984) Plasticity of substance P in mature and aged sympathetic neurons in culture. *Science*, 225: 1499–1500.

Alm, P., Björklund, A., Owman, C. and Thorbert, G. (1979) Tyrosine hydroxylase and dopa decarboxylase activities in the guinea-pig uterus: further evidence for functional adrenergic denervation in association with pregnancy. *Neuroscience*, 4: 145–154.

Armett, C. J. and Ritchie, J. M. (1960) The action of acetylcholine on conduction in mammalian non-myelinated fibres and its prevention by anticholinesterase. *J. Physiol. (Lond.)*, 152: 141–158.

Björklund, H., Hökfelt, T., Goldstein, M., Terenius, L. and Olson, L. (1985) Appearance of the noradrenergic markers tyrosine hydroxylase and neuropeptide Y in cholinergic nerves of the iris following sympathectomy. *J. Neurosci.*, 5: 1633–1643.

Black, I. B., Adler, J. E., Dreyfus, C. F., Jonakait, G. M., Katz, D. M., La Gamma, E. F. and Markey, K. M. (1984) Neurotransmitter plasticity at the molecular level. *Science,* 225: 1266–1270.

Bloom, F. E. (1970) The fine structural localization of biogenic monoamines in nervous tissue. *Int. Rev. Neurobiol.,* 13: 27–66.

Bruns, R. F. (1981) Adenosine antagonism by purines, pteridines and benzopteridines in human fibroblasts. *Biochem. Pharmacol.,* 30: 325–333.

Burn, J. H. and Rand, M. J. (1959) Sympathetic postganglionic mechanism. *Nature (Lond.),* 184: 163–165.

Burn, J. H. and Rand, M. J. (1960) Sympathetic postganglionic cholinergic fibres. *Brit. J. Pharmacol.,* 15: 56–66.

Burn, J. H. and Rand, M. J. (1965) Acetylcholine in adrenergic transmission. *Ann. Rev. Pharmacol.,* 5: 163–182.

Bunge, R., Johnson, M. and Ross, C. D. (1978) Nature and nurture in development of the autonomic neuron. *Science,* 199: 1409–1416.

Campbell, G., Gibbons, I. L., Morris, J. L., Furness, J. B., Costa, M., Oliver, J. R., Beardsley, A. M. and Murphy, R. (1982) Somatostatin is contained in and released from cholinergic nerves in the heart of the toad *Bufo marinus. Neuroscience,* 7: 2013–2023.

Carlson, S. W., Wagner, J. A. and Kelly, R. B. (1978) Purification of synaptic vesicles from elasmobranch electric organ and the use of biophysical criteria to demonstrate purity. *Biochemistry,* 17: 1188–1199.

Choi, D. and Fischbach, G. D. (1981) GABA conductance of chick spinal cord and dorsal root ganglion neurons in cell culture. *J. Neurophysiol.,* 45: 605–620.

Cohen, M. W., Greschner, M. and Tucci, M. (1984) *In vivo* development of cholinesterase at a neuromuscular junction in the absence of motor activity in *Xenopus laevis. J. Physiol. (Lond.),* 348: 57–66.

Cohen, R. A. (1984) Neurogenic coronary contractions due to accumulation by adrenergic nerves of 5-hydroxytryptamine released from platelets. *Physiologist,* 27: Abstract 21.10.

Crain, S. M. and Peterson, E. R. (1974) Development of neural connections in culture. *Ann. N.Y. Acad. Sci.,* 228: 6–34.

Cuello, A. C. (ed.) (1982) *Co-Transmission,* The MacMillan Press Ltd., London.

De Champlain, J., Olson, L., Malmfors, T. and Sachs, C. (1970) Fluorescence morphology of the developing peripheral adrenergic nerves in the rat. *Acta physiol. Scand.,* 80: 276–288.

Dun, N. J., Kiraly, M. and Ma, R. C. (1984) Evidence for a serotonin-mediated slow excitatory potential in the guinea-pig coeliac ganglia. *J. Physiol. (Lond.),* 351: 61–76.

Duval, N., Hicks, P. E. and Langer, S. Z. (1984) Reserpine-resistant responses to nerve stimulation in the cat nictitating membrane are due to newly synthesized transmitter. *Brit. J. Pharmacol.,* 83: 406B.

Eccles, J. C. (1976) From electrical to chemical transmission in the central nervous system. *R. Soc. Notes and Records,* 30: 219–230.

Eränkö, O. and Härkönen, M. (1965) Effect of axon division on the distribution of noradrenaline and acetylcholinesterase in sympathetic neurons of the rat. *Acta physiol. Scand.,* 63: 411–412.

Ferry, C. B. (1963) The sympathomimetic effect of acetylcholine on the spleen of the cat. *J. Physiol. (Lond.),* 167: 487–504.

Ferry, C. B. (1966) Cholinergic link hypothesis in adrenergic neuroeffector transmission. *Physiol. Rev.,* 46: 420–456.

Fukada, K. (1980) Hormonal control of neurotransmitter choice in sympathetic neuron cultures. *Nature (Lond.),* 287: 553–555.

Furshpan, E. J., MacLeish, P. R., O'Lague, P. H. and Potter, D. D. (1976) Chemical transmission between rat sympathetic neurons and cardiac myocytes developing in microcultures: Evidence for cholinergic, adrenergic and dual-function neruons. *Proc. nat. Acad. Sci. USA,* 73: 4225–4229.

Furshpan, E. J., Potter, D. D. and Landis, S. C. (1982) On the transmitter repertoire of sympathetic neurons in culture. *Harvey Lect.,* 76: 149–191.

Furshpan, E. J., Landis, S. C., Matsumoto, S. G. and Potter, D. D. (1986a) Synaptic functions in rat sympathetic neurons in microcultures. I. Separation of norepinephrine and acetylcholine. *J. Neurosci.* (in press).

Furshpan, E. J., Potter, D. D. and Matsumoto, S. G. (1986b) Synaptic functions in rat sympathetic neurons in microcultures. III. A purinergic effect on cardiac myocytes. *J. Neurosci.* (in press).

Gershon, M. and Ross, L. L. (1966) Location of sites of 5-hydroxytryptamine storage and metabolism by autoradiography. *J. Physiol. (Lond.),* 186: 477–492.

Grzanna, R. and Coyle, J. T. (1978) Dopamine-β-hydroxylase in rat submandibular ganglion cells which lack norepinephrine. *Brain Res.,* 151: 206–214.

Härkönen, M. (1964) Carboxylic esterases, oxidative enzymes and catecholamines in the superior cervical ganglion of the rat and the effect of pre- and postganglionic nerve division. *Acta physiol. Scand.,* 63, Suppl. 237: 1–94.

Higgings, D., Iacovitti, L., Joh, T. H. and Burton, H. (1981) The immunocytochemical localization of tyrosine hydroxylase within rat sympathetic neurons that release acetylcholine in culture. *J. Neurosci.,* 1: 126–131.

Hökfelt, T., Efin, L. G., Elde, R., Schultzberg, M., Goldstein, M. and Luft, R. (1977) Occurrence of somatostatin-like immunoreactivity in some peripheral sympathetic noradrenergic neurons. *Proc. nat. Acad. Sci. USA,* 74: 3587–3591.

Hökfelt, T., Johansson, O., Ljüngdahl, A., Lundberg, J. M. and Schultzberg, M. (1980) Peptidergic neurones. *Nature (Lond.),* 284: 515–521.

Hökfelt, T., Johansson, O. and Goldstein, M. (1984) Chemical anatomy of the brain. *Science,* 225: 1326–1334.

Holmstedt, B. and Sjöqvist, F. (1959) Distribution of acetylcholinesterase in the ganglion cells of various sympathetic ganglia. *Acta physiol. Scand.*, 47: 284–296.

Iacovitti, L., Joh, T. H., Park, D. H. and Bunge, R. P. (1981) Dual expression of neurotransmitter synthesis in cultured automatic neurons. *J. Neurosci.*, 1 685–690.

Ip, N. Y., Baldwin, C. and Zigmond, R. E. (1984) Acute stimulation of ganglionic tyrosine hydroxylase activity by secretin, VIP and PHI. *Peptides*, 5: 309–312.

Jaeger, C. B., Ruggiero, D. A., Albert, V. R., Park, D. H., Joh, T. H. and Reis, D. J. (1984) Aromatic L-amino acid decarboxylase in the rat brain: immunocytochemical localization in neurons of the brain stem. *Neuroscience*, 11: 691–713.

Jaim-Etcheverry, G. and Zieher, L. M. (1980) Stimulation-depletion of serotonin and noradrenaline from vesicles of synmpathetic nerves in the pineal gland of the rat. *Cell Tiss. Res.*, 207: 13–20.

Johnson, M. I. (1978) Adult rat dissociated sympathetic neurons in culture: morphological and cytochemical studies. *Soc. Neurosci. Abstr.*, 8: Abstract 343.

Johnson, M. I., Ross, D. Meyers, M., Rees, R., Bunge, R. Wakshull, E. and Burton, H. (1976) Synaptic vesicle cytochemistry changes when cultured sympathetic neurons develop cholinergic interactions. *Nature (Lond.)*, 262: 308–310.

Johnson, M. I., Ross, C. D., Meyers, M., Spitznagel, E. L. and Bunge, R. P. (1980) Morphological and biochemical studies on the development of cholinergic properties in cultured sympathetic neurons. I. Correlative changes in choline acetyltransferase and synaptic vesicle cytochemistry. *J. Cell Biol.*, 84: 680–691.

Katz, D. M., Markey, K. A., Goldstein, M. and Black, I. B. (1983) Expression of catecholaminergic characteristics by primary sensory neurons in the normal adult rat *in vivo*. *Proc. nat. Acad. Sci. USA*, 80: 3526–3531.

Kawaski, H. and Takasaki, K. (1984) Vasoconstrictor response induced by 5-hydroxytryptamine released from vascular adrenergic nerves by periarterial nerve stimulation. *J. Pharmacol. exp. Ther.*, 229: 816–822.

Kessler, J. A. (1984) Environmental regulation of peptide neurotransmitter phenotypic expression. *Soc. Neurosci. Abstr.*, 10: Abstract 8.1.

Koevary, S. B., Azmitia, E. C. and McEvoy, R. C. (1983) Rat pancreatic serotinergic nerves: morpholic, pharmacologic and physiologic studies. *Brain Res.*, 265: 328–332.

Langer, S. Z. and Pinto, J. E. B. (1976) Possible involvement of a transmitter different from norephinephrine in the residual responses to nerve stimulation of the cat nictitating membrane after pretreatment with reserpine. *J. Pharmacol. exp. Ther.*, 196: 697–713.

Landis, S. C. (1976) Rat sympathetic neurons and cardiac myocytes developing in microcultures: correlation of the fine structure of endings with neurotransmitter function in single neurons. *Proc. nat. Acad. Sci. USA*, 73: 4220–4224.

Landis, S. C. (1980) Developmental changes in neurotransmitter properties of dissociated sympathetic neurons: a cytochemical study of the effects of medium. *Develop. Biol.*, 77: 349–361.

Landis, S. C. (1983) Development of cholinergic sympathetic neurons: Evidence for neurotransmitter plasticity *in vivo*. *Fed. Proc.*, 42: 1633–1638.

Landis, S. C. and Keefe, D. (1983) Evidence for neurotransmitter plasticity *in vivo*: Developmental changes in properties of cholinergic sympathetic neurons. *Develop. Biol.*, 98: 349–372.

Landis, S. C., Jackson, P. C. and Fredieu, J. R. (1983) Catecholaminergic properties of neurons and preganglionic axons in the rat ciliary ganglion. *Soc. Neurosci. Abstr.*, 9: 937.

Leblanc, G., and Landis, S. C. (1985) Development of choline acetyltransferase in the sympathetic innervation of rat sweat glands. *J. Neurosci.* (in press).

LeDouarin, N. M. (1980) The ontogeny of the neural crest in avian embryo chimaeras. *Nature (Lond.)*, 268: 663–669.

Lundberg, J. M. (1981) Evidence for coexistence of vasoactive intestinal polypeptide (VIP) and acetylcholine in neurons of cat exocrine glands. Morphological, biochemical and functional studies. *Acta physiol. Scand.*, Suppl. 496: 1–75.

Lundberg, J. M. and Hökfelt, T. (1983) Coexistence of peptides and classical neurotransmitters. *Trends Neurosci.*, 6: 325–333.

Lundberg, J. M., Hökfelt, T., Schultzberg, M., Uvnas-Wallensten, K., Kohler, C. and Said, S. I. (1979) Occurrence of vasoactive intestinal polypeptide (VIP)-like immunoreactivity in certain cholinergic neurons of the cat: evidence from combined immunohistochemistry and acetylcholinesterase staining. *Neuroscience*, 4: 1539–1559.

Malmfors, T. and Sachs, C. (1965) Direct demonstration of the system of terminals belonging to an individual adrenergic neuron and their distribution in the rat iris. *Acta physiol. Scand.*, 64: 377–382.

Matsumoto, S. G., Sah, D., Potter, D. D. and Furshpan, E. J. (1986) Synaptic functions in rat sympathetic neurons in microcultures. IV. A slow, excitatory effect on cardiac myocytes and the variety of multiple transmitter states (submitted).

McGuire, B. A., Hornung, J.-P., Gilbert, C. D. and Wiesel, T. N. (1984) Patterns of synaptic input to layer 4 of cat striate cortex. *J. Neurosci.*, 4: 3021–3033.

O'Lague, P. H., Potter, D. D. and Furshpan, E. J. (1978) Studies on rat synmpathetic neurons developing in cell culture. III. Cholinergic transmission. *Develop. Biol.*, 67: 424–443.

Patterson, P. H. (1978) Environmental determination of autonomic neurotransmitter functions. *Ann. Rev. Neurosci.*, 1: 1–17.

Patterson, P. H. and Chun, L. L. Y. (1977) The induction of acetylcholine synthesis in primary cultures of dissociated rat sympathetic neurons. II. Developmental aspects. *Develop. Biol.*, 60: 473–481.

Pittman, R. N. (1983) Spontaneously released proteins from cultures of sensory ganglia include plasminogen activator and a calcium dependent protease. *Abstracts Soc. Neurosci.*, 9: Abstract 5.4.

Potter, D. D., Furshpan, E. J. and Landis, S. C. (1981) Multiple-transmitter status and "Dale's Principle". *Neurosc. Comment.*, 1: 1–9.

Potter, D. D., Furshpan, E. J. and Landis, S. C. (1983) Transmitter status in cultured rat sympathetic neurons: plasticity and multiple function. *Fed. Proc.*, 42: 1626–1632.

Potter, D. D., Landis, S. C., Matsumoto, S. G. and Furshpan, E. J. (1986) Synaptic functions in rat sympathetic neurons in culture. II. Adrenergic/cholinergic dual status and plasticity. *J. Neurosci.* (in press).

Rosenfeld, M. G., Mermod, J.-J., Amara, S. G., Swanson, L. W., Sawchenko, P. E., Rivier, J., Vale, W. W. and Evans, R. M. (1983) Production of a novel neuropeptide encoded by the calcitonin gene via tissue-specific RNA processing. *Nature (Lond.)*, 304: 129–135.

Ross, C. A., Ruggiero, D. A., Meeley, M. P., Park, D. H. and Reis, D. J. (1984) A new group of neurons in hypothalamus containing phenylethanolamine N-methyl transferase (PNMT) but not tyrosine hydroxylase. *Brain Res.*, 306: 349–353.

Sah, D. and Matsumoto, S. G. (1986) Evidence for serotonin uptake and release in some dissociated rat sympathetic neurons in culture. *J. Neurosci.* (submitted).

Sawchenko, P. E. and Swanson, L. W. (1985) Localization, colocalization and plasticity of corticotropin-releasing factor immunoreactivity in rat brain. *Fed. Proc.*, 44: 221–227.

Siegel, R. E., Schwab, M., and Landis, S. C. (1982) Developmental changes in the neurotransmitter properties of cholinergic sympathetic neurons *in vivo*. *Neuroscience Abstr.*, 8: #6.6.

Silinsky, E. M. (1975) On the association between transmitter secretion and the release of adenine nucleotides from mammalian motor nerve terminals. *J. Physiol. (Lond.)*, 247: 145–162.

Sjöberg, N.-O., Johansson, E. D. B., Owman, C., Rosengren, E. and Wallas, B. (1977) Cyclic fluctuation in noradrenaline transmitter of the monkey oviduct. *Acta obstet. gynec. Scand.*, 56: 139–143.

Sjöstrand, N. O. and Swedin, G. (1976) Influences of age, growth, castration and testosterone treatment on the noradrenaline levels of the ductus deferens and the auxiliary male reproductive glands of the rat. *Acta physiol. Scand.*, 98: 323–338.

Thoa, N. B., Eccleston, D. and Axelrod, J. (1969) The accumulation of ^{14}C-serotonin in the guinea-pig vas deferens. *J. Pharmacol. exp. Ther.*, 169: 68–73.

Thorbert, G., Alm, P., Björklund, A. B., Owman, C. and Sjöberg, N.-O. (1979) Adrenergic innervation of the human uterus. Disappearance of the transmitter and transmitter-forming enzymes during pregnancy. *Amer. J. Obstet. Gynec.*, 135: 223–226.

Tranzer, J. P., Thoenen, H., Snipes, R. L. and Richards, J. G. (1969) Recent developments on the ultrastructural aspect of adrenergic nerve endings in various experimental conditions. *Prog. Brain Res.*, 31: 33–46.

Tuček, S., Kostirova, D. and Gutman, E. (1976) Testosterone-induced changes of choline acetyltransferase and cholinesterase activities in rat levator ani muscle. *J. neurol. Sci.*, 27: 353–362.

Verbeuren, T., Jordaens, F. H. and Herman, A. G. (1983) Accumulation and release of [^{3}H]-5-hydroxytryptamine in saphenous veins and cerebral arteries of the dog. *J. Pharmacol. exp. Ther.*, 226: 579–588.

Verhofstad, A. A. J., Steinbusch, H. W. M., Penke, B., Varga, J. and Joosten, H. W. J. (1981) Serotonin-immunoreactive cells in the superior cervical ganglion of the rat. Evidence for the existence of separate serotonin- and catecholamine-containing small ganglionic cells. *Brain Res.*, 212: 39–49.

Wakshull, E., Johnson, M. I. and Burton, H. (1979) Postnatal rat sympathetic neurons in culture. II. Synaptic transmission by postnatal neurons. *J. Neurophysiol.*, 42: 1426–1436.

Walicke, P. A., Campenot, R. B. and Patterson, P. H. (1977) Determination of transmitter function by neuronal activity. *Proc. nat. Acad. Sci. USA*, 74: 5767–5771.

Wolinsky, E. and Patterson, P. H. (1983) Tyrosine hydroxylase activity decreases with induction of cholinergic properties in cultured sympathetic neurons. *J. Neurosci.*, 3: 1495–1500.

Yodlowski, M. L., Fredieu, J. R. and Landis, S. C. (1984) Neonatal 6-hydroxydopamine treatment eliminates cholinergic sympathetic innervation and induces sensory sprouting in rat sweat glands. *J. Neurosci.*, 4: 1535–1548.

Zigmond, R. E. (1980) The long-term regulation of ganglionic tyrosine hydroxylase by preganglionic nerve activity. *Fed. Proc.*, 39: 3003–3008.

T. Hökfelt, K. Fuxe and B. Pernow (Eds.),
Progress in Brain Research, Vol. 68

CHAPTER 8

Impulse activity differentially regulates co-localized transmitters by altering messenger RNA levels

I. B. Black, J. E. Adler and E. F. LaGamma

Cornell University Medical College, 515 East 71st Street, New York, NY 10021, U.S.A.

Introduction

Concepts of the combinatorial potential of neural communication have undergone a revolution with the realization that neurons use multiple transmitters simultaneously. The coexistence of multiple modulators and transmitters vastly expands our insights concerning the theoretical precision, specificity and flexibility of synaptic interactions.

We have been examining a specific aspect of this problem, the mechanisms by which neurons change phenotypic expression and metabolism of multiple transmitters over time. Our observations indicate that multiple extracellular signals govern the transmitter status of a neuron at any given time. Moreover, our studies suggest that this plasticity is mediated, at least in part, by alteration of neuronal gene read-out. To summarize, our studies indicate that transmitter plasticity occurs during maturity as well as development, and centrally as well as peripherally.

In the present chapter we focus on the role of depolarization in the regulation of transmitter plasticity. Specifically, experiments employing rat sympathetic neurons and adrenomedullary chromaffin cells as models in vivo and in vitro are reviewed. Initially, mechanisms by which depolarization regulates transmitter metabolism and expression in sympathetic neurons is discussed. Evidence indicates that plasticity persists into adulthood. Regulation in the adrenomedullary chromaffin cell is then examined, since the availability of appropriate cDNA probes has helped to identify molecular loci governing plasticity attendant to depolarization.

Results and discussion

Peptides and plasticity in sympathetic neurons

Conventional wisdom had maintained that the traditional sympathetic neuron used either acetylcholine or norepinephrine (NE) as transmitters. However, recent studies from our laboratory, as well as others (see Potter et al., this volume), indicate that individual sympathetics may use a variety of transmitters. We focus on the putative peptide transmitter, substance P (SP) in some detail, to illustrate this point.

In initial studies we found that the adult rat superior cervical sympathetic ganglion (SCG) contained low, but detectable levels of SP, and that ganglion denervation (decentralization) elicited significant elevation of the peptide (Kessler and Black, 1982). Moreover, pharmacologic blockade of ganglionic transmission reproduced the effects of denervation, suggesting that trans-synaptic impulses, through the interaction of acetylcholine with postsynaptic nicotinic receptors and depolarization, normally decreased SP (Kessler and Black, 1982). Conversely, as expected, agents that reflexly increased sympathetic impulse flow significantly depressed ganglion SP below normal, basal levels.

To elucidate underlying molecular mechanisms, ganglia were explanted to culture, allowing experimentation without the confounding, uncontrolled variables encountered in vivo. Explantation (and consequent denervation) resulted in a striking, 20-fold rise in SP by 24 h, and a 50-fold rise after 48 h (Kessler et al., 1981). The marked elevation in SP provided a unique opportunity to localize SP in the SCG. In fact, immunocytochemical examination indicated that the vast majority of the principal sympathetic neurons expressed SP (Kessler et al., 1981; Bohn et al., 1984). These neurons simultaneously expressed the noradrenergic and SP phenotypes (Bohn et al., 1984).

Having localized SP to the sympathetic neurons, we were in a position to examine mechanisms underlying the rise in culture. Inhibition of protein synthesis completely blocked the elevation of SP upon explantation, while inhibition of RNA synthesis partially inhibited the increase. Consequently, it appears that both protein- and RNA-synthesis were necessary for the elevation of SP (Kessler et al., 1981, 1983).

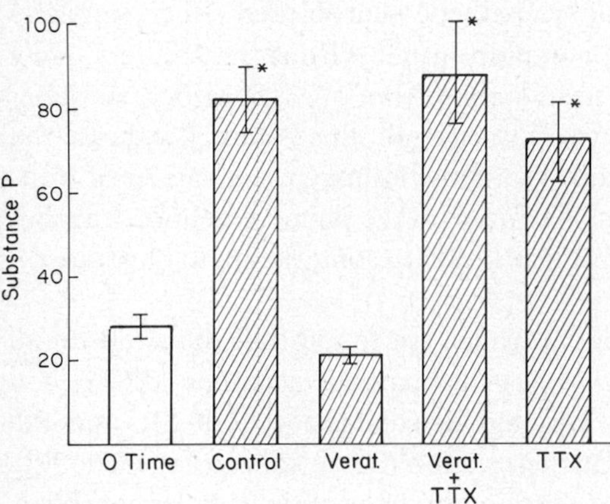

Fig. 1. Effect of membrane depolarization on SP content of adult rat ganglia. Ganglia were cultured in serum-supplemented medium in the presence of veratridine (Verat.) (5×10^{-5} M) or tetrodotoxin (TTX) (10^{-7} M) or both. After 48 h the ganglia were examined for SP content, which is expressed as mean pg/ganglion ± standard error for eight ganglia. Statistical analysis was performed by one-way ANOVA and the Newman-Keuls test. * $p < 0.01$ vs. zero time and Verat. groups. (Data derived from Adler and Black, 1984.)

The above studies were performed with neonatal ganglia, since immature ganglia are more conveniently cultured than mature ganglia. However, we were particularly interested in determining whether mature and developing neurons exhibit similar plastic regulatory mechanisms. We succeeded in culturing mature ganglia, and investigated regulation of SP (Adler and Black, 1984). To determine whether depolarization inhibited the increse of SP, ganglia were cultured in the presence of veratridine, which increases sodium ion influx by binding to sodium channels (Ulbricht, 1964). The alkaloid completely blocked the increase in SP (Fig. 1), reproducing the effects of impulse activity in vivo. Further, addition of tetrodotoxin, which antagonizes the effect of veratridine on sodium channels (Catterall and Nirenberg, 1973; Evans, 1973), blocked the effects of veratridine on SP. Similar results were obtained with neonatal ganglia (Kessler et al., 1981). These observations suggest that depolarization, through the mediation of sodium ion influx suppresses SP in sympathetic neurons. Previous studies had indicated that this effect was not simply due to release of the peptide (Kessler et al., 1983), but rather to inhibition of net synthesis (synthesis less catabolism).

In summary, our in vivo and culture studies, viewed in conjunction, indicate that (a) presynaptic impulse activity, (b) release of acetylcholine, (c) interaction with nicotinic receptors, (d) depolarization and (e) sodium ion influx suppress net synthesis of SP in neonatal and mature sympathetic neurons.

Plasticity in aged sympathetic neurons

The ability to culture ganglia of different ages allowed us to examine the effect of aging itself on peptidergic plasticity. We examined ganglia from 2-year-old (aged) rats and compared them to those from adults. Basal SP content in the aged ganglia was indistinguishable from that in 6-month-old adult controls, 30 pg per ganglion. However, in striking contrast to mature (or neonatal) ganglia, those from aged rats did not exhibit a significant increase in SP after explantation (Fig. 2). Since total protein, neurite elaboration and even zero-time bas-

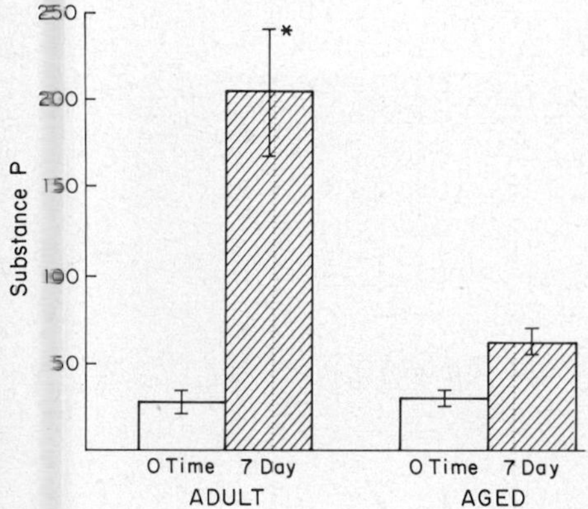

Fig. 2. Accumulation of SP in adult and aged ganglia. Sixteen ganglia were removed from rats aged 6 months (ADULT) or greater than 24 months and were grown in serum-supplemented medium for 7 days. SP is expressed as in Fig. 1 and groups were subjected to the same statistical analysis. * Differs from all other groups at $p < 0.01$. (Data derived from Adler and Black, 1984.)

al SP was normal, as indicated above, the deficit appears to be relatively specific for SP plasticity per se. Although the molecular basis for deranged plasticity remains to be defined, it is now apparent that altered mutability of co-localized transmitters may represent one deficit in the aging process.

Peptidergic and catecholaminergic plasticity

The foregoing studies indicate that trans-synaptic impulse activity decreases SP in sympathetic neurons. In marked contrast, it has long been known that impulse activity biochemically induces key catecholamine (CA) biosynthetic enzymes in the same cells. For example, extensive studies indicate that tyrosine hydroxylase (TH), the rate-limiting enzyme in CA biosynthesis, is trans-synaptically induced (Mueller et al., 1969a, b). Consequently, impulse activity apparently has opposite effects on different transmitter systems within the same neuron.

While we are presently studying molecular genetic mechanisms underlying SP plasticity, we already have relevant information concerning TH induction. Such insights may delineate fundamental cellular mechanisms through which environmental signals regulate plasticity of co-localized transmitters. The availability of a cDNA Probe (Lewis et al., 1983), complementary to TH messenger RNA (mRNA) has allowed us to approach this problem directly. To summarize, our studies have indicated that trans-synaptic induction of rat sympathetic TH in vivo is accompanied by a comparable, 3-fold rise in TH mRNA (Black et al., 1986). Moreover, denervation of the ganglion prevented TH induction and also prevented the increase in mRNA coding for TH. These results suggest that trans-synaptic increases in impulse activity may induce TH by increasing cellular levels of TH mRNA. It is not yet clear whether increased TH mRNA is due to enhanced transcription and/or to stabilization of the mRNA. Nevertheless, it is now apparent that membrane depolarization, or some sequelae thereof, may elicit transmitter plasticity by altering levels of specific species of mRNA. To determine whether analogous mechanisms govern peptide regulation, we examined the rat adrenal medulla, a model system that contains peptides for which cDNA probes are available.

Plasticity in the adrenal medulla

In initial studies we found that CA and opiate peptides, which are co-localized and co-released by adrenomedullary cells (Viveros et al., 1979; Govoni et al., 1981; Nilson et al., 1982), are differentially regulated in these same cells in vivo and in vitro (LaGamma et al., 1984). For example, denervation, or pharmacologic blockade of impulses to the adrenal in adult rats, resulted in more than a 2-fold increase in the opiate peptide, leucine-enkephalin (leu-enk), without altering activity of CA biosynthetic enzymes (LaGamma et al., 1984). Further, explanation of medullae to culture (with consequent denervation) increased leu-enk 50-fold within 4 days, without increasing the CA enzymes (LaGamma et al., 1984). Exposure of the medullae in culture to depolarizing agents completely prevented the increase in leu-enk, and this effect was blocked by tetrodotoxin. These observations suggested that impulse activity exerted differential regulatory effects on co-localized neurohumours in the same medullary cells.

To characterize molecular mechanisms mediating the rise, medullae were cultured for 2.5 days in basal medium, and then exposed to specific metabolic inhibitors for 12 h. Control medullae, maintained in basal medium from 2.5 to 3 days, exhibited the expected 10-fold increase in leu-enk during this period. In contrast, inhibition of protein synthesis with cycloheximide completely prevented the increase in leu-enk (Fig. 3). Inhibition of RNA synthesis with either actinomycin-D or α-amanitin (Chambon, 1975), partially blocked the rise (Fig. 3), whereas inhibition of DNA synthesis with cytosine-arabinoside had no effect (Ara-C); consequently ongoing protein and RNA, but not DNA synthesis, were necessary for the increase.

To begin examining mechanisms underlying the rise in leu-enk in culture, we used a cDNA probe, clone pHPE-9, derived from human pheochromocytoma, located at the Pst I site of pBR322. This

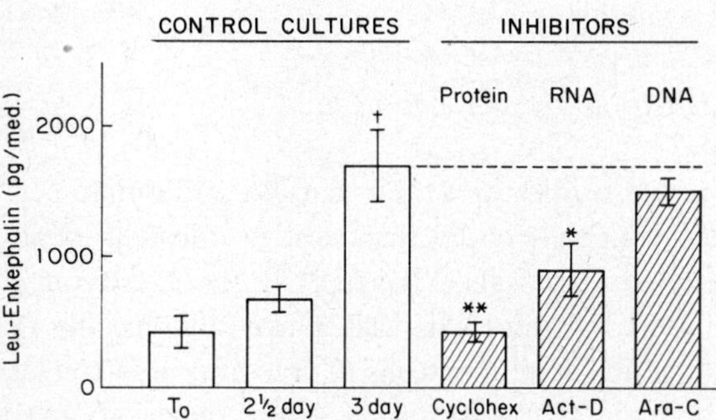

Fig. 3. Effects of metabolic inhibitors on medullary leu-enkephalin content. Groups of 8 medulla were cultured for 2½ days as described in Methods. Control 2½-day medullae were then removed and frozen at −20°C along with zero time samples. In the remaining four groups, the medium was changed and either control medium or medium plus metabolic inhibitors were added as indicated: Cycloheximide (2 mg/ml), Actinomycin-D (1 mg/ml) and Arabinosylcytosine (Ara-C, 10^{-5} M). After 12 h incubation, explants were harvested and leu-enkephalin content was determined by radioimmunoassay. Values represent mean ± S.E.M. of duplicate samples for groups of 8 medullae. * $p < 0.005$ and ** $p < 0.001$ compared to 3-day samples; + $p < 0.001$ compared to zero time or 2½-day samples by analysis of variance and Neuman-Keuls tests. (Data derived from LaGamma et al., 1986.)

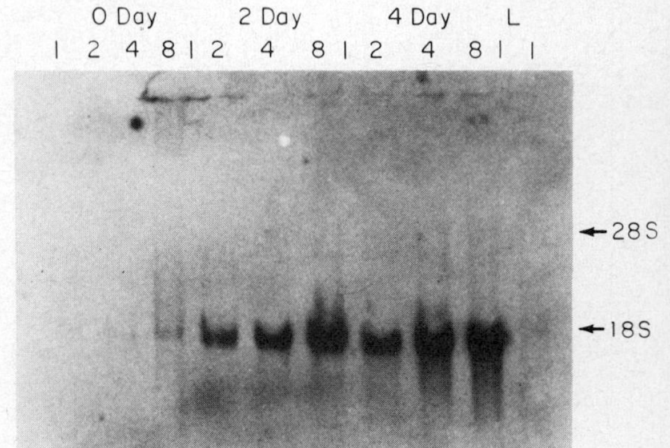

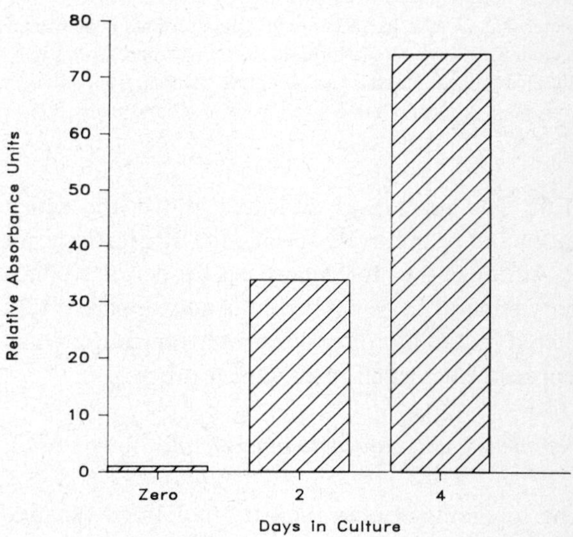

Fig. 4. Top: Time course of increase in preproenkephalin mRNA in cultured medullae. Groups of 10 medullae were grown in culture for zero, 2 or 4 days and then processed for analysis. Two, 4, or 8 μg of extracted nucleic acids were separated on a denaturing gel, transferred to Gene Screen-Plus membrane and hybridized to the preproenkephalin cDNA probe. Prior to autoradiography at −70°C, the RNA blot was washed (2 × SSC 55°C containing 1% SDS) three times at room temperature for 30 min. In each of the culture groups a striking proportional increase in a single 1.5 kb hybridizable species of RNA was detected. At zero time this band was seen only at the highest concentration employed. However, the band was not detected in nucleic acids extracted from non-neuronal tissue controls (liver). Bottom: Quantitation of preproenkephalin mRNA by densitometric scanning: densitometric analysis of the above autoradiogram revealed 34- and 74-fold increases in hybridized material after 2 and 4 days in culture, compared to zero time. (Data derived from LaGamma et al., 1986.)

clone was kindly provided by Dr. E. Herbert (Comb et al., 1982). To determine whether the increase in leu-enk was associated with a rise in mRNA coding for the opiate peptide precursor molecule, preproenkephalin mRNA levels were determined after 4 days in culture. RNA dot hybridization demonstrated a striking increase in preproenkephalin mRNA, compared to freshly dissected (zero time) medullae.

To characterize the apparent increase in preproenkephalin mRNA in greater detail, northern blot analysis was performed on zero time, 2- and 4-day cultured medullae (Fig. 4). Three different concentrations of RNA were employed for each group. At zero time, a faintly positive, approximately 1.4 kb band was detectable only at the highest concentration at the exposure time used (Fig. 4). The cDNA probe hybridized only to this 1.4 kb band in all medullae. However, after explantation there was a striking increase in preproenkephalin mRNA: densitometric analysis revealed a 34-fold

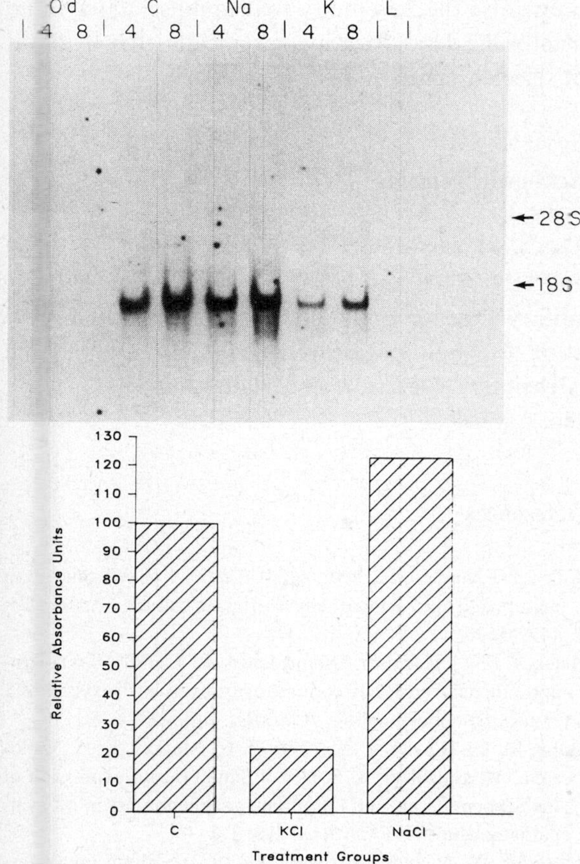

Fig. 5. Top: Effect of KCl depolarization on medullary preproenkephalin mRNA in culture. Groups of 10 medullae were grown for 2 days under standard conditions. In two groups, potassium chloride (50 mM) or 50 mM NaCl were added directly to the medium. Medullae were harvested and processed as in Fig. 2. A single hybridizable species of preproenkephalin mRNA was identified under all culture conditions: 4-day control (C), NaCl (Na), KCl (K). No preproenkephalin mRNA was detected in zero time (0 days) medullae at the exposure used, or in non-neuronal control tissue (liver, L). Numbers above lanes indicate amount (μg) of nucleic acids loaded on the gel. Bottom: Quantitation of preproenkephalin mRNA after depolarization: Densitometric analysis of the above autoradiogram indicated that K^+ treatment resulted in a 78% inhibition of the increase in mRNA; while the preproenkephalin mRNA content of the Na^+-treated control cultures were essentially not different from the untreated control group. (Data derived from LaGamma et al., 1986.)

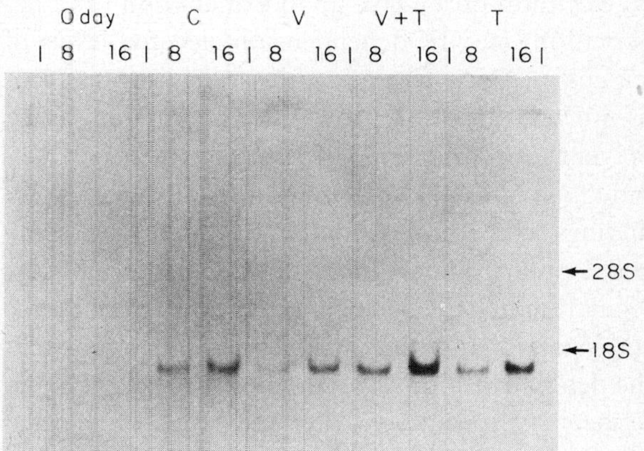

Fig. 6. Effect of veratridine-induced depolarization on medullary preproenkephalin mRNA in culture. Groups of 10 medullae were grown for 2 days under standard conditions. Veratridine (V, 10^{-5} M), tetrodotoxin (T, 10^{-7} M) or both drugs (V+T) were added to the medium at zero time. Control cultures (C) had no drug added. Medullae were harvested and processed as in Fig. 2. Densitometric scanning revealed that veratridine treated cultures had 66% of the hybridizable mRNA compared to the 2 day untreated control cultures. Tetrodotoxin prevented the effect of veratridine on preproenkephalin mRNA without inhibiting its rise when added alone. Zero time medullae (0 day) showed no hybridizable RNA at the exposure time used. Numbers above lanes indicate amount (μg) of nucleic acids loaded on the gel. (Data derived from LaGamma et al., 1986.)

rise after 2 days, and a 74-fold increase after 4 days of culture (Fig. 4). No preproenkephalin mRNA was detected in liver controls or adrenal cortex (not shown) at the exposure time employed.

To determine whether depolarization altered levels of preproenkephalin mRNA, medullae were cultured in the presence of 50 mM potassium chloride. Exposure to elevated potassium inhibited the increase in mRNA at 2 days (Fig. 5). Moreover, the depolarizing agent veratridine (see above) reproduced the effects of potassium, inhibiting the rise in preproenkephalin mRNA (Fig. 6). Tetrodotoxin, which antagonizes the effects of veratridine on sodium ion channels, prevented the effects of veratridine on preproenkephalin mRNA.

In summary, our observations indicate that the normal increase in leu-enk is dependent on ongoing mRNA synthesis, and that the rise in specific message coding for the enkephalin precursor precedes the actual increase in neurohormone. Consequently, elevation of leu-enk upon explanation (and denervation) may be dependent on elevated levels of leu-enk mRNA. Further, our studies suggest that membrane depolarization and sodium ion influx prevent accumulation of specific message. Although additional information is required, these findings raise the possibility that impulse activity and depolarization regulate read-out. Alternatively, regulation may be occurring at the level of message stabilization. In either instance, it is apparent that the depolarization of the neuroendocrine cell membrane may specifically alter the levels of selected species of mRNA encoding co-localized neurohumours.

Summary and conclusions

Our studies of sympathetic neurons during development as well as maturity, indicate that co-localized transmitter molecules are profoundly plastic. Different co-localized transmitter systems are differentially regulated by extraneuronal stimuli such as trans-synaptic impulse traffic and depolarization. Moreover, the use of cDNA probes in sympathetic neurons and adrenal medulla has revealed that membrane depolarization and sodium ion influx specifically and differentially alter levels of mRNA coding for transmitter molecules. These observations raise the possibility that impulse activity and membrane depolarization specifically alter read-out of selected genes.

Acknowledgements

This work was supported by NIH grants NS 10259 and HD 12108 and aided by grants from the Hereditary Disease Foundation, the American Federation for Aging Research (AFAR), Inc. and the Alzheimer's Disease and Related Disorders Assn., Inc.

References

Adler, J. E. and Black, I. B. (1984) Plasticity of substance P in mature and aged sympathetic neurons in culture. *Science,* 225: 1499–1500.

Black, I. B., Chikaraishi, D. and Lewis, E. J. (1986) Trans-synaptic increase in RNA coding for tyrosine hydroxylase in a rat sympathetic ganglion. *Brain Res.* (in press).

Bohn, M. C., Kessler, J. A., Adler, J. E., Markey, K. A., Goldstein, M. and Black, I. B. (1984) Simultaneous expression of the SP-peptidergic and noradrenergic phenotypes in rat sympathetic neurons. *Brain Res.,* 298: 378–381.

Catterall, W. A. and Nirenberg, M. (1973) Sodium uptake associated with activation of action potential ionophores of cultured neuroblastoma and muscle cells. *Proc. nat. Acad. Sci. USA,* 70: 3759–3763.

Chambon, P. (1975) Eukaryotic nuclear RNA polymerases. *Ann. Rev. Biochem.,* 44: 613–638.

Comb, M., Seeburg, P. H., Adelman, J., Eiden, L. and Herbert, E. (1982) Primary structure of the human Met- and Leu-enkephalin precursor and its mRNA. *Nature (Lond.),* 295: 663–666.

Evans, M. H. (1973) Tetrodotoxin, saxitoxin, and related substances: their applications in neurbiology. *Int. Rev. Neurobiol.,* 15: 83–166.

Govoni, S., Hanbauer, I., Hexum, T. D., Yang, H.-Y. T., Kelly, G. D. and Costa, E. (1981) In vivo characterization of the mechanisms that secrete enkephalin-like peptides stored in dog adrenal medulla. *Neuropharmacology,* 20: 639–645.

Kessler, J. A. and Black, I. B. (1982) Regulation of substance P in adult rat sympathetic ganglia. *Brain Res.,* 234: 182–187.

Kessler, J. A., Adler, J. E., Bohn, M. C. and Black, I. B. (1981) Substance P in principal sympathetic neurons: regulation by impulse activity. *Science*, 214: 335–336.

Kessler, J. A., Adler, J. E., Bell, W. O. and Black, I. B. (1983) Substance P and somatostatin metabolism in sympathetic and special sensory ganglia in vitro. *Neuroscience*, 9: 309–318.

LaGamma, E. F., Adler, J. E. and Black, I. B. (1984) Impulse activity differentially regulates leu-enkephalin and catecholamine characters in the adrenal medulla. *Science*, 224: 1102–1104.

LaGamma, E. F., White, J. D., Adler, J. E., Krause, J. E., McKelvy, J. F. and Black, I. B. (1986) Depolarization regulates adrenal preproenkephalin mRNA. *Proc. nat. Acad. Sci. USA*, 82: 8252–8255.

Lewis, E. J., Tank, A. W., Weiner, N. and Chikaraishi, D. M. (1983) Regulation of tyrosine hydroxylase mRNA by glucocorticoid and cyclic AMP in a rat pheochromocytoma cell line. Isolation of a cDNA clone for tyrosine hydroxylase mRNA. *J. Biol. Chem.*, 258: 14632–14637.

Livett, B. G., Dean, D. M., Whelan, L. G., Udenfriend, S. and Rossier, J. (1981) Co-release of enkephalin and catecholamines from cultured adrenal chromaffin cells. *Nature (Lond.)*, 289: 317–319.

Mueller, R. A., Thoenen, H. and Axelrod, J. (1969a) Increase in tyrosine hydroxylase activity after reserpine administration. *J. Pharmacol. exp. Ther.*, 169: 74–79.

Mueller, R. A., Thoenen, H. and Axelrod, J. (1969b) Inhibition of trans-synaptically increased tyrosine hydroxylase activity by cycloheximide and actinomycin D. *Molec. Pharmacol.*, 5: 463–469.

Ulbrecht, W. (1964) The effect of veratridine on excitable membranes of nerve and muscle. *Ergebn. Physiol.*, 61: 18–70.

Viveros, O. H., Diliberto, E. J., Hazum, E. and Chang, K.-J. (1979) Opiate-like materials in the adrenal medulla: evidence for storage and secretion with catecholamines. *Molec. Pharmacol.*, 16: 1101–1108.

Wilson, S. P., Chang, K.-J. and Viveros, O. H. (1982) Proportional secretion of opioid peptides and catecholamines from adrenal chromaffin cells in culture. *J. Neurosci.*, 2: 1150–1156.

T. Hökfelt, K. Fuxe and B. Pernow (Eds.),
Progress in Brain Research, Vol. 68

CHAPTER 9

Coexistence during ontogeny and transplantation

M. Schultzberg[1], G. A. Foster[2], F. H. Gage[3], A. Björklund[4] and T. Hökfelt[5]

[1]*Astra Pharmaceuticals, Södertälje, Sweden,* [2]*Department of Physiology, University College, Cardiff, U.K.,* [3]*Salk Institute, San Diego, U.S.A.,* [4]*Department of Histology, Lund University, Lund, Sweden and* [5]*Department of Histology, Karolinska Institute, Stockholm, Sweden*

The discovery of more than one putative transmitter substance in one and the same neurone has become an abundant phenomenon during the past decade. The first evidence found in the mammalian nervous system was the presence of somatostatin-like immunoreactivity in noradrenergic principal ganglion cells in prevertebral sympathetic ganglia (Hökfelt et al., 1977). Since then, many cases of coexistence, mostly between neuropeptides and "classical" neurotransmitters, have been found both in the central and peripheral nervous system (for review see Hökfelt et al., 1982).

The ontogeny of different transmitter-identified neuronal populations has been extensively investigated. Knowledge of a transmitter's ontogeny may be useful in several circumstances. For example, the relation between the first appearance of a transmitter and the start of a physiological process can be elucidated. It also aids in deciding at what stage, and the exact border of a region from which tissue should be taken for culture studies or transplantations. Furthermore, in the case when neuroactive substances are co-localized, the relationship between the ontogenesis may provide information on their plasticity and factors regulating their transmitter phenotypy. The development of neurones containing catecholamines (Olson and Seiger, 1972, 1973), and their synthetic enzymes (Specht et al., 1981a, b; Foster et al., 1985e), 5-hydroxytryptamine (5-HT) (Olson and Seiger, 1972; Seiger and Olson, 1973), somatostatin (Shiosaka et al., 1982), neurotensin (Hara et al., 1982), enkephalin (Palmer et al., 1982; Senba et al., 1982), substance P (SP) (Inagaki et al., 1982), cholecystokinin (CCK) (Kiyama et al., 1983), α-melanocyte stimulating hormone (Loh et al., 1980) and insulin (Dorn et al., 1984) has been described. In this chapter, a brief account of the embryonic ontogeny of neuropeptide Y (NPY) (Foster and Schultzberg, 1984) is given, and its relationship to the development of tyrosine hydroxylase (TH)-containing neurones is described in view of the coexistence of NPY and catecholamines (Everitt et al., 1984). The relationship between TH- and phenylethanolamine *N*-methyltransferase (PNMT)-containing neurones during foetal life will also be discussed.

The plasticity of transmitter phenotypic expression in co-storing neurones from the central nervous system was also studied in a transplantation model. Ever since the beginning of the century, grafting of neuronal tissue into the mammalian central nervous system has been attempted (Saltykow, 1905; Dunn, 1917; Tidd, 1932). It is only over the last decade, however, that conditions for reliable survival of the transplanted cells have been characterized. Several studies with a variety of experimental models indicate that the transplanted tissue survives and may reverse some lesion-induced, age-induced or genetic behavioural syndromes (Perlow et al., 1979; Björklund and Stenevi, 1979; Gash et al., 1980; Dunnett et al., 1981a,b, 1982, 1985; Krieger et al., 1982; Gage et al., 1983, 1984b), or partly compensate specific neurochemical deficits (Freed et al., 1980; Schmidt et al., 1982, 1983; Björklund et al., 1983).

In the present study two "coexistence systems" were analyzed, i.e. the mesencephalic dopamine (DA) neurones, some of which contain CCK-like immunoreactivity (Hökfelt et al., 1980), and the 5-HT neurones in the raphé nucleus, of which some contain SP- and/or thyrotropin-releasing hormone (TRH)-like immunoreactivity (Hökfelt et al., 1978; Johansson et al., 1981). The mesencephalic CA/CCK neurones were transplanted either as solid grafts placed above the striatum (Schultzberg et al., 1984) or as cell suspensions injected directly into the brain. The latter method was employed also for the raphé neurones (Foster et al., 1985a,b,c,d).

Methods

The method for solid grafting was carried out according to Björklund et al. (1980). Small pieces of mesencephalon from the ventral tegmental area of 16 to 17-day rat embryos were placed in preformed cavities in the cerebral cortex above the striatum of the adult rat. The dopaminergic innervation was depleted by a previous injection of 8 μg 6-hydroxydopamine (Marshall and Ungerstedt, 1977; Björklund et al., 1980). The cell suspension technique was based on that described by Björklund et al. (1983). This technique provides a situation where the influence of the host environment on individual cells is likely to be more marked than in the solid grafts. Therefore, this method may be favourable when the aim is to evaluate the possible effects that the surrounding host brain has on the anatomical and neurochemical development of the transplanted neurones. Another advantage with this technique is that it makes it feasible to implant the cells in most brain regions, whereas the solid tissue grafting is limited to outer areas or to the ventricles. Cell suspensions were made from 13 to 15 days embryonic tissue from the ventral tegmental area, and the mesencephalic and medullary raphé nuclei, respectively. The cells were injected stereotaxically into various sites, after previous lesion by neurotoxins. The serotoninergic innervation was depleted by 150 μg 5,7-dihydroxytryptamine given intraventricularly (Baumgarten et al., 1973). The cells from the ventral tegmental area were injected into the caudate nucleus, both rostrally and caudally, and into the nucleus accumbens. The cells from the raphé nuclei were implanted into the spinal cord, hippocampus or rostral and caudal caudate nucleus.

Two to 12 months after transplantation the rats were taken for immunohistochemistry. Some were given colchicine, either into the lateral ventricle or directly into the relevant area of the central nervous system, 24 h prior to perfusion with 4% paraformaldehyde containing 0.2% picric acid (Zamboni and de Martino, 1967). After rinsing in 10% sucrose in 0.1 M Sörensen phosphate buffer (pH 7.4), the tissues were processed for immunohistochemistry according to the method of Coons and collaborators (1958). The grafts from ventral tegmentum were studied with antisera to CCK and TH, and SP, 5-HT, TRH and TH antisera were applied to the raphé transplants.

The rat embryos used for studies on ontogeny were removed from anaesthetized pregnant females at various gestational ages. The dissection of brain and spinal cord was performed under the surface of the fixation solution, and then immersed in the same fixative, i.e. Zamboni's fixative (see above) or 0.4% parabenzoquinone (PBQ) in 0.1 M cacodylate buffer. The immunohistochemical procedure for adult brain tissue was followed. Antibodies to NPY, TH and PNMT were used.

Figs. 1 and 2. Schematic representation of NPY-(✱) and TH-(●)-like immunoreactive cell bodies in the rat brain on day 17 of gestation (Fig. 1 A–D) and newborn (0 days) (Fig. 2 A–D). The symbol (✪) is used where TH- and NPY-like immunoreactivity were found in the same cell. Each symbol represents 1–3 cells per 14 μm thick section, taken in the frontal plane. Neuroanatomical nomenclature and abbreviations for the various areas of the brain were based on that of Paxinos and Watson (1982). Bar indicates 1.0 mm.

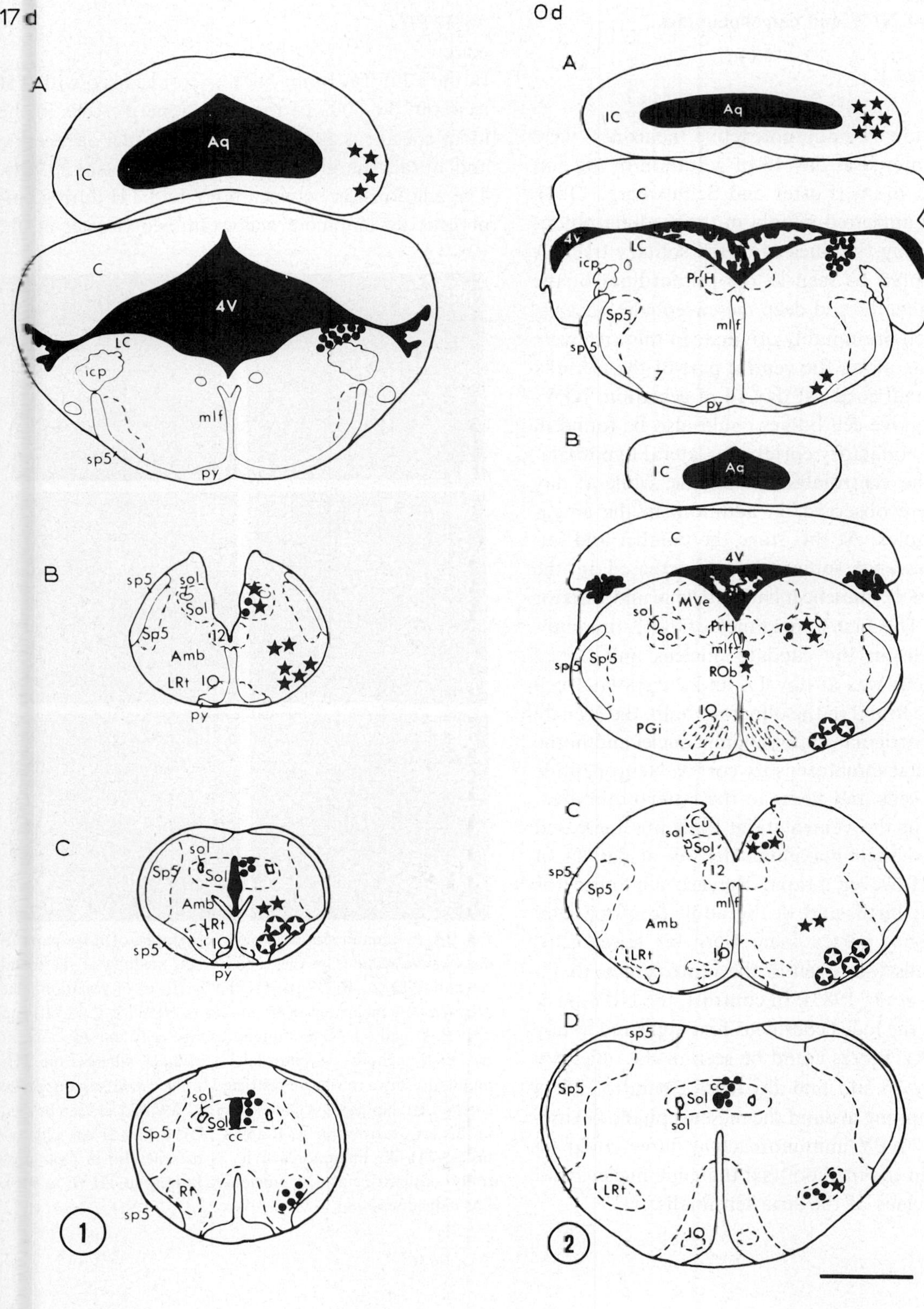

17 d
A
IC
Aq
C
4V
LC
icp
mlf
sp5
py
B
sp5
sol
Sol
Sp5
12
Amb
LRt
IO
py
C
sol
Sp5
Sol
Amb
LRt
IO
sp5
py
D
sol
Sol
Sp5
cc
Rt
sp5
1
Od
A
IC
Aq
C
4V
LC
icp
PrH
Sp5
sp5
mlf
7
py
B
IC
Aq
C
4V
MVe
sol
Sol
PrH
sp5
Sp5
mlf
ROb
IO
PGi
C
Cu
sol
Sol
12
sp5
Sp5
mlf
Amb
LRt
IO
D
sp5
Sp5
Sol
cc
sol
LRt
IO
2

Ontogeny of NPY and catecholamines

Neuropeptide Y

Neuropeptide Y-immunoreactive neurones were first encountered at day 13 of gestation in the embryonic rat brain (Foster and Schultzberg, 1984). These cells appeared mainly in the medulla oblongata, including the nucleus of the solitary tract. A few cells could be seen in the primordium of the inferior colliculus and deep mesencephalic nucleus. Fibres which presumably originate in this area were seen running along the ventral part of the medulla into the spinal cord. At day 14 of gestation, NPY-immunoreactive cell bodies could also be found in the primary olfactory cortex, the lateral hypothalamus and the ventrolateral thalamus, while at day 16 cells were observed, in addition, in the amygdaloid complex. At this stage the number and immunofluorescence intensity had increased in the thalamus, deep mesencephalic nucleus and inferior colliculus. The first appearance of NPY-immunoreactive cells in the caudate nucleus and dorsal raphé nucleus was at day 17, and 2 days later cell bodies were found in the olfactory bulb, the arcuate and paraventricular hypothalamic nuclei and in the frontoparietal somatosensory cortex. Neuropeptide Y-positive cells and fibres in the latter brain area, as well as in the ventrolateral thalamus increased and reached their maximum density at day 21 of gestation. However, a rapid decrease in number was observed at birth, and in the adult frontoparietal somatosensory cortex there were far fewer cells, while no cells were seen in the ventrolateral thalamus (Allen et al., 1983). In contrast, the NPY-positive cells in the locus coeruleus first appeared at day 21 (Fig. 2A). Fibres could be seen in the olfactory bulb at day 16 and one day later a band of fibres was seen running around the mesencephalic flexure. At day 19, NPY-immunoreactive fibres could be visualized in the mediodorsal thalamic nucleus and the bed nucleus of the stria terminalis.

NPY/TH

In the adult rat brain NPY is co-localized with TH in about 30–50% of the noradrenergic cells in the locus coeruleus as well as in many other adrenergic and noradrenergic neurones (Everitt et al., 1984). The relationship between NPY and TH during embryonic development was examined (Foster et al., 1984).

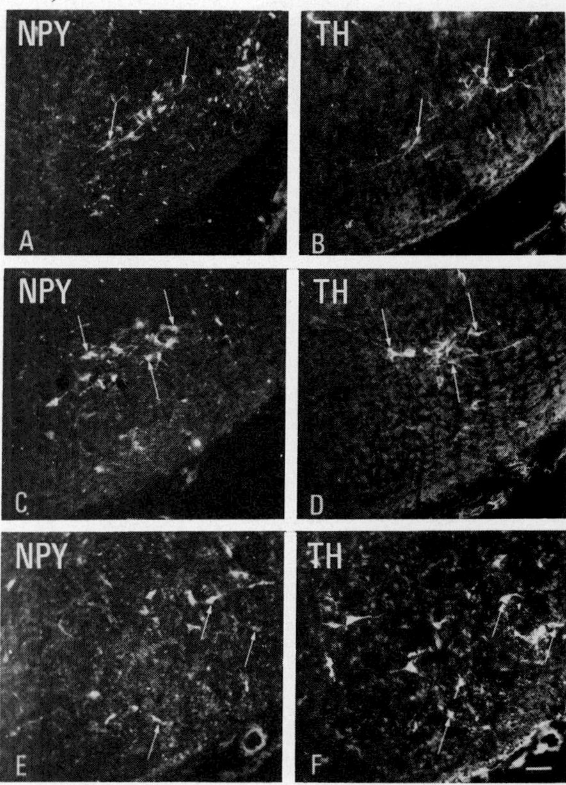

Fig. 3A–F. Immunofluorescence micrographs of three pairs of consecutive sections of the ventrolateral medulla of the foetal rat at day 13 (A, B), 17 (C, D) and 21 (E, F) of gestation. The sections were incubated with antisera to NPY (A, C and E) and TH (B, D and F). NPY-immunoreactive cells first appeared at day 13 thoughout the ventrolateral medulla, whereas the TH-immunoreactive cells were restricted to the caudal region, in the caudal LRt. Numerous cells co-storing NPY and TH can be seen in this area (arrows in A, B and C, D). In the 21-day-old embryos, TH-like immunoreactivity is present also in more rostrally localized neurones, previously lacking in TH (E and F). Bar indicates 50 μm.

As mentioned above, NPY-immunoreactive neurones appeared in the solitary tract nucleus at day 13 of gestation. A few TH-positive cells could also be seen at this stage, none of which contained NPY-like immunoreactivity. Both types of neurones increased in number, but even at day 21 there was no evidence of cells co-storing NPY and TH (Figs. 1 and 2). However, a few such neurones could be found in the solitary tract nucleus at the day of birth.

Cells containing NPY- and/or TH-like immunoreactivity became demonstrable in and around the lateral reticular nucleus at day 13 of gestation. The number of NPY-positive neurones increased until day 15, while the number of TH-positive cells continued to increase until after birth. An increase in the number of NPY/TH cells was also observed, and at day 21 there was an almost total coexistence of the two substances in this brain region (Figs. 1, 2 and 3).

The situation was different in the locus coeruleus, where TH-positive neurones occurred at day 13 of gestation, but NPY-immunoreactive cells did not become visible until day 21 (Figs. 1 and 2). The NPY-like immunoreactivity appeared in the TH-positive cells, but these co-storing cells constituted less than 10% of the total number of cells, which is a smaller proportion than observed in adults.

TH/PNMT

The foetal development of the C1-C3 groups of adrenergic neurones and the A1-A2 groups of noradrenergic neurones in the medulla oblongata was investigated (Foster et al., 1985e). Many TH-immunoreactive cells occurred in the medulla oblongata, presumably constituting the A1-A2 group, at day 11 of gestation, and increased until day 13. The PNMT-immunoreactive neurones first appeared at day 13 in a region rostral to the TH-positive neurones. One day later the noradrenergic (and only TH-positive) cells were localized in the medial and ventrolateral caudal medulla, whereas the PNMT-positive cells occurred more rostrally quite separate from the noradrenergic neurones. Interestingly, no TH-like immunoreactivity could be seen in the PNMT-storing neurones. At day 16 of gestation, TH-like immunoreactivity started to appear in PNMT-positive cells in the caudal part of the C1 group. Progressively more and more rostrally located PNMT-containing neurones of the C1 group were TH-immunoreactive in later embryonic stages, until the day of birth when almost all of them stored both substances (Fig. 4A–F). Such a caudo-rostral wave of appearance of TH-like immunoreactivity was not observed in the C2 group, although an increasing proportion of cells were co-storing.

Cells of the C3 group showed PNMT-, but not TH-like immunoreactivity, for the first time at day 16. Also in this cell group a caudo-rostral wave of TH occurrence could be seen, and at day 20 virtually all PNMT-positive neurones were TH-positive.

Transplantation of CCK/DA neurones

Cell bodies

Solid grafts of the ventral tegmental area of the embryonic mesencephalon were placed in a cavity on top of the rostral caudate nucleus. A typical graft attached well, grew and was found at the bottom of the cavity mostly in close association with the surrounding brain tissue (Fig. 5A–B). The immunohistochemical analysis showed that three types of cells survived the procedure of grafting (Schultzberg et al., 1984). Tyrosine hydroxylase-immunoreactive cells, i.e. DA-containing, and CCK-immunoreactive cells were found, and in addition cells immunoreactive to both TH and CCK could be seen (Fig. 5A–B). The DA neurones were most numerous, comprising about 50% of all cells counted. The cells co-storing TH- and CCK-like immunoreactivity consisted of 35% and the solely CCK-immunoreactive cells made up 15%. These relative proportions were similar to those observed in the ventral tegmentum of the adult rat brain (Hökfelt et al., 1980). Survival of all three types of cells could also be seen when cell suspensions of the

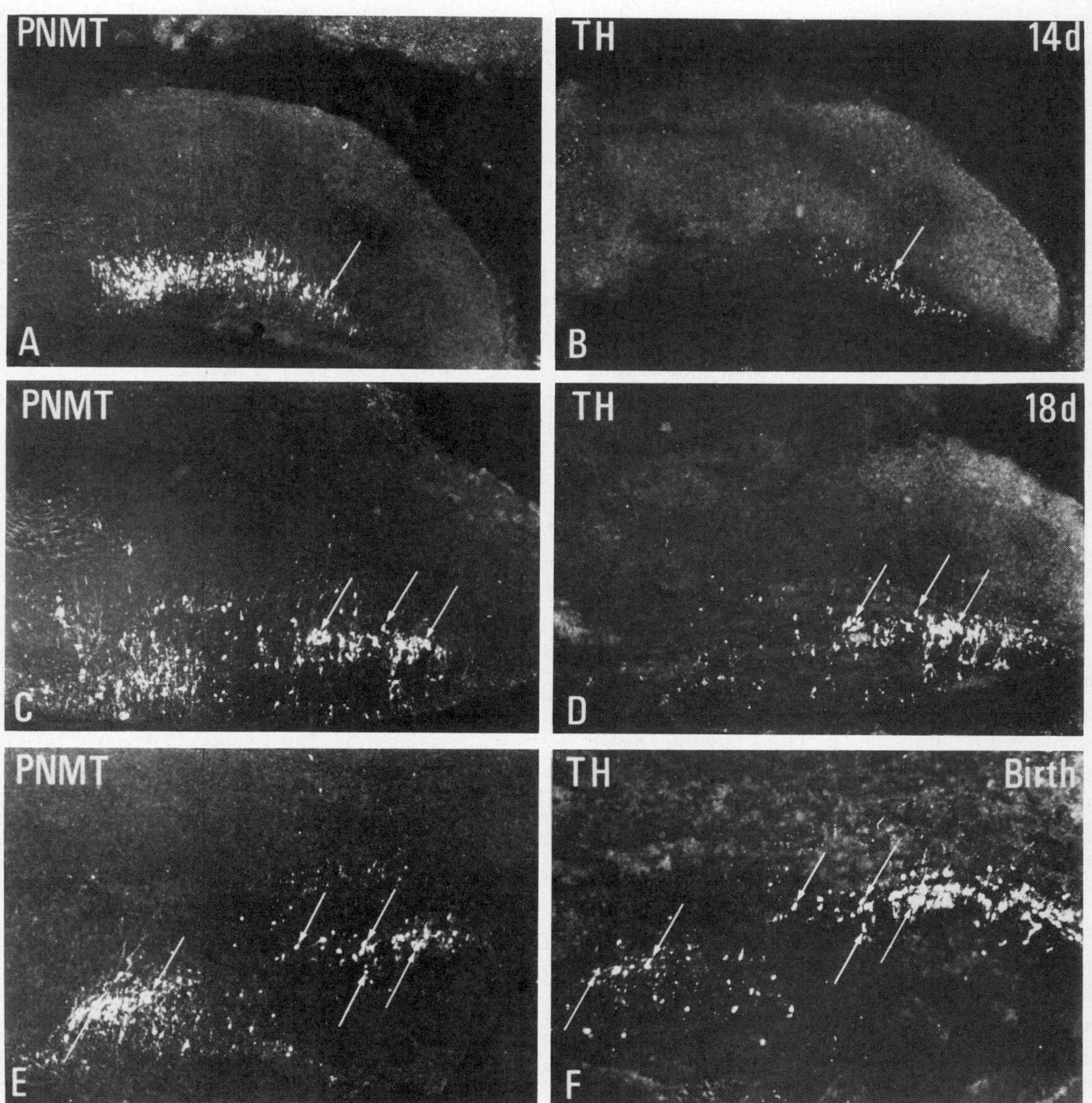

Fig. 4A–F. Immunofluorescence micrographs of three pairs of consecutive sections of the medulla oblongata in the sagittal plane at days 14 (A, B), and 18 (C, D) of gestation and at birth (E, F). The sections were incubated with antibodies to PNMT (A, C and E) and TH (B, D and F). Arrows indicate cells co-storing PNMT- and TH-like immunoreactivity. Note the appearance of TH-like immunoreactivity in a gradually more rostral region. Bar indicates 50 μM.

embryonic tissue were injected into the caudate and nucleus accumbens (Fig. 6A,B).

Outgrowth of fibres

After transplantation of solid grafts and extensive growth of TH-immunoreactive fibres into the surrounding striatum was seen (Fig. 5B), in agreement with earlier findings by Björklund et al. (1980) and Perlow et al. (1979), where the DA fibres were visualized by formalin-induced histofluorescence. However, although there was a fairly dense network of

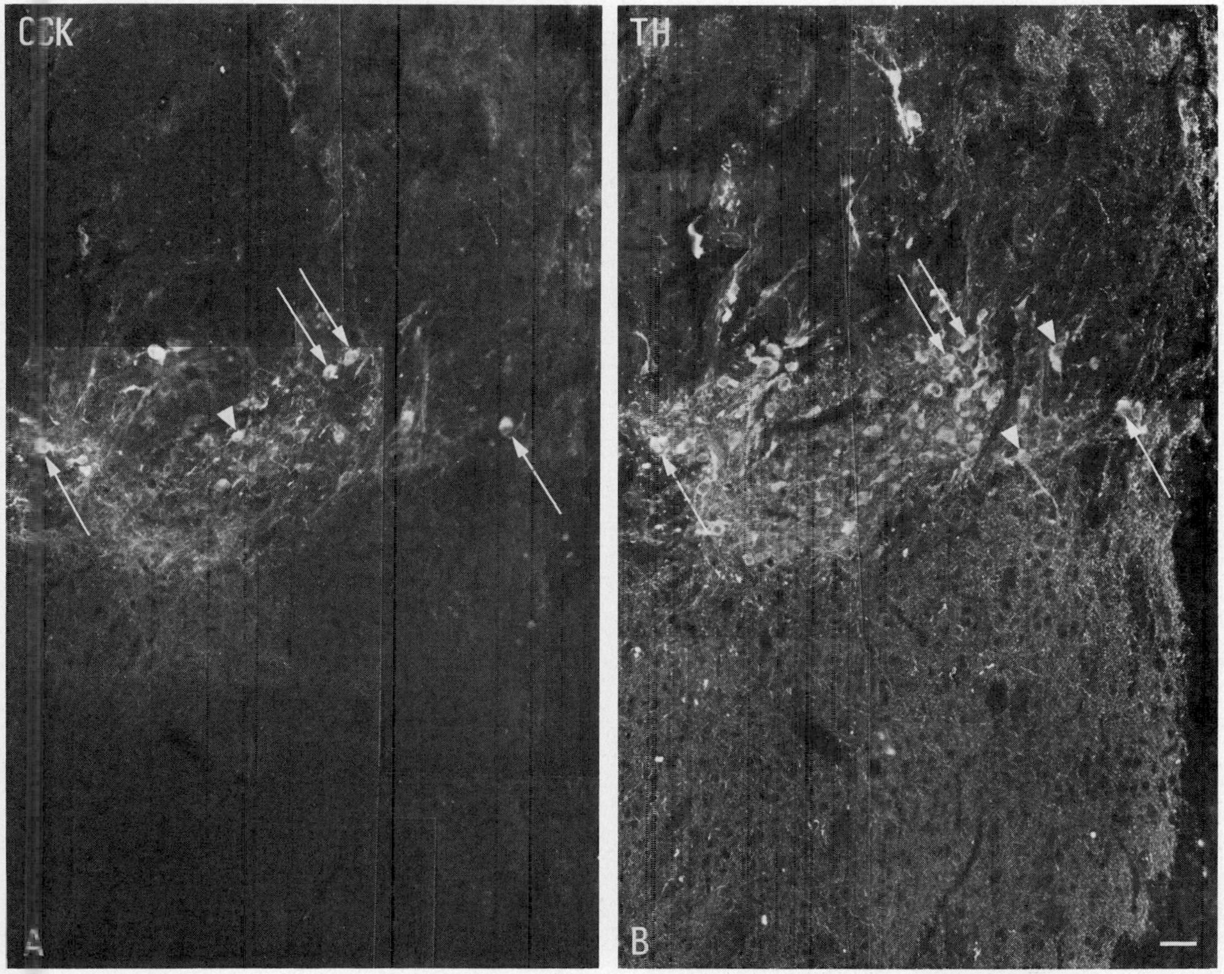

Fig. 5A–B. Immunofluorescence micrographs of a section of an embryonic ventral mesencephalic transplant to the striatum after incubation with antisera to CCK (A) and TH (B). After elution of the CCK-like immunoreactivity according to Tramu et al. (1978), the section was restained with TH antibodies (B). A large number of cells immunoreactive to both CCK and TH can be seen (arrows in A and B). Cells with only one of the two substances are also present (arrow heads). A dense network of outgrowing TH-immunoreactive fibres extend well into the host striatum (B). Many CCK-positive fibres are seen within the graft, but only a limited outgrowth is seen in surrounding striatum (A). Bar indicates 50 μm.

CCK-immunoreactive fibres within the transplants, they extended only a comparatively short distance into the host striatum (Fig. 5A). This may be due to the fact that the dorsal caudate nucleus probably is not the projection area for the DA/CCK neurones in the ventral tegmental area of the mesencephalon (Hökfelt et al., 1980). Instead, retrograde tracing with fluorescent dyes combined with immunohistochemistry have demonstrated that these neurones have terminals, for example, in the nucleus accumbens. Also the tail of the caudate nucleus may represent a target area for DA/CCK neurones. Therefore, outgrowth of the various fibres was studied after injection of cell suspensions of the ventral tegmental area to these sites. The outgrowth of TH-immunoreactive fibres from grafts in the nu-

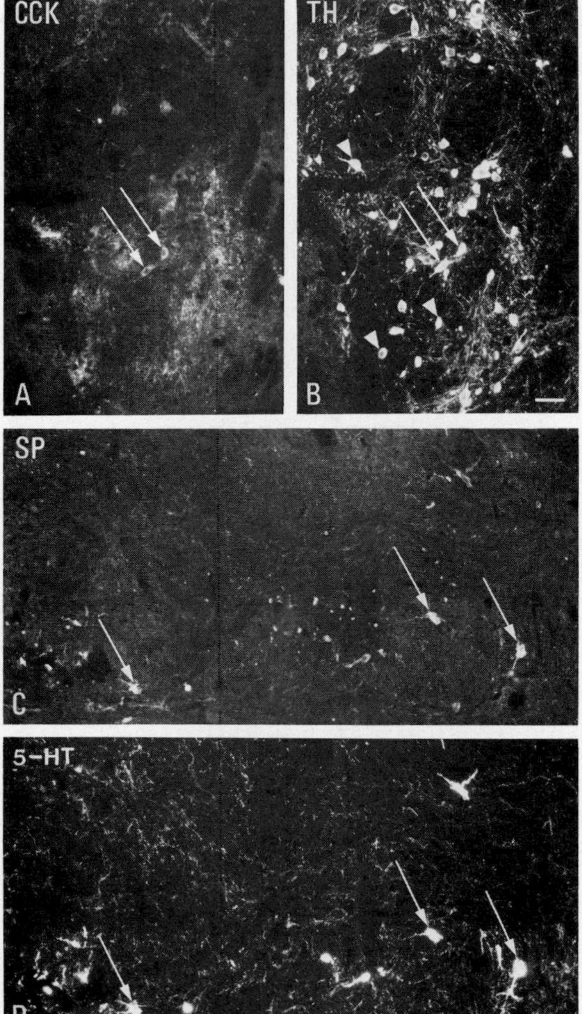

Fig. 6A–D. Immunofluorescence micrographs of sections of a cell suspension of embryonic ventral mesencephalon injected into the adult rat striatum (A, B), and of medullary raphé neurones injected into the spinal cord (C, D). The sections were incubated with antisera to CCK (A), TH (B), SP (C) and 5-HT (D). B is the same section as A after elution and restaining. A large number of TH-positive cells are seen (B), with (arrows in A and B) and without (arrow head in B) CCK-like immunoreactivity. Many cells co-storing SP- and 5-HT-like immunoreactivity are observed in the transplant of medullary raphé to the spinal cord (arrows in C and D). Bars indicate 50 μm.

cleus accumbens and the tail of the caudate nucleus was as extensive as in the dorsal striatum. A very sparse network of weakly fluorescent CCK-immunoreactive fibres emanated from the transplant in the nucleus accumbens, but the evaluation was made difficult by the fact that the 6-OH-DA treatment did not result in a complete disappearance of DA fibres. More numerous and more intensely fluorescent fibres were, however, projecting from the graft in the tail of nucleus caudatus. It appears therefore as if the environment is essential for outgrowth of the CCK-immunoreactive fibres, i.e. they need their proper target area, or otherwise the outgrowth may be inhibited. In fact, several reports have demonstrated that axonal outgrowth from mesencephalic CA neurones is regulated, at least in part, by the target tissue, both in vitro (Appel, 1981; Hemmendinger et al., 1981; Prochiantz et al., 1981) and from neural grafts in vivo (Björklund et al., 1976; 1980; Dunnett et al., 1981; Olson et al., 1979; Schmidt et al., 1981). A further conclusion from our studies is that although the milieu seems to be important for outgrowth of nerve processes, the transmitter phenotypy appears unaffected by it. The principles that govern the fibre outgrowth and transmitter phenotypy in other neurone populations, is further discussed below.

Transplantation of 5-HT/SP/TRH neurones

Embryonic neurones from the medullary and mesencephalic raphé nucleus were implanted into three different regions, i.e. the spinal cord, the hippocampus and the striatum (Foster et al., 1985a, b, c, d). The two former tissues are projection areas for the 5-HT neurones in the mesencephalic raphé nucleus, and the spinal cord is innervated by medullary 5-HT neurones (Fig. 7). A proportion of the serotoninergic neurones in the medullary raphé nucleus has been shown to contain SP-like immunoreactivity (Hökfelt et al., 1978) and some of the cells were subsequently shown to exhibit TRH-like immunoreactivity (Johansson et al., 1981). Such co-containing neurones have so far only been found in the medullary raphé, and therefore mesencephalic raphé tissue has in these transplantation experi-

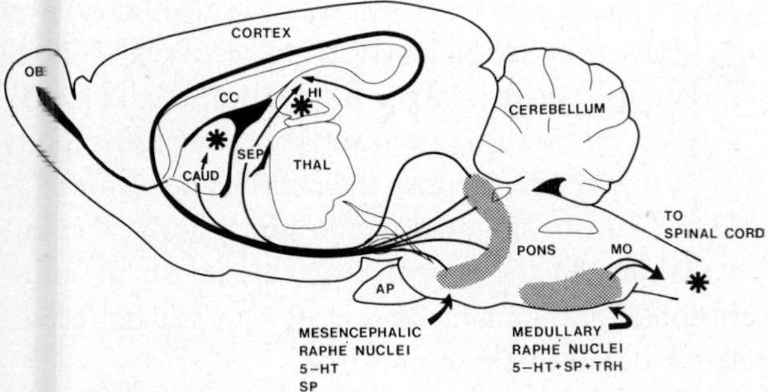

Fig. 7. Schematic drawing of a sagittal section through the adult rat brain. The mesencephalic and medullary raphé nuclei are indicated, and the major serotoninergic projections from these nuclei are delineated as shown by Parent et al. (1984). Neurones containing either 5-HT, SP and/or TRH have been demonstrated in the medullary raphé nucleus. AP = area postrema; CAUD = caudate nucleus; CC = corpus callosum; HI = hippocampus; MO = medulla oblongata; OB = olfactory bulb; SEP = septum; THAL = thalamus.

ments served as a source of 5-HT cells apparently not containing either of these two peptides (SP and TRH). The results have been summarized in Table I.

Spinal cord

Similar to the mesencephalic tissue from the ventral tegmental area, the raphé implants conglomerated to form clusters in the host tissue. In the spinal cord these clusters usually lay within the grey matter. Many intensely fluorescent 5-HT-immunoreactive neurones could be seen in the grafted raphé tissue (Figs. 6D and 8) (Foster et al., 1985b), in agreement with the abundance of serotoninergic neurones in the brain of 14-day rat embryos (Olson and Seiger, 1972; Lauder and Bloom, 1974), i.e. at the time of grafting. The number of 5-HT-immunoreactive cells in the medullary and mesencephalic raphé grafts did not seem to reflect the ratio of serotoninergic neurones found in the respective nuclei in situ. From estimates of the number of serotonin neurones in medullary raphé (Lorez et al., 1978; Descarries et al., 1979) and mesencephalic raphé (Nygren and Olson, 1977; Bowker et al., 1981) of the adult rat brain, there are about 2–2.5 times more cells in the mesencephalic raphé nucleus. In contrast, there were approximately three times as

TABLE I

The occurrence of various types of cells in transplants of medullary and mesencephalic raphé to different implantation sites (for cell types present in the adult rat raphé nuclei see footnote)

Origin	Medullary raphé[a]			Mesencephalic raphé[b]		
Transplantation site	Spinal cord	Hippocampus	Striatum	Spinal cord	Hippocampus	Striatum
Immunohistochemical markers						
5-HT	+	+	+	+	+	+
SP	+	+	+	+	+	+
TRH	+	+	+	–	–	+
5-HT + SP	+	+	+	–	+	+
5-HT + TRH	+	–	–	–	–	–
5-HT + SP + TRH	+	+	+	–	–	–

[a] Medullary raphé: 5-HT; SP; TRH; 5-HT+SP; 5-HT+TRH; 5-HT+SP+TRH; SP+TRH.
[b] Mesencephalic raphé: 5-HT; SP.

many 5-HT-immunoreactive cells to be seen in the medullary raphé grafts as in the mesencephalic transplants. In proportion to the potential number of viable 5-HT neurones that could have been injected at each site, there was a 25% (medullary) and 4% (mesencephalic) survival, respectively. The results suggest that a larger proportion of the 5-HT-positive cells in the mesencephalic raphé transplants failed to survive, or lost their ability to express 5-HT, when transplanted to the spinal cord. The unavailability of the proper target tissue for the mesencephalic raphé neurones may be a reason for selective death of those neurones.

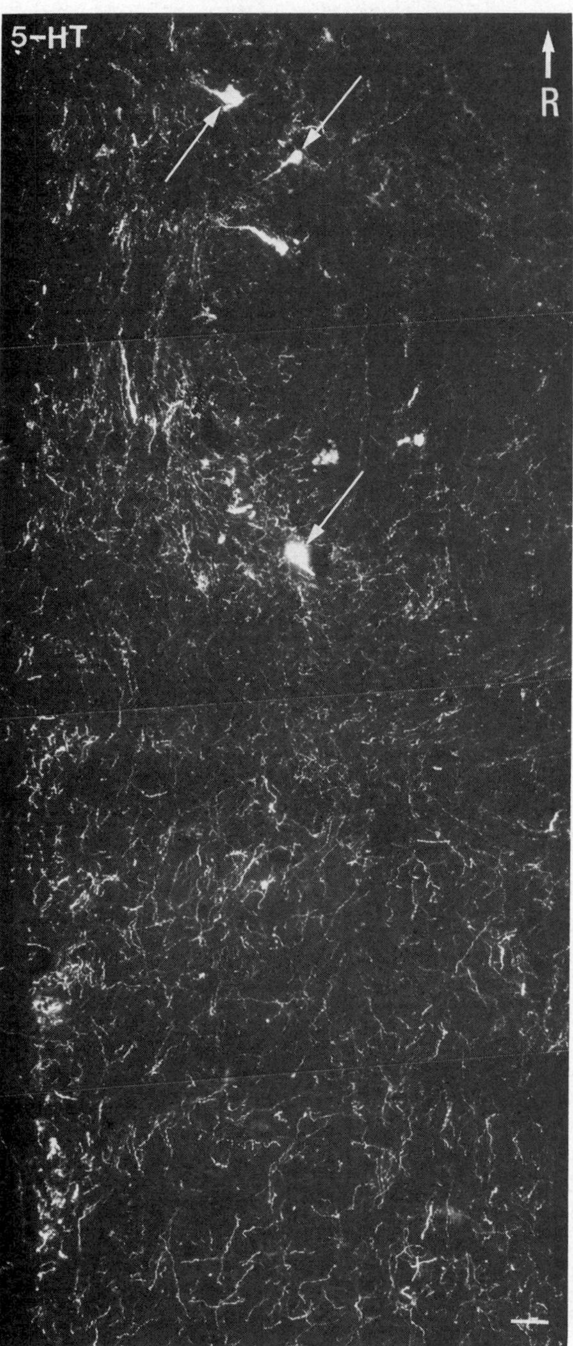

Many of the grafted cells, both medullary and mesencephalic, contained SP-like immunoreactivity (Fig. 6C), whereas TRH-like immunoreactivity only appeared in cells of the medullary raphé transplants. This finding reflects the situation in the adult rat brain, where SP- and TRH-immunoreactive cells are found in the medulla oblongata (Ljungdahl et al., 1978; Johansson et al., 1981), and only SP-immunoreactive cells in the mesencephalon (Ljungdahl et al., 1978). In the medullary raphé transplants many cells contained both 5-HT- and SP-like immunoreactivity, the proportion of which was similar to that found in situ (Hökfelt et al., 1978; Johansson et al., 1981). A small number of cells displayed all three substances. The SP-positive cells in the mesencephalic grafts were never 5-HT-positive. Thus, on the whole, the transmitter phenotype seems to be conserved after grafting to the spinal cord, whether the origin of the tissue was medullary or mesencephalic.

A dense outgrowth of 5-HT-immunoreactive fibres could be seen from both types of transplants (see Fig. 8) and the varicose fibres were seen as far as 1.5 cm away from the border of the graft. The fibres were growing in both rostral and caudal direction,b ut were mostly limited to the grey matter. A special feature was observed of the outgrowth

Fig. 8. Immunofluorescence micrograph of a horizontal section of the rat spinal cord with a graft of embryonic raphé neurones. The section was incubated with 5-HT antiserum. Some 5-HT-immunoreactive neurones can be seen in the transplant (arrows), and an extensive network of fibres are observed growing into the host spinal cord. These fibres are confined mainly to the grey matter. Bar indicates 50 μm.

from medullary raphé implants, namely a basket-like arrangement of varicose 5-HT-immunoreactive fibres surrounding motoneurones in the ventral horn. This innervation pattern was previously observed in animals with solid grafts of raphé neurones to the spinal cord (Nygren et al., 1977), and it resembled the descending innervation of motoneurones in the normal animal. The outgrowth of SP- and TRH-immunoreactive fibres was sparser than the serotoninergic innervation, but followed the same general pattern, with highest density within the graft. The SP-immunoreactive fibres extended only about 2–3 mm from the transplant, and the TRH-immunoreactive fibres even less a distance. In animals with implants of mesencephalic raphé neurones, the fibres were mostly confined to the cluster formed by the injected cell suspension.

Hippocampus

The cells injected into the hippocampus did not aggregate into spheroid clumps, but were distributed as a band approximately parallel to the hippocampal fissure (Fig. 9) (Foster et al., 1985c). The displacement of the cells with respect to the injection needle tract may, in part, be a result of some mechanical interaction with the host hippocampus, such as cleavage at the fissure. There is also a possibility that cellular migration occurred, since the band of implanted cells was often not in the fissure itself, but ventral (0–300 μm) to it.

Immunohistochemical analysis of the transplants showed that many cells contained 5-HT-like immunoreactivity (Fig. 9B). Their number was dependent on site of origin; thus the grafts from mesencephalic raphé contained about 2–2.5 times as many 5-HT-immunoreactive cells as the grafts from the medullary raphé. However, taking into account the number of serotoninergic cells in the normal adult animal, the survival was about 20% for both nuclei. The hippocampus does not appear to exert a similar repressive effect on transplanted embryonic cells from the medullary raphé nucleus as does the spinal cord on the mesencephalic raphé neurones (see above), despite the fact that the hippocampus is not the proper innervation target for the medullary 5-HT neurones.

Many SP- and TRH-immunoreactive cells were found in the medullary raphé grafts (Fig. 9B,C), whereas neurones containing SP-like but not TRH-like immunoreactivity could be seen in the transplants of the mesencephalic raphé. This agrees

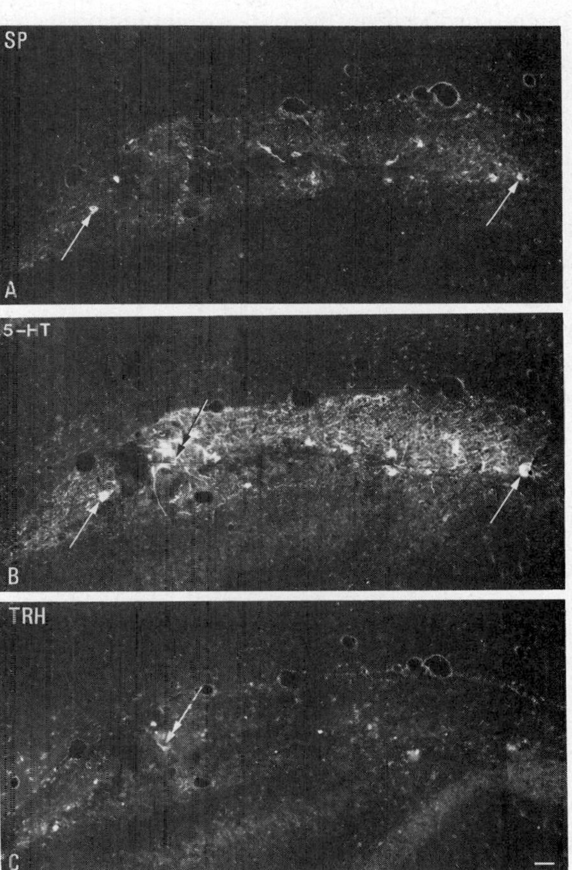

Fig. 9A–C. Immunofluorescence micrographs of consecutive sections of a cell suspension of the embryonic medullary raphé nucleus injected into the adult rat hippocampus, after incubation with antisera to SP (A), 5-HT (B) and TRH (C). The implanted cells have become reorganized in a graft parallel to the hippocampal fissure. Cells co-storing SP and 5-HT (arrows in A and B) and 5-HT and TRH (double arrows in B and C) can be seen. Many additional 5-HT-immunoreactive neurones as well as some SP-positive neurones are present. Numerous 5-HT-positive fibres emanating from the transplant extend far into the host hippocampus, preferentially the dentate gyrus. A sparse network of SP-positive fibres can be seen within the graft. Bar indicates 50 μm.

with the situation in the normal adult raphé regions, where SP- and TRH-immunoreactive cells are found in the medulla oblongata, and SP- but not TRH-immunoreactive neurones occur in the mesencephalon (Hökfelt et al., 1978; Ljungdahl et al., 1978; Johansson et al., 1981). The survival of SP- and TRH-positive cells in medullary grafts was 28 and 6%, respectively, of the potential number roughly deduced on the basis of figures presented by Johansson et al. (1981) of SP and TRH cells that were implanted. These values parallel the recoveries of SP- and TRH-immunoreactive neurones from the same suspensions, but implanted into the spinal cords of the same rats (Foster et al., 1985b). However, the proportionate survival of the medullary serotoninergic neurones differs from that of the peptidergic neurones. Although this phenomenon may be due to a lack of sensitivity of our immunohistochemical technique, it may more probably reflect an actual difference in survival, or a change in the transmitter phenotype. An indication of the latter appeared from the analysis of SP-like immunoreactivity in the transplants of mesencephalic raphé. In these, a small proportion of the 5-HT-positive neurones were also SP-immunoreactive, a co-localization which has not been observed in the mesencephalon of the normal rat (Hökfelt et al., 1978; Johansson et al., 1981; Steinbusch, 1981). Considering the fact that when the same cell suspension was transplanted to the spinal cord we failed to demonstrate a similar phenomenon, it would seem that the hippocampus provides an environment that may contain a factor(s), which either induces SP synthesis, or inhibits its repression. Kessler and Black (1982) reported a similar de novo appearance of SP in neurones of the superior cervical ganglion after deafferentation.

The outgrowth of 5-HT-immunoreactive fibres was extensive from both medullary (Fig. 9B) and mesencephalic raphé transplants to the hippocampus, although somewhat less dense from the former grafts. The proliferation of 5-HT-positive fibres into the dentate gyrus, from both types of grafts was particularly rich, while there was a sparser network in the CA1 and CA3 regions. In fact, the density of the 5-HT fibres growing into the dentate gyrus and CA4 was greater than that found in the normal hippocampus (cf. Steinbusch, 1981). It is notable that the 5-HT fibres were apparently directed towards the appropriate hippocampal regions, and even the correct laminae, but there did not seem to be any specificity with regard to the origin of the serotoninergic cells from which they arose. A sparse network of weakly immunofluorescent SP and TRH fibres could be seen within the transplants, but essentially no processes had grown into the surrounding hippocampus.

Striatum

The implants of raphé cell suspensions into the striatum formed clusters along the injection needle tract (Fig. 10). Staining with antibodies to TH visualized the border between the transplant almost completely lacking dopaminergic fibres and the host striatum with its rich dopaminergic innervation (Fig. 10A).

Numerous 5-HT-positive neurones were observed in the grafts from both medullary and mesencephalic raphé tissue (Fig. 10B) (Foster et al., 1985d). A large number of SP-immunoreactive cells could be seen both in the medullary and mesencephalic raphé transplants. In the medullary grafts a large proportion of the 5-HT-immunoreactive cells also contained SP-like immunoreactivity and such cells occurred even in the mesencephalic transplants, although to a lesser extent. Thus, the striatum appears to have a similar effect on transmitter phenotypy as the hippocampus in inducing the production of SP-like immunoreactivity in 5-HT neurones which normally seem to lack the peptide. In the medullary raphé transplants, TRH-like immunoreactivity occurred in some of the SP/5-HT cells, and in separate cells. Cells with TRH-like immunoreactivity (only) were also seen in the grafts from mesencephalic raphé. These are additional to the types of cells present normally in the mesencephalic raphé.

Extensive proliferation of 5-HT-immunoreactive fibres was observed from the mesencephalic raphé

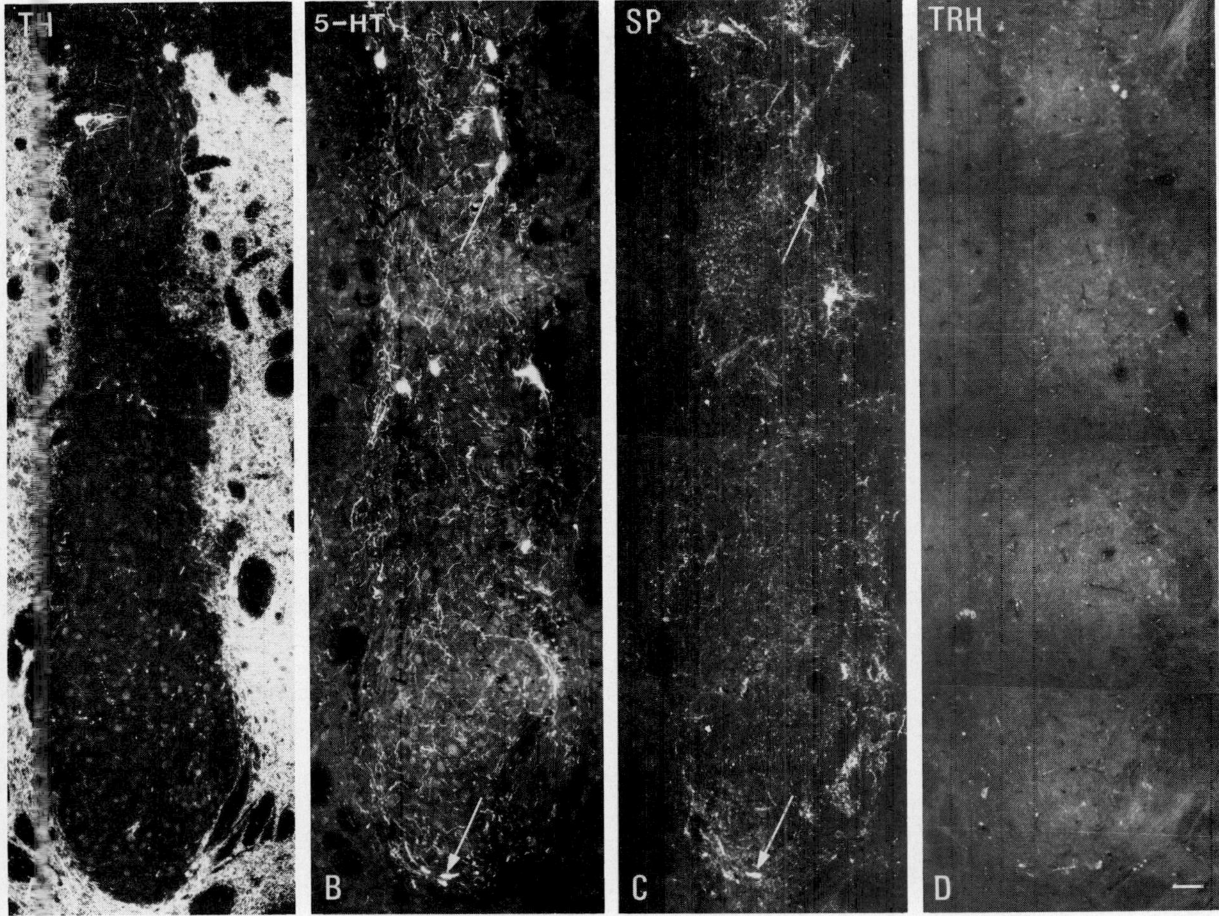

Fig. 10A–D. Immunofluorescence micrographs of consecutive sections of a suspension of embryonic cells from the medullary raphé nucleus injected into the adult rat striatum, after incubation with antisera to TH (A), 5-HT (B), SP (C) and TRH (D). The cells form a cluster, with the borders clearly seen in A where the dense network of dopaminergic fibres of the striatum is interrupted. SP-, 5-HT- and TRH-immunoreactive cells are seen, and cells co-storing SP and 5-HT are indicated by arrows (B and C). A dense network of SP- and 5-HT-immunoreactive fibres can be seen within the graft. Bar indicates 50 μm.

tissue implanted into the striatum. A sparser outgrowth was, however, seen from the medullary grafts, which may indicate that the striatum has a negative influence on these neurones since it is not their proper projection area. The mesencephalic neurones, on the other hand, do project to the striatum, and the extensive outgrowth would therefore be expected.

Nerve fibres showing SP- and TRH-like immunoreactivity, respectively, were moderately numerous within the transplants from both raphé nuclei. A sparse network was seen immediately outside the grafts, but was lacking further into the host striatum.

Conclusions

The present studies on development of different neurone populations during foetal life suggests that central neurones have a certain plasticity with regard to their transmitter phenotype. Thus, some neurones were observed to produce NPY at an early gestational stage, and then later apparently ceased to exhibit NPY-like immunoreactivity. Similar findings have been reported for the peripheral nervous system (Kessler and Black, 1982). In neurones that contain more than one neuroactive substance, there seem to be different factors regulating the synthesis of each substance. This is indicated, for example, by the differential appearance of NPY and TH in neurones in the medulla oblongata. Furthermore, different enzymes involved in the synthesis of one transmitter, such as adrenaline, may be controlled independently.

The plasticity of co-storing neurones was apparent also from the transplantation experiments. Thus, 5-HT neurons from the mesencephalic raphé nucleus appear to express an additional neuroactive substance, namely SP, when placed in the hippocampus and striatum, but not the spinal cord, and some neurones of the same origin became TRH-positive, although no TRH-immunoreactive cells could be visualized in the adult. These results suggest that the environment can influence transmitter phenotypic expression. An effect of the environment on the outgrowth of nerve fibres is indicated by the results obtained from grafting of ventral mesencephalic neurones. These CCK-immunoreactive neurones seem to require their proper target area in order to grow further into the host brain. Similarly, the outgrowth of fibres from the serotoninergic neurones from the medullary raphé nucleus is hampered when placed in the striatum, whereas they grow extensively into the spinal cord. However, the outgrowth is also extensive when these neurones are implanted into the hippocampus, although they do not normally project to this area. These findings indicate a complex and multifactorial control of expression of messenger molecules. To what extent coexisting peptides are involved in regulation of expression of transmitter phenotypy and/or in the control of growth regulation cannot be ascertained at the present stage.

Acknowledgements

The results described in this chapter have been published or will be reported in articles in press or in preparation. The studies were supported by grants from the Swedish Medical Research Council (04X-2887; 04X-3874; 14X-07161; 12P-6965), Alice och Knut Wallenbergs Stiftelse, Karolinska Institutets Fonder, Magnus Bergvalls Stiftelse and by NINCDS (06801) and NIMH (02714) grants. The immunohistochemical studies were made possible by the generous gifts of antibodies from Drs. A. C. Cuello, G. J. Dockray, M. Goldstein, L. Terenius, A. A. J. Verhofstad and T. J. Visser. We are grateful to Ms. A. Folin, Ms. W. Hiort, Ms. A. Peters and Ms. G. Stridsberg for excellent technical assistance. G. A. F. was a NATO Overseas Research Fellow.

References

Allen, Y. S., Adrian, T. E., Allen, J. M., Tatemoto, K., Crow, T. J., Bloom, S. R. and Polak, J. M. (1983) Neuropeptide Y distribution in the rat brain. *Science*, 221: 877–879.

Appel, S. H. (1981) A unifying hypothesis for the cause of amyotrophic lateral sclerosis, parkinsonism and alzheimer disease. *Ann. Neurol.*, 10: 499–505.

Baumgarten, H. G., Björklund, A., Lachemayer, L. and Nobin, A. (1973) Evaluation of the effects of 5,7-dihydroxytryptamine on serotonin and catecholamine neurons in the rat CNS. *Acta physiol. Scand.*, Suppl. 391: 1–19.

Björklund, A. and Stenevi, U. (1979) Reconstruction of the nigrostriatal dopamine pathway by intracerebral nigral transplants. *Brain Res.*, 177: 555–560.

Björklund, A., Stenevi, U. and Svendgaard, N.-Aa. (1976) Growth of transplanted monoaminergic neurones into the adult hippocampus along the perforant path. *Nature (Lond.)*, 262: 787–790.

Björklund, A., Gage, F. H., Schmidt, R. H., Stenevi, U. and Dunnett, S. B. (1983) Recovery of choline acetyltransferase activity and acetylcholine synthesis in the denervated hippocampus reinnervated by septal suspension implants. *Acta physiol. Scand.*, Suppl. 522: 59–66.

Bowker, R. M., Westlund, K. N. and Coulter, J. D. (1981) Origins of serotonergic projections to the spinal cord in rat: an immunocytochemical-retrograde transport study. *Brain Res.*, 226: 187–199.

Coons, A. H. (1958) Fluorescent antibody methods. In J. F. Danielli (Ed.), *General Cytochemical Methods*, Academic Press, New York, pp. 399–422.

Descarries, L., Beaudet, A., Watkins, K. C. and Gracia, S. (1979) The serotonin neurons in the nucleus raphé dorsalis of adult rat. *Anat. Rec.*, 193: 520.

Dorn, A., Reiser, M. and Bernstein, H. G. (1984) Insulin-like immunoreactivity in the rat brain during post-natal ontogenesis. *J. Hirnforsch.*, 25: 439–444.

Dunn, E. H. (1917) Primary and secondary findings in a series of attempts to transplant cerebral cortex in the albino rat. *J. comp. Neurol.*, 27: 565–572.

Dunnett, S. B., Björklund, A., Stenevi, U. and Iversen, S. D. (1981a) Behavioural recovery following transplantation of substantia nigra in rats subjected to 6-OHDA lesions of the nigrostriatal pathway. I. Unilateral lesion. *Brain Res.*, 215: 147–161.

Dunnett, S. B., Björklund, A., Stenevi, U. and Iversen, S. D. (1981b) Grafts of embryonic substantia nigra reinnervating the ventrolateral striatum ameliorate sensorimotor impairments and akinesia in rats with 6-OHDA lesions of the nigrostriatal pathway. *Brain Res.*, 229: 209–217.

Dunnett, S. B., Low, W. C., Iversen, S. D., Stenevi, U. and Björklund, A. (1982) Septal transplants restore maze learning in rats with fornix-fimbria lesion. *Brain Res.*, 251: 335–348.

Dunnett, S. B., Björklund, A., Gage, F. H. and Stenevi, U. (1985) Transplantation of mesencephalic dopamine neurones to the striatum of adult rats. In A. Björklund and U. Stenevi (Eds.), *Transplantation in the Mammalian CNS,* Elsevier Biomedical Press, Amsterdam, pp. 451–469.

Everitt, B. J. Hökfelt, T., Terenius, L., Tatemoto, K., Mutt, V. and Goldstein, M. (1984) Differential co-existence of neuropeptide Y (NPY)-like immunoreactivity with catecholamines in the central nervous system of the rat. *Neuroscience,* 11: 443–462.

Foster, G. A. and Schultzberg, M. (1984) Immunohistochemical analysis of the ontogeny of neuropeptide Y immunoreactive neurones in the foetal rat brain. *Int. J. dev. Neurosci.*, 2: 387–407.

Foster, G. A., Schultzberg, M. and Goldstein, M. (1984) Differential and independent manifestation within co-containing neurones of neuropeptide Y and tyrosine hydroxylase during ontogeny of the rat central nervous system. *Neurochem. Int.*, 6: 761–771.

Foster, G. A., Schultzberg, M., Björklund, A., Gage, F. H. and Hökfelt, T. (1985a) Fate of embryonic mesencephalic and medullary raphé neurones transplanted to the striatum, hippocampus and spinal cord of the adult rat: analysis of 5-hydroxytryptamine-, substance P- and thyrotropin releasing hormone-immunoreactive cells. In A. Björklund and U. Stenevi (Eds.), *Neural Grafting in the Mammalian CNS,* Elsevier Biomedical Press, Amsterdam, pp. 179–189.

Foster, G. A., Schultzberg, M., Gage, F. H., Björklund, A., Hökfelt, T., Nornes, H., Cuello, A. C., Verhofstad, A. A. J. and Visser, T. J. (1985b) Transmitter expression and morphological development of foetal medullary and mesencephalic raphé neurones after transplantation to the adult rat nervous system. I. Grafts to the spinal cord. *Exp. Brain Res.*, 60: 427–444.

Foster, G. A., Schultzberg, M., Gage, F. H., Björklund, A., Hökfelt, T., Cuello, A. C., Verhofstad, A. A. J. and Visser, T. J. (1985c) Transmitter expression and morphological development of embryonic medullary and mesencephalic raphé neurones after transplantation to the adult rat central nervous system. II. Grafts to the hippocampus. *Exp. Brain Res.* (in press).

Foster, G. A., Schultzberg, M., Gage, F. H., Björklund, A., Hökfelt, T., Cuello, A. C., Verhofstad, A. A. J. and Visser, T. J. (1985d) Transmitter expression and morphological development of embryonic medullary and mesencephalic raphé neurones after transplantation to the adult rat central nervous system. III. Grafts to the striatum. *Exp. Brain Res.* (submitted).

Foster, G. A., Schultzberg, M., Goldstein and Hökfelt, T. (1985e) Ontogeny of phenylethanolamine N-methyltransferase- and tyrosine hydroxylase-like immunoreactivity in presumptive adrenaline neurones of the foetal rat central nervous system. *J. comp. Neurol.*, 236: 348–381.

Freed, W. J., Perlow, M. J., Karoum, F., Seiger, Å., Olson, L., Hoffer, B. J. and Wyatt, R. J. (1980) Restoration of dopaminergic function by grafting of fetal substantia nigra to the caudate nucleus: long-term behavioral, biochemical and histochemical studies. *Ann. Neurol.*, 8: 510–526.

Gage, F. H., Dunnett, S. B., Stenevi, U. and Björklund, A. (1983) Aged rats: recovery of motor impairments by instrastriatal nigral grafts. *Science,* 221: 966–969.

Gage, F. H., Björklund, A., Stenevi, U., Dunnett, S. B. and Kelly, P. A. T. (1984) Intrahippocampal septal grafts ameliorate learning impairment in aged rats. *Science,* 225: 533–536.

Gash, D. M., Sladek, J. R., Jr. and Sladek, C. D. (1980) Functional development of grafted vasopressin neurons. *Science,* 210: 1367–1369.

Hara, Y., Shiosaka, S., Senba, E., Sakanaka, M., Inagaki, S., Takagi, H., Kawai, Y., Takatsuki, K., Matzusaki, T. and Tohyama, M. (1982) Ontogeny of the neurotensin-containing neuron system of the rat: immunohistochemical analysis-I. Forebrain and diencephalon. *J. comp. Neurol.*, 208: 177–195.

Hemmendinger, L. M., Garber, B. B., Hoffman, P. C. and Heller, A. (1981) Target neuron-specific process formation by embryonic mesencephalic dopamine neurons *in vitro. Proc. nat. Acad. Sci. USA,* 78: 1264–1268.

Hökfelt, T., Elfvin, L.-G., Elde, R., Schultzberg, M., Goldstein, M. and Luft, R. (1977) Occurrence of somatostatin-like immunoreactivity in some peripheral sympathetic noradrenergic neurons. *Proc. nat. Acad. Sci. USA,* 74: 3587–3591.

Hökfelt, T., Ljungdahl, Å., Steinbusch, H., Verhofstad, A., Nilsson, G., Brodin, E., Pernow, B. and Goldstein, M. (1978) Immunohistochemical evidence of substance P-like immunoreactivity in some 5-hydroxytryptamine-containing neurons in the rat central nervous system. *Neuroscience,* 3: 517–538.

Hökfelt, T., Lundberg, J. M., Skirboll, L., Johansson, O., Schultzberg, M. and Vincent, S. R. (1982) Coexistence of classical transmitters and peptides in neurones. In A. C. Cuello (ed.), *Co-Transmission,* MacMillan Press Ltd, London, pp. 77–125.

Hökfelt, T., Skirboll, L., Rehfeld, J. F., Goldstein, M., Markey, K. and Dann, O. (1980) A subpopulation of mesencephalic dopamine neurons projecting to limbic area contains a cholecystokinin-like peptide: evidence from immunohistochemistry combined with retrograde tracing. *Neuroscience*, 5: 2093–2124.

Inagaki, S., Sakanaka, M., Shiosaka, S., Senba, E., Takatsuki, K., Takagi, H., Kawai, Y., Minagawa, H. and Tohyama, M. (1982) Ontogeny of substance P-containing neuron system of the rat: and immunohistochemical analysis-I. Forebrain and upper brain stem. *Neuroscience*, 7: 251–277.

Johansson, O., Hökfelt, T., Pernow, B., Jeffcoate, S. L., White, N., Steinbusch, H. W. M., Verhofstad, A. A. J., Emson, P. C. and Spindel, E. (1981) Immunohistochemical support for three putative transmitters in one neuron: coexistence of 5-hydroxytryptamine-, substance P- and thyrotropin releasing hormone-like immunoreactivity in medullary neurones projecting to the spinal cord. *Neuroscience*, 6: 1857–1881.

Kessler, J. A. and Black, I. B. (1982) Regulation of substance P in adult rat sympathetic ganglia. *Brain Res.*, 234: 182–187.

Kiyama, H., Shiosaka, S., Kutoba, Y., Cho, H. J., Takagi, H., Tateishi, K., Hasimura, E., Hamaoka, T. and Tohyama, M. (1983) Ontogeny of cholecystokinin-8 containing neuron system of the rat: an immunohistochemical analysis-II. Lower brain stem. *Neuroscience*, 10: 1341–1359.

Krieger, D. T., Perlow, M. J., Gibson, M. J., Davies, T. F., Zimmerman, E. A., Ferin, M. and Charlton, H. M. (1982) Brain grafts reverse hypogonadism of gonadotropin-releasing hormone deficiency. *Nature (Lond.)*, 298: 468–471.

Lauder, J. M. and Bloom, F. E. (1974) Ontogeny of monoamine neurones in the locus coeruleus, raphé magnus and substantia nigra of the rat. I. Cell differentiation. *J. comp. Neurol.*, 155: 469–482.

Ljungdahl, Å., Hökfelt, T. and Nilsson, G. (1978) Distribution of substance P-like immunoreactivity in the central nervous system of the rat. I. Cell bodies and nerve terminals. *Neuroscience*, 3: 861–943.

Loh, Y. P., Eskay, R. L. and Brownstein, M. (1980) α-MSH-like peptides in rat brain: identification and changes in level during development. *Biochem. biophys. Res. Commun.*, 94: 916–923.

Lorez, H. P., Saner, A. and Richards, J. G. (1978) Evidence against a neurotoxic action of halogenated amphetamines on serotoninergic B9 cells. A morphometric fluorescence histochemical study. *Brain Res.*, 146: 189–194.

Nygren, L.-G. and Olson, L. (1977) Intracisternal neurotoxins and monoamine neurons innervating the spinal cord: Acute and chronic effects on cell and axon counts and nerve terminal densities. *Histochemistry*, 52: 281–306.

Nygren, L.-G. Olson, L. and Seiger, Å. (1977) Monoaminergic reinnervation of the transected spinal cord by homologous fetal brain grafts. *Brain Res.*, 129: 227–235.

Olson, L. and Seiger, Å. (1972) Early prenatal ontogeny of central monoamine neurons in the rat: fluorescence histochemical observations. *Z. Anat. Entwickl.-Gesch.*, 137: 301–316.

Olson, L., Seiger, Å., Hoffer, B. and Taylor, D. (1979) Isolated catecholaminergic projections from substantia nigra and locus coeruleus to caudate, hippocampus and cerebral cortex formed by intraocular segmental double brain grafts. *Exp. Brain Res.*, 35: 47–67.

Palmer, M. R., Miller, R. J., Olson, L. and Seiger, Å. (1982) Prenatal ontogeny of neurons with enkephalin-like immunoreactivity in the rat central nervous nervous system: an immunohistochemical mapping investigation. *Med. Biol.*, 60: 61–88.

Parent, A., Poitras, D. and Dubé, L. (1984) Comparative anatomy of central monoaminergic systems. In A. Björklund and T. Hökfelt (Eds.), *Vol. 2*, Elsevier Science Publ., Amsterdam, pp. 409–439.

Paxinos, G. and Watson, C. (1982) *The Rat Brain in Stereotaxic Coordinates*, Academic Press, Sydney.

Perlow, M. J., Freed, W. J., Hoffer, B. J., Seiger, Å., Olson, L. and Wyatt, R. J. (1979) Brain grafts reduce abnormalities produced by destruction of nigrostriatal dopamine system. *Science*, 204: 643–647.

Prochiantz, A., Daguet, M. C., Herbert, A. and Glowinski, J. (1981) Specific stimulation of *in vitro* maturation of mesencephalic dopaminergic neurons by striatal membranes. *Nature (Lond.)*, 293: 570–572.

Saltykow, S. (1905) Versuche über Gehirnreplantation, zugleich ein Beitrag zur Kenntniss reaktiver Vorgänge an den zelligen Gehrinelementen. *Arch. Psychiatr.*, 40: 239–256.

Schmidt, R. H., Björklund, A. and Stenevi, U. (1981) Intracerebral grafting of dissociated CNS tissue suspensions: a new approach for neuronal transplantation to deep brain sites. *Brain Res.*, 218: 347–356.

Schmidt, R. H., Ingvar, M., Lindvall, O., Stenevi, U. and Björklund, A. (1982) Functional activity of substantia nigra grafts reinnervating the striatum: neurotransmitter metabolism and ^{14}C-2-deoxy-D-glucose autoradiography. *J. Neurochem.*, 38: 737–748.

Schultzberg, M., Dunnett, S. B., Björklund, A., Stenevi, U., Hökfelt, T., Dockray, G. J. and Goldstein, M. (1984) Dopamine and cholecystokinin immunoreactive neurones in mesencephalic grafts reinnervating the neostriatum: evidence for selective growth regulation. *Neuroscience*, 12: 17–32.

Seiger, Å. and Olson, L. (1973) Late prenatal ontogeny of central monoamine neurons in the rat: fluorescence histochemical observations. *Z. Anat. Entwickl.-Gesch.*, 140: 281–318.

Senba, E., Shiosaka, S., Hara, Y., Inagaki, S., Kawai, Y., Takatsuki, K., Sakanaka, M., Iida, H., Takagi, H., Minagawa, H. and Tohyama, M. (1982) Ontogeny of the leucine-enkephalin neuron system of the rat: immunohistochemical analysis. I. Lower brain stem. *J. comp. Neurol.*, 205: 341–370.

Shiosaka, S., Takatsuki, K., Sakanaka, M., Inagaki, S., Takagi, H., Senba, E., Kawai, Y., Iida, H., Minagawa, H., Hara, Y., Matsuzaki, T. and Tohyama, M. (1982) Ontogeny of somatostatin-containing neuron system in the rat: immunohistochemical analysis. II. Forebrain and diencephalon. *J. comp. Neurol.*, 204: 211–224.

Specht, L. A., Pickel, V. M., Joh, T. H. and Reis, D. J. (1981a) Light-microscopic immunocytochemical localization of tyrosine hydroxylase in pre-natal rat brain. I. Early ontogeny. *J. comp. Neurol.*, 199: 233–253.

Specht, L. A., Pickel, V. M., Joh, T. H. and Reis, D. J. (1981b) Light-microscopic immunocytochemical localization of tyrosine hydroxylase in pre-natal rat brain. II. Late ontogeny. *J. comp. Neurol.*, 199: 255–276.

Steinbusch, H. W. M. (1981) Distribution of serotonin immunoreactivity in the central nervous system of the rat — cell bodies and terminals. *Neuroscience*, 6: 557–618.

Tidd, C. W. (1932) The transplantation of spinal ganglia in the white rat. A study of the morphological changes in surviving cells. *J. comp. Neurol.*, 55: 531–543.

Tramu, G., Pillez, A. and Leonardelli, J. (1978) An efficient method of antibody elution for the successive or simultaneous location of two antigens by immunocytochemistry. *J. Histochem. Cytochem.*, 26: 322–324.

Zamboni, L. and de Martino, C. (1967) Buffered picric-acid formaldehyde: a new rapid fixative for electron-microscopy. *J. Cell Biol.*, 35: 148A.

SECTION IV

Multiple Peptide Systems

T. Hökfelt, K. Fuxe and B. Pernow (Eds.),
Progress in Brain Research, Vol. 68

CHAPTER 10

Genetic background for multiple messengers

Floyd E. Bloom

Division of Preclinical Neuroscience and Endocrinology, Scripps Clinic and Research Foundation, 10666 North Torrey Pines Road, La Jolla, CA 92037, U.S.A.

Introduction

Molecular discovery in the neurosciences has until recently largely focussed on neurotransmitters and hypothalamic hypophysiotrophic hormones. Historically we can view transmitter discovery as having had a "classical" period and a "modern" period. The "classical" period began with the discoveries of Dale, Loewi, Elliott and their contemporaries and persists into the present. Currently, we are in transition to an era in which powerful molecular biological methods maintain the pace of discovery after all the "easy" transmitter discoveries were already made. In this Chapter I review the advances made in these molecular biological efforts on transmitters that coexist, and consider some of the opportunities and puzzles that lie ahead.

Strategies of transmitter discovery

As we look back upon the growing list of consensus transmitters (see Iversen, 1983; Palkovits, 1984 for recent listings), those discovered in the classical period can attribute their discovery to one of two strategies, depending on whether the factor was discovered before or after the biological actions for which it is now recognized.

In the "factor first-function later" strategy are substances that bear mainly chemical names: acetylcholine, gamma-amino butyrate, dopamine, glutamate, aspartate, glycine or taurine. They earned chemical names because it was their chemical structure for which they were exclusively identified as biological products, without functional inferences.

In the "assay first-factor later" strategy, the development of a bio-assay for an unknown regulatory factor became the starting point for a purification-isolation process. This was the classical approach of Starling and the early gastrointestinal regulatory peptides, for insulin and glucagon, and for the "sympathin" era of Cannon and colleagues. All of the largely peptidic messengers resulting from this approach carry functional names rather than chemical names: gastrin, cholecystokinin, prostaglandin, substance P, angiotensin, oxytocin, vasopressin, as well as more conventional small molecules like the biogenic amines, adrenaline, histamine and serotonin.

This methodology reached its zenith under the skilled prodding of Guillemin, Schally, McCann and others who pushed their colleagues to detect the hypophysiotrophic factors conceived by Geoffery Harris in the mid-1940's and early 1950's (Guillemin, 1978; Krieger, 1983), requiring the development of sensitive new methods for peptide isolation, purification, and sequence analysis, as well as very large amounts of freshly dissected cattle brains. From this effort came the "assay first", functional names for thyrotropin-releasing hormone, somatostatin, gonadotropin-releasing hormone, and prolactin, and including the last two of the originally postulated hypophysiotrophic factors predicted, corticotropin-releasing factor (Vale et al., 1981) and growth hormone releasing factor (Guillemin et al., 1982) have been solved. This neo-classical approach proved its value time and time again as others used the methods to isolate factors based on rather unpredictable assays: the loss of blood pressure that lead to neurotensin (McDonald et al., 1983), the opiate-like effects in vitro assays that lead to the endorphins (see Snyder, 1984), and the gut vascular effects that lead to vasoactive intestinal polypeptide and gastric inhibitory peptide (Mutt, 1976). The success of the "assay first" strategy may also be gauged by the degree to which it is being exploited still for the possibility that other endogenous ligands for sites at which drugs act could yield the identity of the factors accounting for benzodiazepine actions (see Costa, this volume).

Two modern strategies of transmitter discovery

Two series of developments over the past half decade have made their impressive effects on the emerging list of transmitters recognized. Both derive from the recognition of common chemical principles, but use different ways to exploit the general feature. Mutt and colleagues (Tatemoto and Mutt, 1980, 1981) looked at the frequent occurrence of C-terminally amidated peptides that functioned as messengers. By identifying other important molecules with this common structure they found new peptide members of the glucagon-VIP family and the pancreatic polypeptide family.

The second new approach is based on the central dogma of molecular biology — all peptides are synthesized under the direction of a specific messenger RNA (mRNA) encoded by the gene for that peptide. With the emergence of recombinant DNA technologies, restriction endonucleases and nucleotide sequencing a new opportunity for molecular discovery became available. Nakanishi et al. (1979) were the first to determine the precise sequence of the pro-hormone for "opio-cortin" and to discover that it contained an unanticipated third biologically relevant peptide, deduced solely from the mRNA sequence on the basis of its structural analogy to alpha and beta melanocyte-stimulating hormone (MSH).

Subsequently, the recombinant DNA approach has been employed to obtain the pro-hormone structural sequences, and some of the genomic sequences for almost every one of the previously identified neuropeptides: all of the major branches of the endorphin family (Nakanishi et al., 1979; Gubler et al., 1982; Kakidani et al., 1982; Noda et al., 1982); somatostatin (Goodman et al., 1982; Montimny et al., 1984); VIP (Itoh et al., 1983), Neuropeptide Tyrosine (Minth et al., 1984); oxytocin, and vasopressin (Ivell and Richter, 1984; Schmale and Richter, 1984); corticotropin-releasing factor (Furutani et al., 1983), growth hormone-releasing factor (Gubler et al., 1983; Mayo et al., 1983), substance P (Nawa et al., 1983) cholecystokinin (Deschenes et al., 1984; Gubler et al., 1984), luteinizing hormone-releasing hormone (Seeburg and Adelman, 1984) and the amphibian skin pro-thyrotrophin releasing hormone (Richter et al., 1984). Potentially new, previously unsuspected co-expressed peptides were suggested from these mRNA sequences to predict a new form of VIP (Itoh et al., 1983), and substance P (Nawa et al., 1983). Moreover, pursuit of the pro-hormone for calcitonin, led Rosenfeld and Evans and their collaborators to the recognition that rearrangements of parts of the mRNA domains of the pro-calcitonin, could give rise to a "calcitonin-gene related peptide" (Rosenfeld et al., 1983) which in fact was found in special segments of the rat CNS and had unsuspected biological activity.

Another possible general strategy for transmitter discovery

The appearance of the report suggesting that propiocortin might actually be pro-opio-melanocortin gave rise to the idea that better analysis of brain mRNAs could disclose the existence of possible biologically important cleavage products. Believing that such an approach might not only yield neurotransmitters but might also yield information important to the complete characterization of the properties of neurons and their cell assemblies, my colleagues and I began an effort to employ recombinant DNA methods as a broad open-ended approach to characterizing important but unpredicted agonists and response systems of the brain. The continuous stream of results (Milner and Sutcliffe, 1983; Sutcliffe et al., 1983a,b, 1984; Milner et al., 1984; Bloom et al., 1985; Malfroy et al., 1985) suggest that all of our opportunistic wishes may be realizable.

We have used molecular cloning methods to purify randomly chosen copies (cDNAs) of rat brain messenger RNAs (mRNAs). Poly(A)$^+$ RNA was purified from the brains of adult rats, copied into double stranded cDNA, and inserted into the plasmid pBR322 for cloning in E. coli. Clones bearing cDNA inserts that were at least 500 base pairs in length were nick translated and evaluated for their patterns of hybridization to mRNAs isolated from brain, liver and kidney. Those clones that hybridize to brain mRNAs, but not to mRNAs extracted from other organs, we define as being brain-specific.

This categorization has been extremely productive since such basic quantitative characterizations had not previously been available. For example, (Milner and Sutcliffe, 1983) from the sizes of the mRNAs in brain, their relative abundances and the total complexity of the brain mRNA population, it may be calculated that the rat's brain expresses about 30,000 mRNAs, of which most are "brain-specific" by our standards. Furthermore, the brain-specific mRNAs tend to be larger and more rare than the mRNAs found in other major organ systems, suggesting that genetic messages in brain may encode for more complex translation products.

In addition, this phase of our research quickly yielded a wholly unanticipated finding: a very small, highly repetitive endogenous RNA, BC1, about 160 nucleotides in length, to which several clones of much greater length hybridized (see Sutcliffe et al., 1984). This small RNA target is found specifically in cytoplasmic extracts of brain. This sequence is present in approximately 100,000 copies in the rat genome and we view it as an identifier or "ID" sequence that is necessary, but not sufficient for the tissue-specific expression of brain-specific genetic messages (Sutcliffe and Milner, 1984; Sutcliffe et al., 1984).

Biochemical studies

One of the brain-specific cDNA clones (p1B236) that we have studied in detail by this approach (see Sutcliffe et al., 1983a,b; Bloom et al., 1985) is highly pertinent to the topic of this conference. This clone corresponds to a mRNA present in brain with an abundance of approximately 0.01% but not detectable in liver or kidney.The nucleotide sequence of p1B236 provided the novel 318 amino acid carboxy terminal sequence of the corresponding protein 1B236. One of the notable features of the 1B236 amino acid sequence was the presence of several pairs of basic amino acids (Arg-Arg-Lys-Lys, Lys-Arg, Arg-Arg, Lys-Arg) in its C-terminal region known to demarcate neuropeptides or other peptide hormones in their precursor proteins and have been shown to be the sites of proteolytic processing to generate bioactive peptides. In this respect, 1B236 — a wholly novel protein — appeared to resemble known neuropeptide or peptide hormone precursors.

Based on this structural similarity, we postulated that the 1B236 protein might be proteolytically processed in vivo to generate physiologically relevant neuropeptides and suggested that the most likely cleavage products would be the peptides P5, P6, and P7. To detect and characterize the 1B236 protein and at the same time to test this hypothesis, we selected these peptides for synthesis and antibody production. These antibodies were used for immunocytochemical localization of 1B236 and detected immunoreactive material in neuronal cells and fibers distributed throughout the rat CNS. Immunoreactivity was prominent in hindbrain, particularly spinal cord and cerebellum, midbrain structures such as hippocampus, and cingulate and somatosensory cortex. The patterns were distinct from any other previously characterized neuronal system (see below).

Recently we examined brain extracts for material detected by the specific radioimmunoassay (RIAs) we developed with the antibodies against the synthetic peptide fragments of 1B236. Our data (see Malfroy et al., 1985) provide evidence for the existence of both high molecular weight and peptide forms of 1B236, suggesting that this protein is indeed subjected to extensive proteolytic processing in vivo and providing further support for the hypothesis that the 1B236 molecule is the precursor for a novel family of co-existing neuropeptides.

A different pattern emerged when rat brains were heated rapidly by microwave irradiation immediately after dissection and before salt or detergent-salt extraction. The most noticeable difference was that low molecular weight P5 immunoreactive material could now be consistently detected: similar amounts were found with or without detergent. Furthermore, low molecular weight P7 immunoreactive material could now be detected in extracts in the absence of detergent.

To assay for the effects of endogenous peptidases on the stability and recovery of 1B236-derived peptides, small, known amounts of unlabelled synthetic peptides were incubated with brain homogenates prepared under various conditions and their recovery was evaluated by RIA after different times. All three of the synthetic peptides were rapidly degraded in Tris/NaCl homogenates of fresh brains but were completely stable either in an acid homogenate or in a Tris/NaCl homogenate from a microwave-irradiated brain for at least an hour at room temperature.

Thus, there would appear to be several forms of the brain-specific polypeptide 1B236, detected using RIAs against three non-overlapping peptide regions of this protein. The high molecular weight material is found predominantly in a form requiring detergent for solubilization but a fraction also exists as a soluble protein. Low molecular weight 1B236 species of peptide size can also be reproducibly detected under conditions where endogenous protease activity is abolished. This material probably corresponds to peptides present in vivo.

The multiplicity of 1B236 molecular forms demonstrated here, together with evidence that 1B236 is glycosylated, indicates that this molecule undergoes extensive post-translational modification, including proteolytic processing to generate a novel family of brain-specific peptides. Isolation of these peptides, determination of their exact relationship to the other forms of 1B236, and the demonstration that they are physiologically relevant are currently planned extensions of this line of our research.

Immunocytochemical studies

In immunocytochemical mapping, the same antisera employed in the assays described above were also used for immunocytochemical mapping studies. With antisera to each of three non-overlapping peptides, we were able to develop three independent sets of mapping data on normal and on colchicine-treated adult rats, and more recently on developing rats, and adult primates. The studies on the adult rat brain have progressed the furthest and are reported in detail elsewhere (Bloom et al., 1985) so that a survey will suffice to draw out some general conclusions about the approach and its possible insight into the questions of peptide and other transmitter co-existences.

Our three sets of mapping data with three independently directed sets of antisera, gave three virtually superimposable maps of intense immunoreactivity within a few specific neuronal systems, being most intense in the olfactory, limbic, somatosensory and extrapyramidal motor systems (Table I; Bloom et al., 1985). If these synthetic fragments are in fact natural-processing products of the 1B236 peptide, as our neurochemical evidence favors, then it is equally relevant to be aware that P5 and P6 have already been observed to exhibit biological activity on the cellular and behavioral

TABLE I

Peptide 236 distribution by immunocytochemistry

Region	Neuropil		
	Peptide 5	Peptide 6	Peptide 7
Olfactory bulb			
Internal granule cell layers	++++	++++	++++
Forebrain			
Anterior olfactory nuclei	++++	++++	++++
Olfactory tubercle	++++	++++	++++
Bed nucleus stria terminalis	++++	++++	++++
Lateral septal nuclei	++++	++++	++++
Primary olfactory cortex	+++	+++	+++
Caudate/putamen	++++	++++	++++
Parietal cortex	++++	++++	++++
Cingulate gyrus (mid-post.)	++++	++++	++++
Subiculum	++++	++++	++++
Hippocampus (CA3 ≫ CA1)	++++	++++	++++
Amygdala (Baso-Lat., Med-Cort.)	+++	+++	+++
Diencephalon			
Pre-optic area	++++	++++	++++
Dorsomedial N., ventro lateral and ventro posterolateral Thal.	+++	+++	+++
Paraventricular N., hypothal.	+++	+++	+++
Medial forebrain bundle	+++	+++	+++
Arcuate	++	++	++
Inferior colliculi	+++	+++	+++
Superior colluli	++	++	++
Periaqueductal grey	++	++	++
Brain stem			
Substantia nigra	+	+	+
Locus coeruleus	+	+	+
Central grey	+++	+++	+++
Dorsal, pontine raphe	+	+	+
Dorsal cochlear nucl.	+++	+++	+++
Motor V, VII, IX, X, XII	+++	+++	+++
Inferior olive	++	++	++
Medial trapezoid nucleus	++	++	++
Cerebellum			
Granular cell layer	++++	++++	++++
Molecular layer (proximal)	++	++	++
Deep cerebellar nuclei	+++	0	0

Region	Neuropil		
	Peptide 5	Peptide 6	Peptide 7
Spinal cord			
Dorsal horn (II–III)	+++	+++	+++
Ventral horn	+++	+++	+++
Central grey	++	++	++

The density of immunoreactive neuropil in each indicated rat brain structure was evaluated in untreated rats with antisera to P5, P6, or P7, and rated on a scale of 1 (least) to 4 (most), as indicated by the number of + symbols. Areas in which neuropil was non-reactive are not included. Note that with the rare exceptions noted in the text, the pattern of intensities of immunoreactivity across these regions varies identically with antisera directed against the adjacent, but non-homologous peptide fragments of the polypeptide structure deduced from the 1B236 mRNA.

levels (S. J. Henriksen and G. F. Koob, personal communication).

Given these correlative observations, which neuronal systems were found to exhibit the most intensive immunoreactivity for 1B236 peptides? The immunoreactivity was especially dense in olfactory bulb, specific preoptic, and diencephalic nuclei, and also in the neostriatum, limbic and neocortical regions. Neuropil staining was also prominent within selected thalamic and cranial nerve nuclei, as well as in cerebellum and spinal cord. Maps constructed from the optimally reactive antisera for each of the three C-terminal fragments of 1B236 gave virtually identical patterns with some minor exceptions (see Bloom et al., 1985, and below). The following descriptions summarize the major patterns of immunoreactivity within regions showing prominent staining in both neuropil components (normal rats) and perikarya (colchicine-treated rats) in two selected sets of neurons: the olfactory bulb-penduncle, and the neocortex, as examples of the data derived from this detailed analysis. Immunoreactivity is also striking in specific zones of hippocampus.

Olfactory bulb and peduncle

Intense immunoreactivity was seen within the perimeters of the glomeruli, where immunoreactive periglomerular neurons were observed in colchicine-pretreated rats. The external plexiform layer and mitral cell layer showed no immunoreactivity, while extensive fiber staining was observed surrounding the unreactive granule cells in the internal plexiform layer. In favorable sections, isolated, small, short-axon cells could be resolved in the outer third of the internal plexiform layer. Preliminary electron microscope localization of immunoreactivity for P5 in the olfactory bulb confirmed the reactivity within dendrites and perikarya of the periglomerular neurons, and in fine nerve terminals synapsing on small dendritic spines within the internal plexiform layer. In immunoreactive terminals, the reaction product was associated exclusively with the cytoplasmic face of the synaptic vesicles.

In the olfactory peduncle, extensive neuropil immunoreactivity was observed in all nuclear fields and transition zones. Both fibers of passage and finer processes with relatively few varicosities were observed to collect at the lateral ventral pole of the peduncle, and entering the inner surface of the lateral olfactory tract. Fiber-like staining was not seen within the anterior commissure. In colchicine-pretreated rats, large and medium sized multipolar neurons were also seen in all nuclear fields of the peduncle, as well as within and around the nucleus of the anterior commissure and the nucleus of the lateral olfactory tract. Such neurons constitute up to 25% of the total neuronal population visualized in these fields by general cytoplasmic counter-staining.

Cerebral cortex

In cerebral cortex, neuropil immunoreactivity for P5, P6, and P7 showed virtually identical region-specific patterns when compared over the major cortical regions. Based upon published topographic and cytological criteria for rat cortical regions it was possible to correlate 1B236 immunoreactivity with presumptive functionally defined regions of rat cerebral cortex. Somatosensory cortex was the predominant region of cortical immunoreactivity; posterior cingulate cortex showed intermediate immunoreactivity, with motor, temporal (auditory) fields, and the occipital (visual) cortex, showing low density immunoreactivity; anterior cingulate cortex and, in particular, the frontal medial cortex had no immunoreactivity. These regional variations were consistent from antibody to antibody and from animal to animal, whether sectioned frontally or sagitally.

Within the parietal and posterior cingulate cortex, intense radially oriented immunoreactive processes spanned the entire cortical thickness intermingled with fine varicose fiber-like processes, and isolated punctate structures. These patterns were virtually identical for antisera against P5, P6, or P7. All three sera showed similar patterns, with the P6 antisera showing somewhat denser overall immunoreactivity. Thick tangential processes were seen in outer lamina I, just below the pia, with relative modest reactivity within the inner zone of this lamina. The thick radially directed processes were seen most clearly in deep laminae II and III, with dense, but finer, immunoreactive processes clustered around the perikarya in laminae IV, V and mid-VI. Three contrasting bands of higher immunoreactivity in deep layer I and superficial layer II and in the deeper portions of V and VI were reproducible throughout the somatosensory regions of cortex in frontal sections. Some fiber-like immunoreactive processes with distinct varicosities could also be seen within the superficial layers of the subcortical white matter.

Large multipolar neurons were also seen within the deep white matter of the parietal cortex and within the white matter of the anterior commissure and its nucleus. Cells were detected in layers V–VI of somatosensory cortex, as well as in the peripheral white matter just below laminaVI. Sections taken for electron microscopic localization of P5, from mid-lamina IV show immunoperoxidase positive nerve terminals with reactivity associated with small lucent synaptic vesicles.

Interpretations

Regardless of whether 1B236 represents a transmitter or some other class of cell-specific neuronal protein whose function remains to be determined, the distribution of this marker within functional circuits of the rat brain deserves further consideration. The 1B236 protein is clearly not expressed by every neuron within any of these systems, even those that are most heavily labelled. As one traces through the circuitry of the olfactory system, it is clear that the primary olfactory nerves, as well as the primary output cells of the bulb, the mitral cells, are both uncreactive. However, periglomerular cells, short axon cells of the internal plexiform layer, and selected large neurons within almost all regions directly innervated by the lateral olfactory tract, and known to send centrifugal fibers back to the granule cells of the bulb, are all strongly positive. Furthermore, 1B236 immunoreactive afferents to the thalamus, to the piriform and olfactory regions of the forebrain and whose source locations are not yet determined are also strongly positive. Somatosensory and amygdaloid neurons with immunoreactivity for 1B236 could account for these circuits.

The density of the immunoreactivity within elements of the somatosensory and olfactory fields, as well as the more modest representation in segments

TABLE II

Region	Peptide 5	Peptide 6	Peptide 7
Cell staining			
Paraventricular/SON	0	0	+ + + +
Medial trapezoid	+ + +	0	0
Fiber staining			
Deep cerebellar nuclei	+ + + +	0	0

Although most regional and cellular staining patterns were consistent across all three P immunoreactivities, there were consistent differences, as illustrated in this table. These differences may reflect covert cross-reacting epitopes exposed in colchicine-treated rats or variations in post-translational processing of the 1B236 protein (see text).

of the auditory, extrapyramidal, and cranial motor neuron fields, suggests that 1B236 is expressed in systems which are evolutionarily old.

No specific patterns can yet be simply assembled from the immunoreactive elements within known sequential systems. Within the olfactory and limbic structures, the immunoreactive elements alternate with non-immunoreactive elements in the multi-synaptic chains of interconnected neurons that have been well studied for these functional systems. The meaning of such an alternating pattern of expression of a specific marker is not obvious. At one level, it can be directly interpreted as reflecting only that these cells contain the same protein and hence share at least one specific chemical property which may relate these separated cell types functionally.

If 1B236 is eventually found to meet all of the criteria of a transmitter, our catalog of other brain-specific mRNAs of this relative abundance and complexity suggests that there may be several hundred more to be found and studied. Even if 1B236 does not meet the criteria, its existence within neurons linked with specific functional systems whose neuronal elements are far from completely characterized suggests that our strategy may have more fundamental value. Certainly the ability to generate synthetic fragments of an unknown gene product and to raise antisera against it offers a powerful advantage.

As stated, in general, the rat and primate maps with antisera to P5, P6, or P7 were superimposable as to cell and neuropil immunoreactivity, and this result is directly supportive of the existence of a single common pro-hormone form of the deduced gene product, from which immunodetectable forms of the three peptides can all be seen within the same restricted populations of neurons. However, given the rather impressively large proportion of immunoreactive sites that did show common reactivity (Table I) the exceptions to the generally superimposable maps of immunoreactive structures take on some added interest.

Clearly, at this point, the most likely explanation for these rare exceptions (Table II) is that these structures contain a cross-reactive epitope of unknown structure, and thus, that these exceptions have no other biological importance. Alternative explanations, however, with a more substantive meaning can be considered. Regions that exhibit immunoreactivity to P5, but not P6 or P7, such as the neurons of the medial trapezoid nucleus and the nerve terminal-like staining surrounding the neurons of the deep cerebellar nuclei, may represent partial differential processing, with either post-translational destruction of the major immunogens of P6 and P7, or failure to transcribe.

In fact, early results, spurred in part by a second form of 1B236 prominently exhibited during development, has in fact provided support for the view that there is an alternative form of the 1B236 mRNA in which a variant, longer form of P5 is translated but not P6 or P7. However, no simple alternative exists to explain the presence of P7 immunoreactivity in those structures not exhibiting reactivity with antisera to P5 or P6. Although this isolated finding within the magnocellular neurons probably represents only a cross-reacting endogenous epitope read by the P7 antisera, such a result would also be compatible with a recombination of a DNA exon segment for P7 without P5 or P6, analogous to the expression of mRNAs for the calcitonin gene-related peptide (Rosenfeld et al., 1983). No evidence of such mRNA processing alternatives exists, however.

These exceptions serve well to illustrate the confidence level achievable when non-overlapping synthetic fragments are used to generate immune reagents that give superimposable cytological patterns. When these conditions are met, the antisera can provide more information than conventional immunocytochemistry or even monoclonal antibody-based cytochemistry, due to the convergence on the same protein by antisera against adjacent segments. Furthermore, because the present approach has demonstrated that an immunologically identical protein is expressed in different neurons, it is also possible to infer that these cells may share similar chemical properties and perhaps epigenetic states.

With regard to transmitter co-existences, it is striking that within the limbic system, the fornix projection from the medial septum is strongly positive, as is the perforant path input to the outer molecular layer of the dentate gyrus, and possible amygdaloid inputs to the ventral and dorsal subiculum. The former path is considered a consensus cholinergic system (see Ross et al., 1983), while the latter pathway has been linked to several peptide systems, including the pro-enkephalin derived peptides (McGinty et al., 1984).

Open questions

These thoughts then bring us back to the essential open questions that have been contributed to the coexistence enigma by molecular biological research. Even though the questions cannot now be answered, it may prove heuristic to begin to consider them.

(1) *Are there recurrent patterns in peptide, monoamine and amino acid transmitter coexistences that arise from a co-ordinated control of the underlying genome?* If there were some sorts of underlying expression "ties" between the genes coding for messenger molecules as well as other neuronal properties, then consistent patterns might be expected, especially when there are many more markers of neuronal phenotypy to select from.

(2) *What does it mean to have a neuron of a given phenotype?* Clearly transmitter designations per se are inadequate, and even cells in the same location, with a single common transmitter often seem to express in individual clusters variable combinations of co-existing pairs of transmitters. What is the meaning of this variation — is it random, or reflective of some unforeseen property? In any case, it seems likely that neuronal phenotypy is an issue that reveals more properties of a neuron than simply size, shape, location, and connectivity.

(3) *Is there insight to be gained, whether evolutionarily significant or relevant to current functional properties, from analysis of the similarities and differences in the molecular encoding patterns that have emerged for neuropeptides?* Some are C-terminal products, some are N-terminal products, some are neither. Some give rise to only one end product, at least as far as is known now, while other pro-hormones can give rise to multiple potential products (POMC, pro-Dynorphin) all of which have biological properties. The same hypothetical question could be asked at even a more basic level, in terms of gene capacity: while some single product propeptides (like vasopressin/oxytocin) seem to arise from multiple different exons all relating to particular domains of the peptides' packaging and secretion, some multi-product peptides like POMC seem to stem from a single exon.

(4) *Does the common occurrence of a shared exon among cells of different systems imply a common origin or a common function,* as we have asked about

the 1B236 within the olfactory and limbic systems? At least to me, as an interested neuroscientist who does cloning largely by sideline cheer-leading, I am perplexed by the lack of information as to where in the eukaryotic genome the genes occur that are expressed by neurons. Could those genes that control messenger molecules or their receptors be clustered, such that a neuron expresses within its program of post-mitotic differentiation steps a set sequence of transmitters that reflect the changing needs of neurons as shifts in the nature of the hemoglobins coordinate with the environments in which erythrocytes function.

(5) Lastly, perhaps a minor note or two of caution. Without wanting to disturb the elegant trains of momentum that are building upon example after example of co-existing neuropeptide immunoreactivity with other monoamine and amino acid transmitter markers, one must at least be aware that there are precious few sites in the CNS or PNS at which peptides have been shown to mediate the effects of a stimulated nerve on its target cells. Perhaps, as we have done for 1B236 it may be worth considering the possibility that even when processed to smaller forms, those forms may not be actively secreted, but could reflect the nature of the function of the larger molecules from which they are cleaved. As pure speculation, one wonders about the generality of the hypothetical arrangement noted by Hales (1978) that a receptor starts as a form from which small intracellular signals are derived. Perhaps later, these intracellular signals are found also to elicit useful responses on leakage or co-transmission, and are retained for the enrichment they provide in the main process of transmission.

In any case, it seems clear that molecular biologic approaches have much to offer as insight into the nature of co-existing neurotransmitters, and vice versa. We await future developments with great interest.

References

Bloom, F. E., Battenberg, E. L. F., Milner, R. J. and Sutcliffe, J. G. (1985) Immunocytochemical mapping of 1B236, A brain specific neuronal polypeptide deduced from the sequence of a cloned mRNA. *J. Neurosci.*, 5: 1781–1802.

Deschenes, R. J., Lorenz, L. J., Haun, R. S., Roos, B. A., Collier, K. J. and Dixon, J. E. (1984) Cloning and sequence analysis of a cDNA encoding rat preprocholecystokinin. *Proc. natl. Acad. Sci. USA*, 81: 726–730.

Furutani, Y., Morimoto, Y., Shibahara, S., Noda, M., Takahashi, H., Hirose, T., Asai, M., Inayama, S., Hayashida, H., Miyata, T. and Numa, S. (1983) Cloning and sequence analysis of cDNA for ovine corticotropin-releasing factor precursor. *Nature (Lond.)*, 301: 537–540.

Goodman, R. H., Jacobs, J. W., Dee, P. C. and Habener, J. F. (1982) Somatostatin-28 encoded in a cloned cDNA obtained from a rat medullary thyroid carcinoma. *J. biol. Chem.*, 257: 1156–1159.

Gubler, U., Seeburg, P., Hoffman, B. J., Gage, L. P. and Udenfriend, S. (1982) Molecular cloning establishes proenkephalin as precursor of enkephalin-containing peptides. *Nature (Lond.)*, 295: 206–280.

Gubler, U., Monahan, J. J., Lomedico, P. T., Bhatt, R. S., Collier, K. J., Hoffman, B. J., Bohlen, P., Esch, F., Ling, N., Zeytin, F., Brazeau, P., Poonian, M. S. and Gage, L. P. (1983) Cloning and sequence analysis of cDNA for the precursor of human growth hormone-releasing factor, somatocrinin. *Proc. nat. Acad. Sci. USA*, 80: 4311–4314.

Gubler, U., Chua, A. O., Hoffman, B. J., Collier, K. J. and Eng, J. (1984) Cloned cDNA to cholecystokinin mRNA predicts an identical preprocholecystokinin in pig brain and gut. *Proc. nat. Acad. Sci. USA*, 81: 4307–4310.

Guillemin, R. (1978) Peptides in the brain: the new endocrinology of the neuron. *Science*, 202: 390–402.

Guillemin, R., Brazeau, P., Bohlen, P., Esch, F., Ling, N. and Wehrenberg, W. B. (1982) Growth hormones-releasing factor from a human pancreatic tumor that caused acromegaly. *Science*, 218: 585–587.

Hales, C. N. (1978) Proteolysis and the evolutionary origin of polypeptide hormones. *FEBS Lett.*, 94: 10–16.

Itoh, N., Obata, K., Yanaihara, N. and Okamoto, H. (1983) Human preprovasoactive intestinal polypeptide contains a novel PHI-27-like peptide, PHM-27. *Nature (Lond.)*, 304: 547–549.

Ivell, R. and Richter, D. (1984) Structure and comparison of the oxytocin and vasopressin genes from rat. *Proc. nat. Acad. Sci. USA*, 81: 2006–2010.

Iversen, L. L. (1983) Neuropeptides — what next? *Trends Neurosci.*, 9: 293–294.

Kakidani, H., Furutani, Y., Takahashi, H., Noda, M., Morimoto, Y., Hirose, T., Asai, M., Inayama, S., Nakanishi, S. and Numa, S. (1982) Cloning and sequence analysis of cDNA for porcine beta-neo-endorphin/dynorphin precursor. *Nature (Lond.)*, 298: 245–249.

Krieger, D. T. (1983) Brain peptides: What, where, and why? *Science*, 222: 975–985.

Malfroy, B., Bakhit, C., Bloom, F. E., Sutcliffe, J. G. and Milner, R. J. (1985) Brain-specific polypeptide 1B236 exists in multiple molecular forms. *Proc. nat. Acad. Sci. USA*, 82: 2009–2013.

Mayo, K. E., Vale, W., Rivier, J., Rosenfeld, M. G. and Evans, R. M. (1983) Expression-cloning and sequence of a cDNA encoding human growth hormone-releasing factor. *Nature (Lond.)*, 306: 86–88.

McDonald, T. J., Jornvall, H., Tatemoto, K. and Mutt, V. (1983) Identification and characterization of variant forms of the gastrin-releasing peptide (GRP). *FEBS Lett.*, 156: 349–356.

McGinty, J. F., van der Kooy, D. and Bloom, F. E. (1984) The distribution and morphology of opioid peptide immunoreactive neurons in the cerebral cortex of rats. *J. Neurosci.*, 4: 1104–1117.

Milner, R. J. and Sutcliffe, J. G. (1983) Gene expression in rat brain. *Nucleic Acids Res.*, 11: 5497–5520.

Milner, R. J., Bloom, F. E., Lai, C., Lerner, R. A. and Sutcliffe, J. G. (1984) Brain-specific genes have identifier sequences in their introns. *Proc. nat. Acad. Sci. USA*, 81: 713–717.

Minth, C. D., Bloom, S. R., Polak, J. M. and Dixon, J. E. (1984) Cloning, characterization and DNA sequence of a human cDNA encoding neuropeptide tyrosine. *Proc. nat. Acad. Sci. USA*, 81: 4577–4580.

Montminy, M. R., Goodman, R. H., Horovitch, S. J. and Habener, J. F. (1984) Primary structure of the gene encoding rat preprosomatostatin. *Proc. nat. Acad. Sci. USA*, 81: 3337–3340.

Mutt, V. (1976) Further investigations of intestinal hormonal polypeptides. *Clin. Endocrinol.*, 5: 175S–183S.

Nakanishi, S., Inoue, A., Kita, T., Nakamura, M., Chang, A. C. Y., Cohen, S. N. and Numa, S. (1979) Nucleotide sequence of cloned cDNA for bovine corticotropin-B-lipoprotein precursor. *Nature (Lond.)*, 278: 423–427.

Nawa, H., Hirose, T., Takashima, H., Inayama, S. and Nakanishi, S. (1983) Nucleotide sequences of clones cDNAs for two types of bovine brain substance P precursor. *Nature (Lond.)*, 306: 32–36.

Noda, M., Furutani, Y., Takahashi, H., Toyosato, M., Hirose, T., Inayama, S., Nakanishi, S. and Numa, S. (1982) Cloning and sequence analysis of cDNA for bovine adrenal preproenkephalin. *Nature (Lond.)*, 295: 202–206.

Palkovits, M. (1984) Distribution of neuropeptides in the central nervous system: A review of biochemical mapping studies. *Prog. Neurobiol.*, 23: 151–189.

Richter, K., Kawashima, E., Egger, R. and Kreil, G. (1984) Biosynthesis of thyrotropin releasing hormone in the skin of Xenopus laevis: partial sequence of the precursor deduced from cloned cDNA. *EMBO J.*, 3: 617–621.

Rosenfeld, M. G., Mermod, J.-J., Amara, S. G., Swanson, L. W., Sawchenko, P. E., Rivier, J., Vale, W. and Evans, R. M. (1983) Production of a novel neuropeptide encoded by the calcitonin gene via tissue-specific RNA processing. *Nature (Lond.)*, 304: 129–135.

Ross, M. E., Park, D. H. Teitelman, G., Pickel, V. M., Reis, D. J. and Joh, T. H. (1983) Immunohistochemical localization of choline acetyltransferase using a monoclonal antibody: a radioautographic method. *Neuroscience*, 10: 907–922.

Schmale, H. and Richter, D. (1984) Single base deletion in the vasopressin gene is the cause of diabetes insipidus in Brattleboro rats. *Nature (Lond.)*, 308: 705–709.

Seeburg, P. H. and Adelman, J. P. (1984) Characterization of cDNA for precursor of human luteinizing hormone releasing hormone. *Nature (Lond.)*, 311: 666–668.

Snyder, S. H. (1984) Drug and neurotransmitter receptors in the brain. *Science*, 224: 22–31.

Spindel, E. R., Chin, W. W., Price, J., Rees, L. H., Besser, G. M. and Habener, J. F. (1984) Cloning and characterization of cDNAs encoding human gastrin-releasing peptide. *Proc. nat. Acad. Sci. USA*, 81: 5699–5703.

Sutcliffe, J. G., Milner, R. J., Shinnick, T. M. and Bloom, F. E. (1983a) Identifying the protein products of brain-specific genes with antibodies to chemically synthesized peptides. *Cell*, 33: 671–682.

Sutcliffe, J. G., Milner, R. J. and Bloom, F. E. (1983b) Cellular localization and function of the proteins encoded by brain-specific mRNAs. *Cold Spring Harbor Symp.*, 48: 477–484.

Sutcliffe, J. G., Milner, R. J., Gottesfeld, J. M. and Lerner, R. A. (1984) ID sequences are transcribed specifically in brain. *Nature (Lond.)*, 308: 237–241.

Tatemoto, K. and Mutt, V. (1980) Isolation of two novel candidate hormones using a chemical method for finding naturally occurring polypeptides. *Nature (Lond.)*, 285: 417–418.

Tatemoto, K. and Mutt, V. (1981) Isolation and characterization of the intestinal peptide porcine PHI (PHI-27), a new member of the glucagon — secretin family. *Proc. nat. Acad. Sci. USA*, 78: 6603–6607.

Vale, W., Spiess, J., Rivier, C. and Rivier, J. (1981) Characterization of a 41 residue ovine hypothalamic peptide that stimulates secretion of corticotropin and B-endorphin. *Science*, 213: 1394–1397.

T. Hökfelt, K. Fuxe and B. Pernow (Eds.),
Progress in Brain Research, Vol. 68

CHAPTER 11

Multiple chemical messengers in hypothalamic magnocellular neurons

Michael J. Brownstein and Éva Mezey

Laboratory of Cell Biology, NIMH, Bethesda, MD 20205, U.S.A.

Introduction

There are two major groups of large neurosecretory neurons in the hypothalamus, one in the supraoptic nucleus (SON) and the other in the paraventricular nucleus (PVN). Most of these cells send their axons through the internal zone of the median eminence to the posterior lobe of the pituitary where they terminate; a small number seem to project to the external zone of the median eminence as well. It should be noted that some parvocellular neurons also project to the posterior pituitary. Thus putative neurotransmitters detected in the posterior lobe (Table I) may be in processes of magnocellular or parvocellular neurons, or in cells intrinsic to the posterior lobe itself. Few of the "candidates" listed in Table I actually reside in magnocellular cells.

The magnocellular neurons develop from midline (i.e. periventricular) neuroblasts. Those in the SON migrate ventrolaterally and take up residence alongside the optic chiasm. Scattered nests of cells fail to complete this migration and come to rest between the PVN and SON. These nests of neurons are called accessory magnocellular cells and comprise less than 5% of the magnocellular population.

Each of the two supraoptic nuclei contains about 4500 magnocellular neurons. The PVN, on the other hand, has a substantial number of small cells (about 6000) in addition to its large ones (about 11,000). Until fairly recently the former received little attention, but in the last several years the importance of the parvocellular neurons in the PVN has come to be appreciated. Since these cells are discussed by Swanson elsewhere in this volume, the present chapter will deal exclusively with the magnocellular neurons. The data cited are all taken from studies of rat brains.

Several techniques have been used to demonstrate that particular transmitters are present in or absent from magnocellular cells. Studies of the effect of stalk transections or PVN lesions on transmitter levels in the posterior pituitary have helped to show whether neurotransmitters are in non-neuronal cells intrinsic to the posterior lobe or in processes provided by neurons extrinsic to it. Light microscopic examination of immunohistochemically stained serial sections through the PVN and SON or double stained individual sections has allowed colocalization of neurotransmitters in single perikarya. Recently, in situ hybridization cytochemistry, a method for visualizing discrete mRNAs in cells, has been combined with immunohistochemistry to colocalize transmitters (Young, Mezey and Siegel, submitted). Finally, electron microscopic immunohistochemical studies of nerve endings in the posterior pituitary have been used to show that certain molecules share not only the same terminal but also the same storage granule.

The various magnocellular neurons make either vasopressin, the antidiuretic hormone, or oxytocin, the hormone responsible for milk letdown. That these neurons make and release additional chemical

TABLE I

Concentrations of peptides and non-peptide neurotransmitters in the rat posterior pituitary

	fmole/lobe	References
Vasopressin	660,000	Crowley et al., 1978
Oxytocin	750,000	Crowley et al., 1978
α-Neo-endorphin	1,000	Zamir et al., 1984
β-Neo-endorphin	950	Zamir et al., 1984
Dynorphin A	600	Zamir et al., 1984
Dynorphin B	1,200	Zamir et al., 1984
Leu-enkephalin	1,200	Zamir et al., 1984
Met-enkephalin	600	Zamir et al., 1984
Corticotropin-releasing hormone	20	Palkovits et al., 1983
Somatostatin	180	Saavedra et al., 1983
Thyrotropin-releasing hormone	300	Jackson and Reichlin, 1974
Cholecystokinin	200	Beinfeld et al., 1980
Secretin	30	Charlton et al., 1983
Substance P	30	DePalatis et al., 1984
Neurotensin	2	Güllner et al., 1982
Dopamine	4,500	Saavedra et al., 1975
Norepinephrine	500	Saavedra et al., 1975
Epinephrine*	–	Saavedra et al., 1975
Serotonin	2,500	Saavedra et al., 1975
Histamine	10,000	Saavedra et al., 1975
Acetylcholine*	–	Saavedra et al., 1975

* Phenylethanolamine-*N*-methyltransferase and choline acetyltransferase are not detectable in the rat posterior pituitary; presumably epinephrine and acetylcholine are not present there.

messengers was suggested by the discovery of a number of peptide and non-peptide neurotransmitters in the posterior pituitary (see Table I). Some of these are now known to coexist with oxytocin or vasopressin in magnocellular cells. The cases for and against the cotransmitter candidates in Table I will be summarized below.

Opioid peptides

Two families of opioid peptides are present in neuronal processes in the posterior pituitary, the peptides derived from proenkephalin A and proenkephalin B. Proenkephalin A, the products of which are found in large amounts in the bovine adrenal medulla, contains six copies of Met-enkephalin and one copy of Leu-enkephalin. Its processing results in the formation of several unique products: Met-enkephalin-Arg^{6}-Phe^{7}, Met-enkephalin-Arg^{6}-Gly^{7}-Leu^{8}, and ‘synenkephalin,” a 77-residue protein that comprises the N-terminus of the precursor. Proenkephalin B gives rise to a number of Leu-enkephalin-containing peptides including α-neoendorphin, β-neoendorphin, dynorphin A, and dynorphin B. One or more of these appear to be processed further to yield Leu-enkephalin itself.

It is difficult to interpret the results of early attempts to colocalize opioid and neurohypophyseal peptides because antibodies against Met- or Leu-enkephalin were used, and they were not perfectly specific for one pentapeptide or the other. Despite this, a pattern emerged which has been confirmed subsequently — that proenkephalin A and B are made by oxytocinergic and vasopressinergic neurons, respectively (see Martin and Voigt, 1981, 1982). For example, synenkephalin and Met-enkephalin-Arg^6-Phe^7 have been detected in cells that contain oxytocin (Martin et al., 1983; Vanderhaeghen et al., 1983) and dynorphin has been found

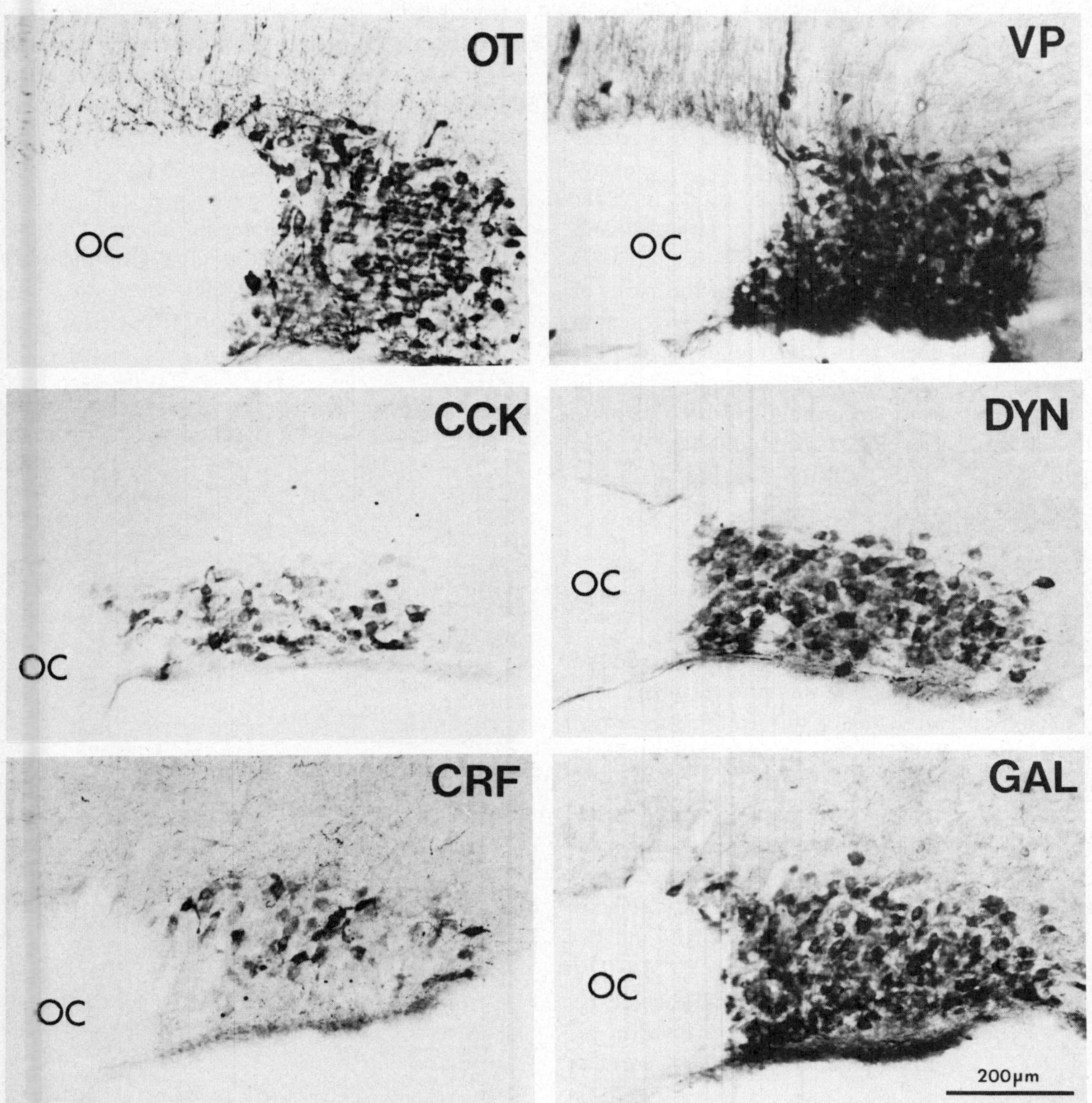

Fig. 1. Neuropeptide staining in the rat SON. The immunostaining was done using 40 μm thick Vibratome sections. To develop this staining the Avidin-Biotin peroxidase method was used. Abbreviations: OT = oxytocin; OC = optic chiasm; VP = vasopressin; CCK = cholecystokinin; DYN = dynorphin; CRF = corticotropin-releasing factor; GAL = galanin.

in cells that stain for vasopressin (Watson et al., 1982; Weber et al., 1982). Indeed dynorphin has been shown to occupy the same secretory granules that house vasopressin in the posterior lobe (Whitnall et al., 1983). In addition, Zamir et al. (1985) have recently shown that the levels of proenkephalin A- and B-derived peptides vary independently in response to physiological manipulations supporting the suggestion that they subserve different functions.

While it is clear that proenkephalin A products are in oxytocinergic nerve endings in the neurohypophysis, these enkephalins may reside in other nerve endings too. Transection of the pituitary stalk deprives the posterior lobe of all of its Met-enkephalin, but combined lesions of all of the axons of PVN and SON neurons only cause a 45% reduction in Met-enkephalin. Perhaps the remaining Met-enkephalin is provided by enkephalinergic neurons in the arcuate nucleus since monosodium glutamate administration causes a substantial fall in Met-enkephalin in the neural lobe (Zamir, personal communication).

Cholecystokinin, galanin, and other "gut" peptides

In 1975, Vanderhaeghen and his colleagues found that a gastrin-like peptide was present in the neuryhypophysis. Subsequently this peptide was shown to be the sulfated octapeptide cholecystokinin (CCK) (Beinfeld et al., 1980). CCK-containing magnocellular neurons have been visualized in the SON and PVN; these same neurons also make oxytocin (Vanderhaeghen et al., 1981) (see Fig. 1). Interestingly, a second population of parvocellular neurons in the PVN contain CCK, CRF, and vasopressin (Mezey et al., 1985). These CCK/CRF/vasopressin cells project to the external zone of the median eminence and appear to be involved in regulating ACTH secretion by pituitary corticotrophs.

Rokaeus and his coworkers (1984) have demonstrated that galanin is present in magnocellular neurons in the rat central nervous system. Fig. 2 shows that galanin coexists with vasopressin in the cells.

Other gut hormones have been detected in the posterior pituitary. The secretin in the neural lobe seems to be of central origin; it disappears after stalk transections and falls by 50% following PVN lesions (Charlton et al., 1982). The cells that make it remain to be found. Similarly, a motilin-like peptide has been reported to be present in the posterior lobe (O'Donohue et al., 1981) and in magnocellular neurons (Jacobowitz et al., 1981), but its precise identity remains to be established.

Tager and his colleagues (1980) have said that antisera against pancreatic glucagon stain magnocellular neurons in vasopressin-rich parts of the PVN and SON. Güllner et al. (1982), on the other hand, have been unable to detect glucagon by radioimmunoassay in extracts of rat posterior lobe.

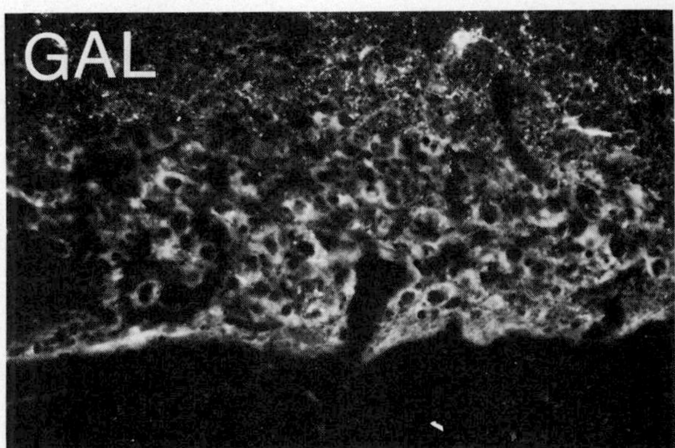

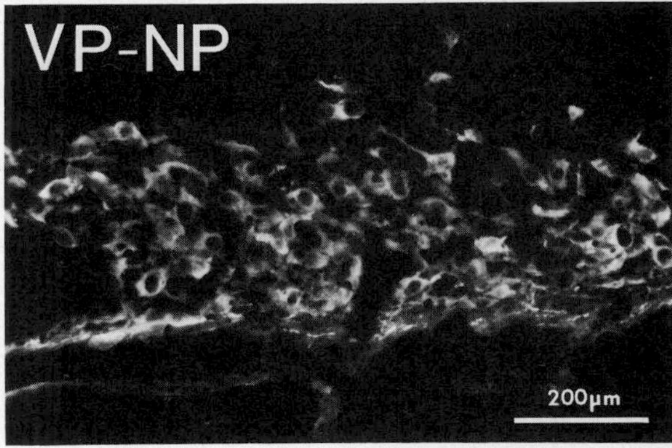

Fig. 2. Coexistence of GAL and VP-NP in the same SON cells. Fluorescence double staining using anti rabbit IgG Rhodamin (GAL) and antimouse IgG FITC (VP-NP) on the same section.

Thus, one cannot yet conclude that glucagon and vasopressin coexist in cells that project to the neurohypophysis.

Corticotropin-releasing factor (CRF) and other hypothalamic hormones

As mentioned above, CRF coexists with CCK and vasopressin in a population of small cells in the PVN. In addition, it is present in large oxytocin-containing neurons in the PVN and SON (Burlet et al., 1983; Swanson et al., 1983; Antoni et al., 1984; Dreyfus et al., 1984) (see Fig. 1) as well as their processes in the internal zone of the median eminence.

Thyrotropin-releasing hormine (TRH) is present in the posterior pituitary (Jackson and Reichlin, 1974), and its levels fall precipitously following stalk transections or PVN lesions (Brownstein et al., 1982). Perhaps the TRH in the posterior lobe is contributed by neurons in the PVN; this nucleus does contain a population of TRH-positive parvocellular cells that project to the external zone of the median eminence. In like manner, the somatostatin in the posterior pituitary is probably in processes of parvocellular cells in the periventricular nucleus. While Dubois and Kolodziejczyk (1975) reported that magnocellular neurons in the SON could be stained with antisomatostatin antibodies, Dierickx and Vandesande (1980) have concluded that this staining was due to cross-reactivity with neurophysin.

Other biologically active peptides

Several other peptides have been said to exist in magnocellular neurons and/or the neurohypophysis. Angiotensin-antibodies stain both small PVN neurons (see Swanson, this volume) and large (vasopressinergic?) cells in the PVN and SON. The staining of magnocellular neurons is not readily blocked by addition of an excess of angiotensin (Lind et al., 1985), and it is not clear whether these neurons really make and secrete the peptide. Renin-positive magnocellular neurons have also been described (Fuxe et al., 1982). These neurons were suggested to be oxytocinergic. No absorption control was done.

Atrial natriuretic factor (ANF) has been visualized in fibers in the posterior pituitary, but ANF-positive magnocellular neurons have not been found (Skofitsch et al., 1985). The same is true of substance P.

Bombesin/GRF- (Chronwall et al., 1985), ranatensin- (Chronwall et al., 1985), and FMRFamide- (O'Donohue et al., 1984) like peptides have been detected in the posterior lobe by RIA, but the immunologically reactive species have not been characterized and their origins are unknown (bombesin and FMRM-like immunoreactivity have been detected in scattered cells in the PVN) (see Roth et al., 1982; Chronwall et al., 1985).

The posterior pituitary of adrenalectomized, but not normal, rats contains fibers that can be stained with antineurotensin antibodies (Mezey, unpublished). Lesion studies have suggested that a significant portion of the neurotensin in the median eminence and posterior lobe comes from cells other than the medium-size neurotensin-positive neurons in the medial PVN.

Neither VIP nor PHI have been detected in processes in the posterior lobe though both have been observed in medium-to-large neurons in the PVN following adrenalectomy (Mezey and Kiss, 1985). These cells probably project to the median eminence.

Monoamines

Tyrosine hydroxylase has been visualized immunocytochemically in magnocellular neurons in the SON and PVN of normal rats (Chan-Palay et al., 1984). The staining is much more intense in Brattleboro (i.e. vasopressin deficient) rats (Kiss and Mezey, submitted). No staining for dopamine-β-hydroxylase or PNMT can be detected (Mezey, unpublished). Thus, the tyrosine hydroxylase positive neurons are probably dopaminergic.

The level of dopamine in the posterior lobe is quite high (see Table I). Whether this dopamine is in processes of magnocellular neurons, arcuate nucleus neurons, or both remains to be determined. Only one-tenth as much norepinephrine as dopamine is present in the posterior lobe; its origin is unknown.

The neurohypophysis receives little if any serotoninergic innervation; transection of the pituitary stalk has no effect on its 5-HT level. The bulk of the 5-HT in the neural lobe is probably in platelets and mast cells (Palkovits et al., 1985b). Most of the histamine in the posterior pituitary is also undoubtedly stored in mast cells.

Since phenylethanolamine-*N*-methyltransferase and choline acetyltransferase are not found in the neurohypophysis (Saavedra et al., 1975), it must not receive an adrenergic or cholinergic imput.

Concluding remarks

Magnocellular neurons may or may not be exceptional in making several chemical messengers. They synthesize and release one major neurosecretory product (vasopressin or oxytocin) and a number of "cotransmitters". The latter seem to be stored in (and, therefore, released from) the same granules that contain vasopressin and oxytocin. The role of the cotransmitters is unclear, however. They are released into the systemic circulation in very small amounts, and it is hard to believe that they have peripheral targets. It seems more likely that they act locally. They could affect the terminals that release them, augmenting or reducing peptide secretion, or they could influence nearby cells — cells in the intermediate or anterior lobe of the pituitary or neurons in the medial basal hypothalamus. They may aid in orchestrating the animal's responses to water imbalance or suckling. Cataloging the cotransmitters only represents the first step toward understanding their actions.

Summary

Vasopressin (VP) and oxytocin (OT) are made by separate populations of magnocellular neurons. There may be a small group of cells that make both VP and OT, but these remain to be identified rigorously. The vasopressinergic magnocellular neurons have been shown to make opioid peptides derived from preproenkephalin B (e.g. Leu-enkephalin, dynorphin). In addition, they seem to contain galanin and dopamine. The case for the latter is incomplete at present.

Oxytocinergic magnocellular neurons appear to make three other peptides: CCK, Met-enkephalin (and other preproenkephalin A derivatives such as Met-enkephalin-Arg^{6}-Phe^{7} and synenkephalin) and CRF.

Glucagon, angiotensin, renin, and pro-opiomelanocortin products (ACTH, β-endorphin) have been suggested to be present in magnocellular elements, but the evidence in support of their coexistence with VP or OT is incomplete or unconvincing. Substance P, neurotensin, TRH and somatostatin in the neural lobe are probably contributed by parvocellular hypothalamic elements. Finally, the histamine there (and most of the serotonin) is likely to be in mast cells. The list of agents in the neural lobe continues to expand and additional "cotransmitters" may be discovered.

References

Antoni, F. A., Palkovits, M., Makara, G. B., Kiss, J. Z., Linton, E. A., Lowry, P. J. and Leranth, C. (1984) Immunoreactive ovine cortitropin releasing factor (oCRF-LI) in the hypothalamohypophyseal tract of the rat. In E. Usdin, R. Kvetnansky and J. Axelrod (Eds.), *Prodeedings of the Third Symposium on Catecholamines and Other Neurotransmitters in Sress*, Gordon and Breach Science Publishers, N.Y., pp. 233–241.

Beinfeld, M. C., Meyer, D. K. and Brownstein, M. J. (1980) Cholecystokinin octapeptide in rat hypothalamo-neurohypophysial system. *Nature (Lond.)*, 288: 376–378.

Brownstein, M. J., Eskay, R. and Palkovits, M. (1982) Thyrotropin releasing hormone in the median eminence is in processes of paraventricular nucleus neurons. *Neuropeptides*, 2: 197–201.

Burlet, A., Tonon, M. C., Tankosic, P., Coy, D. and Vaudry, M. (1983) Comparative immunochemical localization of corticotropin releasing factor (CRF-41) and neurohypophysial peptides in the brain of Brattleboro and Long-Evans rats. *Neuroendocrinology*, 37: 64–72.

Chan-Palay, V., Zaborszky, L., Kohler, C., Goldstein, M. and Palay, S. L. (1984) Distribution of tyrosine-hydroxylase immunoreactive neurons in the hypothalamus of rats. *J. comp. Neurol.*, 227: 467–496.

Charlton, C. G., O'Donohue, T. L., Miller, R. L. and Jacobowitz, D. M. (1982) Secretin in the rat hypothalamo-pituitary system: localization, identification and characterization. *Peptides*, 3: 565–567.

Crowley, W. R., O'Donohue, T. L., George, M. J. and Jacobowitz, D. M. (1978) Changes in pituitary oxytocin and vasopressin during the estrous cycle and after ovarian hormones: evidence for mediation by norepinephrine. *Life Sci.*, 23: 2579–2586.

Chronwall, B. M., Olschowka, J. A. and O'Donohue, T. L. (1984) Histochemical localization of FMRFamide-like immunoreacativity in the rat brain. *Peptides*, 5: 569–584.

Chronwall, B. M., Pisano, J. J., Bishop, J. F., Moody, T. W. and O'Donohue, T. L. (1985) Biochemical and histochemical characterization of ranatensin immunoreactive peptides in rat brain: lack of coexistence with Bombesin/GRP. *Brain Res.* (in press).

DePalatis, L. R., Khorram, O., Ho, R. H., Negro-Vilar, A. and McCann, S. M. (1984) Partial characterization of immunoreactiave substance P in the rat pituitary gland. *Life Sci.*, 34: 225–238.

Dierickx, K. and Vandesande, F. (1980) Immunocytochemical localization of somatostatin-containing neurons in the rat hypothalamus. *Cell Tissue Res.*, 201: 349–359.

Dreyfuss, F., Burlet, A., Tonon, M. C. and Vaudry, H. (1984) Comparative immunoelectron microscopic localization of corticotropin-releasing factor (CRF-41) and oxytocin in the rat median eminence. *Neuroendocrinology*, 39: 284–287.

Dubois, M. P. and Kolodziejczyk, E. (1975) Centres hypothalamiques du rat secretant la somatostatine: repartition des pericaryons en 2 systemes magno et parvocellulaires (etude immunocytologique). *C.R. Acad. Sci. (Paris)*, 281: 1737–1740.

Fuxe, K., Ganten, D., Hokfelt, T., Locatelli, V., Poulsen, K., Stock, G., Rix, E. and Tanger, R. (1980) Renin-like immunocytochemical activity in the rat and mouse brain. *Neurosci. Lett.*, 18: 245–250.

Güllner, H.-G., Kwakowski, E. C. and Unger, R. H. (1982) Somatostatin is decreased in the neurohypophysis of the Brattleboro rat and may play a role in the regulation of vasopressin secretion. *Ann. N.Y. Acad. Sci.*, 394: 142–146.

Jackson, I. and Reichlin, S. (1974) Thyrotropin-releasing hormone (TRH): distribution in hypothalamic and extrahypothalamic brain tissues of mammalian and submammalian chordates. *Endocrinology*, 95: 854.

Jacobowitz, D. M., O'Donohue, T. L., Chay, W. Y. and Chang, T.-M. (1981) Mapping of motilin immunoreactive neurons of the rat brain. *Peptides*, 2: 479–487.

Kiss, J. and Mezey, E. (1985) Tyrosine hydroxylase (TH) immunoreactivity in magnocellular hypothalamic neurons (submaitted).

Lind, R. W., Swanson, L. W. and Ganten, D. (1985) Organization of angiotensin II immunoreactive cells and fibers in the rat central nervous system. *Neuroendocrinology*, 40: 2–24.

Martin, R. and Voigt, K. H. (1981) Enkephalins co-exist with oxytocin and vasopressin in nerve terminals of rat neurohypophysis. *Nature (Lond.)*, 289: 502–504.

Martin, R. and Voigt, K. H. (1982) Leucine-enkephalin-like immunoreactivity in vasopressin terminals is enhanced by treatment with peptidases. *Life Sci.*, 31: 1728–1732.

Martin, R., Geis, R., Holl, R., Schafer, M. and Voigt, K. H. (1983) Co-existence of unrelated peptides in oxytocin and vasopressin terminals of rat neurohypophysis: immunoreactive methionine[5]-enkephalin, leucine[5]-enkephalin, and cholecystokinin-like substances. *Neuroscience*, 8: 213.

Mezey, E. and Kiss, J. Z. (1985) Vasoactive intestinal peptide-containing neurons in the paraventricular nucleus may participate in regulating prolactin secretion. *Proc. nat. Acad. Sci. USA*, 82: 245–247.

Mezey, E., Reisine, T., Skirboll, L., Beinfeld, M. C. and Kiss, J. Z. (1985) Role of cholecystokinin in ACTH release: coexistence with vasopressin and CRF in cells of the rat hypothalamic paraventricular nucleus. *Proc. nat. Acad. Sci. USA* (submitted).

O'Donohue, T. L., Beinfeld, M. C., Chay, W. Y., Chang, T., Nilaver, G., Zimmerman, E. A., Yajima, H., Adachi, H., Poth, M., McDevitt, R. C. and Jacobowitz, D. M. (1981) Identification, characterization and distribution of motilin immunoreactivity in the rat central nervous system. *Peptides*, 2: 467–477.

O'Donohue, T. L., Bishop, J. F., Chronwall, B. M., Watson, W. H. and Groome, J. R. (1984) Characterization and distribution of FMRFamide immunoreactivity in the rat central nervous system. *Peptides*, 5: 563–568.

Palkovits, M., Brownstein, M. J. and Vale, W. (1985a) Distribution of corticotropin-releasing factor in rat brain. *Fed. Proc.*, 44: 215–219.

Palkovits, M., Mezey, E., Chieuh, M., Krieger, D., Gallantz, K. and Brownstein, M. J. (1985b) Serotonin-containing elements of the rat pituitary intermediate lobe. *Neuroendocrinology* (in press).

Rõkaeus, A., Melander, T., Hökfelt, T., Lundberg, J. M., Tatemoto, K., Carlquist, M. and Mutt, V. (1984) A galanin-like peptide in the central nervous system and intestine of the rat. *Neurosci. Lett.*, 47: 161–166.

Roth, K. A., Weber, E. and Barchas, J. D. (1982) Distribution of gastrin releasing peptide-Bombesin-like immunostaining in rat brain. *Brain Res.*, 251: 277–282.

Saavedra, J. M., Palkovits, M., Kiser, J. S., Brownstein, M. J. and Zivin, J. A. (1975) Distribution of biogenic amines and related enzymes in the rat pituitary gland. *J. Neurochem.*, 25: 257–260.

Skofitsch, G., Jacobowitz, D. M., Eskay, R. L. and Zamir, N. (1985) Distribution of atrial natriuretic factor-like immunoreactive neurons in the rat brain. *Neuroscience* (in press).

Swanson, L. W., Sawchenko, P. E., Rivier, J. and Vale, W. W. (1983) Organization of ovine corticotropin-releasing factor immunoreactive cells and fibers in the rat brain: an immunohistochemical study. *Neuroendocrinology,* 36: 165–186.

Tager, H., Hohenboken, M., Markese, J. and Dinerstein, R. J. (1980) Identification and localization of glucagon-related peptides in the rat brain. *Proc. nat. Acad. Sci. USA,* 77: 6229–6233.

Vanderhaeghen, J. J., Signeau, J. C. and Gepts, W. (1975) New peptide in vertebrate CNS reacting with antigastrin antibodies. *Nature (Lond.),* 257: 604–605.

Vanderhaeghen, J. J., Lofstra, F., Vandesande, F. and Dierickx, K. (1981) Coexistence of cholecystokinin and oxytocin-neurophysin in some magnocellular hypothalamo-hypophyseal neurons. *Cell Tissue Res.,* 221: 227–231.

Vanderhaeghen, J. J., Lofstra, F., Liston, D. R. and Rossier, J. (1983) Proenkephalin, (Met)enkephalin and oxytocin immunoreactivities are colocalized in bovine hypothalamic magnocellular neurons. *Proc. nat. Acad. Sci. USA,* 80: 5139–5143.

Watson, S. J., Akil, H., Fiaschli, W., Goldstein, A., Zimmerman, E., Nilaver, G. and vanWimersma Greidanus, T. B. (1982) Dynorphin and vasopressin: common localization in magnocellular neurons. *Science,* 216: 85–87.

Weber, E., Evans, C. J. and Barchas, J. D. (1982) Mapping of hypothalamic opioid peptide neurons by a novel immunohistochemical technique: relation to α-neo-endorphin and vasopressin systems. *Advanc. Biochem. Psychopharmacol.,* 33: 519–526.

Whitnall, M. H., Gainer, H., Cox, B. M. and Molineaux, C. J. (1983) Dynorphin-A-(1-8) is contained within vasopressin neurosecretory vesicles in rat pituitary. *Science,* 222: 1137.

Young, III, W. S., Mezey, E. and Siegel, R. E. Differential localization of mRNA and encoded neuropeptides in the brain: proopiomelanocortin system (submitted).

Zamir, N. (1985) On the origin of Leu-enkephalin and Met-enkephalin in the rat neurohypophysis (submitted).

Zamir, N., Zamir, D., Eiden, L. E., Palkovits, M., Brownstein, M. J. Eskay, R. L., Weber, E., Faden, A. I. and Feuerstein, G. (1985) Methionine and leucine enkephalin in rat neurophypophysis: different responses to osmotic stimuli and T_2 toxin. *Science,* 228: 606–608.

T. Hökfelt, K. Fuxe and B. Pernow (Eds.),
Progress in Brain Research, Vol. 68

CHAPTER 12

Regulation of multiple peptides in CRF parvocellular neurosecretory neurons: implications for the stress response

L. W. Swanson, P. E. Sawchenko and R. W. Lind

The Salk Institute for Biological Studies, La Jolla, CA, 92037, U.S.A.

Introduction

In this chapter we shall outline current views about the organization of neural circuitry underlying the integration of stress responses, with special emphasis on the hypothalamic regulation of ACTH release from the anterior pituitary. The adrenal gland has long been known to play a major role in such responses; the release of glucocorticoid hormones from the adrenal cortex is influenced by ACTH, while the release of catecholamines from the adrenal medulla is mediated primarily by the sympathetic nervous system. The most influential unifying hypothesis in this field was advanced by Hans Selye (1976), who proposed that most stressors induce two classes of response. One, which he called the stress response, is common to all stressors, and involves the release of ACTH and adrenal catecholamines, which may have different time courses and lead to different functional consequences (Henry, 1980). The other consists of responses that are appropriate for individual stressors. For example, exposure to a hot or a cold environment are both followed by ACTH and adrenal catecholamine release, as well as by a set of unique endocrine, autonomic, and behavioral responses that are appropriate for maintaining a relatively constant body temperature.

The brain is involved in processing all classes of stimuli that can be regarded as stressors, and is responsible for coordinating groups of appropriate autonomic, endocrine, and behavioral responses. Furthermore, it is widely held that the hypothalamus plays a critical role in the integration of these responses. However, only since the characterization of hypothalamic corticotropin-releasing factor (CRF) by Vale and his colleagues (1981) have major new insights into the organization of specific neural pathways mediating ACTH release emerged.

Our own work has focussed on the organization of circuits that mediate responses to one type of stress, hypovolemia. This is a particularly advantageous model since a great deal is known about the physiology of body water regulation. As outlined in Table I, an integrated series of well-defined autonomic, endocrine, and behavioral responses are elicited by hemorrhage. The visceral (autonomic and endocrine) responses act to maintain blood pressure with available body water, while the behavioral response, drinking (and the associated sensation of thirst) constitutes a major strategy the animal uses to replenish lost body water. According to Selye's model, some of the neural pathways involved in this integrated set of responses should be common to all stress responses, while others are con-

Address for correspondence: Dr. L. W. Swanson, The Salk Institute, P.O. Box 85800, San Diego, CA, 92138, U.S.A.

TABLE I

Major responses to hemorrhage

(A)	*Autonomic*
	(1) Baroreceptor reflex
(B)	*Endocrine*
	(1) Adrenal catecholamine release (via sympathetic system)
	(2) Adrenal glucocorticoid release (via CRF and ACTH)
	(3) Vasopressin release (antidiuretic hormone)
	(4) Angiotensin II release (via renin from kidney)
	(5) Adrenal aldosterone release (via angiotensin II)
(C)	*Behavioral*
	(1) Thirst (partly via central actions of angiotensin II)

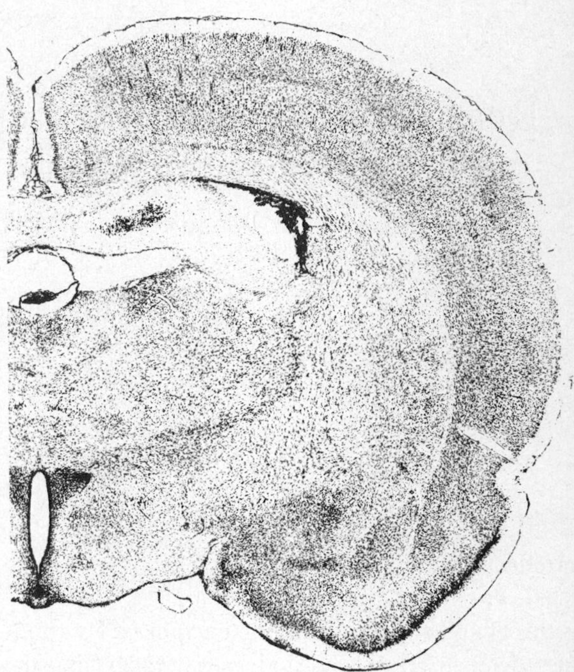

Fig. 1. Low-power photomicrograph of a Nissl-stained frontal section through the forebrain of the rat to show the location and appearance of the PVH, the dark, wingshaped region adjacent to the top of the third ventricle (lower left). ×8.

cerned specifically with hypovolemia. By examining the circuitry underlying responses to this stimulus, the hope would be to gain insight into pathways subserving specific responses, as well as pathways involved in the more general aspects of stress.

Following the production of antisera to CRF, it became clear from immunohistochemical studies, described below, that the paraventricular nucleus of the hypothalamus (PVH) plays a critical role as the final common pathway in the neuroendocrine limb of the stress response. Therefore, the projections and cellular compartmentalization of the PVH will be reviewed first, and this will be followed by a consideration of the endocrine and neural factors that appear to be involved specifically in modulating CRF neurons in the nucleus. Since the most detailed morphological work has been carried out in the rat, attention will be focussed on this species.

Output of the paraventricular nucleus

The PVH is a densely-packed, wing-shaped nucleus that lies on either side of the third ventricle in rostral parts of the hypothalamus (Fig. 1), and contains about 10,000 neurons (Swanson and Sawchenko, 1983). It is undoubtedly the best understood cell group in the hypothalamus from a functional point of view since, along with the supraoptic nucleus and scattered accessory neurons between, it contains the magnocellular neurosecretory neurons that synthesize vasopressin (antidiuretic hormone) and oxytocin, and release them into the general circulation from terminals in the posterior pituitary (see Dierickx, 1980 for review). The axons that transport these nonapeptide hormones together constitute the paraventriculoneurohypophyseal tract, which courses laterally around the fornix, then ventrally over the supraoptic nucleus, and finally medially through the internal lamina of the median eminence to the posterior lobe.

About a decade ago, two other projections from the PVH were identified. One consisted of vasopressin (and oxytocin) immunoreactive fibers to the external lamina (neurohemal zone) of the median eminence that were postulated to influence the secretion of one or another of the anterior pituitary hormones (Vandesande et al., 1977). The other consisted of descending fibers to cell groups in the brainstem and spinal cord (Conrad and Pfaff, 1976; Saper et al., 1976). As indicated in Fig. 2, these fibers preferentially innervate regions associated with the autonomic nervous system, including the Edinger-Westphal nucleus, parabrachial nucleus, nucleus of the solitary tract, dorsal motor nucleus of the vagus nerve, and intermediolateral column, as well as the periaqueductal gray, pedunculopontine nucleus, locus coeruleus, marginal zone of the sensory trigeminal nuclei and spinal gray matter, and spinal central gray (see also Swanson and McKellar, 1979; Swanson and Hartman 1980; Swanson et al., 1984).

This evidence clearly suggested that the PVH may be viewed best as a visceral motor nucleus whose neurons can release hormones into the general circulation from the posterior pituitary, influence the secretion of hormones from the anterior pituitary by way of the hypophyseal portal system, and modulate neural activity in preganglionic neurons of both the sympathetic and parasympathetic systems. In addition, they may influence (a) the central relay of vagal and glossopharyngeal visceral sensory information through projections to the nucleus of the solitary tract and the parabrachial nucleus (see Swanson and Sawchenko, 1983); (b) the central relay of nociceptive or thermal sensory information through projections to the marginal zone; and (c) behavior through projections to the pedunculopontine nucleus, which has been referred to as the mesencephalic locomotor region (see Swanson et al., 1984).

This evidence raised several interesting questions. First, do individual neurons in the PVH send axon collaterals to each of these functionally distinct terminal fields, or are separate populations of cells involved? The answer to this question has important implications for understanding mechanisms underlying the integration of responses mediated by the PVH. This problem was first approached by placing HRP in the spinal cord, and noting that retrogradely labeled neurons tend to be segregated from magnocellular neurosecretory neurons (Hosoya and Matsushita, 1979). However, a more direct approach was based on the use of a fluorescence

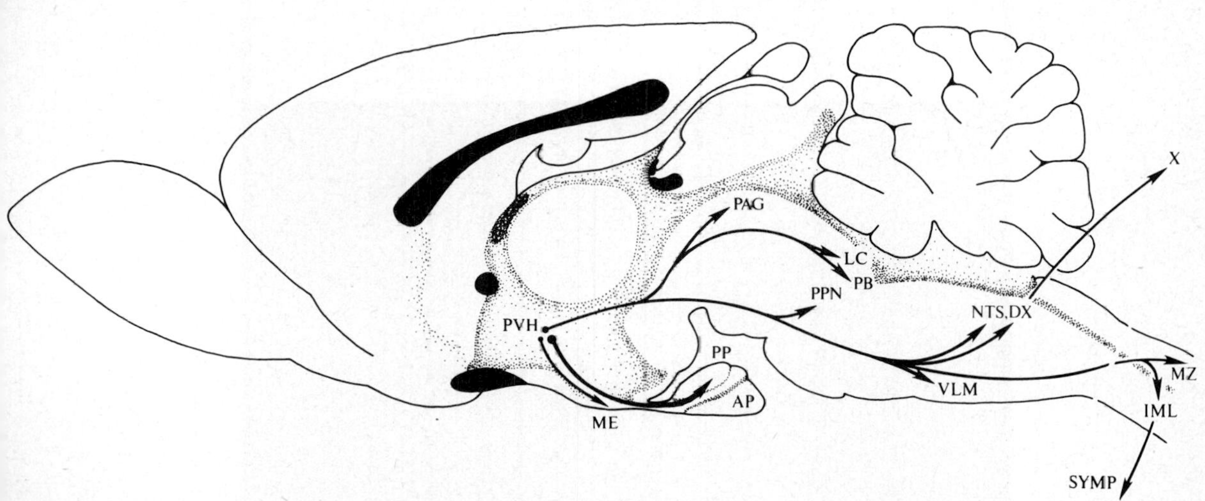

Fig. 2. A summary of the major neuroendocrine and descending projections of the PVH in the rat. AP = anterior pituitary; DX = dorsal motor nucleus of the vagus nerve; IML = intermediolateral column; LC = locus coeruleus; ME = neurohemal zone of the median eminence; MZ = marginal zone; NTS = nucleus of the solitary tract; PAG = periaqueductal gray; PB = parabrachial nucleus; PP = posterior pituitary; PPN = pedunculopontine nucleus; SYMP = sympathetic nervous system; X = vagus nerve.

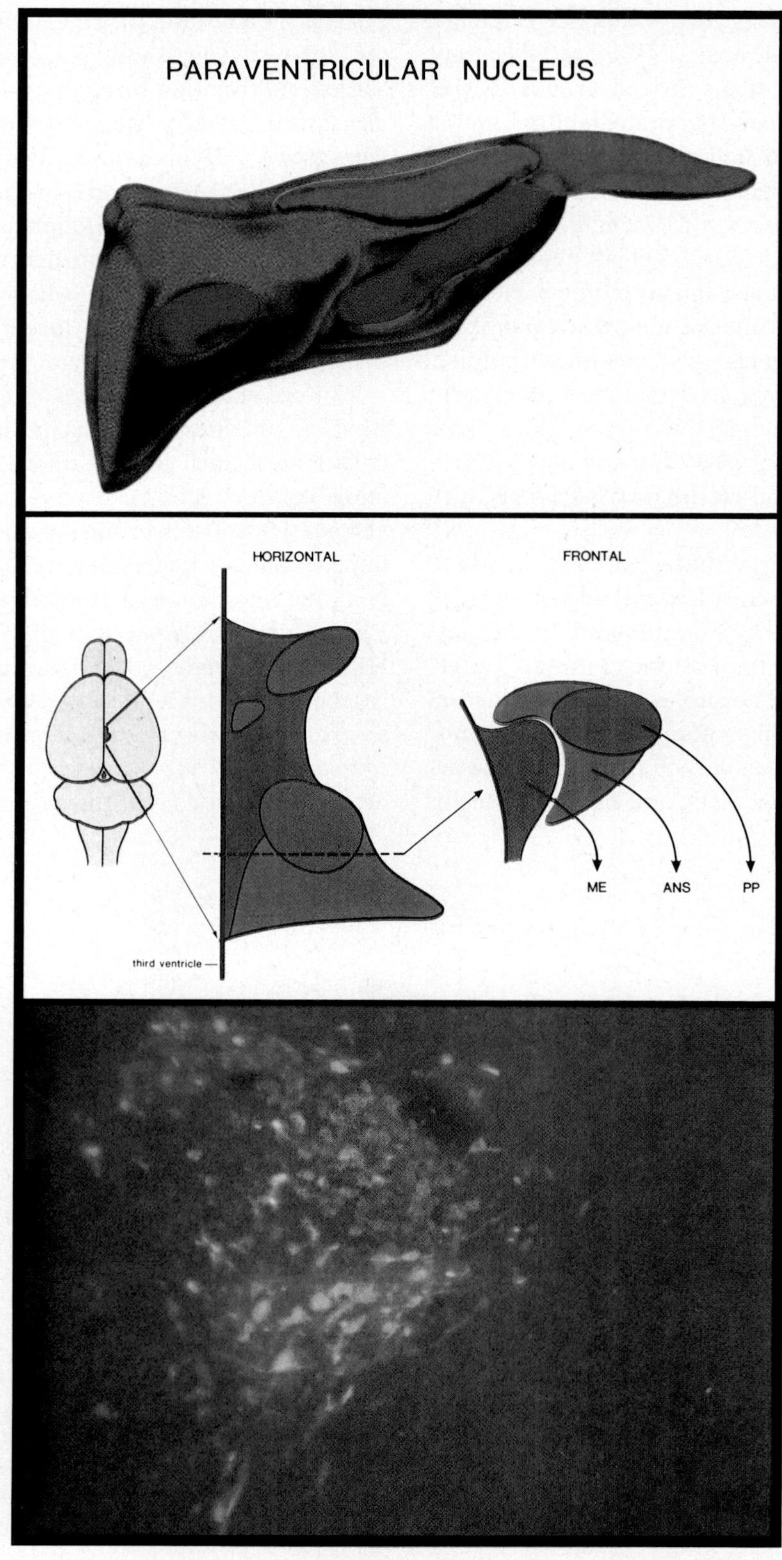
PARAVENTRICULAR NUCLEUS
HORIZONTAL
FRONTAL
third ventricle
ME
ANS
PP

double retrograde labeling method developed by Kuypers and his colleagues. The results of these experiments (Swanson and Kuypers, 1980; Swanson et al., 1980) suggested that essentially separate groups of neurons in the PVH project to the posterior pituitary, median eminence, and autonomic centers (Fig. 3). However, a small population of medium-sized cells projects both to the posterior pituitary and to autonomic centers (see also Zerihun and Harris, 1981), and at least 15% of the neurons in the PVH projecting to the dorsal vagal complex may also send a collateral to the spinal cord. It is important to note that while retrograde tracer experiments demonstrate that neurons projecting to the posterior pituitary, median eminence, and autonomic centers tend to be clustered in separate parts of the PVN (see below), at least a few neurons of each type are found throughout the nucleus; thus, a complete topographic segregation of different cell types does not occur within the nucleus.

And second, it was of interest to identify possible neuroactive substances utilized by neurons within each functional subdivision of the nucleus. The neurosecretory subdivisions will be described below; the population of cells in the PVH that projects to the brainstem and spinal cord, which numbers some 1500 (Swanson and Kuypers, 1980), may be surprisingly heterogeneous as judged by the results of combined retrograde transport-immunofluorescence experiments. Thus, small populations of neurons that appear to contain oxytocin, vasopressin (Swanson 1977; Sawchenko and Swanson, 1980, 1982; Sofroniew and Schrell 1981), dopamine, somatostatin, enkephalin, neurotensin, CRF, or angiotensin (Swanson et al., 1981; Sawchenko and Swanson, 1982, 1985; R. W. Lind and L. W. Swanson, in preparation) have been observed and counted. Interestingly, oxytocin-stained neurons outnumber vasopressin-stained neurons by a ratio of about 3:1, yet oxytocin-stained neurons still account for only about 15% of the PVH neurons with descending projections, and together all of the cell types identified thus far account for less than a third of the total number. This suggests that other, as yet unidentified, neurotransmitters play a major role in this projection. The functional significance of this diversity is unclear, although detailed examination of oxytocin-stained fibers in the spinal cord (most, if not all, of which arise in the PVH) indicates that they innervate specific groups of preganglionic neurons in specific segments of the cord (Swanson and McKellar, 1979). Thus, different cell types in the PVH may preferentially innervate specific groups of preganglionic neurons, modulating sympathetic influences on specific groups of visceral organs. This, of course, remains to be shown experimentally, and it is also worth pointing out that the issue of possible colocalization of neuroactive substances in these preautonomic neurons has not yet been addressed, although clearly oxytocin and vasopressin are synthesized in different neurons.

Compartmentalization in the paraventricular nucleus

The evidence gained from retrograde tracer studies, combined with immunohistochemical results, has led to the concept of PVH cellular compartmentalization illustrated in Fig. 4, which is important for understanding the afferent control of CRF release, and its integration with other responses modulated by the nucleus. The basic conclusion that can be

Fig. 3. Top: A drawing of the PVH as viewed from the lateral aspect, with anterior to the left, and dorsal at the top; red, parvocellular; blue, mediocellular; green, magnocellular. Middle: Schematic views of the PVH to show the general location of cell groups that project to the median eminence (ME), autonomic cell groups (ANS), and the posterior pituitary. Bottom: Photomicrograph of the PVH to show the distribution of magnocellular vasopressin cells (immunostaining labeled with fluorescein), parvocellular CRF cells (immunostaining labeled with rhodamine), and cells that project to the spinal cord (retrogradely labeled with true blue). Triple exposure, ×60.

drawn from retrograde tracer studies is that the PVH can be divided into three functional zones on the basis of efferent projections: a medial, parvocellular, zone related to the neurohemal zone and anterior pituitary; an intermediate, mediocellular, zone related to autonomic centers; and a lateral, magnocellular, zone related to the posterior pituitary.

As shown in Figs. 3 and 4, each zone can be further subdivided. First, immunohistochemical studies have shown that there are three separate parts within the magnocellular zone (Fig. 3), and that the anterior and medial parts contain almost exclusively oxytocinergic neurons, while the posterior part can be divided into an anteromedial oxytocinergic region and a posterolateral vasopressinergic part (Vandesande and Dierickx, 1975; Swaab et al., 1975; McNeill and Sladek 1981; Rhodes et al., 1981; Swanson et al., 1981; Sawchenko and Swanson, 1982). Second, retrograde tracer studies indicate that the mediocellular zone can be divided into a dorsal part, where at least 90% of the cells project to the spinal cord but very few project to the dorsal vagal complex, and a ventral medial part, where cells projecting to the spinal cord, the dorsal vagal complex, or both, are intermixed (Swanson and Kuypers, 1980; Sawchenko and Swanson, 1981a). And third, the parvocellular zone can roughly be divided into three vertical regions, one adjacent to the ventricle that contains somatostatinergic neurons predominantly (see Sawchenko and Swanson, 1982), one just lateral to this in which thyrotropin-releasing hormone (TRH)-synthesizing neurons are concentrated (Lechan and Jackson, 1982), and a far lateral region where CRF neurons are densely aggregated (see Bloom et al., 1982; Bugnon et al., 1982; Kawata et al., 1982; Merchanthaler et al., 1982; Olschowska et al., 1982; Cummings et al., 1982; Swanson et al., 1983). Experimental evidence based on the use of lesions indicates that most, if not all, of the TRH (Brownstein et al., 1982) and CRF (Antoni et al., 1983) terminals in the neurohemal zone of the median eminence arise from cells in the PVH.

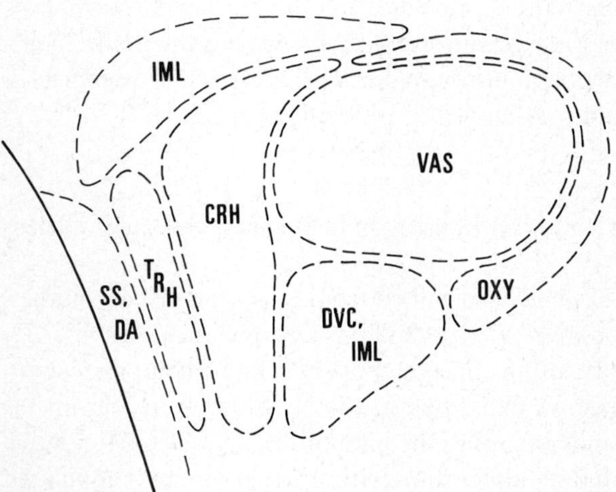

Fig. 4. Major divisions of the PVH based on cell-types in a schematic frontal section at the level shown in Fig. 3. The dashed lines indicate where particular cell-types are concentrated, although there is some overlap, and a few cells of each type may be found in many parts of the nucleus. CRH = parvocellular neurosecretory corticotropin-releasing hormone (factor) cells; DA = dopamine; DVC = to dorsal vagal complex; IML = to intermediolateral column; OXY = magnocellular neurosecretory oxytocin cells; SS = somatostatin; TRH = parvocellular neurosecretory thyrotropin-releasing hormone cells; VAS = magnocellular neurosecretory vasopressin cells.

It is possible to correlate these functional regions with the cytoarchitectonic appearance of the PVH. In our original parcellation (Swanson and Kuypers, 1980), the PVH was divided into a magnocellular division with three parts (anterior, medial, and posterior), and a parvocellular division with five parts (periventricular, anterior, medial, lateral, and dorsal). Since that time it has become clear that two of these parts should be further subdivided: the posterior magnocellular part has a medial (oxytocinergic) and a lateral (vasopressinergic) region (see Hatton et al., 1976), while the medial parvocellular part has a dorsal (neurosecretory) and a ventral (preautonomic) region. Thus, it now seems clear that the PVH has at least 10 cytoarchitectonically recognizable compartments in the rat, and for the sake of completeness, a lateral magnocellular group, which is contiguous with the caudolateral tip of the nucleus as it arches towards and over the fornix (the posterior fornical group of Koh and

Ricardo, 1980), should probably be added. The hormone specificity of the magnocellular division has already been discussed. Within the parvocellular division, the periventricular part contains the majority of somatostatin cells, the dorsal medial part contains TRH and CRF neurons, the ventral, medial and lateral parts send fibers to the dorsal vagal complex and spinal cord, and the dorsal part sends fibers to the spinal cord, but very few to the dorsal vagal complex.

It is also worth pointing out that while the anterior magnocellular and anterior parvocellular, and the periventricular, parts have not always been included within the PVH proper (for historical review see Swanson and Kuypers, 1980), we have chosen to do so for three reasons. First, they are topographically continuous; second, they share functionally similar cell types; and third, they share certain neural inputs. Perhaps the most dramatic is provided by aminergic fibers. Thus, noradrenergic fibers massively and selectively innvervate the PVH as defined here, with relatively few fibers in adjacent areas (see Fig. 5), while the opposite is true of serotonergic fibers (Sawchenko et al., 1983).

Neurosecretory CRF cells

At least 2000 CRF immunoreactive neurons may be counted in the PVH on each side of the brain in

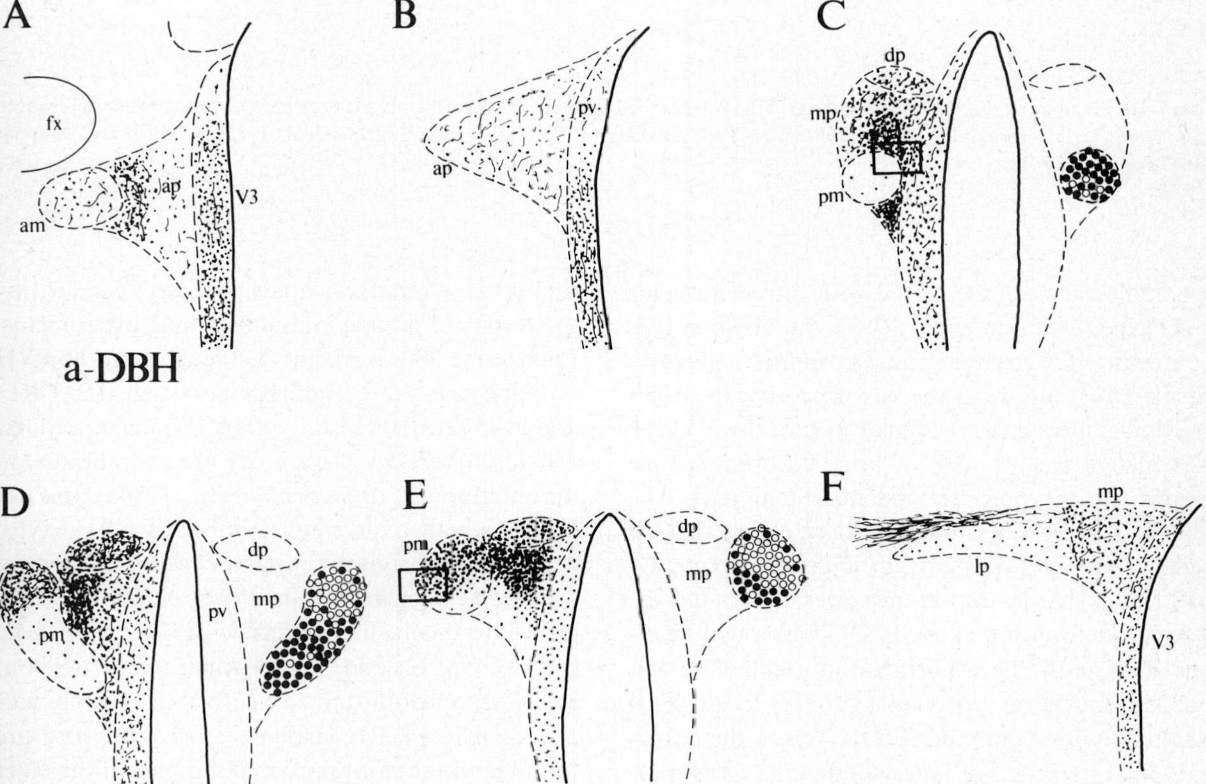

Fig. 5. The distribution of dopamine-β-hydroxylase (DBH)-stained fibers in the PVH (left), compared with the distribution of vasopressin (○) and oxytocin (●) cell bodies. The frontal sections are arranged from rostral (A) to caudal (F). Subdivisons of PVH: am = anterior magnocellular; ap = anterior parvocellular; dp = dorsal parvocellular; lp = lateral parvocellular; mp = medial parvocellular; pm = posterior magnocellular; pv = periventricular. (From Swanson et al., 1981.)

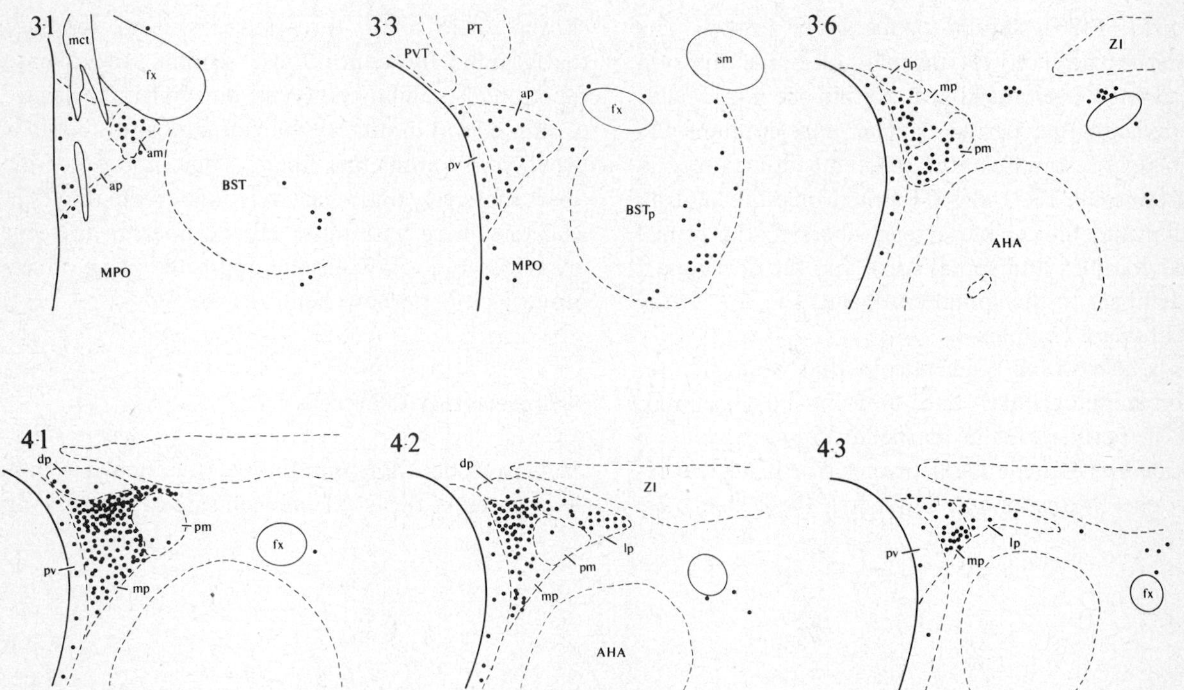

Fig. 6. The distribution of CRF neurons (dots) in the PVH of the normal male rat pretreated with colchicine. Frontal sections arranged from rostral (3.1) to caudal (4.3). Abbreviations for PVH subdivisions: see Fig. 5; from Swanson et al., 1983. For other abbreviations see this reference.

the adult male rat pretreated with intraventricular colchicine (Swanson et al., 1983). As shown in Fig. 6, at least a few such neurons are found in all parts of the PVH, although the vast majority lie within the dorsal medial parvocellular part of the nucleus, just medial to the mass of large vasopressinergic neurons in the posterior magnocellular part. The axons of these CRF neurons take essentially the same course as the paraventriculoneurohypophyseal tract. That is, they course laterally around the fornix (see Swanson et al., 1983). This might be referred to as the paraventriculo-infundibular tract, but it seems more reasonable to refer to all fibers (including those containing TRH) from the paraventricular nucleus that follow this course as the paraventriculohypophyseal tract, which in fact is itself a component of a much larger hypothalamo-hypophyseal tract with the same general course.

CRF-containing neurons in the PVH may also synthesize a variety of other peptides as judged by the results of double immunostaining experiments. First, some 200 oxytocinergic neurons in the PVH of colchicine-treated animals also stain for CRF; about 75% of these lie within the magnocellular division, where a vast majority are concentrated in the anterior part (Sawchenko et al., 1984a). It is not known whether the small number of CRF/oxytocin-stained neurons in the parvocellular division are displaced magnocellular neurons, or whether they project to the median eminence or some other part of the CNS. Second, a very small number (about 30) of vasopressin-stained neurons in such animals also stain for CRF, and a majority of these are found in the anterior parvocellular part of the PVH (Sawchenko et al., 1984a). Third, about 75 CRF-stained neurons in the parvocellular division of the PVH can also be stained with neurotensin antisera in the colchicine-treated male rat, although there are many singly-labeled CRF, as well as neurotensin, neurons in this division (Sawchenko et al., 1984a). Fourth and fifth, extensive colocalization of CRF with enkephalin- and PHI-immunoreactivity has been reported in parvocellular parts of the PVH (Hökfelt et al., 1983). And sixth, cholecystokinin (CCK) has also now been reported in the parvocellular region of the PVH where CRF neurons are concentrated (Kiss et al., 1984).

Thus, it would appear that, in the normal adult male rat, CRF may be coexpressed with at least one or more of six additional peptides in the PVH. Some of this colocalization appears to occur preferentially in specific subpopulations of magnocellular neurosecretory neurons with oxytocin, and this is consistent with reports of CRF-stained fibers in the posterior pituitary (see Bloom et al., 1982). In the dorsal medial parvocellular part of the PVH, which contains most of the parvocellular neurosecretory CRF neurons, it would appear that many CRF neurons may also express neurotensin, enkephalin, PHI, and/or CCK, although clearly this is not a homogeneous population in the sense that comparable levels of each peptide are not synthesized in each cell simultaneously.

Effects of adrenalectomy

It is well known that steroid hormones of the adrenal cortex (glucocorticoids) exert a negative feedback effect on the synthesis and release of ACTH in the anterior pituitary (Schachter et al., 1982), and it also seems likely that these hormones exert similar effects on CRF production and release (Yates and Maran, 1974). It is not surprising, therefore, that adrenalectomy leads after 3–7 days to a dramatic increase in CRF immunostaining in the PVH (Bugnon et al., 1983; Merchenthaler et al., 1983; Paul and Gibbs, 1983; Swanson et al., 1983; Tramu et al., 1983). In the normal male rat that has not been treated with colchicine, only a few lightly-stained CRF neurons are observed in the PVH. Following adrenalectomy, somewhat more than a third as many brightly-stained CRF neurons may be counted in the PVH as compared to colchicine-treated animals (about 750 vs. 2000 cells), and these neurons are centered in the dorsal medial parvocellular part of the nucleus (Swanson et al., 1983).

When colocalization experiments were reported in adrenalectomized animals, several interesting features emerged (Fig. 7). First, a substantial proportion of the CRF-stained parvocellular neurons in the PVH also express vasopressin immunoreactivity (Tramu et al., 1983; Kiss et al., 1984; Sawchenko et al., 1984b); in fact, at least 70% of the CRF neurons can be doubly labeled (Sawchenko et al., 1984). On the other hand, levels of oxytocin in neurons that also stain for CRF do not appear to be influenced by adrenalectomy (Kiss et al., 1984; Sawchenko et al., 1984b). Second, angiotensin II-immunoreactivity can be detected in a substantial proportion of parvocellular CRF neurons after adrenalectomy and colchicine pretreatment (Lind et al., 1984), and triple immunostaining procedures clearly indicate that many individual cells in parvocellular parts of the PVH appear to contain CRF, vasopressin, and angiotensin following this treatment (Fig. 8). Third, these effects are specific in the sense that levels of neurotensin and enkephalin do not appear to be influenced, at least qualitatively, in CRF parvocellular neurons following adrenalectomy (Sawchenko and Swanson, 1984). Fourth, the specificity of these effects has also been shown in steroid replacement experiments (Sawchenko and Swanson, 1984). Thus, increases in CRF and vasopressin staining following adrenalectomy can be reversed completely by dexamethasone, while being only mildly attenuated by comparable levels of mineralocorticoids. The role of adrenal steroids, as opposed to ACTH, is further emphasized by the observation that hypophysectomy results in a pattern of CRF/vasopressin coexpression similar to that found after adrenalectomy (see Sawchenko and Swanson, 1985). And fifth, it is clear that angiotensin (and to a lesser extent vasopressin) immunostaining in magnocellular neurosecretory neurons is actually decreased in adrenalectomized, colchicine-treated animals (R. W. Lind and L. W. Swanson, unpublished observations; see Fig. 8).

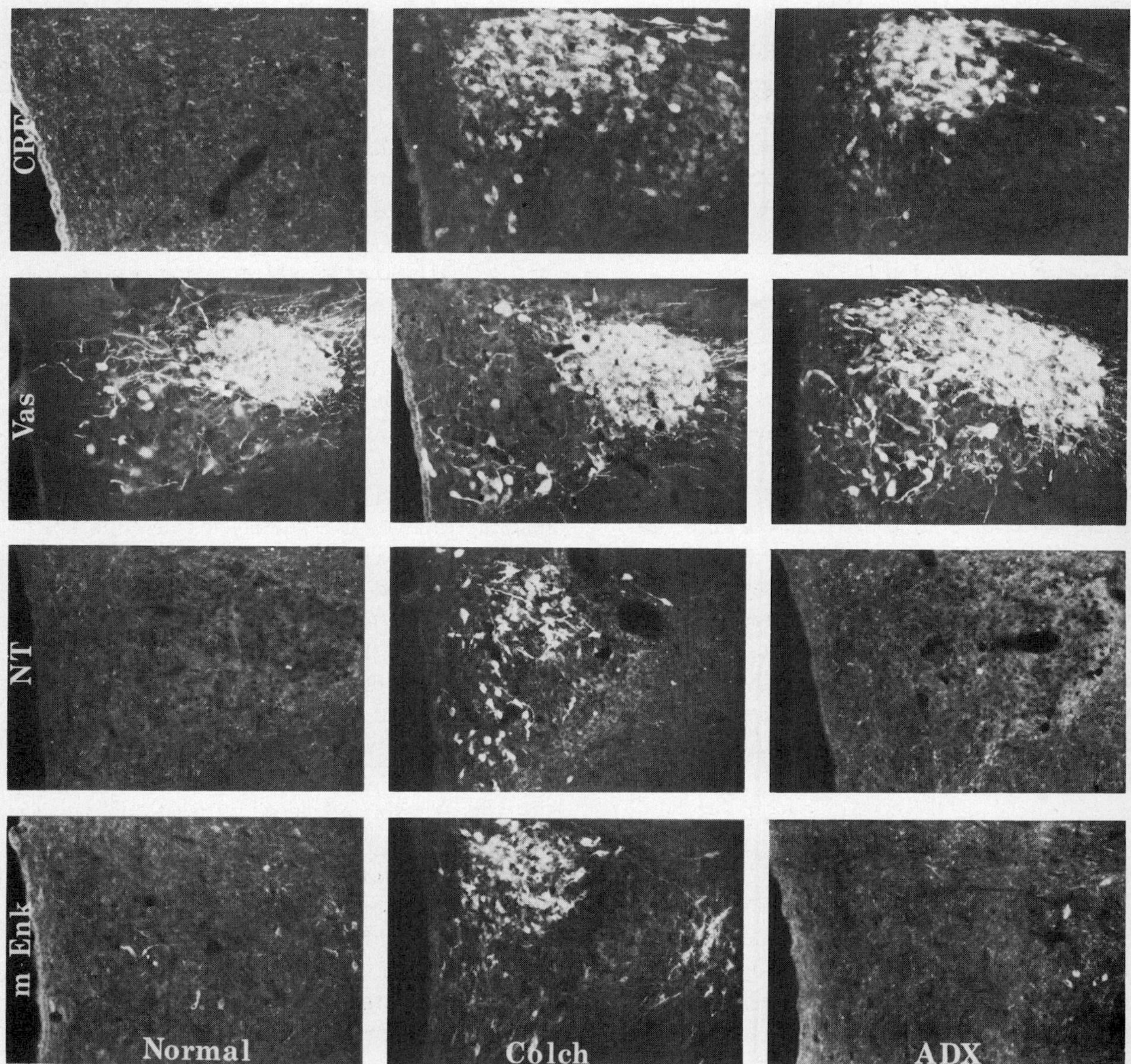

Fig. 7. This montage shows the appearance of immunostaining for four different peptides (CRF, vasopressin, neurotensin, and met-enkephalin) and three different conditions (normal male rat, colchicine pretreated male rat, and adrenalectomized rat — no colchicine). All sections were cut in the frontal plane and are through approximately the same rostrocaudal level of the nucleus. Note especially in the adrenalectomized animal that vasopressin is colocalized extensively with CRF, and that neurotensin and met-enkephalin have the same appearance as in the normal animal. ×40.

The results of this work are summarized in Fig. 9. In the normal male rat, many CRF neurons in the dorsal medial parvocellular part of the PVH also appear to synthesize enkephalin, CCK, and neurotensin. However, following adrenalectomy, these same neurons stain much more brightly with antisera to CRF, and also stain brightly with antisera to vasopressin and angiotensin II. The most

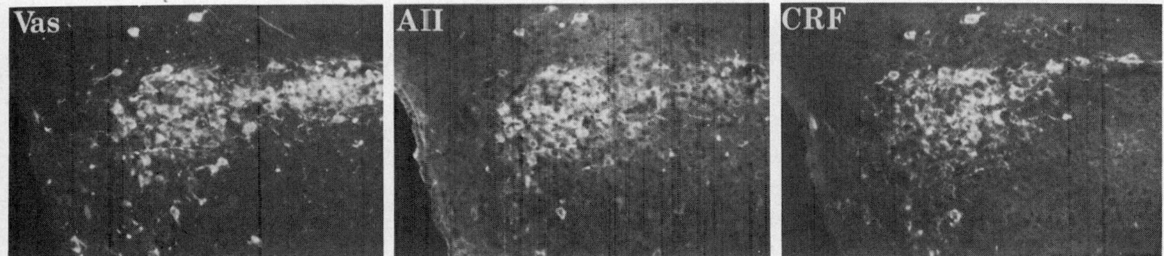

Fig. 8. Immunostaining for vasopressin (Vas), angiotensin II (AII), and CRF in the PVH of an adrenalectomized, colchicine pretreated male rat, as viewed in an individual section. Vasopressin was stained with a monoclonal antibody (rhodamine secondary antiserum) and AII was stained with a rabbit antiserum (fluorescein secondary antiserum). After photography and elution, CRF was stained with a rabbit antiserum and the section was rephotographed. Note the many triply-labeled neurons (three isolated cells in the upper left-hand corner are particularly obvious), as well as singly- and doubly-labeled cells. ×40.

Fig. 9. A summary of peptide immunohistochemical (IHC) staining in "parvocellular CRF" cells and "magnocellular vasopressin" cells in the PVH of the normal and adrenalectomized (ADX) adult male rat. In the ADX animal, the intensity of CRF, vasopressin (VAS), and angiotensin II (AII) staining increases dramatically in parvocellular neurons, while no change is apparent for enkephalin (ENK) and neurotensin (NT); cholecystokinin (CCK) and PHI have not been examined quantitatively (see Fig. 7). In contrast, after ADX, AII and to a lesser extent VAS immunostaining is noticeably decreased in magnocellular neurons. Of the peptides shown, only CRF, VAS and AII are thought to be physiological releasers of ACTH from the anterior pituitary.

straightforward interpretation of the results is that these neurons synthesize increased amounts of the three peptides, all of which are secretagogues for ACTH, and appear to act synergistically (see Vale et al., 1983). On the other hand, immunostaining for enkephalin and PHI, which are not known to stimulate ACTH release at physiological concentrations, does not appear to be influenced significantly by adrenalectomy. And, interestingly, adrenal steroids may have opposite effects on adjacent magnocellular neurosecretory neurons, which also appear to synthesize vasopressin and angiotensin II. Finally, it is worth pointing out that the population of "CRF" neurons in the PVH of the adrenalectomized rat is quite heterogenous with respect to the ratios of peptides in the cell bodies of individual cells at any one time, as judged by the immunohistochemical evidence. In fact, it is tempting to speculate that the ratio of the seven described peptides may be different in every cell in this population; in any event, it is clear that the ratios vary widely from cell to cell. Possible mechanisms underlying this variability will be discussed below.

Neural inputs to CRF cells

The immunohistochemical evidence just reviewed indicates that adrenal steroids influence levels of CRF in the paraventriculo-infundibular system. However, it is not entirely clear where these hormones exert their effects in the brain. Thus, using classical autoradiographic techniques, it has not been possible to demonstrate binding of [^{3}H]corticosterone to cytoplasmic or nuclear receptors in the hypothalamus; instead, high levels of binding are found in parts of the limbic region, especially the hippocampus, as well as in certain regions of the brainstem (see McEwen, 1982). On the other hand, there is evidence to suggest that glucocorticoids act at the level of CRF terminals to inhibit release of the peptide (Edwardson and Bennett, 1974). Therefore, it would appear that glucocorticoids can act to regulate their own secretion at many levels, from the anterior pituitary, to the median eminence, limbic region, and perhaps brainstem as well. Furthermore, it is entirely possible that the hormones act on the plasma membrane or genome of CRF cell bodies in the PVH (see Agnati et al., 1985), although further work is needed to clarify this point.

This evidence does raise the possibility however, that substances released from neural inputs may influence the synthesis of CRF and other peptides in these cells. And since there is no doubt that neural inputs influence the release of CRF, what is currently known about the origin and possible neurotransmitter content of these pathways will now be reviewed.

We have taken advantage of the fact that parvocellular neurosecretory CRF neurons form a dense cluster in the dorsal medial parvocellular part of the PVH to study neural inputs to this region at the light microscopic level. The basic strategy was to identify all neural inputs to the PVH with retrograde axonal transport methods, to counterstain as many of these retrogradely labeled cells as possible with appropriate antisera, and then to determine their distribution within the PVH using anterograde axonal transport methods. The results of this work to date are summarized in Fig. 10. For ease of description, likely inputs to CRF neurons can be divided into four sets.

The first set consists of ascending fibers that appear to relay visceral sensory information from the brainstem. The initial clue to the origin of these inputs came from observations (Swanson et al., 1981) that well-known catecholaminergic inputs to the PVH (e.g. Carlsson et al., 1962) appear to end most densely in the dorsal medial parvocellular ("CRF") part of the nucleus, and that this terminal field consists of both adrenergic and noradrenergic fibers.

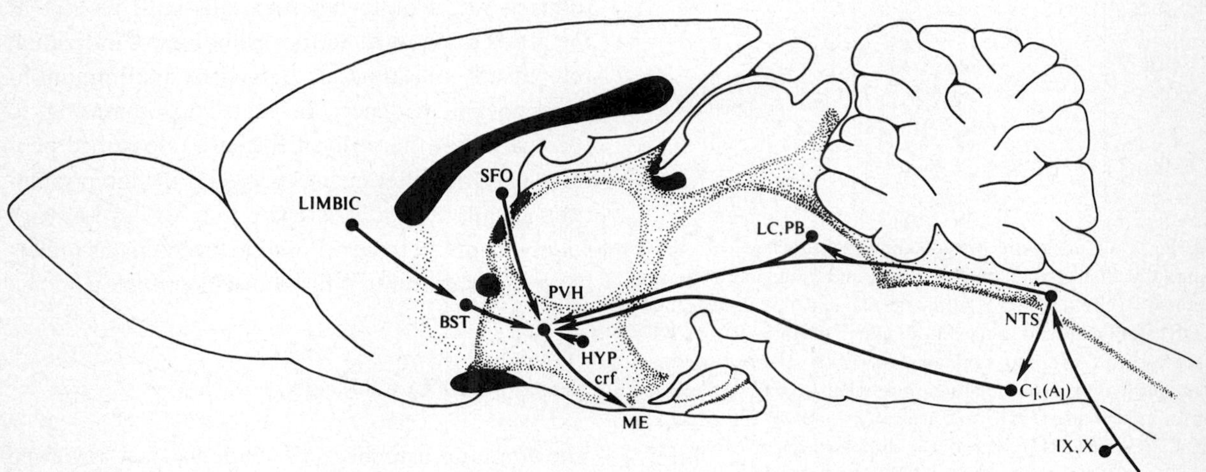

Fig. 10. Summary of major, anatomically-defined neural inputs to the region of parvocellular neurosecretory CRF neurons in the PVH of the rat. BST = bed nucleus of the stria terminalis; A_1, C_1 = noradrenergic and adrenergic groups in ventrolateral medulla; HYP = hypothalamus; LC = locus coeruleus; ME = median eminence; NTS = nucleus of the solitary tract; PB = parabrachial nucleus; SFO = subfornical organ; IX = glossopharyngeal nerve; X = vagus nerve.

Subsequent axonal transport and immunohistochemical studies (Sawchenko and Swanson, 1982) indicated that the noadrenergic fibers to the PVH arise predominantly (about 70% of the participating cell bodies) from the A_1 cell group in the caudal ventrolateral medulla, while on the order of 20% of the cells lie within the nucleus of the solitary tract (the A_2 cell group), and the few remaining are found in the locus coeruleus. Furthermore, autoradiographic evidence suggested that only the A_1 and A_2 groups project in a significant way directly to the region of CRF cell bodies in the PVH. And finally, combined retrograde transport-immuno studies indicated that at least 80% of the neurons in the A_1 and A_2 regions projecting to the PVH are noradrenergic. More recently, similar techniques have been used to show that cells in the C_1, C_2, and C_3 regions all contribute adrenergic fibers to the PVH as well (Sawchenko et al., 1985).

The latter study also characterized a new layer of complexity in the organization of ascending projections to the PVH. Using combined retrograde transport-immuno methods it was shown that the massive NPY input to the PVH (see Olschowka, 1984), which is particularly dense in the CRF region, arises in part from noradrenergic neurons centered in ventral parts of the A_1 region, and in adrenergic neurons of the C_{1-3} groups. Interestingly, very few noradrenergic cells that project to the PVH from the nucleus of the solitary tract, and from more dorsal parts of the A_1 region, contain detectable levels of NPY (see also Everitt et al., 1984).

As summarized in Fig. 10, a great deal of evidence (for references see Sawchenko and Swanson, 1982b; Swanson and Sawchenko, 1983) now suggests that these aminergic pathways to the PVH relay visceral sensory information from the vagus and glossopharyngeal nerves. For example, it now seems clear that these pathways are involved in stimulating the release of CRF and vasopressin in response to hemorrhage (see Caverson and Ciriello, 1984; Blessing and Willoughby, 1985). For the sake of completeness, it should be pointed out that the nucleus of the solitary tract projects massively to the A_1 (and C_1) region by way of non-aminergic fibers (Sawchenko and Swanson, 1982b), as well as to the parabrachial nucleus (Norgren, 1978), which in turn projects substantially to the parvocellular division of the PVH (Saper and Loewy, 1980).

In summary, then, it now seems clear that visceral sensory information is relayed to CRF neurons in the PVH by way of a highly differentiated series of pathways from the lower brainstem. The precise distribution within the PVH of fibers from A_1, A_2 and C_{1-3} groups, and from individual cells within these groups, remains to be determined, but it seems likely that they are not identical. If this is indeed the case, then it is possible that the pattern of neurotransmitter release in the PVH is also highly differentiated, and may contribute to the variable ratios of peptide levels in CRF neurons discussed above. Tantalizing evidence for this was provided by Mezey et al. (1984) who showed that peripheral injections of a phenylethanolamine-*N*-methyltransferase inhibitor, which decrease PVH levels of adrenaline, lead to increased levels of CRF-immunoreactivity in the nucleus. Although the mechanisms underlying this effect are not yet clear, we have recently observed that knife-cuts in the brainstem, which interrupt ascending catecholamine fibers, also lead to modest increases in CRF but not vasopressin immunostaining in the PVH (P. E. Sawchenko, unpublished observations).

A second input to the PVH arises in the subfornical organ (Miselis, 1981; Lind et al., 1982), and consists, at least in part, of fibers that cross-react with antisera to angiotensin II (Lind et al., 1984b). A component of this projection ends in the region of dense CRF cells (Sawchenko and Swanson, 1983), and it has been shown electrophysiologically that neurons in the subfornical organ excite neurons in the region of the PVH projecting to the median eminence (Ferguson et al., 1984a). As reviewed elsewhere (Simpson, 1981; Lind et al., 1985), the subfornical organ pays a critical role in mediating the central effects of circulating angiotensin II, and the evidence just referred to suggests that one of these effects may involve the modulation of CRF release.

A third input to the region of CRF cells in the

PVH arises in ventral parts of the bed nucleus of the stria terminalis (Sawchenko and Swanson, 1983). The possible functional significance of this pathway, whose neurotransmitters have not been identified, is illustrated in Fig. 10. The bed nucleus, which constitutes the ventral division of the septal region, receives massive inputs from the amygdala (Krettek and Price, 1978), and temporal parts of the hippocampal formation (Swanson and Cowan, 1977). Since the limbic region provides the most direct route for neocortical influences on the hypothalamus (for a recent review see Swanson, 1983), the bed nucleus may be thought of as the end of a limbic funnel for cognitive influences on CRF release. And fourth, axonal transport studies indicate that neurons in many parts of the hypothalamus itself may also innervate CRF neurons in the PVH (Sawchenko and Swanson, 1983). The functional significance of these inputs is presently obscure.

Neural inputs to vasopressin and preautonomic cells

In addition to CRF release, hemorrhage leads to baroreceptor reflex activation and vasopressin secretion from the posterior pituitary. Since the PVH appears to exert a tonic inhibitory influence on the baroreceptor reflex (Ciriello and Calaresu, 1980), and contains a substantial population of magnocellular vasopressin cells, we shall now review what is known about neural pathways that may be involved in the coordinate activation of CRF and vasopressin neurons in the PVH, as well as the preautonomic neurons described above.

The anatomical evidence suggests that direct neural inputs to magnocellular vasopressin cells may be less complex than those to CRF neurons. Noradrenergic inputs to the region of vasopressin cell bodies appear to arise almost exclusively from cells in the A_1 region (Sawchenko and Swanson, 1982), some of which may also contain NPY-immunoreactivity (Sawchenko et al., 1986), and to exert a predominantly excitatory influence (Day et al., 1984). Electrical stimulation of the A_2 region leads to an equally potent release of vasopressin (Day et al., 1984), but it is not clear whether this effect is mediated polysynaptically, perhaps through the A_1 region or through cells with recurrent collaterals (Van den Pol, 1982) in parvocellular parts of the PVH. The anatomical evidence suggests that cells in the nucleus of the solitary tract, the parabrachial nucleus, and medullary adrenergic cell groups provide at best a sparse direct input to magnocellular vasopressin neurons in the PVH and supraoptic nucleus (see Sawchenko and Swanson, 1983). There is now good electrophysiological (Caverson and Ciriello, 1984; Day et al., 1984) and physiological (Blessing and Willoughby, 1985) evidence that pressor information in the vagus and glossopharyngeal nerves is relayed to vasopressin neurons by way of a projection from the nucleus of the solitary tract to the A_1 cell group.

Furthermore, the anatomical evidence suggests that the brainstem cell groups projecting to CRF neurons in the PVH (Fig. 10) also end in the preautonomic zone of the PVH (see Saper and Loewy, 1980; Sawchenko and Swanson, 1983; Sawchenko et al., 1985). Taken together, the evidence suggests that baroreceptor and other visceral sensory information is relayed to all functional regions of the PVH by way of a highly differentiated series of projections from the medulla and pons (Fig. 11). From this standpoint, these fibers provide for the feed-forward release of CRF and vasopressin, while concurrently being involved in a long-loop feedback influence on baroreceptor reflex circuitry in the brainstem and spinal cord.

A second major input to the PVH arises in the subfornical organ (see above) and ends partly in the region of magnocellular vasopressin cells (Sawchenko and Swanson, 1983). This pathway may consist in part of angiotensin-immunoreactive fibers (Lind et al., 1985) and appears to be excitatory (Ferguson et al., 1984a). It is now clear that this pathway mediates the vasopressin release elicited by circulating angiotensin II (Knepel et al., 1982).

The subfornical organ also innervates preautonomic cell groups in the PVH (Sawchenko and Swanson, 1983). This is of interest in view of the fact that circulating angiotensin II elicits a pressor

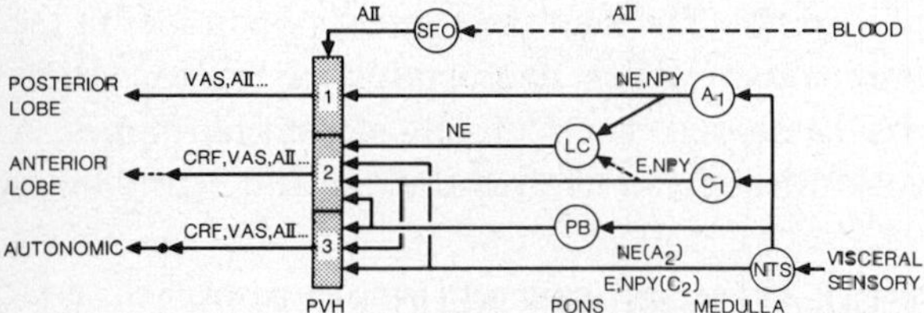

Fig. 11. Flow chart to summarize organization and neurotransmitter content of major known projections from the pons and medulla to the PVH in the rat. This figure stresses how these pathways may be involved in relaying visceral sensory information from the vagus and glossopharyngeal nerves to the PVH, as well as the influence of circulating angiotensin II (AII) on the subfornical organ (SFO), which also projects to all three functional zones of the PVH. A_1 = noradrenergic group in ventrolateral medulla; A_2 = noradrenergic group in NTS; C_1 = adrenergic group in ventrolateral medulla; C_2 = adrenergic group in NTS; E = epinephrine; LC = locus coeruleus; NE = norepinephrine; NTS = nucleus of the solitary tract; PB = parabrachial nucleus; VAS = vasopressin.

response (Mangiapani and Simpson, 1980; Lind et al., 1983) that appears to be mediated at least in part by a pathway from the subfornical organ to preautonomic cell groups in the PVH (Ciriello et al., 1984; Zhang and Ciriello, 1985). Thus, circulating angiotensin II activates neurons in the subfornical organ, some of which in turn project to all three functional regions of the PVH. From this perspective, the subfornical organ constitutes a neuroendocrine sensory nucleus, which provides a feed-forward signal for vasopressin and CRF release, as well as for baroreceptor reflex activation via medullary and spinal cord circuitry (see also Ferguson et al., 1984a,b).

The only other direct input to magnocellular vasopressin cells that has been identified thus far arises in the vicinity of the median preoptic nucleus (Swanson, 1976; Sawchenko and Swanson, 1983), which in turn receives a massive input from the subfornical organ (Miselis, 1981; Lind et al., 1982), consisting in part at least of angiotensin-immunoreactive fibers (Lind et al., 1984c).

There is clear electrophysiological evidence that stimulation of various sites in the limbic region influences vasopressin release from the posterior pituitary. However, axonal transport studies suggest that a vast majority of the fibers arising in the amygdala and septal region end in, or pass through, regions just outside the limits of the PVH and supraoptic nucleus (Sawchenko and Swanson, 1983; Oldfield et al., 1985). Thus, these limbic regions may influence pituitary vasopressin release either by ending on the distal dendrites of magnocellular neurons, or by ending on nearby hypothalamic neurons that in turn project to the PVH or supraoptic nucleus. Recent ultrastructural evidence indicates that a few limbic fibers end on the dendrites of vasopressin neurons in or near the PVH (Oldfield et al., 1985), but it is not clear whether the postsynaptic elements were associated with magnocellular, mediocellular, or parvocellular neurons. On the other hand, it does seem clear that the bed nucleus of the stria terminalis, which appears to innervate CRF cells (see above), also sends fibers to preautonomic parts of the PVH, thus providing a potential avenue for limbic influences on these cells through as yet unidentified chemical messengers.

Thirst

As discussed above, circulating angiotensin II acts on the subfornical organ to influence vasopressin release and baroreceptor reflexes through projections to the PVH, and to stimulate thirst. Little is known about neural circuits that mediate this behavioral response to hypovolemia (Table I), although recent axonal transport studies (Lind and Swanson, 1985) indicate that neurons in the subfornical organ send fibers directly to regions of the forebrain thought to be involved in behavioral arousal, somatomotor control (including locomotion), and cognitive functions (Fig. 12). And in view of the role played by the PVH in stress responses, it is of interest that epinephrine, norepinephrine, and NPY (see Fig. 11) stimulate both drinking and eating when injected directly into the PVH (see Stanley and Leibowitz, 1984), and that the eating response, at least, is mediated in part by descending projections (Sawchenko et al., 1981; McCabe et al.,

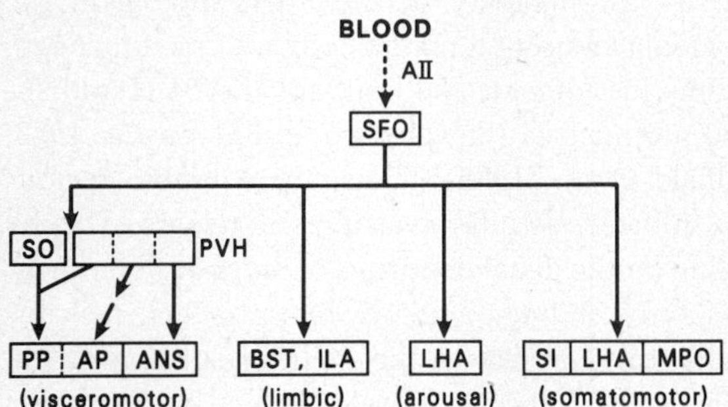

Fig. 12. Summary of major outputs of subfornical organ (SFO) as determined by axonal transport studies with the anterograde tracer PHA-L, and the retrograde tracer, fast blue. ANS = autonomic nervous system; AP = anterior pituitary; BST = bed nucleus of the stria terminalis; ILA = infralimbic area (area 25) of prefrontal cortex; LHA = lateral hypothalamic area; MPO = medial preoptic area; PP = posterior pituitary; SI = substantia innominata (ventral pallidum); SO = supraoptic nucleus.

1984), although the effect depends on the presence of circulating glucocorticoids (Liebowitz et al., 1984). Taken together, the evidence suggests that the circuitry outlined in Figs. 10–12 is involved in mediating endocrine, autonomic, and behavioral responses to certain stressors.

Conclusion

Recent anatomical and physiological evidence is beginning to clarify the organization of specific neural circuits mediating adrenal steroid and catecholamine release during the stress response, as well as the other endocrine, autonomic, and behavioral responses specific to hypovolemia. In this chapter, we have focused on the role of the PVH in this circuitry because it regulates ACTH release from the anterior pituitary, plays an important role in the secretion of vasopressin from the posterior pituitary, and modulates baroreceptor reflexes. The evidence reviewed here suggests that these motor functions of the PVH are mediated by neural inputs relaying visceral and endocrine, as well as cognitive information, and that the content of peptides in the terminals of PVH neuroendocrine motoneurons may be altered by circulating steroid hormones. A working model of likely endocrine and neural influ-

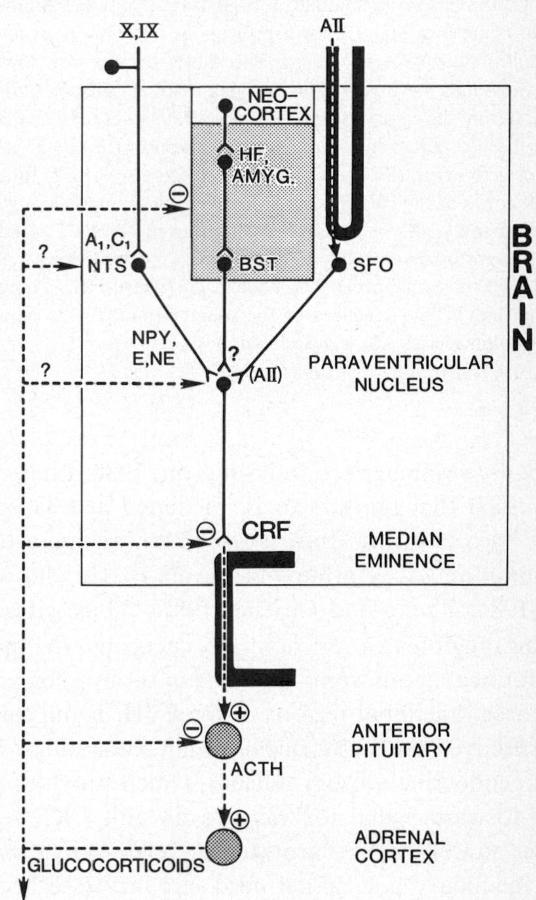

Fig. 13. Model of major neural and hormonal influences on the regulation of CRF neurons in the PVH, based on current evidence reviewed in the text. The exact site of presumed glucocorticoid feedback on neurons in the brainstem (e.g. in or near the NTS, A_1, and C_1 regions) and hypothalamus is not yet clear, although binding of circulating glucocorticoids to parts of the limbic region (stipple, with AMYG, BST, and HF) is well-established. A_1 = noradrenergic group in ventrolateral medulla; AII = angiotensin II; ACTH = adrenocorticotropic hormone; AMYG = amygdala, BST = bed nucleus of the stria terminalis; C_1 = adrenergic group in ventrolateral medulla; E = epinephrine; HF = hippocampal formation; NE = norepinephrine; NTS = nucleus of the solitary tract; SFO = subfornical organ; IX glossapharyngeal nerve; X = vagus nerve.

ences on neurosecretory CRF cells in the PVH is presented in Fig. 13.

Our understanding of this circuitry is still quite incomplete. For example, the extent to which the axons of individual afferent neurons collateralize to innervate different functional cell types within the PVH is unknown, and synaptic relationships between neurochemically specific afferents and functionally distinct cell types within the PVH have not yet been explored. Ultimately, this will require simultaneously identifying the origin and transmitter content of presynaptic terminals, as well as the projections and transmitter content of postsynaptic cells, at the ultrastructural level. Furthermore, it will be necessary to determine the electrophysiological, and perhaps the metabolic, characteristics of these synaptic relationships. And finally, while the broad outlines of the major circuitry associated with the PVH now seem clear, there is no doubt that additional connections and neuroactive substances remain to be elucidated, and it is well-established that the nucleus plays a role in a number of other visceral mechanisms (see Swanson and Sawchenko, 1984).

Perhaps the most interesting feature to emerge from studies of the PVH is the apparently broad variety of peptides that can be expressed by neurosecretory neurons. As reviewed above, immunohistochemical evidence suggests that CRF neurons in the normal rat synthesize at least five peptides encoded by different genes, and following adrenalectomy the number may be increased by at least two. In addition, it has been reported that VIP can be detected in these neurons as well, in the lactating, adrenalectomized rat pretreated with colchicine (Kiss et al., 1984).

These immunohistochemical observations lead to a number of important questions about peptide gene regulation and synthesis in CRF neurons, questions that can be approached with tools provided by cell and molecular biology. First, it will be necessary to determine whether glucocorticoids act directly on CRF neurons through receptors that bind to the genome, and if so, what mechanisms are involved in modulating the differential expression of peptide genes in these cells. The immunohistochemical evidence suggests that glucocorticoids normally depress levels of CRF, vasopressin, and angiotensin, while not affecting levels of enkephalin and neurotensin, but it remains to be shown whether this is due to an inhibition of mRNA transcription, or to effects on post-translational processing and peptide turnover rates. Recent evidence based on in situ hybridization methods indicates that there are increased levels of vasopressin mRNA in parvocellular parts of the PVH after adrenalectomy (Wolfson et al., 1985), but the extent to which higher message levels are localized within neurons that display increased levels of CRF is not yet clear. Nevertheless, this approach, when refined to allow for the simultaneous cellular localization of immunoreactivity, will lead to new insights into the molecular biology of this system.

Second, it will be of interest to clarify whether glucocorticoids can exert effects on peptide metabolism in CRF neurons by acting on the genome of neurons that project to the PVH. If so, this would imply that chemical messengers released from certain afferent fibers may exert genomic effects on postsynaptic neurons in the hypothalamus. An attractive candidate for this type of mechanism is the adrenergic projection from medullary groups C_{1-3} to CRF neurons in the PVH, although recent immuno-autoradiographic evidence suggests that such neurons may not concentrate circulating corticosterone (Duncan and Stumpf, 1985).

And third, the role of membrane-bound glucocorticoid receptors in controlling the release of CRF needs to be clarified. There is evidence suggesting that glucocorticoids act on terminals in the median eminence to inhibit CRF release (Edwardson and Bennett, 1974), and it also seems clear that these hormones can alter the firing rate of neurons in parts of the limbic region that project (through multisynaptic pathways) to CRF neurons in the PVH (see McEwen, 1982). Thus it is possible that glucocorticoids may affect CRF release in at least three distinct ways: first, by influencing secretion from terminals; second, by influencing the firing rate of appropriate neurons; and third, by influencing gene transcription. It will be of particular interest to determine whether other peptides and biogenic amines can exert similar effects. In this regard it is worth pointing out that several hypothalamic-releasing factors (including CRF) have dual actions on cells in the anterior pituitary; they stimulate secretion as well as the transcription of mRNA encoding specific hormones (Baringa et al., 1983; Bruhn et al., 1984). Since these substances are also found in central pathways, it will be of interest to determine whether they exert similar effects through synapses within the brain and spinal cord. Recent evidence indicates that acetylcholine exerts metabolic effects on sympathetic ganglion cells, particularly during development (see Hamill et al., 1983), and that noradrenergic sympathetic fibers influence the production of melatonin in the pineal gland (Ebadi, 1984). It seems reasonable to predict that similar mechanisms may play a role in the function of circuitry in the brain.

These results have helped to clarify the anatomical organization and neurotransmitter content of circuitry involved in mediating the stress response, as well as visceral and behavioral responses specific to hypovolemia. At the same time, they suggest that certain links in this circuitry may be subject to biochemical plasticity, in the sense that circulating steroid hormones, and perhaps certain neural secretagogues as well, may alter the content of peptides in certain neurons. If this is true, then the responses elicited by activation of this presumably fixed anatomical circuitry may vary over time depending, for example, on the endocrine status of the animal. It remains to be determined what functional consequences this might have on responses elicited following acute or chronic stress. Nevertheless, the neurosecretory CRF cell in the PVH is emerging as a popular model for studying multiple gene regulation and post-translational processing in central neurons. It is worth pointing out, however, that a clear definition of these cells is not available. They are centered in the dorsal medial parvocellular part of the PVH, which contains a dense cluster of small neurons, not all of which can be stained immunohistochemically for CRF. Furthermore, the number of "CRF" neurons varies with circulating levels of adrenal steroid hormones, and different CRF neurons in this region can express detectable levels of at least seven other peptides, although rarely do individual neurons show equal proportions, or even the presence of, all of these peptides. Clearly, a great deal remains to be learned about the function, cell biology, and molecular biology of neurosecretory CRF cells, which constitute the final common pathway for the central neural control of ACTH, β-endorphin and glucocorticoid levels in the blood.

References

Agnati, L. F., Fuxe, K., Yu, Z.-Y., Harstiand, A., Okret, S., Wikstrom, A.-C., Goldstein, M., Zoli, M., Vale, W. and Gustafsson, J.-A. (1985) Morphometrical analysis of the distribution of corticotropin releasing factor, glucocorticoid receptor and phenylethanolamine-N-methyltransferase immunoreactive structures in the paraventricular hypothalamic nucleus of the rat. *Neurosci. Lett.*, 54: 147–152.

Antoni, F. A., Palkovits, M., Makara, G. B., Linton, E. A., Lowry, P. J. and Kiss, J. Z. (1983) Immunoreactive corticotropin-releasing hormone in the hypothalamoinfundibular tract. *Neuroendocrinology*, 36: 415–432.

Baringa, M., Yamanoto, G., Rivier, C., Vale, W., Evans, R. and Rosenfeld, M. G. (1983) Transcriptional regulation of growth hormone gene expression by growth hormone-releasing factor. *Nature (Lond.)*, 206: 84–85.

Blessing, W. W. and Willoughby, J. O. (1985) Excitation of neuronal function in rabbit caudal ventrolateral medulla elevates plasma vasopressin. *Neurosci. Lett.* (in press).

Bloom, F. E., Battenberg, E. L. F., Rivier J. and Vale, W. (1982) Corticotropin releasing factor (CRF) immunoreactive neurons and fibers in rat hypothalamus. *Regul. Peptides*, 4: 43–48.

Brownstein, M. J., Eskay, R. L. and Palkovits, M. (1982) Thyrotropin releasing hormone in the median eminence is in processes of paraventricular nucleus neurons. *Neuropeptides*, 2: 197–201.

Bruhn, T. O., Sutton, R. E., Rivier, C. L. and Vale, W. W. (1984) Corticotropin-releasing factor regulates proopiomelanocortin messenger ribonucleic acid levels in vivo. *Neuroendocrinology*, 39: 170–175.

Bugnon, C., Fellman, D., Gouget, A. and Cardot, J. (1982) Corticoliberin in rat brain: immunocytochemical identification and localization of a novel neuroglandular system. *Neurosci. Lett.*, 30: 25–30.

Bugnon, C., Fellman, D. and Gouget, A. (1983) Changes in corticoliberin and vasopressin-like immunoreactivities in the zona externa of the median eminence in adrenalectomized rats. *Neurosci. Lett.*, 37: 43–49.

Carlsson, A., Falck, B. and Hillarp, N.-A. (1962) Cellular localization of brain monoamines. *Acta physiol. Scand.*, 56, Suppl. 196: 1–27.

Caverson, M. M. and Ciriello, J. (1984) Electrophysiological identification of neurons in ventrolateral medulla sending collateral axons to paraventricular and suproptic nuclei in the cat. *Brain Res.*, 305: 375–379.

Ciriello, J. and Calaresu, F. R. (1980) Role of paraventricular and supraoptic nuclei in central cardiovascular regulation in the cat. *Amer. J. Physiol.*, 239: R137–R142.

Ciriello, J., Kleine, R. L., Zhang, T.-X. and Caverson, M. M. (1984) Lesions of the paraventricular nucleus alter the development of spontaneous hypertension in the rat. *Brain Res.*, 310: 355–359.

Conrad, L. C. A. and Pfaff, D. W. (1976) Efferents from medial basal forebrain and hypothalamus in the rat. II. An autoradiographic study of the anterior hypothalamus. *J. comp. Neurol.*, 169: 221–262.

Cummings, S., Elde, R., Ells, J. and Lendall, A. (1983) Corticotropin-releasing factor immunoreactivity is widely distributed within the central nervous system of the rat: an immunohistochemical study. *J. Neurosci.*, 3: 1355–1368.

Day, T. A., Ferguson, A. V. and Renaud, L. P. (1984) Facilitatory influence of noradrenergic afferents on the excitability of rat paraventricular nucleus neurosecretory cells. *J. Physiol. (Lond.)*, 355: 237–249.

Dierickx, K. (1980) Immunocytochemical localization of the vertebrate cyclic nonapeptide neurohypophyseal hormones and neurophysins. *Int. Rev. Cytol.*, 62: 119–183.

Duncan, G. E. and Stumpf, W. E. (1985) A combined autoradiographic and immunocytochemical study of ^{3}H-corticosterone target neurons and catecholamine neurons in rat and mouse lower brain stem. *Neuroendocrinology*, 40: 262–271.

Ebadi, M. (1984) Regulation of the synthesis of melatonin and its significance to neuroendocrinology. In R. J. Reiter (Ed.), *The Pineal Gland*, Raven Press, New York, pp. 1–37.

Edwardson, J. A. and Bennett, G. W. (1974) Modulation of corticotrophin-releasing factor release from hypothalamic synaptosomes. *Nature (Lond.)*, 251: 425–427.

Everitt, B. J., Hökfelt, T., Terenius, L., Tatemoto, K., Mutt, V. and Goldstein, M. (1984) Differential co-existence of neuropeptide Y (NPY)-like immunoreactivity with catecholamines in the central nervous system of the rat. *Neuroscience*, 11: 443–462.

Ferguson, A. V., Day, T. A. and Renaud, L. P. (1984a) Subfornical organ efferents influence the excitability of neurohyophyseal and tuberoinfundibular paraventricular nucleus neurons in the rat. *Neuroendocrinlogy*, 39: 423–248.

Ferguson, A. V., Day, T. A. and Renaud, L. P. (1984b) Subfornical organ stimulation excites paraventricular neurons projecting to dorsal medulla. *Amer. J. Physiol.*, 247: R1088–R1092.

Hamill, R. W., Cochard, P. and Black, I. B. (1983) Long-term effects of spinal transection on the development and function of sympathetic ganglia. *Brain Res.*, 266: 21–27.

Hatton, G. I., Hutton, U. E., Hoblitzell, E. R. and Armstrong, W. E. (1976) Morphological evidence for two populations of magnocellular elements in the rat paraventricular nucleus. *Brain Res.*, 108: 187–193.

Henry, J. P. (1980) Present concept of stress theory. In E. Usdin, R. Kvetnansky and I. J. Kopin (Eds.), *Catecholamines and Stress; Recent Advances*, Elsevier, Amsterdam, pp. 557–570.

Hökfelt, T., Fahrenkrug, J., Tatemoto, K., Mutt, V., Werner, S., Hultings, A.-L. Terenius, L. and Chang, K. J. (1983) The PHI (PHI-27) corticotropin-releasing factor/enkephalin immunoreactive hypothalamic neuron: possible morphological basis for integrated control of prolactin, corticotropin, and growth hormone secretion. *Proc. nat. Acad. Sci. USA*, 80: 895–898.

Hosoya, Y. and Matsushita, M. (1979) Identification and distribution of the spinal and hypophysial projection neurons in the paraventricular nucleus of the rat. A light and electron microscopic study with the horseradish peroxidase method. *Exp. Brain Res.*, 35: 315–331.

Kawata, M., Hashimoto, K., Takahara, J. and Sano, Y. (1982) Immunohistochemical demonstration of corticotropin-releasing factor containing neurons in the hypothalamus of mammals including primates. *Anat. Embryol.*, 165: 303–313.

Kiss, J. Z., Williams, T. H. and Palkovitz, M. (1984) Distribution and projections of cholecystokinin-immunoreactive neurons in the hypothalamic paraventricular nucleus of rat. *J. comp. Neurol.*, 227: 173–181.

Knepel, W., Nutto, D. and Meyer, D. K. (1982) Effect of transection of subfornical organ efferent projections on vasopressin release induced by angiotensin or isoprenalin in the rat. *Brain Res.*, 248: 180–184.

Koh, E. T. and Ricardo, J. A. (1980) Paraventricular nucleus of the hypothalamus: evidence of ten functionally discrete subdivisions. *Soc. Neurosci. Abstr.*, 6: 521.

Krettek, J. E. and Price, J. L. (1978) Amygdaloid projections to subcortical structures within the basal forebrain and the brainstem in the rat and cat. *J. comp. Neurol.*, 178: 225–254.

Lechan, R. M. and Jackson, I. M. D. (1982) Immunohistochemical localization of thyrotropin-releasing hormone in the rat hypothalamus and pituitary. *Endocrinology*, 111: 55–65.

Leibowitz, S. F., Roland, C. R., Hor, L. and Squillari, V. (1984) Noradrenergic feeding elicited via the paraventricular nucleus is dependent upon circulating corticosterone. *Physiol. Behav.*, 32: 857–864.

Lind, R. W. and Swanson, L. W. (1985) New afferent and efferent neural connections of the subfornical organ. *Soc. Neurosci. Abstr.*, 11: 555.

Lind, R. W., Van Hoesen, G. W. and Johnson, A. K. (1982) An HRP study of the connections of the subfornical organ of the rat. *J. comp. Neurol.*, 210: 265–277.

Lind, R. W., Ohman, L. E., Lansing, M. B. and Johnson, A. K.

(1983) Transection of subfornical organ neural connections diminishes the pressor response to intravenously infused angiotensin II. *Brain Res.*, 275: 361–364.

Lind, R. W., Swanson, L. W., Chin, D. A., Bruhn, T. O. and Ganten, D. (1984a) Angiotensin II: an immunohistochemical study of its distribution in the paraventriculo-hypophysial system and its co-localization with vasopressin and CRF in paravocellular neurons. *Soc. Neurosci. Abstr.*, 10: 88.

Lind, R. W., Swanson, L. W. and Ganten, D. (1984b) Angiotensin II immunoreactive pathways in the central nervous system of the rat: evidence for a projection from the subfornical organ to the paraventricular nucleus of the hypothalamus. *Clin. Exp. Hypertension,* A6: 1915–1920.

Lind, R. W., Swanson, L. W. and Genten, D. (1984c) Angiotensin II immunoreactivity in the neural afferents and efferents of the subfornical organ of the rat. *Brain Res.*, 321: 209–215.

Lind, R. W., Swanson, L. W. and Ganten, D. (1985) Organization of angiotensin II immunoreactive cells and fibers in the rat central nervous system. *Neuroendocrinology*, 40: 2–24.

Mangiapane, M. L. and Simpson, J. B. (1980) Subfornical organ: forebrain sites of pressor and dipsogenic action of angiotensin II. *Amer. J. Physiol.*, 239: R382–R389.

McCabe, J. T., DeBellis, M. and Leibowitz, S. F. (1984) Clonidine-induced feeding: Analysis of central sites of action and fiber projections mediating this response. *Brain Res.*, 309: 85–104.

McEwen, B. (1982) Glucocorticoids and hippocampus: Receptors in search of a function. In D. Ganten and D. Pfaff (Eds.), *Current Topics in Neuroendocrinology, Vol. 2,* Springer-Verlag, Berlin, pp. 23-47.

McNeill, T. H. and Sladek, J. R. (1980) Simultaneous monoamine histofluorescence and neuropeptide immunocytochemistry. II. Correlative distribution of catecholamine varicosities and magnocellular neurosecretory neurons in the rat supraoptic and paraventricular nuclei. *J. comp. Neurol.*, 193: 1023–1033.

Merchenthaler, I., Vigh, S., Petrusz, P. and Schally, A. V. (1982) Immunocytochemical localization of corticotropin-releasing factor (CRF) in the rat brain. *Amer. J. Anat.*, 165: 385–396.

Merchenthaler, I., Vigh, S., Petrusz, P. and Schally, A. V. (1983) The paraventriculoinfundibular corticotropin releasing factor (CRF) pathway as revealed by immunocytochemistry in long--term hypophysectomized or adrenalectomized rats. *Regul. Peptides,* 5: 295–305.

Mezey, E., Kiss, J. Z., Skirboll, L. R., Goldstein, M. and Axelrod, J. (1984) Increase of corticotropin-releasing factor staining in rat paraventricular nucleus neurones by depletion of hypothalamic adrenaline. *Nature (Lond.),* 310: 140–141.

Miselis, R. R. (1981) The efferent projections of the subfornical organ of the rat: A circumventricular organ within a neural network subserving water balance. *Brain Res.*, 230: 1–23.

Norgren, R. (1978) Projections from the nucleus of the solitary tract in the rat. *Neuroscience,* 3: 207–218.

Oldfield, B. J., Hou-Yu, A. and Silverman, A.-J. (1985) A combined electron microscopic HRP and immunocythochemical study of the limbic projections to rat hypothalamic nuclei containing vasopressin and oxytocin neurons. *J. comp. Neurol.*, 231: 221–231.

Olschowka, J. A. (1984) Neuropeptide Y innervation of the rat paraventricular and supraoptic nuclei. *Soc. Neurosci. Abstr.*, 10: 437.

Olschowka, J. A., O'Donohue, T. L., Mueller, G. P. and Jacobowitz, D. M. (1982) The distribution of corticotropin releasing factor-like immunoreactive neurons in rat brain. *Peptides,* 3: 995–1015.

Paull, W. K. and Gibbs, F. P. (1983) The corticotropin releasing factor (CRF) neurosecretory system in intact, adrenalectomized, and adrenalectomized-dexamethasone treated trats. *Histochemistry*, 78: 303–316.

Rhodes, C. H., Morrell, J. I. and Pfaff, D. W. (1981) Immunohistochemical analysis of magnocellular elements in rat hypothalamus: Distribution and numbers of cells containing neurophysin, oxytocin, and vasopressin. *J. comp. Neurol.*, 198: 45–64.

Saper, C. B. and Loewy, A. D. (1980) Efferent connections of the parabrachial nucleus in the rat. *Brain Res.*, 197: 291–317.

Saper, C. B., Loewy, A. D., Swanson, L. W. and Cowan, W. M. (1976) Direct hypothalamo-autonomic connections. *Brain Res.*, 117: 305–312.

Sawchenko, P. E. and Swanson, L. W. (1980) Immunohistochemical identification of paraventricular hypothalamic neurons which project to the medulla or spinal cord in the rat. *Soc. Neurosci. Abstr.*, 6: 520.

Sawchenko, P. E. and Swanson, L. W. (1981) A method for tracing biochemically defined pathways in the central nervous system using combined fluorescence retrograde transport and immunohistochemical techniques. *Brain Res.*, 210: 31–51.

Sawchenko, P. E. and Swanson, L. W. (1982a) Immunohistochemical identification of neurons in the paraventricular nucleus of the hypothalamus that project to the medulla or to the spinal cord in the rat. *J. comp. Neurol.*, 205: 260–272.

Sawchenko, P. E. and Swanson, L. W. (1982b) The organization of noradrenergic pathways from the brainstem to the paraventricular and supraoptic nuclei in the rat. *Brain Res. Rev.*, 4: 275–325.

Sawchenko, P. E. and Swanson L. W. (1983) The organization of forebrain afferents to the paraventricular and supraoptic nuclei of the rat. *J. comp. Neurol.*, 218: 121–144.

Sawchenko, P. E. and Swanson, L. W. (1984) Adrenalectomy-induced enhancement of CRF- and vasopressin-immunoreactivity in parvocellular neurosecretory neurons: anatomic, peptide and steroid specificity. *Soc. Neurosci. Abstr.*, 10: 83.

Sawchenko, P. E. and Swanson, L. W. (1985) Localization, colocalization, and plasticity of corticotropin-releasing factor immunoreactivity in rat brain. *Fed. Proc.*, 44: 221–227.

Sawchenko, P. E., Gold, R. M. and Leibowitz, S. F. (1981) Evidence for vagal involvement in the eating elicited by adrenergic stimulation of the paraventricular nucleus. *Brain Res.*, 225: 249–269.

Sawchenko, P. E., Swanson, L. W., Steinbusch, H. W. M. and Verhofstad, A. A. J. (1983) The distribution and cells of origin of serotonergic inputs to the paraventricular and supraoptic nuclei of the rat. *Brain Res.*, 277: 355–360.

Sawchenko, P. E., Swanson, L. W. and Vale, W. W. (1984a) Corticotropin-releasing factor: coexpression within distinct subsets of oxytocin-, vasopressin-, and neurotensin-immunoreactive neurons in the hypothalamus of the male rat. *J. Neurosci.*, 4: 1118–1129.

Sawchenko, P. E., Swanson, L. W. and Vale, W. W. (1984b) Co-expression of corticotropin-releasing factor and vasopressin immunoreactivity in parvocellular neurosecretory neurons of the adrenalectomized rat. *Proc. nat. Acad. Sci. USA*, 81: 1883–1877.

Sawchenko, P. E., Swanson, L. W., Grzanna, R., Howe, P. R. C., Polak, J. M. and Bloom, S. R. (1985) Co-localization of neuropeptide Y-immunoreactivity in brainstem catecholaminergic neurons that project to the paraventricular nucleus of the hypothalamus. *J. comp. Neurol.*, 241: 138–153.

Schachter, B. S., Johnson, L. K., Baxter, J. D. and Roberts, J. L. (1982) Differential regulation by glucocorticoids of proopiomelanocortin mRNA levels in the anterior and intermediate lobes of the rat pituitary. *Endocrinology*, 110: 1442–1444.

Selye, H. (1976) *Stress in Health and Disease*, Butterworth, Boston.

Simpson, J. B. (1981) The circumventricular organs and the central actions of angiotensin *Neuroendocrinology*, 32: 248–256.

Sofroniew, M. V. and U. Schrell (1981) Evidence for a direct projection from oxytocin and vasopressin neurons in the hypothalamic paraventricular nucleus to the medulla oblongata: Immunohistochemical visualization of both the horseradish peroxidase transported and peptide produced by the same neurons. *Neurosci. Lett.*, 22: 211–217.

Stanley, B. G. and Leibowitz, S. F. (1984) Neuropeptide Y: stimulation of feeding and drinking by injection into the paraventricular nucleus. *Life Sci.*, 35: 2635–2642.

Swaab, D. F., Pool, C. W. and Nijveldt, F. (1975) Immunofluorescence of vasopressin and oxytocin in the rat hypothalamo-neurohypophyseal system. *J. Neural Trans.*, 36: 195–215.

Swanson, L. W. (1976) An autoradiographic study of the efferent connections of the preoptic region in the rat. *J. comp. Neurol.*, 167: 227–256.

Swanson, L. W. (1977) Immunohistochemical evidence for a neurophysin-containing autonomic pathway arising in the paraventricular nucleus of the hypothalamus. *Brain Res.*, 128: 356–363.

Swanson, L. W. (1983) The hippocampus and the concept of the limbic system. In W. Seifert (Ed.), *Neurobiology of the Hippocampus*, Academic Press, New York, pp. 3–20.

Swanson, L. W. and Cowan, W. M. (1977) An autoradiographic study of the organization of the efferent connections of the hippocampal formation in the rat. *J. comp. Neurol.*, 172: 49–84.

Swanson, L. W. and Hartman, B. K. (1980) Biochemical specificity in central pathways related to peripheral and intracerebral homeostatic function. *Neurosci. Lett.*, 16: 55–60.

Swanson, L. W. and Kuypers, H. G. J. M. (1980) The paraventricular nucleus of the hypothalamus: Cytoarchitectonic subdivisions and the organization of projections to the pituitary, dorsal vagal complex and spinal cord as demonstrated by retrograde fluorescence double labeling methods. *J. comp. Neurol.*, 194: 555–570.

Swanson, L. W. and McKellar, S. (1979) The distribution of oxytocin- and neurophysin-stained fibers in the spinal cord of the rat and monkey. *J. comp. Neurol.*, 188: 87–106.

Swanson, L. W. and Sawchenko, P. E. (1983) Hypothalamic integration: organization of the paraventricular and supraoptic nuclei. *Ann. Rev. Neurosci.*, 6: 275–325.

Swanson, L. W., Sawchenko, P. E., Wiegand, S. J. and Price, J. L. (1980) Separate neurons in the paraventricular nucleus project to the median eminence and to the medulla or spinal cord. *Brain Res.*, 197: 207–212.

Swanson, L. W., Sawchenko, P. E., Bérod, A., Hartman, B. K., Helle, K. B. and Van Orden, D. E. (1981) An immunohistochemical study of the organization of catecholaminergic cells and terminal fields in the paraventricular and supraoptic nuclei of the hypothalamus. *J. comp. Neurol.*, 196: 271–285.

Swanson, L. W., Sawchenko, P. E., Rivier, J. and Vale, W. W. (1983) Organization of ovine corticotropin-releasing factor immunoreactive cells and fibers in the rat brain: an immunohistochemical study. *Neuroendocrinology*, 36: 165–186.

Swanson, L. W., Mogenson, G. J., Gerfen, C. R. and Robinson, P. (1984) Evidence for a projection from the lateral preoptic area and substantia innominata to the "mesencephalic locomotor region" in the rat. *Brain Res.*, 295: 161–178.

Tramu, G., Croix, C. and Pillez, A. (1983) Ability of the CRF immunoreactive neurons of the paraventricular nucleus to produce a vasopressin-like material. *Neuroendocrinology*, 37: 467–469.

Vale, W., Spiess, J., Rivier, C. and Rivier, J. (1981) Characterization of a 41-residue ovine hypothalamic peptide that stimulates secretion of corticotropin and β-endorphin. *Science*, 213: 1394–1397.

Vale, W., Rivier, C., Brown, M. R., Spiess, J., Koob, G., Swanson, L., Bilezikjian, L., Bloom, F. and Rivier, J. (1983) Chemical and biological characterization of corticotropin releasing factor. *Rec. Prog. Hor. Res.*, 39: 245–270.

Van Den Pol, A. N. (1982) The magnocellular and parvocellular paraventricular nucleus of the rat: Intrinsic organization. *J. comp. Neurol.*, 206: 317–345.

Vandesande, F. and Dierickx, K. (1975) Identification of the vasopressin producing and of the oxytocin producing neurons in the hypothalamic neurosecretory system of the rat. *Cell Tiss. Res.*, 164: 153–162.

Vandesande, F., Dierickx, K. and J. DeMey (1977) The origin of the vasopressinergic and oxytocinergic fibres of the external region of the median eminence of the rat hypophysis. *Cell Tiss. Res.*, 180: 443–452.

Wolfson, B., Manning, R. W., Davis, L. G., Arentzen, R. and Baldino, F. (1985) Colocalization of corticotropin releasing factor and vasopressin mRNA in neurons after adrenalectomy. *Nature (Lond.)*, 315: 59–61.

Yates, F. G. and Maran, J. W. (1974) Stimulation and inhibition of adrenocorticotropin release. In E. Knubil and H. W. Sawyer (Eds.), *Handbook of Physiology, Section 7, Endocrinology, Vol. IV: The Pituitary Gland and Its Neuroendocrine Control, Part 2,* Am. Physiol. Soc., Washington, D.C., pp. 367–404.

Zerihun, L. and Harris, M. (1981) Electrophysiological identification of neurons of paraventricular nucleus sending axons to both the neurohypophysis and the medulla in the rat. *Neurosci. Lett.*, 23: 157–160.

Zhang, T.-X. and Ciriello, J. (1985) Effect of paraventricular nucleus lesions on arterial pressure and heart rate after aortic baroreceptor denervation in the rat. *Brain Res.* (in press).

SECTION V

Peripheral Systems

T. Hökfelt, K. Fuxe and B. Pernow (Eds.),
Progress in Brain Research, Vol. 68

CHAPTER 13

Purines as cotransmitters in adrenergic and cholinergic neurones

G. Burnstock

Department of Anatomy and Embryology and Centre for Neuroscience, University College London, Gower Street, London WCIE 6BT, U.K.

Introduction

When I posed the question in a Neuroscience Commentary in 1976 "Do some nerve cells release more than one transmitter?" (Burnstock, 1976), after examining data from a wide variety of preparations in vertebrates and invertebrates, I had to admit that this did not constitute strong supporting evidence. However, less than 10 years later, there is abundant experimental support for cotransmission, and it begins to appear that few nerves contain only one transmitter — indeed the indications are that most nerve fibres utilise several transmitter substances that vary in proportions during development and under the influence of environmental factors such as hormones, disease and compensatory demands following trauma.

In this chapter, my task is to focus on the evidence for ATP as a cotransmitter in adrenergic and cholinergic neurones.

ATP as a cotransmitter with noradrenaline in sympathetic nerves

Evidence for cotransmission in different tissues

Vas deferens

Although we did not realise it at the time, when Mollie Holman and I first recorded excitatory junction potentials (ejps) in smooth muscle cells of the vas deferens in response to stimulation of sympathetic nerves (Burnstock and Holman, 1960) we were observing responses to ATP rather than to noradrenaline (NA). Since ejps were abolished by the sympathetic neurone blocking agents, bretylium and guanethidine, drugs that prevent nerve-mediated release of transmitter, we were correct in assuming they were produced by transmitter released from sympathetic nerves. However, it is now clear that ejps are not blocked by adrenoceptor antagonists such as phentolamine or prazosin or by depletion of NA with reserpine (Sneddon et al., 1982; Sneddon and Westfall, 1984). They are, however, blocked by the ATP receptor (P_2-purinoceptor) antagonist, arylazido aminopropionyl-ATP (ANAPP$_3$) and also following selective desensitisation of the P_2-purinoceptor with the stable analog of ATP, α,β-methylene ATP (Sneddon and Westfall, 1984; Stjärne and Åstrand, 1984; Sneddon and Burnstock, 1984a). Furthermore, local pressure ejection of ATP mimicks the ejp, while NA does not (Sneddon and Burnstock, 1984a). More recently it was shown that "discrete events" recorded in the vas deferens measure single quanta of ATP secreted from the sympathetic nerves in the vas deferens (Cunnanne and Stjärne, 1984; Stjärne and Åstrand, 1984).

The mechanical response of the vas deferens to stimulation of the sympathetic nerves is biphasic, a rapid twitch contraction followed by a slower tonic contraction: both phases are abolished by guanethidine. The slow tonic component is blocked by α-adrenoceptor agonists and reserpine depletion and is due to NA (Ambache and Zar, 1971), but the twitch component is insensitive to these drugs. It is, however, blocked by $ANAPP_3$ (Fedan et al., 1981) and by ATP receptor desensitisation with α,β-methylene ATP (Meldrum and Burnstock, 1983). Evidence has also been presented that ATP is stored and released from sympathetic nerves supplying the guinea-pig vas deferens (Westfall et al., 1978; Fedan et al., 1981; Levitt et al., 1984).

Taken together, this represents compelling evidence that ATP is a cotransmitter together with NA in sympathetic nerves supplying the vas deferens. The two transmitters act in different ways to produce contraction of the smooth muscle. ATP produces ejps that sum and facilitate, until at a critical depolarisation threshold, spikes are initiated which lead to contraction; this then is achieved by a mechanism of electro-mechanical coupling, and since the Ca^{2+}-channel blocker, nifedepine, antagonises this component of the sympathetic response, it appears to involve a voltage-dependent Ca^{2+} channel (Stone, 1981a). In contrast, NA can produce contraction without production of spikes, although some slow depolarisation can be elicited upon perfusion; this suggests that NA can act by a type of pharmaco-mechanical, or at least spike-free coupling, involving receptor-operated Ca^{2+} channels (Burnstock and Sneddon, 1984).

Figure 1 summarises these events and also indicates the roles of NA, ATP and its breakdown product, adenosine, as neuromodulators in the cotransmission process. Firstly, ATP can act as a *postjunctional* modulator, potentiating the action of NA (Holck and Marks, 1978; Kazic and Milosavljevic, 1980). Secondly, ATP, after rapid breakdown following its release by ectoenzymes to adenosine, largely acts as a prejunctional modulator on adenosine receptors (P_1-purinoceptors) on the nerve terminals to reduce the release of NA (Sneddon et al., 1984).

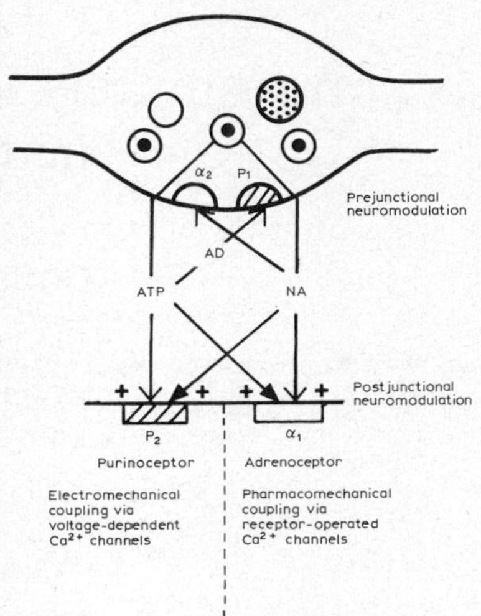

Fig. 1. ATP and noradrenaline (NA) are released from the sympathetic nerves supplying the vas deferens. ATP acts on P_2-purinoceptors on the smooth muscle to initiate ejps, action potentials and the phasic contraction. NA acts on α_1-adrenoceptors to produce the second phase of the contraction by a different mechanism. Prejunctional α_2- and P_1-receptors can reduce transmitter release when activated by noradrenaline and adenosine (AD), respectively. (From Burnstock, 1983 with permission of the publisher.)

Guinea-pig taenia coli

An early indication that ATP might be released from adrenergic nerves was the demonstration that stimulation of periarterial adrenergic nerves led to release of tritium from taenia coli preincubated in [^{3}H]adenosine (which is taken up and converted to [^{3}H]ATP); both the release of tritium and NA were blocked by guanethidine (Su et al., 1971).

Cat nictitating membrane

Langer and Pinto (1976) suggested that the substantial residual non-adrenergic, non-cholinergic response of the cat nictitating membrane following depletion of NA by reserpine, may be due to release of the ATP remaining in adrenergic nerves. More recently, Langer and his colleagues have shown that α,β-methylene ATP administered intra-arterially through the lingual artery, inhibited the residual responses evoked by sympathetic nerve stimulation in reserpinised cats, without modifying the contractions evoked by exogenous (i.a.) NA (Duval et al., 1985).

Blood vessels

Using tritium-labelled adenosine and NA, ATP has been shown to be released together with NA from sympathetic nerves supplying the rabbit aorta and portal vein (Su, 1975, 1978; Levitt and Westfall, 1982). Coexistence of NA and ATP has also been demonstrated in rabbit ear artery (Head et al., 1977), dog basilar artery (Muramatsu et al., 1981) and rabbit pulmonary artery (Katsuragi and Su, 1980, 1982). ATP, as well as NA, release from guinea-pig portal vein has been shown to be abolished following sympathectomy (Burnstock et al., 1979). Fluorescence in nerves of the rat portal vein following incubation in quinacrine, which binds strongly to ATP (Olson et al., 1976; Da Prada et al., 1978), is also abolished by sympathectomy.

More recently, ejps recorded in smooth muscle cells of the rat tail artery (Cheung, 1982) and rabbit ear artery (Suzuki, 1985) have been shown to be blocked by α,β-methylene ATP, but not by prazosin, and local application of ATP (but not NA) mimicks them (Sneddon and Burnstock, 1984b; Allcorn et al., 1985). α,β-Methylene ATP inhibits the vasoconstriction of tail arteries to periarterial field stimulation in spontaneously hypertensive, but not normotensive, rats suggesting that cotransmitter release of ATP has a more important role in spontaneously hypertensive than in normotensive arteries (Hicks et al., 1985). Skeletal muscle vasodilatation produced by hypothalamic stimulation in anaesthetised rabbits has been claimed to be mediated by ATP released from sympathetic nerves (Shimada and Stitt, 1984). A contribution of ATP to sympathetic vasopressor responses of the pithed rabbit has also been demonstrated (Grant et al., 1985).

Frog heart

Transmural stimulation of the intrinsic nerves supplying the frog atrium produces inhibition of heart contractions; when this response is blocked with atropine, an excitatory response is revealed which has two components. The slow second component is mimicked by adrenaline (the sympathetic transmitter in anuran amphibians) and is blocked by the β-adrenoceptor antagonist, propranolol; while the first faster component is mimicked by ATP and blocked by α,β-methylene ATP (Hoyle and Burnstock, 1986). Since both excitatory components are abolished by guanethidine, the sympathetic nerves controlling the frog heart also appear to utilise ATP and catecholamines as cotransmitters.

Cultured sympathetic neurones

Co-transmission in sympathetic nerves has also been elegantly demonstrated in tissue culture (Potter et al., 1983). By growing isolated single sympathetic neurones on a matrix of cultured cardiac muscle cells, they were able to show that NA, acetylcholine (ACh) and purines were stored and released in variable proportions from different neurones; some nerves released largely NA, others released largely ACh and some were predominantly purinergic.

Sympathetic neurone-related and other cell types

It has been known for a number of years that ATP is stored and released together with catecholamines from adrenal chromaffin cells (Douglas and Poisner, 1966; Douglas, 1968; Stevens et al., 1972; Smith, 1972). It has also been suggested that medullary granule-associated nucleotides may act locally as "co-agonists" with biogenic amines and may additionally provide a circulatory pool of purines for use by heart and lungs (Van Dyke et al., 1977).

Other cell types that show positive reaction to quinacrine, and where ATP is bound together with a monoamine in large granular vesicles that can be released by exocytosis, include platelets, mast cells, pancreatic islet cells, melanophores, Merkel cells, carotid chief cells, juxtaglomerular cells and megakaryocytes (Leitner et al., 1975; Da Prada et al., 1978, 1982; Crowe and Whitear, 1978; Ålund and Olson, 1979; Ålund, 1980; Böck, 1980).

Modulatory actions of purine nucleotides and nucleosides on adrenergic transmission

Prejunctional actions

Adenine nucleosides and nucleotides have been shown to inhibit NA release from adrenergic nerves supplying a variety of visceral and vascular tissues including vas deferens, spleen, kidney, heart, subcutaneous adipose tissue and saphenous, tibial, portal, pulmonary and mesenteric vessels (see Burnstock, 1982; Kitzen et al., 1983; Fredholm et al., 1983a; Snyder, 1985). Adenosine has also been shown to modulate depolarisation or field stimulation-induced release of NA from slices of rat brain neocortex (Harms et al., 1978; Fredholm et al., 1983b). The presynaptic receptor that mediates these actions is the P_1-purinoceptor, since the inhibitory actions of both ATP and adenosine are blocked by methylxanthines and because slowly degradable analogs of ATP are ineffective (De Mey et al., 1979). In most tissues the effect appears to be mediated by P_1-purinoceptors of the A_1-subtype to which the analog L-phenylisopropyl adenosine (L-PIA) shows a high affinity (Fredholm et al., 1983a), although the A_2-subtype appears to be dominant in the rat portal vein (Kennedy and Burnstock, 1984). It has been suggested that occupation of P_1-purinoceptors leads to decrease in Ca^{2+} influx and subsequent reduction in NA release (Wakade and Wakade, 1978). Diminished purinergic modulation of vascular adrenergic neurotransmission has been claimed in spontaneously hypertensive rats (Kamikawa et al., 1980).

Postjunctional actions

ATP can act directly on P_2-purinoceptors in the membranes of smooth muscles supplied by sympathetic nerves (see Burnstock, 1981a). It may also have modulatory actions on the postjunctional actions of NA. AMP and adenosine were shown to enhance contractile responses to NA in the guinea-pig vas deferens (Hedqvist and Fredholm, 1976), and it has been suggested that there is a mutual interaction between purinergic and α-adrenoceptor mechanisms (Holck and Marks, 1978). Guanine nucleotides are known to enhance β-adrenoceptor activation (Mukherjee and Lefkowitz, 1976). Conversely, NA potentiates the responses to ATP in the vas deferens and seminal vesicle (Nakanishi and Takeda, 1973; Holck and Marks, 1978).

ATP as a cotransmitter with acetylcholine in motor and parasympathetic nerves

Evidence for cotransmission in different tissues

Electric organ of fish

Cholinergic vesicles isolated from the electric organ of various elasmobranch fish contain ATP in addition to the principal transmitter ACh: *Torpedo marmorata* (Dowdall et al., 1974; Israel et al., 1979; Zimmermann and Bokor, 1979; Zimmermann et al., 1979); *Narcine brasiliensis* (Boyne, 1976); and *Electrophonis electricus* (Zimmermann and Denston, 1976). The ACh:ATP molar ratio in all three species is 4–10:1. The major nucleotide in these vesicles is ATP (83% of the total), with ADP (15%) and traces of AMP also being present (Dowdall et al., 1974; Zimmermann, 1978, 1982). ^{31}P-NMR analysis suggests that synaptic vesicles from electric organ of *Torpedo* store ATP together with ACh and Mg^{2+} essentially in free solution at an acidic pH (Füldner and Stadler, 1982).

Studies of the turnover of adenine nucleotides in cholinergic synaptic vesicles have shown that ATP and ACh are depleted to the same extent (about 50%) during nerve stimulation, that adenosine is an effective precursor of vesicular adenine nucleotides and that the new population of vesicles that appear following nerve stimulation has a high turnover rate for both ATP and ACh (Zimmermann and Denston, 1977; Zimmermann, 1978, 1979). Simultaneous release of ACh and ATP from synaptosome preparations from electric organ of *Torpedo* has also been demonstrated during depolarisation, although the ratio of ACh:ATP released was much higher (45:1) than that released from vesicle preparations (5:1) (Morel and Meunier, 1981).

Synaptosomes isolated from the electric organ

contain activity of both Mg^{2+}-activated ATPase and 5′-nucleotidase at the extracellular face of the plasma membrane, which leads to breakdown to adenosine nucleotides released during exocytosis of synaptic vesicle contents (Keller and Zimmermann, 1983). A saturable uptake system for adenosine into nerve terminals isolated from the *Torpedo* electric organ with a K_m value of 1 μM has been reported, which is comparable with that of the high affinity choline uptake system (Dowdall, 1978; Tomas et al., 1982). Evidence for axonal flow of ATP, as for ACh, in organelles other than mitochondria has also been reported (Davies, 1978).

Israel and his co-workers have presented evidence to suggest that ATP may be released from postsynaptic sites as a result of the depolarisation produced by ACh (Meunier et al., 1975; Israel et al., 1976). They showed that depolarisation of postsynaptic membranes by K^+ led to ATP release, but experiments by this group have also shown that ATP can be released by K^+ depolarisation from nerve terminals isolated from electric tissue (Meunier, 1978).

Frog gastrocnemius

Close arterial injection of small amounts of ATP (0.08×10^{-6} M) produced tetanus-like contractions comparable to those produced by ACh (Buchthal and Folkow, 1944). This action also occurs on curarised or denervated muscle (Buchthal and Folkow, 1948).

Rat diaphragm

Considerable quantities of ATP (up to 0.1 mM) have been reported to be released from the endings of phrenic nerves in the rat diaphragm during stimulation (Silinsky and Hubbard, 1973; Silinsky, 1975). This compares well with the levels of ATP released on stimulation of some regions of the cortex (Heller and McIlwain, 1973; Pull and McIlwain, 1973; Wu and Phillis, 1978).

Developing chick myotube

Although no evidence for an action of ATP on striated muscle of adult animals has been claimed, recent work on the developing chick myotube suggests that receptors for ATP are present as well as those for ACh (Kolb and Wakelam, 1983; Häggblad et al., 1985). In patch clamp studies of cultured chick myoblasts, external ATP in micromolar concentrations activated cation selective channels. Using biochemical methods, ATP was shown to induce an inward flux of ^{86}Rb into cultured chick myotubes that was additional to carbachol influx and, in contrast to the latter, it was not blocked by α-bungarotoxin (Häggblad et al., 1985).

Bladder

Ejps in response to stimulation of pelvic nerves, which gave a mixture of atropine-sensitive and atropine-resistant responses, are unaffected by atropine, but are blocked by α,β-methylene ATP (Hoyle and Burnstock, 1985).

Botulinum neurotoxin virtually abolished the atropine-resistant response of the guinea-pig bladder to field stimulation, suggesting that ATP, which is a strong contender for the non-cholinergic transmitter to this preparation (Burnstock et al., 1978; Westfall et al., 1983) is being released as a cotransmitter with ACh (MacKenzie et al., 1982). Hoyes et al. (1975) presented ultrastructural evidence which supports this view.

Brain

Release of [^{3}H]adenine derivatives has been shown to occur in the cholinergic septal system, which were considered as possible cotransmitters with ACh (Rose and Schubert, 1977).

Modulatory actions of purine nucleotides and nucleosides on cholinergic transmission

Prejunctional actions

ATP and adenosine have been shown to act on presynaptic purinergic receptors leading to modulation of the release of ACh from cholinergic motor nerves in skeletal muscle of rat diaphragm, frog sartorius, fish electric organ, brain and intestine (see Burnstock, 1982; Vizi et al., 1983; Kitzen et al., 1983; Pedata et al., 1983; Fredholm et al., 1983a;

Snyder, 1985). These responses are blocked by methylxanthines, indicating that they are mediated by P_1-purinoceptors. ATP does not usually act by way of P_2-purinoceptors, but is rapidly broken down to AMP and adenosine which occupy the P_1-purinoceptors on the cholinergic nerve terminals (Moody and Burnstock, 1982). It has been suggested that occupation of the presynaptic P_1-purinoceptors leads to decrease in the entry of Ca^{2+}, with consequent reduction in release of transmitter (Ribeiro, 1979; Dowdle and Maske, 1980; Israel et al., 1980; Hayashi et al., 1981).

Evidence that the actions of adenosine (and ATP) are presynaptic at the motor endplates in both rat diaphragm and frog sartorius is that, while the frequency of miniature endplate potentials (mepps), representing spontaneous release of ACh, is reduced and the amplitude of the nerve-evoked endplate potentials is reduced, the mean amplitude of the mepps is not reduced (Ginsborg and Hirst, 1972; Ribeiro and Walker, 1975). Neither adenosine nor ATP modifies the action potential in frog sciatic nerve (Okamoto et al., 1964; Ribeiro and Dominguez, 1978). Furthermore, ATP in concentrations sufficient to produce modulatory effects (0.01–0.2 mM), which are comparable to the amounts collected during nerve stimulation, has no postsynaptic action (Ribeiro, 1977), although at high concentrations, ATP potentiated the postjunctional action of ACh (see below). Reduction of evoked excitatory postsynaptic potentials (epsps) in brain to half control values by way of presynaptic receptors to low concentrations of adenosine (or ATP) have also been reported (Kuroda et al., 1976; Scholfield, 1978). Two types of adenosine receptors may be present at cholinergic nerve endings in frog skeletal muscle, one mediating depression and the other enhancing ACh release (Silinsky, 1980). It has been suggested that activation of extracellular adenosine receptors inhibits ACh release from motor nerve endings in frog skeletal muscle by reducing the affinity for Ca^{2+} of an intracellular component of the secretory apparatus (Silinsky, 1984).

Postjunctional actions

Apart from the direct action of ATP on P_2-purinoceptors on postjunctional cells (see Burnstock, 1981b; Stone, 1981b), ATP can act as a postjunctional modulator of the action of ACh. Increase of ACh receptor sensitivity by ATP has been demonstrated (Buchthal and Kahlson, 1944; Saji et al., 1975; Ewald, 1976; Ribeiro, 1977; Akasu et al., 1981; see Stone, 1981b). The amplitude of the current induced by ionophoretic application of ACh to the frog skeletal muscle endplate is increased in the presence of ATP, and kinetic analysis has suggested that ATP increases ACh sensitivity by acting on the allosteric site of the receptor-ionic channel complex without changing the affinity of ACh for its recognition site.

Summary

(1) Evidence has been presented that ATP is released as a cotransmitter with NA from sympathetic nerves supplying the vas deferens, taenia coli, nictitating membrane, a number of blood vessels and frog heart. It seems likely that the proportion of ATP to NA varies considerably in sympathetic nerves supplying different organs and in different species. It is also likely that various peptides coexist with ATP and NA in different sympathetic nerves, particularly neuropeptide Y (Lundberg et al., 1982a, 1985), but also somatostatin (Hökfelt et al., 1982), enkephalin (Schultzberg et al., 1983), vasoactive intestinal polypeptide (Lundberg et al., 1982b) and vasopressin-like peptide (Hanley et al., 1984). The precise roles and interactions of these substances contained in sympathetic nerves remains to be resolved.

(2) Co-transmission of ATP and NA seems to involve different postjunctional mechanisms: ATP produces contractions via an electromechanical coupling mechanism involving voltage-dependent Ca^{2+} channels; while NA produces contractions via a spike-independent mechanism involving receptor-

operated Ca^{2+} channels. ATP and NA act synergistically potentiating each others actions, and they help each other terminate neurotransmission by acting on prejunctional receptors to inhibit release of transmitter.

(3) Prejunctional modulation of neurotransmitter release takes place via prejunctional purinoceptors on sympathetic nerve terminal varicosities. Prejunctional purinoceptors are predominantly of the P_1-purinoceptor type, although some P_2-purinoceptors also appear to be involved at close (20 nm) neuromuscular junctions. Postjunctional facilitation of the actions of NA by ATP also occurs during sympathetic co-transmission and vice versa.

(4) While there is evidence for both storage and release of ATP with ACh from motor nerves, evidence is only available to date for a cotransmitter role involving postjunctional ATP receptors in the developing striated muscle of the chick myotube. Both prejunctional and postjunctional modulation of cholinergic transmission via P_1- and P_2-purinoceptors occurs.

(5) It is proposed that ATP is a primitive neurotransmitter that has been retained as the principal transmitter in some nerves, and that, during evolution, it has been utilised as a cotransmitter to variable extents in other nerve types.

References

Akasu,T., Hirai, K. and Koketsu, K. (1981) Increase of acetylcholine receptor sensitivity by adenosine triphosphate; a novel action of ATP on ACh-sensitivity. *Br. J. Pharmacol.*, 74: 505–507.

Allcorn, R. J., Cunnane, T. C., Muir, T. C. and Wardle, K. A. (1985) Does contraction in the rabbit ear artery require excitatory junction potentials (e.j.p.'s) and spikes? *J. Physiol. (Lond.)*, 362: 30p.

Ålund, M. (1980) Juxtaglomerular cell activity during haemorrhage and ischemia as revealed by quinacrine histofluorescence. *Acta physiol. Scand.*, 110: 113–121.

Ålund, M. and Olson, L. (1979) Quinacrine affinity of endocrine cell systems containing dense core vesicles as visualised by fluorescence microscopy. *Cell Tiss. Res.*, 204: 171–186.

Ambache, N. and Zar, M. A. (1971) Evidence against adrenergic motor transmission in the guinea-pig vas deferens. *J. Physiol. (Lond.)*, 216: 359.

Böck, P. (1980) Adenine nucleotides in the carotid body. *Cell Tiss. Res.*, 206: 279–290.

Boyne, A. F. (1976) Isolation of synaptic vesicles from *Narcine brasiliensis* electric organ — some influences on release of vesicular acetylcholine and ATP. *Brain Res.*, 114: 481–491.

Buchthal, F. and Folkow, B. (1944) Close arterial injection of adenosine triphosphate and inorganic triphosphate into frog muscle. *Acta physiol. Scand.*, 8: 312–316.

Buchthal, F. and Folkow, B. (1948) Interaction between acetylcholine and adenosine triphosphate in normal, curarised and denervated muscle. *Acta physiol. Scand.*, 15: 150–160.

Buchthal, F. and Kahlson, G. (1944) The motor effect of adenosine triphosphate and allied phosphorus compounds on smooth mammalian muscle. *Acta physiol. Scand.*, 8: 325–334.

Burnstock, G. (Ed.) (1981a) *Purinergic Receptors. Receptors and Recognition, Series B, Vol. 12,* Chapman & Hall, London.

Burnstock, G. (1981b) Neurotransmitters and trophic factors in the autonomic nervous system. *J. Physiol. (Lond.)*, 313: 1–35.

Burnstock, G. (1982) The co-transmitter hypothesis, with special reference to the storage and release of ATP with noradrenaline and acetylcholine. In A. C. Cuello (Ed.), *Co-Transmission,* MacMillan Press, London, pp. 151–163.

Burnstock, G. (1983) Recent concepts of chemical communication between excitable cells. In N. N. Osborne (Ed.), *Dale's Principle and Communication Between Neurones,* Pergamon Press, Oxford, pp. 7–35.

Burnstock, G. and Holman, M. E. (1960) Autonomic nerve-smooth muscle transmission. *Nature (Lond.)*, 187: 951–952.

Burnstock, G. and Sneddon, P. (1984) Electrical events underlying contractile responses to sympathetic nerve stimulation in rat tail artery. *J. Physiol. (Lond.)*, 357: 130P.

Burnstock, G., Cocks, T., Kasakov, L. and Wong H. (1978) Direct evidence for ATP release from non-adrenergic, non-cholinergic ("Purinergic") nerves in the guinea-pig taenia coli and bladder. *Europ. J. Pharmacol.*, 49: 145–149.

Burnstock, G., Crowe, R. and Wong, H. K. (1979) Comparative pharmacological and histochemical evidence for purinergic inhibitory innervation of the portal vein of the rabbit, but not guinea-pig. *Brit. J. Pharmacol.*, 65: 377–388.

Cheung, D. W. (1982) Two components in the cellular response of rat tail arteries to nerve stimulation. *J. Physiol. (Lond.)*, 328: 461–468.

Crowe, R. and Whitear, M. (1978) Quinacrine fluorescence of Merkel cells in Xenopus laevis. *Cell Tiss. Res.*, 190: 273–283.

Cunnane, T. C. and Stjärne, L. (1984) Transmitter secretion from individual varicosities of guinea-pig and mouse vas deferens: highly intermittent and monoquantal. *Neuroscience*, 13: 1–20.

Da Prada, M., Richards, J. G. and Lorez, H. P. (1978) Blood platelets and biogenic monoamines: biochemical, pharmacological and morphological studies. In G. de Gaetano and S. Garattini (Eds.), *Platelets: a Multidisciplinary Approach,* Raven Press, New York, pp. 331–353.

Da Prada, M. Lorez, H. P. and Richards, J. G. (1982) Platelet granules. In Poisner and Trifaro (Eds.), *The Secretory Granule,* Elsevier Biomedical Press, Amsterdam, pp. 279–316.

Davies, L. P. (1978) ATP in cholinergic nerves — evidence for axonal-transport of a stable pool. *Exp. Brain Res.,* 33: 149–157.

De Mey, J., Burnstock, G. and Vanhoutte, P. M. (1979) Modulation of the evoked release of noradrenaline in canine saphenous vein via presynaptic receptors for adenosine but not ATP. *Europ. J. Pharmacol.,* 55: 401–405.

Douglas, W. W. (1968) Stimulus-secretion coupling: the concept and clues from chromaffin and other cells. *Brit. J. Pharmacol.,* 34: 451–474.

Douglas, W. W. and Poisner, A. M. (1966) On the relation between ATP splitting and secretion in the adrenal chromaffin cell: extrusion of ATP (unhydrolysed) during release of catecholamines. *J. Physiol. (Lond.),* 183: 249–256.

Dowdall, M. J. (1978) Adenine nucleotides in cholinergic transmission: presynaptic aspects. *J. Physiol. (Paris),* 74: 497–501.

Dowdall, M. J., Boyne, A. F. and Whittaker, V. P. (1974) Adenosine triphosphate: a constituent of cholinergic synaptic vesicles. *Biochem. J.,* 140: 1–12.

Dowdle, E. B. and Maske, R. (1980) The effects of calcium concentration on the inhibition of cholinergic neurotransmission in the myenteric plexus of guinea-pig ileum by adenine nucleotides. *Brit. J. Pharmacol.,* 71: 245–252.

Duval, N., Hicks, P. E. and Langer, S. Z. (1985) Inhibitory effects of α,β-methylene ATP on nerve-mediated contractions of the nictitating membrane in reserpinised cats. *Europ. J. Pharmacol.,* 110: 373–377.

Ewald, D. A. (1976) Potentiation of postjunctional cholinergic sensitivity of rat diaphragm muscle by high-energy-phosphate adenine nucleotides. *J. Membr. Biol.,* 29: 47–65.

Fedan, J. S., Hogaboom, G. K., O'Donnell, J. P., Colby, J. and Westfall, D. P. (1981) Contributions by purines to the neurogenic response of the vas deferens of the guinea-pig. *Europ. J. Pharmacol.,* 69: 41–53.

Fredholm, B. B., Gustafsson, L. E., Hedqvist, P. and Sollevi, A. (1983a) Adenosine in the regulation of neurotransmitter release in the peripheral nervous system. In R. M. Berne, T. W. Rall and R. Rubio (Eds.), *Regulatory Function of Adenosine,* Martinus Nijhoff, The Hague–Boston–London, pp. 479–495.

Fredholm, B. B., Jonzon, B. and Lindgren, E. (1983b) Inhibition of noradrenaline release from hippocampal slices by a stable adenosine analogue. *Acta physiol. Scand.,* Suppl. 515: 7–10.

Füldner, H. H. and Stadler, H. (1982) ^{31}P-NMR analysis of synaptic vesicles. Status of ATP and internal pH. *Europ. J. Biochem.,* 121: 519–524.

Ginsborg, B. L. and Hirst, G. D. S. (1972) The effect of adenosine on the release of the transmitter from the phrenic nerve of the rat. *J. Physiol. (Lond.),* 224: 629–645.

Grant, T. L., Flavahan, N. A., Greig, J., McGrath, J. C., McKean, C. E. and Reid, J. L. (1985) Attempts to uncover subtypes of α-adrenoceptors and associated mechanisms by using sequential administration of blocking drugs. *Clin. Sci.,* 68, Suppl. 10: 10s–25s.

Häggblad, J., Eriksson, H. and Heilbronn, E. (1985) ATP-induced cation influx in myotubes is additive to cholinergic agonist action. *Acta physiol. Scand.,* 125: 389–394.

Hanley, M. R., Benton, H. P., Lightman, S. L., Todd, K., Bone, E. A., Fretten, P., Palmer, S., Kirk, C. J. and Michell, R. H. (1984) A vasopressin-like peptide in the mammalian sympathetic nervous system. *Nature (Lond.),* 309: 258–261.

Harms, H. H., Wardeh, G. and Mulder, A. H. (1978) Adenosine modulates depolarization-induced release of ^{3}H-noradrenaline from slices of rat-brain neocortex. *Europ. J. Pharmacol.,* 49: 305–308.

Hayashi, E., Yamada, S. and Shinozuka, K. (1981) The influence of extracellular Ca^{2+} concentration on the inhibitory effect of adenosine in guinea-pig ileal longitudinal muscles. *Jap. J. Pharmacol.,* 31: 141–143.

Head, R. J., Stitzel, R. E., de la Land, I. S. and Johnson, S. M. (1977) Effect of chronic denervation on the activities of monoamine-oxidase and catechol-O-methyltransferase and on the contents of noradrenaline and adenosine-triphosphate in the rabbit ear artery. *Blood Vessels,* 14: 229–239.

Hedqvist, P. and Fredholm, B.B. (1976) Effects of adenosine on adrenergic neurotransmission; prejunctional inhibition and postjunctional enhancement. *Naunyn-Schmiedeberg's Arch. Pharmacol.,* 293: 217–223.

Heller, I. H. and McIlwain, H. (1973) Release of (^{14}C)adenine derivatives from isolated subsystems of the guinea-pig brain: actions of electrical stimulation and of papaverine. *Brain Res.,* 53: 105–116.

Hicks, P. E., Langer, S.Z. and Vidal, M. J. (1985) α,β-Methylene ATP inhibits the vasoconstriction to periarterial field stimulation in SHR but not WKY tail arteries in vitro. *Brit. J. Pharmacol.,* 85: 225P.

Hökfelt, T., Lundberg, J. M., Skirboll, L., Johansson, O., Schultzberg, M. and Vincent, S. R. (1982) Co-existence of classical transmitters and peptides in neurones. In A. C. Cuello (Ed.), *Co-Transmission,* Macmillan Press, London, pp. 77–125.

Holck, M. I. and Marks, B. H. (1978) Purine nucleoside and nucleotide interactions on normal and subsensitive α-adrenoreceptor responsiveness in guinea-pig vas deferens. *J. Pharmacol. exp. Ther.,* 205: 104–117.

Hoyes, A. D., Barber, P. and Martin, B. G. H. (1975) Comparative ultrastructure of nerves innervating muscle of body of bladder. *Cell Tiss. Res.,* 164: 133–144.

Hoyle, C. H. V. and Burnstock, G. (1985) Atropine-resistant excitatory junction potentials in rabbit bladder are blocked by α,β-methylene ATP. *Europ. J. Pharmacol.,* 114: 239–240.

Hoyle, C. H. V. and Burnstock, G. (1986) Evidence that ATP is a neurotransmitter in the frog heart. *Europ. J. Pharmacol.* (in press).

Israel, M., Lesbats, B., Meunier, F. M. and Stinnakre, J. (1976) Postsynaptic release of adenosine triphosphate induced by single impulse transmitter action. *Proc. roy. Soc. Lond. B.*, 193: 461–468.

Israel, M., Dunant, Y., Lesbats, B., Manaranche, R., Marsal, J. and Meunier, F. (1979) Rapid acetylcholine and adenosine triphosphate oscillations triggered by stimulation of the *Torpedo* electric organ. *J. exp. Biol.*, 81: 63–73.

Israel, M., Lesbats, B., Manaranche, R., Meunier, F. M. and Franchon, P. (1980) Retrograde inhibition of transmitter release by ATP. *J. Neurochem.*, 34: 923–932.

Kamikawa, Y., Cline, J. R. and Su, C. (1980) Diminished purinergic modulation of the vascular adrenergic neurotransmission in spontaneously hypertensive rats. *Europ. J. Pharmacol.*, 66: 347–353.

Katsuragi, T. and Su, C. (1980) Purine release from vascular adrenergic nerves by high potassium and a calcium ionophore A-23187. *J. Pharmacol. exp. Ther.*, 215: 685–690.

Katsuragi, T. and Su, C. (1982) Augmentation by theophylline of (^{3}H) purine release from vascular adrenergic nerves: evidence for presynaptic autoinhibition. *J. Pharmacol. exp. Ther.*, 220: 152–156.

Kazic, T. and Milosavljevic, D. (1980) Interaction between adenosine triphosphate and noradrenaline in the isolated vas deferens of the guinea-pig. *Brit. J. Pharmacol.*, 71: 93–98.

Keller, F. and Zimmermann, H. (1983) Ecto-adenosine triphosphate activity at the cholinergic nerve endings of the *Torpedo* electric organ. *Life Sci.*, 33: 2635–2641.

Kennedy, C. and Burnstock, G. (1984) Evidence for an inhibitory prejunctional P_1-purinoceptor in the rat portal vein with characteristics of the A_2 rather than of the A_1 subtype. *Europ. J. Pharmacol.*, 100: 363–368.

Kitzen, J. M., Schwenkler, M. A., Moeller, J. E., Hellyer, L. D. and Wilson, S. J. (1983) Effects of N^6-cyclohexyladenosine (CHA) on responses to adrenergic and cholinergic nerve stimulation in the peripheral autonomic nervous system. *Drug Dev. Res.*, 3: 319–330.

Kolb, H.-A. and Wakelam, M. J. O. (1983) Transmitter-like action of ATP on patched membranes of cultured myoblasts and myotubes. *Nature (Lond.)*, 303: 621–623.

Kuroda, Y., Saito, M. and Kobayashi, K. (1976) Concomitant changes in cyclic AMP level and postsynaptic potentials of olfactory cortex slices induced by adenosine derivatives. *Brain Res.*, 109: 196–201.

Langer, S. Z. and Pinto, J. E. B. (1976) Possible involvement of a transmitter different from norepinephrine in residual responses to nerve stimulation of cat nictitating membrane after pretreatment with reserpine. *J. Pharmacol. exp. Ther.*, 196: 697–713.

Leitner, J. W., Sussman, K. E., Vatter, A. E. and Schneider, F. H. (1975) Adenine nucleotides in the secretory granule fraction of rat islets. *Endocrinology*, 96: 662–677.

Levitt, B. and Westfall, D. P. (1982) Factors influencing the release of purines and norepinephrine in the rabbit portal vein. *Blood Vessels*, 19: 30–40.

Levitt, B., Head, R. J. and Westfall, D. P. (1984) High-pressure chromatographic-fluorometric detection of adenosine and adenine nucleotides: application to endogenous content and electrically-induced release of adenyl purines in guinea-pig vas deferens. *Anal.Biochem.*, 137: 93–100.

Lundberg, J. M., Terenius, L., Hökfelt, T., Martling, C. R., Tatemoto, K., Mutt, V., Polak, J., Bloom, S. and Goldstein, M. (1982a) Neuropeptide-Y (NPY)-like immunoreactivity in peripheral noradrenergic neurons and effects of NPY on sympathetic function. *Acta physiol. Scand.*, 116: 477–480.

Lundberg, J. M., Hökfelt, T., Änggård, A., Terenius, L., Elde, R., Markey, K., Goldstein, M. and Kimmel, J. (1982b) Organisational principles in the peripheral sympathetic nervous system: subdivision by coexisting peptides (somatostatin-, avian pancreatic polypeptide-, and vasoactive intestinal polypeptide-like immunoreactive materials). *Proc. nat. Acad. Sci. USA*, 79: 1303–1307.

Lundberg, J. M., Saria, A., Franco-Cereceda, A., Hökfelt, T., Terenius, L. and Goldstein, M. (1985) Differential effects of reserpine and 6-hydroxydopamine on neuropeptide Y (NPY) and noradrenaline in peripheral neurons. *Naunyn-Schmiedeberg's Arch. Pharmacol.*, 328: 331–340.

MacKenzie, I., Burnstock, G. and Dolly, J. O. (1982) The effects of purified botulinum neurotoxin Type A on cholinergic, adrenergic and non-adrenergic, atropine-resistant autonomic-neuromuscular transmission. *Neuroscience*, 7: 997–1006.

Meldrum, L. A. and Burnstock, G. (1983) Evidence that ATP acts as a cotransmitter with noradrenaline in sympathetic nerves supplying the guinea-pig vas deferens. *Europ. J. Pharmacol.*, 92: 161–163.

Meunier, F. M. (1978) Effet de la dépolarisation sur la liberation d'ATP pre- et postsynaptique. Nucleotides and neurotransmission. *Conf. Neurobiologie de Gif.*, p. 15.

Meunier, F. M., Israel, M. and Lesbats, B. (1975) Release of ATP from stimulated nerve electroplaque junctions. *Nature (Lond.)*, 257: 407–408.

Moody, C. and Burnstock, G. (1982) Evidence for the presence of P_1-purinoceptors on cholinergic nerve terminals in the guinea-pig ileum. *Europ. J. Pharmacol.*, 77: 1–9.

Morel, N. and Meunier, F.-M. (1981) Simultaneous release of acetylcholine and ATP from stimulated cholinergic synaptosomes. *J. Neurochem.*, 36: 1766–1773.

Mukherjee, C. and Lefkowitz, R. J. (1976) Desensitization of β-adrenergic receptors by β-adrenergic agonists in a cell-free system: resensitization by guanosine 5'-(β,γ-imino) triphosphate and other purine nucleotides. *Proc. nat. Acad. Sci. USA*, 73: 1494–1498.

Muramatsu, I., Fujiwara, M. Miura, A. and Sakakibara, Y. (1981) Possible involvement of adenine nucleotides in sympathetic neuroeffector mechanisms of dog basilar artery. *J. Pharmacol. exp. Ther.*, 216: 401–409.

Nakanishi, H. and Takeda, H. (1973) The possible role of adenosine triphosphate in chemical transmission between the hypogastric nerve terminal and seminal vesicle in the guinea-pig. *Jap. J. Pharmacol.*, 23: 479–490.

Okamoto, M., Askari, A. and Kuperman, A. S. (1964) The stabilizing actions of adenosine triphosphate and related nucleotides on calcium-deficient nerve. *J. Pharmacol. exp.Ther.*, 144: 229–235.

Olson, L., Ålund, M. and Norberg, K.-A. (1976) Fluorescence microscopical demonstration of a population of gastro-intestinal nerve fibres with a selective affinity for quinacrine. *Cell Tiss. Res.*, 171: 407–423.

Pedata, F., Antonelli, T., Lambertini, L., Beani, L. and Pepeu, G. (1983) Effect of adenosine, adenosine triphosphate, adenosine deaminase, dipyridamole and aminophylline on acetylcholine release from electrically-stimulated brain slices. *Neuropharmacology*, 22: 609–614.

Potter, D. D., Furshpan, E. J. and Landis, S. C. (1983) Transmitter status in cultured rat sympathetic neurons: plasticity and multiple function. *Fed. Proc.*, 42: 1626–1632.

Pull, I. and McIlwain, H. (1973) Output of (^{14}C)adenine nucleotides and their derivatives from cerebral tissues: Tetrodotoxin resistant and calcium ion requiring components. *Biochem. J.*, 136: 893–901.

Ribeiro, J. A. (1977) Potentiation of postjunctional cholinergic sensitivity of rat diaphragm muscle by high energy-phosphate adenine nucleotides. *J. Membr. Biol.*, 33: 401–402.

Ribeiro, J. A. (1979) Purinergic modulation of transmitter release. *J. Theor. Biol.*, 80: 259–270.

Ribeiro, J. A. and Dominguez, M. L. (1978) Mechanisms of depression of neuromuscular transmission by ATP and adenosine. *J. Physiol. (Paris)*, 74: 491–496.

Ribeiro, J. A. and Walker, J. (1975) The effects of adenosine triphosphate and adenosine diphosphate on transmission at the rat and frog neuromuscular junctions. *Brit. J. Pharmacol.*, 54: 213–218.

Rose, G. and Schubert, P. (1977) Release and transfer of (^{3}H)adenosine derivatives in cholinergic septal system. *Brain Res.*, 121: 353–357.

Saji, Y., Escalona de Motta, G. and del Castillo, J. (1975) Depolarization and potentiation of responses to acetylcholine elicited by ATP on frog muscle. *Life Sci.*, 16: 945–954.

Scholfield, C. N. (1978) Depression of evoked potentials in brain-slices by adenosine compounds. *Brit. J. Pharmacol.*, 63: 239–244.

Schultzberg, M., Hökfelt, T., Lundberg, J. M., Dalsgaard, C. J. and Elfvin, L.-G. (1983) Transmitter histochemistry of autonomic ganglia. In L.-G. Elfvin (Ed.), *Autonomic Ganglia*, John Wiley & Sons, Chichester, pp. 205–233.

Shimada, S. G. and Stitt, J. T. (1984) An analysis of the purinergic component of active muscle vasodilatation obtained by electrical stimulation of the hypothalamus in rabbits. *Brit. J. Pharmacol.*, 83: 577–589.

Silinsky, E. M. (1975) On the association between transmitter secretion and the release of adenine nucleotides from mammalian motor nerve terminals. *J. Physiol. (Lond.)*, 247: 145–162.

Silinsky, E. M. (1980) Evidence for specific adenosine receptors at cholinergic nerve endings. *Brit. J. Pharmacol.*, 71: 191–194.

Silinsky, E. M. (1984) On the mechanism by which adenosine receptor activation inhibits the release of acetylcholine from motor nerve endings. *J. Physiol. (Lond.)*, 346: 243–256.

Silinsky, E. M. and Hubbard, J. I. (1973) Release of ATP from rat motor nerve terminals. *Nature (Lond.)*, 243: 404–405.

Smith, A. D. (1972) Subcellular localisation of noradrenaline in sympathetic neurones. *Pharmacol. Rev.*, 24: 435–440.

Sneddon, P. and Burnstock, G. (1984a) Inhibition of excitatory junction potentials in guinea-pig vas deferens by α,β-methylene-ATP: further evidence for ATP and noradrenaline as cotransmitters. *Europ. J. Pharmacol.*, 100: 85–90.

Sneddon, P. and Burnstock, G. (1984b) ATP as a neurotransmitter in rat tail artery. *Europ. J. Pharmacol.*, 106: 149–152.

Sneddon, P. and Westfall, D. P. (1984) Pharmacological evidence that adenosine triphosphate and noradrenaline are cotransmitters in the guinea-pig vas deferens. *J. Physiol. (Lond.)*, 347: 561–580.

Sneddon, P., Westfall, D. P. and Fedan, J. S. (1982) Co-transmitters in the motor nerves of the guinea-pig vas deferens: electrophysiological evidence. *Science*, 218: 693–695.

Sneddon, P., Meldrum, L. and Burnstock, G. (1984) Control of transmitter release in guinea-pig vas deferens by pre-junctional P_1-purinoceptors. *Europ. J. Pharmacol.*, 105: 293–299.

Snyder, S. H. (1985) Adenosine as a neuromodulator. *Ann. Rev. Neurosci.*, 8: 103–124.

Stevens, P., Robinson, R. L., Van Dyke, K. and Stitzel, R. (1972) Studies on the synthesis and release of adenosine triphosphate-8-^{3}H in the isolated perfused cat adrenal gland. *J. Pharmacol. exp. Ther.*, 181: 463–471.

Stjärne, L. and Åstrand, P. (1984) Discrete events measure single quanta of ATP secreted from sympathetic nerves of guinea-pig and mouse vas deferens. *Neuroscience*, 13: 21–28.

Stone, T. W. (1981a) Differential blockade of ATP, noradrenaline and electrically evoked contractions of the rat vas deferens by nifedipine. *Europ. J. Pharmacol.*, 74: 373–376.

Stone, T. W. (1981b) Physiological roles for adenosine and adenosine 5′-triphosphate in the nervous system. *Neuroscience*, 6: 523–555.

Su, C. (1975) Neurogenic release of purine compounds in blood-vessels. *J. Pharmacol. exp. Ther.*, 195: 159–166.

Su, C. (1978) Modes of vasoconstrictor and vasodilator neurotransmission. *Blood Vessels*, 15: 183–189.

Su, C., Bevan, J. A. and Burnstock, G. (1971) [^{3}H]Adenosine triphosphate: release during stimulation of enteric nerves. *Science*, 173: 337–339.

Suzuki, H. (1985) Electrical responses of smooth muscle cells of the rabbit ear artery to adenosine triphosphate. *J. Physiol. (Lond.)*, 359: 401–415.

Tomas, J., Marsal, J., Esquerda, J. E. and Solsona, C. (1982) Ionic dependence of adenosine uptake by isolated nerve endings from *Torpedo* electric organ. *Neurochem. Int.*, 4: 513–521.

Van Dyke, K., Robinson, R., Urquilla, P., Smith, D., Taylor, M., Trush, M. and Wilson, M. (1977) Analysis of nucleotides and catecholamines in bovine medullary granules by anion-exchange high pressure liquid chromatography and fluorescence evidence that most of catecholamines in chromaffin granules are stored without associated ATP. *Pharmacology,* 15: 377–391.

Vizi, E. S., Somogyi, G. T. and Magyar, K. (1983) Presynaptic control by adenosine of acetylcholine release: inhibitory effect of norepinephrine and opioid peptides as an independent action. In J. W. Daly, Y. Kuroda, J. W. Phillis, H. Shimizu and M. Ui (Eds.), *Physiology and Pharmacology of Adenosine Derivatives,* Raven Press, New York, pp. 209–217.

Wakade, A. R. and Wakade, T. D. (1978) Inhibition of noradrenaline release by adenosine. *J. Physiol. (Lond.),* 282: 35–49.

Westfall, D. P., Stitzel, R. E. and Rowe, J. N. (1978) The postjunctional effects and neural release of purine compounds in guinea-pig vas deferens. *Europ. J. Pharmacol.,* 50: 27–38.

Westfall, D. P., Fedan, J. S., Colby, J., Hogaboom, G. K. and O'Donnell, J. P. (1983) Evidence for a contribution by purines to the neurogenic response of the guinea-pig urinary bladder. *Europ. J. Pharmacol.,* 87: 415–422.

Wu, P. H. and Phillis, J. W. (1978) Distribution and release of adenosine-triphosphate in rat-brain. *Neurochem. Res.,* 3: 563–571.

Zimmermann, H. (1978) Turnover of adenine nucleotides in cholinergic synaptic vesicles of the *Torpedo* electric organ. *Neuroscience,* 3: 827–836.

Zimmermann, H. (1979) Commentary: vesicles recycling and transmitter release. *Neuroscience,* 4: 1773–1803.

Zimmermann, H. (1982) Co-existence of adenosine 5′-triphosphate and acetylcholine in the electromotor synapse. In A. C. Cuello (Ed.) *Co-Transmission,* Macmillan Press, London, pp. 243–259.

Zimmermann, H. and Bokor, J. T. (1979) 5′-Triphosphate recycles independently of acetylcholine in cholinergic synaptic vesicles. *Neurosci. Lett.,* 13: 319–324.

Zimmermann, H. and Denston, C. R. (1976) Adenosine triphosphate in cholinergic vesicles isolated from the electric organ of *Electrophorus electricus. Brain Res.,* 111: 365–376.

Zimmermann, H. and Denston, C. R. (1977) Separation of synaptic vesicles of different functional states from the cholinergic synapses of the *Torpedo* electric organ. *Neuroscience,* 2: 715–730.

Zimmermann, H., Dowdall, M. J. and Lane, D. A. (1979) Purine salvage at the cholinergic nerve-endings of the *Torpedo* electric organ—central role of adenosine. *Neuroscience,* 4: 979–993.

T. Hökfelt, K. Fuxe and B. Pernow (Eds.),
Progress in Brain Research, Vol. 68

CHAPTER 14

The LHRH family of peptide messengers in the frog nervous system

W. D. Branton, H. S. Phillips and Y. N. Jan

Department of Physiology, School of Medicine, University of California, San Francisco and Howard Hughes Medical Institute, San Francisco, CA 94143, U.S.A.

Introduction

The diversity of peptides found in the nervous systems is striking. At present, more than 30 peptides are considered as putative neurotransmitters. Most likely, many more will be found in the future. The complexity is compounded by the fact that the discovery of a peptide, often leads to finding of a family of related peptides and associated with each family of peptides are often multiple types of receptors.

At present, it is not understood why the nervous system utilizes so many different transmitters and receptors. A detailed analysis of the action of neuropeptides may reveal characteristics unique to peptidergic transmissions and shed light on the functional significance of the multiple of peptide transmitters. For this purpose, we have been studying the functional roles of LHRH-like peptides in the frog.

We were initially attracted to this system because of the finding that a LHRH-like peptide mediates a slow synaptic potential in frog sympathetic ganglia (Jan et al., 1979). Sympathetic ganglia have provided a good system for this study because of their simple anatomy. Neurons in these ganglia are unipolar and have no dendrites. Preganglionic fibers make synaptic contacts almost exclusively on the ganglionic cell bodies. This arrangement facilitates analysis of the physiological effects of neurotransmitters and allows accurate anatomical description of synaptic connections. By studying the actions of the LHRH-like peptide in these ganglia, we came upon some novel features of peptidergic transmission (for review see Jan et al., 1983).

More recently, it became clear that there are at least two forms of LHRH-like peptide in the frog nervous system (Branton et al., 1982; Eiden et al., 1982). LHRH-I is apparently identical to mammalian pituitary LHRH (Rivier at al., 1981) and seems to be the predominant form in adult frog brain. LHRH-II represents either a single peptide or a group of peptides closely related to teleost LHRH. It is the predominant form in frog sympathetic ganglia and it is also found in the central nervous system (CNS) (Branton et al., 1982). Since LHRH is a well-characterized peptide hormone in the CNS and the action of the LHRH-like peptide in sympathetic ganglia is fairly well understood, a careful analysis of the differential distribution and function of those peptides in the frog nervous system could prove useful in understanding the functional roles and possible interactions of members of a peptide family.

To study the functions of a peptide family, one needs to localize individual members of the peptide family as well as the various subtypes of receptors. Toward this goal, we describe in this chapter the use of antibodies that distinguish between LHRH-

I and LHRH-II to delineate the distribution of the different LHRH-like peptides in the frog nervous systems.

Materials and methods

Antisera

HP1, HP3 and HP5 were generated in rabbits against synthetic salmon LHRH (Peninsula Labs) coupled to bovine serum albumin (BSA) with glutaraldehyde. HPDB1 was generated in the same way but with $DLys^6$ mammalian LHRH (Peninsula) and DB1 was generated in rabbit against $Ornithine^8$ mammalian LHRH coupled to BSA with Dimethyl Suberimidate (Pierce). $Ornithine^8$ LHRH was a gift of Karoly Nickolics, Antiserum 1076 was a gift from Robert Millar, L-5 from Wylie Vale, and R42 from Terry Nett.

High pressure liquid chromatography (HPLC)

Tissue was removed from MS222-anesthetized animals, frozen on dry ice and lyophylized. Dry tissue was extracted overnight in dry acetone, homogenized in hot 3N acetic acid and the solubilized material extracted with ethyl ether. The aqueous phase was lyophylized and re-dissolved in 0.25 M triethyl ammonium formate (TEAF) at pH 6.5. A sample was applied to a supellco DBC18 column (0.46 × 25 cm) and eluted with a gradient of acetonitrile in 0.25 M TEAF pH 6.5. Fractions were assayed for LHRH immunoreactivity by RIA with Nett R42 antiserum.

Immunocytochemistry

Animals were anesthetized in MS222 and fixed by cardiac perfusion with 4% paraformaldehyde in 0.1 M phosphate buffer pH 7.2. Tissue was removed and post-fixed overnight at 4°C in the same solution. Sections were either cut by vibratome (Oxford) or infiltrated with 30% sucrose and cut on a cryostat (Slee) at −25°C. The sections were incubated overnight at 4°C in various dilutions of primary antibody. The incubation solutions contained 0.1 M Tris HCl pH 7.2, 0.9% NaCl, 0.1% Triton and 4% normal goat serum. Bound antibody was labeled by sequential incubation (1 h, 25°C) with biotinylated anti-rabbit IgG and avidin-biotinylated-peroxidase complex (Vector Labs ABC Kit) after the method of Hsu et al. (1981). Peroxidase staining was visualized by incubation with diaminobenzidine and H_2O_2. Staining reported was dependent on the presence of the primary antibody, and was not seen when the antibody was pre-incubated with the peptide (10^{-5} M) against which it was made. Primary antibody dilutions were as follows: 1076, 1:4000; DB1 1:4000; HPDB1 1:2000; HP1, HP3, HP5, 1:2000; L-5 1:1000. For figures 6C and 7C affinity purified HP1 was utilized at a concentration of 1 μg/ml.

Retrograde label

Frogs were anesthetized in MS222 and cooled on ice. The 8th sympathetic ramus was cut near the 8th paravertebral ganglion and the central end exposed to 50% HRP (Sigma type VI) for 12 h at 0°C. The excess HRP was removed; the animal was closed, and allowed to survive 2 days. At the end of the survival period the animal was perfused and fixed as for immunocytochemistry. HRP was visualized by reaction with tetramethyl benzidine and H_2O_2.

Results

Action of LHRH-like peptide in bullfrog sympathetic ganglia — a brief review

An LHRH-like peptide is the transmitter mediating the late slow excitatory post-synaptic potential (epsp)

Acetylcholine (ACh) has been known for years to be a transmitter contained in the preganglionic fibers. Three types of synaptic responses are mediated by ACh: (1) the nicotinic fast epsp's which last for about 30–50 msec; (2) the muscarinic slow epsp's lasting 30–60 sec; and (3) the muscarinic slow inhibitory post-synaptic potential of 1–2 sec duration. In 1968, a fourth synaptic potential was discovered by Nishi and Koketsu and named the late slow epsp. This response lasts for several minutes and is not mediated by ACh. From studies done in the last few years, we believe that the late slow epsp is mediated by a LHRH-like peptide because it met essentially all criteria commonly used for identifying a substance as a transmitter: an LHRH-like peptide is *present* in the appropriate preganglion fibers. This peptide is *released* into the extracellular medium when the appropriate preganglionic fibers are stimulated, the physiologic effects of the endogeneous transmitters are *mimicked* by LHRH and its agonists, and finally, the late slow epsp is *blocked by antagonists* of LHRH (Jan et al., 1979; Jan and Jan, 1982).

The LHRH-like peptide and ACh are probably contained and released from the same preganglionic fibers

Since the pioneering work of Hökfelt and his colleagues (1980), there is now considerable evidence that a neuron may use more than one transmitter. The frog sympathetic ganglion has lent itself to a rigorous test of the idea of coexistence and corelease of more than one transmitter, because in this system the substances in question actually could be shown to function as transmitters.

The innervation of the last two ganglia of the Lumbar chain, the 9th and 10th ganglia are summarized in Fig. 1. There are two types of sympathetic neurons. B cells are in synaptic contact with preganglionic B fibers arising from the 3rd, 4th, and 5th spinal nerves, whereas C cells are in synaptic contact with preganglionic C fibers, arising from the 7th and 8th spinal nerves. Stimulation of 3rd, 4th and 5th spinal nerves generate cholinergic synaptic potentials in B cells only. Stimulation of the 7th and 8th spinal nerves generate peptidergic synaptic potentials in both B cells and C cells, as well as cholinergic responses in C cells. Several lines of evidence suggest that the same preganglionic C fibers contains both ACh and a LHRH-like peptide (Jan and Jan, 1983):

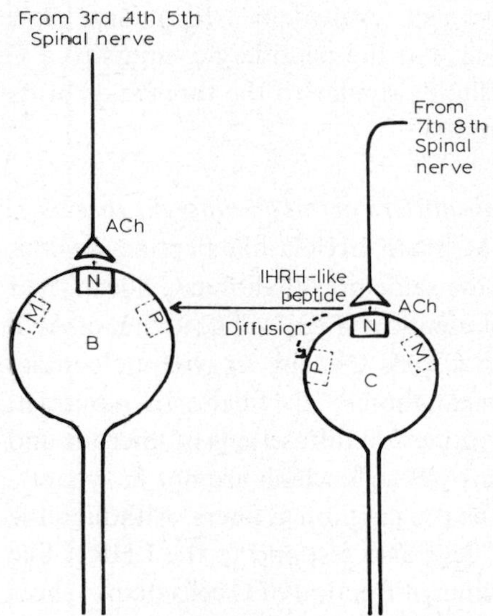

Fig. 1. Scheme of innervation of neurons in the 9th and 10th ganglia, the last two ganglia in the sympathetic chain. B cells are larger, whereas C cells are smaller. Cholinergic axons for B neurons arise from the 3rd, 4th, and 5th spinal nerves, whereas preganglionic fibers for C cells come through the 7th and 8th spinal nerves. LHRH-positive nerve terminals are present only on C cells. Most likely, both the LHRH-like peptide and ACh are contained and released from the same preganglionic fibers for C cells. (N) Nicotinic cholinergic receptors; (M) muscarinic cholinergic receptors; (P) LHRH receptors. Of the three types of receptors, only the nicotinic cholinergic receptors have been localized. They are situated right in apposition to the synaptic boutons. (Reprinted with permission from Jan and Jan, 1982.)

(1) Essentially all (>95%) terminals of preganglionic C fibers contain the LHRH-like peptide. Since at least some of these terminals must also contain ACh, at least some of the terminals of preganglionic C fibers must contain both ACh and LHRH-like peptide.

(2) Physiological experiments indicate that each preganglionic C fiber probably releases both ACh and the LHRH-like peptide: a sympathetic C neuron typically receives several cholinergic inputs with different thresholds for stimulation, so that one may raise the stimulation strength gradually to recruit cholinergic preganglionic fibers one by one. In doing so, we found that each time a cholinergic fiber is recruited, repetitive stimulation at that stimu-

lation strength also resulted in a larger late slow epsp, indicating that the peptidergic inputs to a C cell have thresholds similar to the thresholds of its cholinergic inputs.

Coexisting transmitters act upon different targets

Although ACh and LHRH-like peptide are contained within the same preganglionic C fibers, their targets are not identical (Fig. 1). The action of ACh is restricted to C cells that are in synaptic contact with the preganglionic C fiber. In contrast, LHRH-like peptide can diffuse tens of microns and act on the nearby B cells which are not in synaptic contact with the preganglion C fibers. Although the majority of C cells also respond to the LHRH-like peptide, a significant fraction of C cells do not show membrane potential change to LHRH or the nerve-released LHRH-like peptide, despite the fact that they are in synaptic contact with LHRH-like peptide-containing fibers. Figure 2 is an example of a recording from a B cell and an adjacent C cell. The B cell responded vigorously to both endogenous and applied LHRH-like peptide, whereas the C cell did not respond to either. This example illustrates that the morphologically defined synaptic connection may be misleading in identifying target neurons for a peptide transmitter whereas localization of peptide receptors might be the most important criterion.

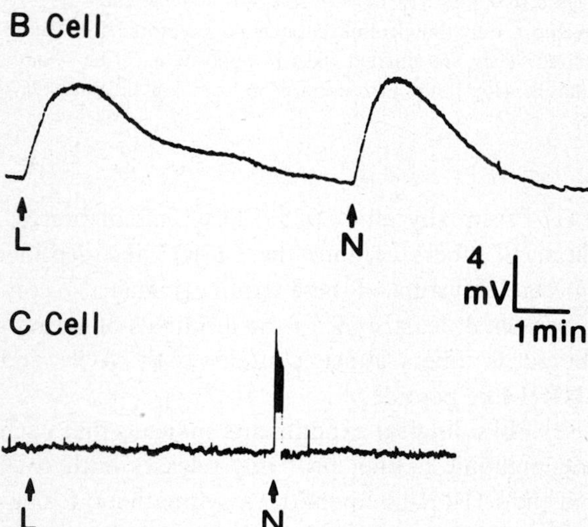

Fig. 2. Intracellular recording from two adjacent cells: a B cell and a C cell. LHRH was delivered to the cell body with a brief (3 sec) pulse or LHRH via pressure ejection. Nerve stimulation was elicited by stimulating the 7th and 8th spinal nerve with a brief train (10 sec, 5 Hz).

Selective communication using diffusible peptides as chemical messengers thus will not necessarily involve the precise circuitry of synaptic contacts. Instead, different neurons in a given region may express different subsets of receptors, so that a peptide transmitter released in the vicinity will influence only those neurons that have the appropriate receptors on their surfaces (Fig. 1). For this type of interneuronal communication to be used extensively without cross-talk between parallel pathways, a necessary requirement is that many different molecules are used as transmitters. Perhaps this is one reason for the multiplicity of putative peptide transmitters (Jan et al., 1983).

Multiple forms of LHRH-like peptides in frog nervous system

Frog sympathetic ganglia contain LHRH-II, which is different from mammalian LHRH

The LHRH-like transmitter in frog sympathetic ganglia is immunologically similar to, but not identical to mammalian LHRH (Jan et al., 1979; Eiden and Eskay, 1980). Based on immunological and chromatographical criteria, it was proposed that LHRH-II is identical to teleost hypothalamic LHRH which differs from mammalian hypothalamic LHRH (i.e. LHRH-I) by two amino acids at positions 7 and 8 (Sherwood et al., 1983). This hypothesis is supported by electrophysiological experiments (Jan et al., 1983; Jones et al., 1984) in that teleost LHRH is much more potent than mammalian LHRH-I in mimicking the late slow epsp in sympathetic ganglia. Thus, it seems likely that LHRH-II is either very similar or identical to teleost LHRH. Whether LHRH-II is identical to teleost LHRH can only be determined by obtaining the sequence of LHRH-II.

The frog brain contains both LHRH-I and LHRH-II

The adult frog brain contains a large amount of LHRH-I (Fig. 3). By a variety of criteria, including amino acid analysis of LHRH-like peptides purified from frog brains, LHRH-I is most likely identical to mammalian LHRH. In addition to LHRH-I, the frog brain also contains LHRH-II, as revealed by HPLC extracts of frog brain (Fig. 3). In this experiment, Nett R42 antiserum was used to detect LHRH-immunoreactivity. This antiserum is highly specific for LHRH-like structures, and it requires both intact N- and C-termini of LHRH. It recognizes teleost LHRH about 50% as well as mammalian LHRH. As shown on Fig. 3, the brain extract contains a large peak of LHRH-I and a smaller LHRH-II peak. The elution time of brain LHRH-II is comparable to that of LHRH-II from sympathetic ganglia.

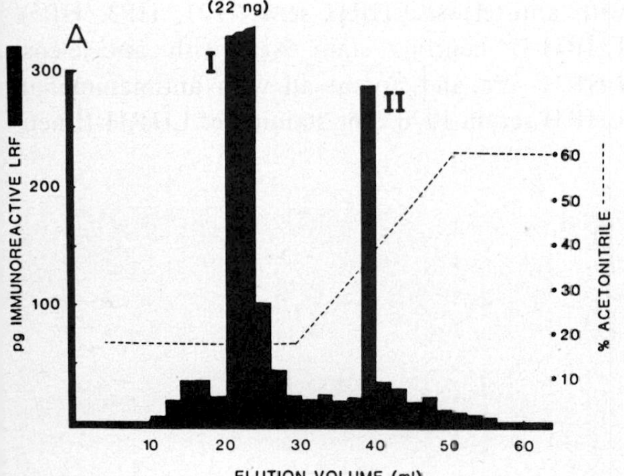

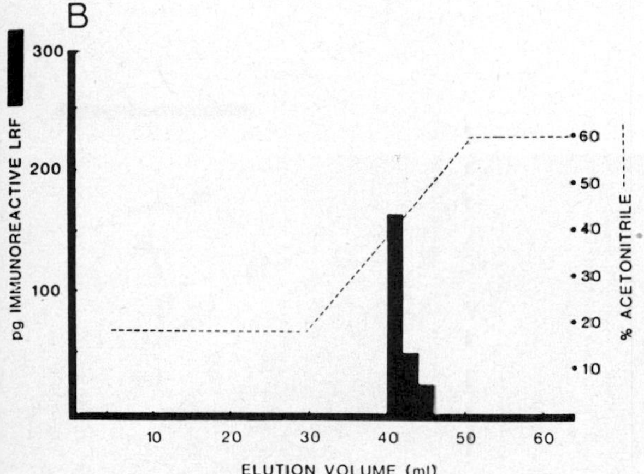

Fig. 3. HPLC of extracts of frog brain and sympathetic ganglia. Samples were loaded on a C18 column in 0.25 M TEAF pH 6.5, and eluted with a gradient of acetonitrile (dashed line). Fractions were collected and assayed for LHRH immunoreactivity by radioimmunoassay with antiserum R42. (A) Frog brain extract displays two peaks of immunoreactivity. LHRH-I represents mammalian LHRH, and LHRH-II corresponds in elution position to the LHRH-II of sympathetic ganglion. (B) Sympathetic ganglia extract showing only one immunoreactive region corresponding to LHRH-II in frog brain.

LHRH-I and II have very different developmental profiles. In adult frog brain, LHRH-I is the predominant form. In contrast, in early tadpole stages, LHRH-II is the predominant form found in the brain. The relative amount of LHRH-I increases greatly near the climax stage of metamorphosis (Branton et al., 1982). More detailed characterization of LHRH-I and II and their development profiles will be published elsewhere (Branton et al., in preparation).

Given that the structure and developmental profile of LHRH-I are different from that of LHRH-II, and since LHRH-II functions as a transmitter in sympathetic ganglia, while LHRH-I most likely functions as a releasing factor, we hypothesized that in frog CNS, LHRH-II and LHRH-I-containing systems have distinct distribution and function. To approach this problem, we need to be able to differentiate LHRH-I and LHRH-II and localize them separately at the single cell level. This is made possible by antisera that can distinguish the two forms.

Distribution of LHRH-I and LHRH-II in frog nervous system

Antibodies that can differentiate both LHRH-I and LHRH-II

The antisera can be divided into three categories:

(1) Antisera generated against teleost LHRH (HP1, HP3, HP5). These antisera gave intense

staining of preganglionic terminals on C cells (Fig. 4A) where LHRH-II is the only form of LHRH present. These antisera stain LHRH-I and mammalian LHRH poorly (Fig. 4C).

(2) Antiserum specific for LHRH-I (Millar, 1076). This antiserum stains structures containing LHRH-I intensely (Fig. 4B) and fails to stain frog sympathetic ganglia at all (fig. 4D).

(3) Antisera generated against mammalian LHRH that cross-react with LHRH-II (DB1, HPDB1, L5).

Criteria for identification of LHRH-I and LHRH-II-containing perikarya

Utilizing the antisera described above, we have identified two populations of neurons in the frog nervous system. LHRH-I neurons stain intensely with all of the sera generated against mammalian LHRH (1076, L5, HPDB1, DB1) and only weakly with anti-teleost LHRH sera (HP1, HP3, HP5). LHRH-II neurons stain well with anti-teleost LHRH sera and not at all with antimammalian LHRH serum 1076. The staining of LHRH-II neu-

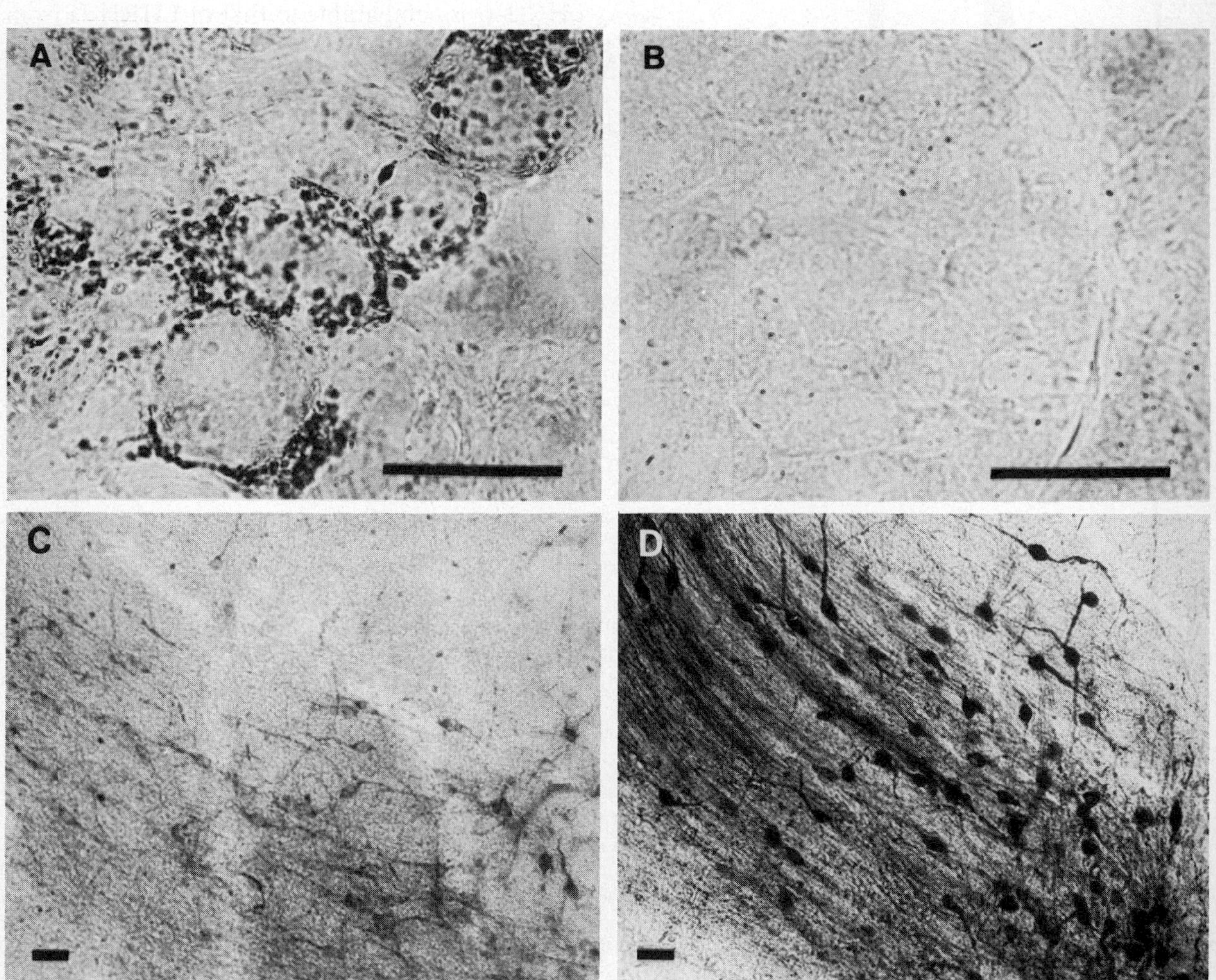

Fig. 4. Specificity of immunocytochemistry for LHRH-I and LHRH-II-type neurons. (A) Section of 9th ganglion showing LHRH-II terminals stained with serum HP1. (B) Similar section as in (A), but stained with serum 1076. Note the complete absence of staining. (C) Median septal nucleus of frog brain stained with serum HP1. (D) Similar section to C with LHRH-I cells and fibers intensely stained with serum 1076. Bar = 50 μm in (A,B), 30 μm in (C,D).

rons is abolished by preadsorption of anti-teleost LHRH serum with teleost LHRH but not with mammalian LHRH.

LHRH-I-containing system

Most of the LHRH-I system has been previously described (Alpert et al., 1976; Nozaki et al., 1979). A large group of neurons located in what has been described as the median septal nucleus (MSN), project heavily to the median eminence (Fig. 5A,B). Occasional LHRH-I neurons are found along the path of this projection and in the neural lobe of the pituitary. This system of neurons apparently serves the same role as their mammalian counterparts in the control of pituitary LH release. Large numbers of positive fibers were seen in the septal region surrounding the cell bodies, and some fibers appear to project caudally from this region, including fibers which invest the optic tectum. LHRH-I cells are also found to extend rostrally along the midline of the septum. Small clusters of LHRH-I cell bodies populate the ventral lateral edge of the olfactory

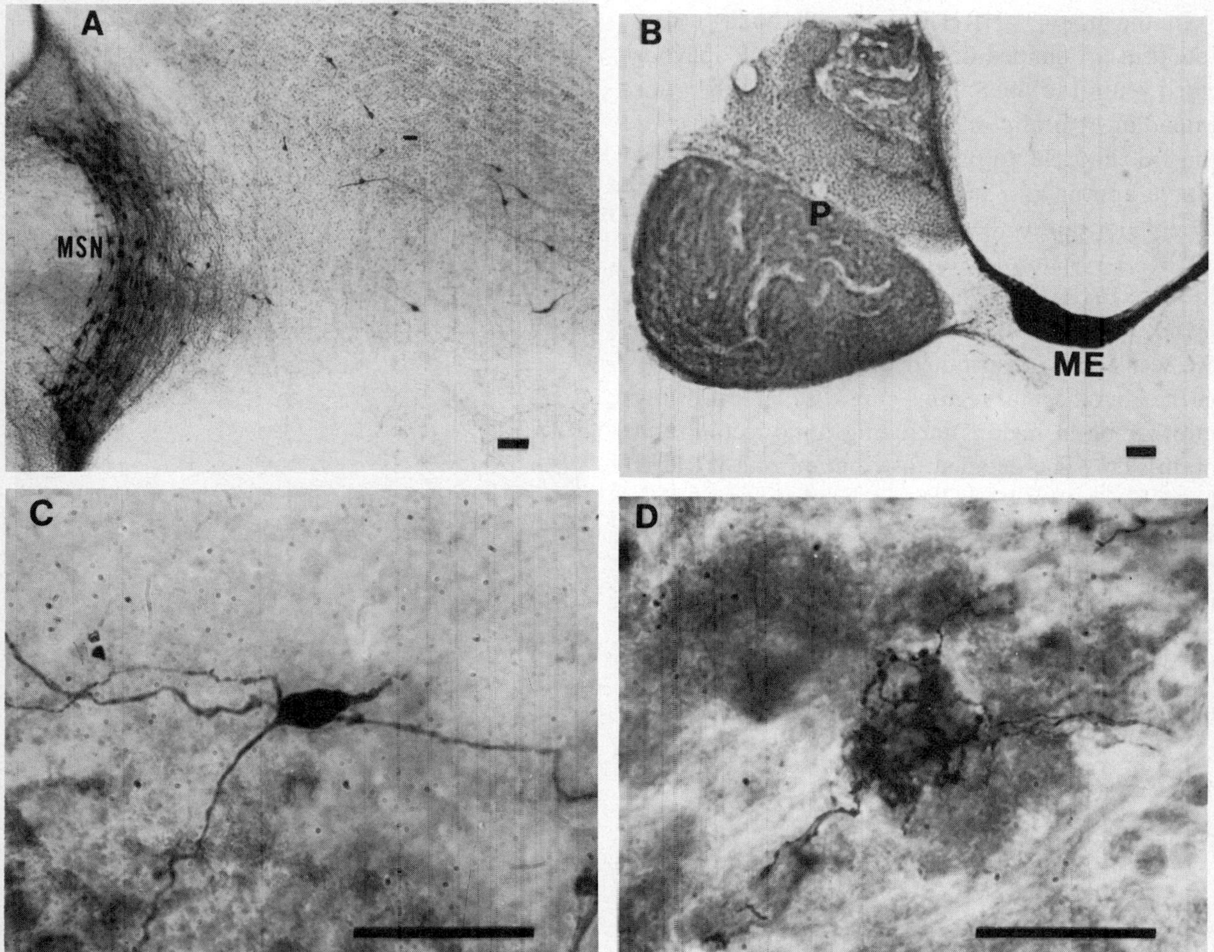

Fig. 5. LHRH-I cells and terminals in frog brain stained with antiserum DB1. (A) Midline parasagittal section showing the median septal region including the median septal nucleus (MSN) and cells along the anterior septal midline. (B) Midline parasagittal section showing dense staining of LHRH-I in median emminence (ME) (P = pituitary). (C) LHRH-I cells stained along the ventrolateral border of the olfactory bulbs. (D) LHRH-I fibers investing an olfactory glomerulus. Bar = 100 μm in (A,B), 50 μm in (C,D).

bulbs (Fig. 5C). The olfactory nerves and selected olfactory glomeruli were heavily invested with LHRH-I fibers and terminals (Fig. 5D).

LHRH-II-containing system

In the 9th and 10th sympathetic ganglia, intensely-stained LHRH-II terminals are seen on C cells (Fig. 6A). Immunocytochemical staining of spinal cord with anti-teleost LHRH serum demonstrates LHRH-II type neurons in the interomediolateral column that are indistinguishable from C type preganglionic neurons labeled by retrograde transport from 7th and 8th rami (Fig. 6B,C).

In the brain, LHRH-II type cell bodies, were found in a v-shaped distribution with the apex located ventral to the Sylvian aqueduct and the arms extending rostrally and dorsally on either side of the 3rd ventricle. In parasagittal section, these perikarya appear as a band extending from the mesencephalon into the caudal diencephalon (Fig. 7A,B). A system of neurons apparently analogous to these LHRH-II cells has been reported in fishes (Münz et al., 1980). LHRH-II fibers and terminals are seen widely distributed through diencephalon, in the lateral septal regions (Fig. 7C), and possibly in other brain regions including optic tectum and brain stem. The detailed distribution of LHRH-II fibers has not yet been defined, partly because antisera HP1, HP3, and HP5 cross-react slightly with mammalian LHRH (i.e. rat median eminence) and weakly stain some LHRH-I type neurons. We presume this is because of the very large amounts of LHRH-I present in these cells, but we can not completely rule out the possibility that the LHRH-I cells may contain small amounts of LHRH-II.

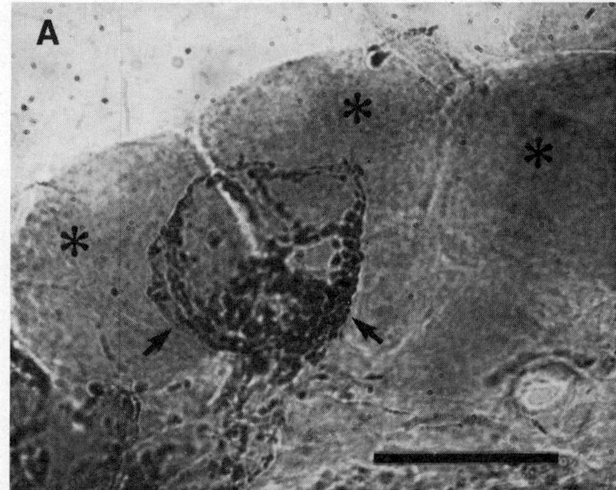

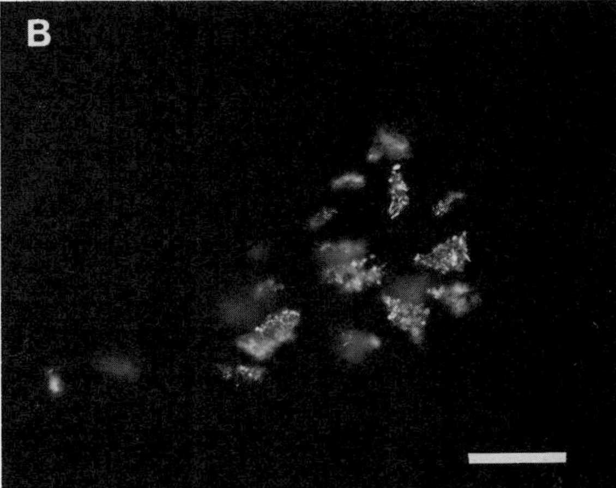

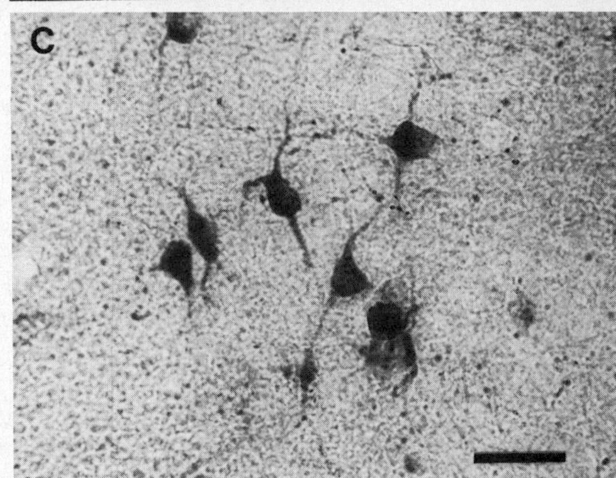

Fig. 6. LHRH-II system in sympathetic ganglion and spinal cord. (A) Staining of terminals surrounding a C cell (arrows) in the 9th ganglion with antiserum HP1. Note the absence of terminals on neighboring B cells (asterisks). (B) Crystals of TMB reaction product in retrogradely labeled C-type preganglionic cells in intermediolateral columns of spinal cord (crossed polarization) (C) Similar section as (B), stained with HP1. Bar = 50 μm.

Discussion

Two types of LHRH-like peptides are found in the frog nervous system. A schematic diagram of the LHRH-containing cell bodies is shown in Fig. 8. LHRH-I is most likely identical to mammalian LHRH, because it resembles mammalian LHRH immunologically and chromatographically and has

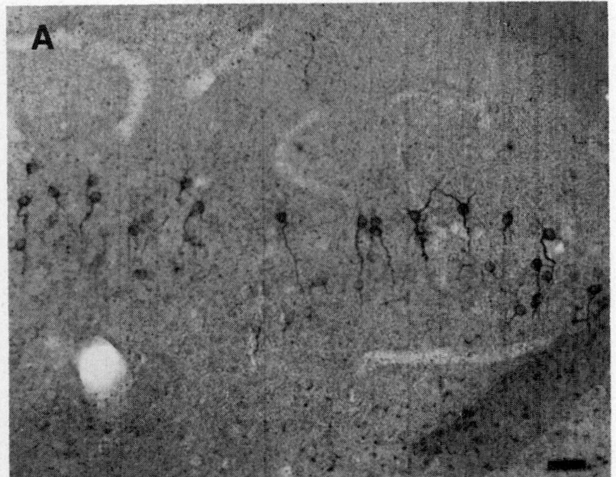

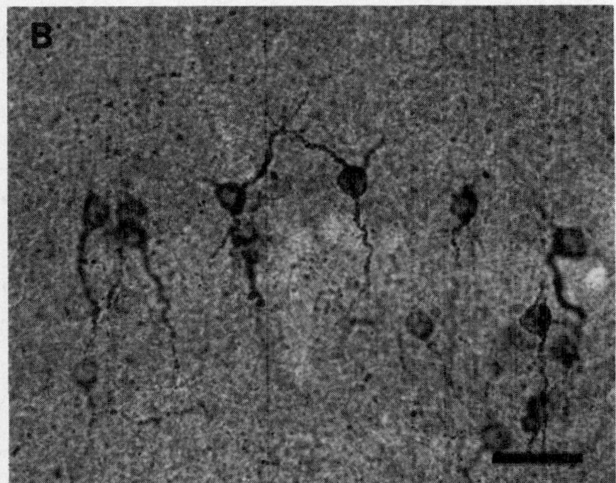

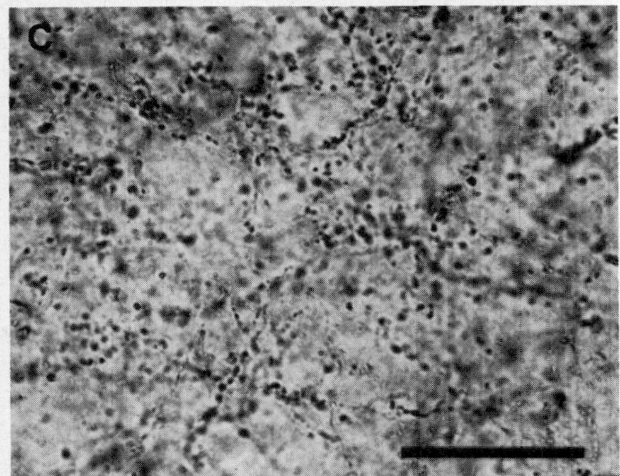

Fig. 7. LHRH-II cells and terminals in frog brain. (A) Parasagittal section stained with HP1, showing a band of LHRH-II cells along the 3rd ventricle. (B) Increased magnification of (A). (C) Example of LHRH-II terminals and fibers distributed in lateral septum stained with serum HP1. Bar = 50 μm.

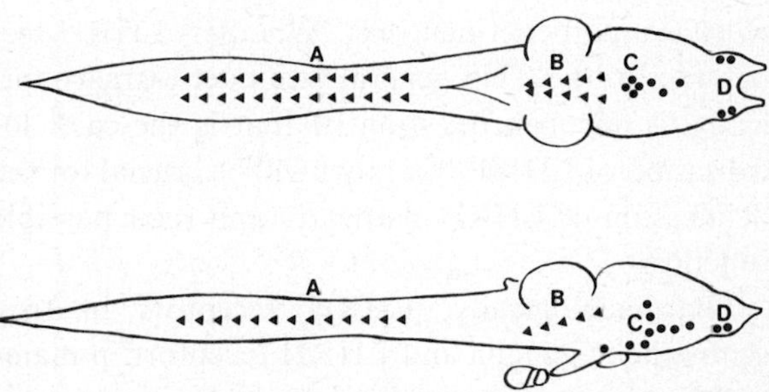

Fig. 8. Schematic diagram of the distribution of LHRH-I and LHRH-II cells in frog brain and spinal cord, Horizontal above, sagittal below. ●, LHRH-I cells; ▲, LHRH-II cells. LHRH-II cells are distributed in intermediolateral columns of spinal cord (A), and in a paired mesencephalic nucleus (B). LHRH-I cells are located primarily in the median septal region (C) and at the ventral-lateral border of the olfactory bulbs (D).

the same amino acid composition. The distribution of LHRH-I in the frog CNS is analogous to that of LHRH in mammalian CNS. The location of LHRH-I-type neurons and their projections strongly suggests that LHRH-I in frog, and LHRH in mammals share the same functions. Thus, LHRH-I is probably the frog-releasing factor.

LHRH-II is distinguishable from mammalian LHRH immunologically and chromatographically. Based on these criteria, LHRH-II is likely to be identical to teleost LHRH, or a group of closely related peptides (Sherwood et al., 1983). LHRH-II is found in the periphery in paravertebral sympathetic ganglia in coexistence with ACh and functions as a neurotransmitter. The preganglionic cell bodies reside in the intermediolateral cell column of the spinal cord. LHRH-II-type cell bodies in brain form a band of cells which extends from the diencephalon to mesencephalon. There is a widely distributed network of LHRH-II-containing varicosities and terminals in the frog brain, consistent with a global function.

As a releasing factor, LHRH is carried by the portal circulation and acts upon targets at a distance. LHRH-II in sympathetic ganglia can also diffuse for tens of microns and induce late slow epsp's extrasynaptically, even though it is found in preganglionic terminals forming classical synapses with sympathetic neurons. Whether LHRH-like peptides in the CNS generally can act extrasynaptically, is an open question. If that is the case, localization of LHRH receptors will be crucial for the delineation of LHRH pathways and their possible functions.

Pharmacologically, LHRH receptors in frog sympathetic ganglia and LHRH receptors in mammalian pituitary show distinct specificities appropriate to their endogenous ligand (Jan et al., 1983; Sherwood et al., 1983). It is possible that more than one type of LHRH receptor is involved in the frog CNS. It would be interesting to find out how various functions are correlated with the different forms of LHRH and receptors.

Evolutionarily, the LHRH-I system probably arose in amphibia from a portion of an early fish LHRH system and assumed functions including that of a releasing factor. The distribution of LHRH in fish CNS corresponds to that of both LHRH-I-type and LHRH-II-type neurons in the frog, while the distribution of LHRH in mammalian CNS lacks the LHRH-II component but corresponds to the LHRH-I-type neurons in the frog (Münz et al., 1980, see Demski, 1984). What happened to those neurons that are LHRH-positive in fish and amphibia but not in mammals? Do they contain a LHRH-like peptide that cross-reacts poorly with antibodies against the known forms of LHRH? Current evidence suggests there is only one gene encoding mammalian LHRH in mammals (Seeburg and Adelman, 1984). We wonder whether there are other genes encoding a LHRH-II-derived peptide or group of peptides in mammals. Analysis of genes encoding LHRH-I and LHRH-II in the frog might lead to the discovery of a mammalian member of the LHRH-II family, and of additional LHRH neurons in mammals analogous to those found in lower vertebrates.

Acknowledgements

We would like to thank Dr. L. Y. Jan for critical reading of the manuscript and Mr. L. Ackerman for helping with the illustrations. This work is supported by Howard Hughes Medical Institute and a grant from National Institutes of Health (NS-15757). D. B. and H. P. are NIH postdoctoral fellows and Y. N. J. is an investigator of Howard Hughes Medical Institute.

References

Alpert, L. C., Brawer, J. R., Jackson, M. D. and Reichlin, S. (1976) Localization of LHRH in neurons in frog brain (Rana pipiens & Rana catesbeiana), *Endocrinology,* 98: 910–921.

Branton, W. D., Jan, L. Y. and Jan, Y. N. (1982) Non-mammalian lutenizing hormone-releasing factor (LRF) in tadpole and frog brain. *Soc. Neurosci. Abstr.,* 8: 14.

Demski, L. S. (1984) The evolution of neuroanatomical substrates of reproductive behavior: sex steroid and LHRH specific pathways including the terminal nerve. *Amer. Zool.,* 24: 809–830.

Eiden, L. E. and R. L. Eskay. (1980) Characterization of LRF-like immunoreactivity in the frog sympathetic ganglia: Nonidentity with LRF decapeptide. *Neuropeptides,* 1: 29.

Eiden, L. E., Loumaye, E., Sherwood, N. and R. L. Eskay. (1982) Two chemically and immunologically distinct forms of lutenizing hormone-releasing hormone are differentially expressed in frog neural tissue. *Peptides,* 3: 323.

Hökfelt, T., Johannson, O., Ljungdahl, A., Lundberg, J. M. and Schultzberg, M. (1980) Peptidergic neurons. *Nature (Lond.),* 284: 515.

Hsu, S. M., Raine, L. and Fanger, H. (1981) Use of avidin-biotin-peroxidase complex (ABC) in immunoperoxidase techniques. *J. Histochem. Cytochem.,* 29: 577.

Jan, L. Y. and Jan, Y. N. (1982) Peptidergic transmission in sympathetic ganglia of the frog. *J. Physiol. (Lond.),* 327: 219.

Jan, Y. N. and Jan, L. Y. (1983) Coexistence and co-release of acetylcholine and the LHRH-like peptide from the same preganglionic fibers in frog sympathetic ganglia. *Fed. Proc.,* 42: 2929.

Jan, Y. N., Jan, L. Y. and Kuffler, S. W. (1979) A peptide as a possible transmitter in sympathetic ganglia of the frog. *Proc. nat. Acad. Sci. USA,* 76: 1501.

Jan, Y. N., Bowers, C. W., Branton, D. B., Evans, L. and Jan, L. Y. (1983) Peptides in neuronal function: studies using frog autonomic ganglia. *Cold Spring Harbor Symp. Quant. Biol.,* 48: 363.

Jones, S. W., Adams, P. R., Brownstein, M. J. and Rivier, J. E. (1984) Teleost luteinizing hormone-releasing hormone: action on bullfrog sympathetic ganglia is consistent with role as neurotransmitter. *J. Neurosci.,* 4: 420–429.

Münz, H., Stumpf, W. E. and Jennes, L. (1980) LHRH systems in the brain of platyfish. *Brain Res.,* 221: 1–13.

Nishi, S. and Koketzu, K. (1968) Early and late after-discharges of amphibian sympathetic ganglion cells. *J. Neurophysiol.*, 31: 109.

Nozaki, M. and Kobayashi, H. (1979) Distribution of LHRH-like substance in the vertebrate brain as revealed by immunohistochemistry. *Arch. Histol. (Jap.)*, 42: 201.

Rivier, J., River, C., Branton, D., Millar, R., Spiess, J. and Vale W. (1981) HPLC purification of ovine CRF, rat extra hypothalamic brain somatostatin and frog brain nRH. In D. H. Rich and E. Gross (Eds.), *Peptides: Synthesis-Structure-Function*, Pierce Chemical Co., Rockford, Ill., pp. 771–776.

Seeburg, P. H. and Adelman, J. P. (1984) Characterization of cDNA for precursor of human luteinizing hormone releasing hormone. *Nature (Lond.)*, 311: 666.

Sherwood, N., Eiden, L., Brownstein, M., Spiess, J., Rivier, J. and Vale, W. (1983) Characterization of a teleost gonadotropin-releasing hormone. *Proc. nat. Acad. Sci. USA*, 80: 2794.

T. Hökfelt, K. Fuxe and B. Pernow (Eds.),
Progress in Brain Research, Vol. 68

CHAPTER 15

Chemical coding of enteric neurons

M. Costa, J. B. Furness and I. L. Gibbins

Departments of Physiology and Anatomy and Histology, and the Centre for Neuroscience, School of Medicine, Flinders University of South Australia, Bedford Park, SA 5042, Australia

Introduction

In the mammalian enteric nervous system there are as many neurons as in the spinal cord, and there are numerous different enteric neurons characterized by the substances they contain, their shapes and their projections. Moreover, there are distinct functional types of neurons, i.e. enteric motor neurons to muscle, interneurons, sensory neurons, vasomotor neurons and secretomotor neurons as well as extrinsic sensory and motor neurons. The discovery of coexistence of chemical messengers in neurons prompted our systematic immunohistochemical investigation of the patterns of coexistence of messengers in enteric neurons. The methods for the simultaneous localization of two antigens, and the problems encountered, are discussed and some of the applications of studies of coexistence of multiple messengers are demonstrated. The results point to the principle that the enteric neurons, and other autonomic neurons, are subdivided into groups with well-defined combinations of chemical messengers (chemical coding), well-defined projections (i.e. origins, terminations, and connections) and well-defined functions. This principle of organization of the enteric nervous system provides an extremely valuable framework in working out its circuitry and assists in identifying the possible roles of the multiple chemical messengers in individual neurons. We propose a re-evaluation of terminology and notation to encompass the realization that every neuron has multiple chemical messengers and that each neuron may transmit multiple messages.

Most gastrointestinal functions, that is, motility with its vast repertoire of behavior, blood flow, and secretion and absorption of water and electrolytes, are known to be controlled or influenced by autonomic nerves. As may be expected, there is an extensive system of neurons devoted to these functions, but, it must come as some surprise to many neuroscientists that these neurons are embedded within the wall of the gastrointestinal tract and that their number is of the same order of magnitude as that of the neurons present in the spinal cord of the same species (Furness and Costa, 1980). These neurons are arranged in two ganglionated plexuses, one, discovered by Meissner (1857), in the submucosa and the other, discovered by Auerbach (1862), between the muscle layers. The enteric nervous system consists of these neurons and nerve fibres of extrinsic origin (sensory, sympathetic and parasympathetic). The general organization of the enteric nervous system has been reviewed in some detail (Gabella, 1976; Llewellyn-Smith et al., 1983; Furness et al., 1986).

In this chapter we will describe observations which lead to the view that there is a precise multiple neurochemical coding of the subpopulations of enteric neurons which form the intricate neuronal circuits that control intestinal functions. Earlier observations obtained with classical neurohistological techniques simply showed that the enteric plexuses were a complicated but seemingly homogeneous network of nerve cells and fibres. With staining by methylene blue, silver, and osmium, the early neurohistologists could not identify the origins and projections of specific populations of enteric neurons (see reviews by Schabadasch, 1930; Stöhr, 1930, 1952; Schofield, 1968). Extending the techniques to their limits, Kuntz interpreted some morphological observations as evidence that there were enteric neurons organized into intrinsic reflex pathways (1953). The presence of distinct shapes of enteric neurons, which was first shown elegantly in whole mount preparations stained with methylene blue by Dogiel (1899), led him to postulate that the differences in morphology represented differences in function. Thus Dogiel suggested that his Type I cells (each with a flattened cell body and numerous flat, short, stubby dendrites and a long, irregular axonal process) were motor, while the Type II cells (each with a smooth cell body and 3 to 10 long smooth branching processes) were sensory. This distinction was not fully accepted and a variety of opposing views continued to be proposed up until recently (see Hill, 1927; Schofield, 1968; Gabella, 1976).

Histochemistry of the enteric nervous system

It is only in the last 20 years, with the advent of specific histochemical techniques, that the complexities of the enteric nervous system have begun to be unravelled. The fluorescence histochemical technique for catecholamines developed by Falck and Hillarp (Falck et al., 1962) allowed Norberg (1964) to identify with certainty the terminal axons of postganglionic sympathetic neurons and thus resolve a long-standing controversy as to the site of action of sympathetic inhibition of intestinal motility (see Furness and Costa, 1974). It was only very recently that enteric cholinergic neurons could be revealed by immunohistochemistry (Furness et al., 1983b).

Since the first report by Hökfelt et al. (1975) of somatostatin (SOM) in enteric nerves, every review on the subject has seen a steady increase in the number of neuropeptides found in intestinal nerves (Schultzberg et al., 1980; Sundler et al., 1980; Furness and Costa, 1980; Costa and Furness, 1982). Despite the difficulties and uncertainties in the identification of the molecular forms of the peptides visualized by immunohistochemical methods (Hökfelt et al., 1980; Walsh, 1981; Furness et al., 1982a; Furness and Costa, 1982b), there is good evidence in intestinal nerves for the presence of cholecystokinin (CCK) 1-8, dynorphin (DYN) 1-8 and 1-17, met and leu-enkephalin, galanin, gastrin-releasing peptide (GRP) 1-27 and a shorter form; neuropeptide Y (NPY), peptide HI (PHI), SOM 1-14, substance K, substance P (SP) and vasoactive intestinal peptide (VIP) (Furness et al., 1986)*. The strong suspicion that serotonin is contained in intestinal nerves (Gershon, 1981) has been confirmed by the immunohistochemical demonstration of a population of enteric neurons with serotonin immunoreactivity (Costa et al., 1982; Griffith and Burnstock, 1983; Legay et al., 1984). The evidence that GABA is present in enteric neurons depends on autoradiographic demonstration of a specific neuronal uptake of radiolabelled GABA (Krantis and Kerr, 1981; Jessen et al., 1983).

A further level of complexity was added to this increasing number of potential transmitter substances found in enteric neurons when the pattern of projections of the different populations of histochemically identified enteric neurons began to be unveiled. Instrumental in this recent advancement in the analysis of the circuitry of the enteric nervous system was the development of two methodologies: immunohistochemistry in whole mount preparations of the different layers of the gut, making possible a full view of large areas of enteric plexuses with the nerve cells and their processes intact (Costa et al., 1980a; Costa and Furness, 1983b); and microsurgical procedures for interrupting the nerve

* In this article, the terminology is simplified so that we will use, for example, VIP containing neurons or VIP neurons instead of neurons with VIP-like immunoreactivity.

TABLE I

Projections of enteric neurons

Guinea-pig small intestine intrinsic projections	SOM	Costa et al., 1980c
		Keast et al., 1984
	SP	Costa et al., 1981
		Keast et al., 1984
	Serotonin	Furness and Costa, 1982a
	VIP	Furness and Costa, 1979
		Costa and Furness, 1983a
		Keast et al., 1984
	NPY	Furness et al., 1983a, 1985
		Keast et al., 1984
	CCK	Keast et al., 1984
	GRP	Costa et al., 1984
	CGRP	Furness et al., 1985
	DYN	Costa et al., 1985b
Guinea-pig caecum intrinsic projections	VIP	Furness et al., 1981
Guinea-pig small intestine projections to coeliac ganglion	VIP	Costa and Furness, 1983a
	GRP	Costa et al., 1984
	CCK	Macrae et al., 1986
	DYN	Macrae et al., 1986
	ENK	Macrae et al., 1986
Rat small intestine projections to coeliac ganglion	GRP	Schultzberg and Dalsgaard, 1983
Guinea-pig large intestine projections to inferior mesenteric ganglion	GRP	Dalsgaard et al., 1983a
	CCK	Dalsgaard et al., 1983a
	VIP	Dalsgaard et al., 1983a
	DYN	Dalsgaard et al., 1983b
Rat small intestine intrinsic projections	GRP	Ekblad et al., 1984
Extrinsic nerves projecting to the intestine	NA in numerous species	see Furness and Costa, 1974
	SP in different species	Costa et al., 1981
		Hayashi et al., 1982
		Lindh et al., 1983
		Sharkey et al., 1984
	NPY	Furness et al., 1983a
	SOM	Costa and Furness, 1984
	CGRP	Gibbins et al., 1985

pathways within the enteric plexuses (Furness and Costa, 1979).

The application of these techniques led to the analysis of pathways and projections of most histochemically identified enteric neurons in the guinea-pig small intestine (Table I). The total number of individual projections defined by a single histochemical marker in the guinea-pig small intestine is now over 50. However, the discovery of coexistence of substances in enteric neurons (see below) shows that the number of neurochemical identified subpopulations of enteric neurons is actually much fewer than this.

Functional types of enteric neurons

As a counterpart to the intricacy of the neuronal network in the enteric nervous system, which is associated with a large variety of histochemically distinct neuronal types, there is also a multiplicity of types of enteric neurons demonstrated by functional studies (Kosterlitz and Lees, 1964; Hirst, 1979; Furness and Costa, 1980; North, 1981). These functionally defined types of neurons are as follows:

Intrinsic motor neurons to the muscle
- excitatory cholinergic
- excitatory non-cholinergic (probably utilizing SP)
- inhibitory apamin-sensitive
- inhibitory apamin-insensitive
  (Niel et al., 1983; Costa et al., 1986)

Intrinsic secretomotor neurons
- cholinergic
- non-cholinergic
  (Cooke, 1984)

Intrinsic vasomotor neurons
- vasodilator neurons of unknown nature

Interneurons in myenteric ganglia
- excitatory cholinergic
- excitatory non-cholinergic
- inhibitory of unknown nature

Interneurons in submucous ganglia
- cholinergic excitatory (Hirst and McKirdy, 1975)
- non-cholinergic excitatory (Surprenant, 1984)
- inhibitory (North and Surprenant, 1985)

Intrinsic sensory neurons

Extrinsic neurons
- sympathetic noradrenergic neurons
  (a) inhibitory to myenteric ganglia
  (b) inhibitory to submucous ganglia
  (c) excitatory to blood vessels
- visceral afferent nerves from dorsal root ganglia

Intestinofugal neurons
- excitatory enteric cholinergic neurons projecting to prevertebral ganglia (Szurszewski, 1976)

From this list it is apparent that there is a functional complexity in the enteric nervous system which matches its neurochemical complexity. If one considers that the enteric nervous system controls a number of coordinated behaviours of the gastrointestinal tract such as propulsion of food by peristalsis, mixing of food by different patterns of motility and the migration of a motor complex in the interdigestive period, it is then easy to predict that more functionally different enteric sensory and interneurons are likely to be present.

The unravelling of the neuronal circuitry and the functional identification of enteric neurons appears, therefore, to be a vital key to the understanding of the working of the enteric nervous system.

Coexistence of messengers in enteric neurons

The finding of coexistence of neuropeptides and amine transmitters in the same neurons in the central and peripheral nervous system by Hökfelt and collaborators (Hökfelt et al., 1980, 1984) has opened a new era in the studies of the neurochemical coding of neurons. In the enteric nervous system the initial observation by Schultzberg et al. (1980) that SOM and CCK coexisted in some submucous neurons prompted us to investigate the extent of coexistence in other enteric neurons.

A multiplicity of strategies was used:

(1) histochemical techniques for localizing two substances in the same cell;
(2) identification of subgroups of enteric neurons by establishing their projections;
(3) identification of subgroups of enteric neurons by specific chemical lesions;
(4) combinations of these techniques, and of physiological investigations.

Double staining techniques

Three main methods are available to study the coexistence of substances in neurons histochemically:

(1) immunohistochemical staining of different antigens in adjacent sections;
(2) sequential immunohistochemical staining of two antigens with chemical elution of the first of the two antibodies;
(3) simultaneous staining of two antigens using two different fluorescent labels.

For the study of coexistence in enteric neurons in whole mount preparations we have used the third technique which is described in greater detail below.

The double staining immunohistochemical technique

This technique is an extension of the indirect immunofluorescence procedure in which a tissue antigen is bound by a first antiserum raised against the antigen. A second antiserum raised against γ-globulins of the same host species as the first antiserum and labelled with a fluorescent tag is used. The second antiserum binds to the first antiserum and thus the tissue antigen is visualized indirectly (Coons, 1954; Sternberger, 1974). The indirect technique is used successfully in many laboratories to visualize single antigens in both sections and whole mount preparations. Discussion of the different procedures for fixation of tissue antigens, and to determine antibody specificity is beyond the scope of this chapter.

We have used successfully for double staining the procedures for fixation and antibody penetration which were developed for single staining of neuronal antigens in whole mount preparations (Costa et al., 1980a; Costa and Furness, 1983b).

Figure 1 shows the principles of double staining fluorescence techniques and Figs. 2–7 show examples of applications to enteric neurons. In the Appendix, tests required to ensure the correct interpretation of the results are summarized.

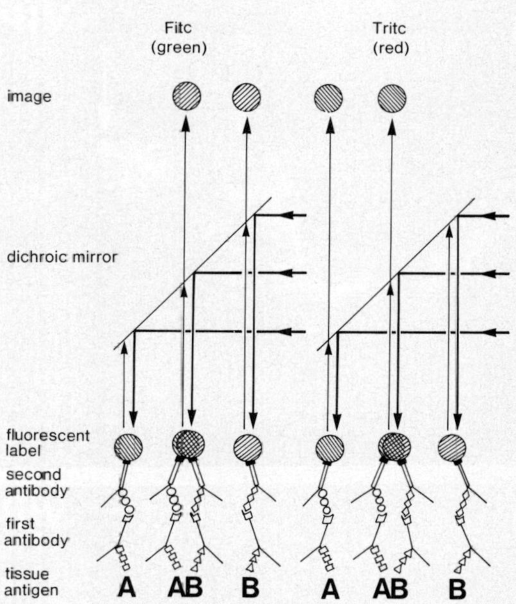

Fig. 1. Diagram summarizing the method for visualizing two antigens in the same preparation (double staining technique). Two antigens (A and B) which coexist in some cells (AB) are visualized by using specific antibodies raised in different species against each of the antigens. The first antibodies bind to their respective antigens. Two second antibodies, each raised in a third species against the γ-globulins of the species in which the first antibody was raised, bind to the respective first antibodies. One of the two second antibodies is labelled with fluorescein isothiocyanate (Fitc), the other with tetramethyl rhodamine isothiocyanate (Tritc). When illuminated via the appropriate dichroic mirror in the filter block (epi-illumination) the fluorophore emits a longer wavelength which is collected by the microscope objective. By changing the filter block, the green light of the Fitc or the red light of the Tritc reaches the observer. Structures with only one of the two antigens will only be seen in one colour. Structures with both antigens will be both red and green.

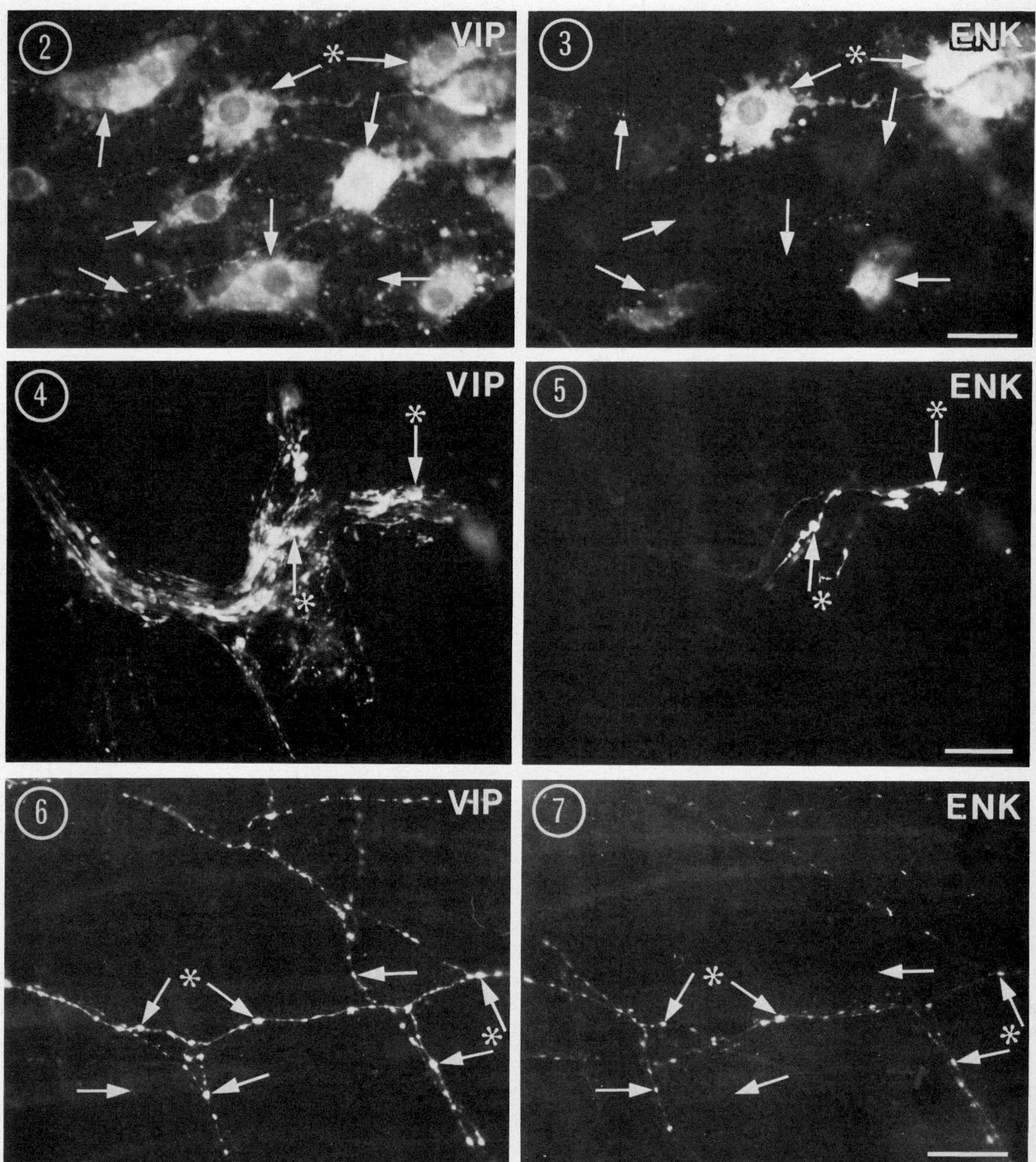

Figs. 2–7. Pairs of microphotographs obtained with the double staining immunofluorescence technique to investigate the coexistence of chemical messengers.

Fluorophores and filters

This technique can only be used at present to visualize two antigens at a time. Appropriate second antibodies with fluorescent labels are available commercially. Fluorescein isothiocyanate (Fitc) is the most common fluorophore used in fluorescence microscopy and two other fluorophores can be used in conjunction with Fitc. These are rhodamine (tetramethylrhodamine isothiocyanate; Tritc) and Texas red. Most fluorescence microscopes with epi-illumination are equipped with facilities for changing the filter blocks, and most manufacturers produce filters suitable for the visualization of each of the fluorophores individually.

Filter systems for double staining must be selective. The emission of one fluorophore most be transmitted, while that of the other fluorophore must be blocked. The problem of selectivity has been discussed in some detail by Haaijman (1983) and can be resolved by a suitable choice of pairs of emission filters. In the Leitz fluorescence microscope system the standard filter blocks do not have a degree of selectivity sufficient to prevent unwanted transmission of fluorescence by the other fluorophores. This problem is particularly acute for the filters for Fitc which also transmit the light emitted by rhodamine.

We have increased the selectivity of the Fitc filters by modifying the Leitz filter block I2 by replacing the emission filter with a band-pass filter BP 515-560 taken from the L2.1 filter block (Furness et al., 1984). In this manner, we could narrow the band of the emission filters to obtain optimal selectivity. There is, however, a lower fluorescent yield which requires longer exposure time for photography (see below). The problem is much less prominent with the filters for viewing rhodamine fluorescence and the standard Leitz filter block N_2 has a sufficient selectivity that no Fitc fluorescence is transmitted. All photographs of double stained preparations shown in this chapter have been obtained with the combination of these two filter blocks. The Nikon company has recently added selective filters to its standard range.

The other fluorophore used in conjunction with Fitc is Texas red. For instance, Lee et al. (1985) have successfully used Fitc and Texas red labelled second antibodies for double staining and have used the Nikon filter systems B and G respectively to achieve very high selectivity.

First antibodies

The two first antibodies must be raised in different species. Most antibodies are raised in rabbits and therefore it is necessary to obtain additional antibodies raised in other species. Because of the range of secondary antibodies available, rats, mice, goats or sheep are suitable hosts. If there is no binding between the first antibodies (see Appendix for tests) sections or whole mounts can be exposed to a mixture of suitable dilutions of the two first antibodies.

Figs. 2 and 3. Whole mount of guinea-pig myenteric plexus incubated in a culture medium with colchicine (10^{-5} M) for 24 h, showing a large number of VIP immunoreactive nerve cell bodies viewed with the filter for Tritc (Fig. 2) and the same field viewed with the filter for Fitc (Fig. 3) showing that some cells (arrows with asterisks) stain for both VIP and ENK, and that many cells only stain for one antigen (arrows). Each arrow is in the same position in corresponding microphotographs.

Fig. 4 and 5. Whole mount preparations of guinea-pig myenteric plexus taken from an animal in which the myenteric plexus was surgically interrupted 2 days before. The photographs show the same field on the oral edge of the lesion. All the swollen fibres with accumulation of ENK immunoreactivity also contain VIP immunoreactivity (arrows point to same structures in both photographs).

Figs. 6 and 7. Whole mount preparation of the myenteric plexus showing the tertiary plexus with fibres with both VIP and ENK immunoreactivity (arrows with asterisks) and fibres with only one antigen (arrows). Magnification bars: Figs. 2, 3, 6 and 7, 30 μm; Figs. 4 and 5, 50 μm.

Second antibodies

The second antisera represent the major cause of unwanted cross-reactivity. These can be tested easily (see Appendix) and only second antibodies free from such cross-reactivities can be used in the double staining. To avoid binding between second antibodies each should be raised, in the same species, against the γ-globulin of the species in which the corresponding first antibody was raised. The two antibodies must be labelled with different fluorophores. Each second antibody must be tested to ensure that it does not recognize the inappropriate first antibody in double staining experiments. In some cases, inappropriate cross-reactivity between first and second antibodies may be restricted to only some first antibodies. For instance, we have found that the rat monoclonal antibody against serotonin (Consolazione et al., 1981; commercially available from Serva) which is excellent in single staining studies, binds to all the anti-rabbit second antibodies we have tested (over 10 brands) even though these anti-rabbit antibodies do not bind to other rat γ-globulins.

Observation of double stained preparations

In many brands of microscopes set up for epi-illumination fluorescence, the filter blocks can be rapidly changed allowing alternative viewing of two fluorophores. In this manner, structures in the tissue, e.g. axon varicosities or nerve cell bodies, can be observed in rapid succession with the two sets of filters. It can be established directly whether some or all the structures which contain one fluorophore also contain the other fluorophore. If there is complete overlapping of staining it may mean that either (1) the two antigens coexist in the same structures; or (2) that there are unwanted cross-reactivities between the two first antibodies or between the second antibodies or between a second antibody and the inappropiate first antibody. It is therefore essential to test for such cross-reactivities (see Appendix). Partial overlap of staining usually indicates that there are no unwanted cross-reactivities of antibodies, and it is likely that where overlap does occur in such preparations there is a true coexistence of the antigens.

There are, however, other potential causes of artefacts in the staining. It is possible that the two first antibodies compete spatially for binding if the two antigens are in very close association. If one of the two antigens is present in greater amounts, or is bound by antibody more effectively, then the other antigen may not be located even though it is present.

Photography

One of the results of increasing the selectivity of filters for the fluorophores by narrowing the emission band, is that the amount of light reaching the eyepieces decreases. In addition, the balance of sensitivity between film and automatic light meters varies with wavelength. We found that, while the red light passing through the Tritc filter to an automatic camera would produce a suitable exposure of a black and white film, the film was underexposed by Fitc fluorescence. This problem can be resolved empirically by changing the automatic camera setting to longer exposure times when photographing Fitc fluorescence.

The use of colchicine to enhance immunoreactivity in nerve cell bodies

Colchicine is widely used by neurohistochemists to enhance the visualization of nerve cell bodies. Usually it is injected into the animal to produce its effect. However, since colchicine is very toxic to the animals, we have experimented with its use in vitro. Incubation of segments of intestine for 24 h in a culture medium containing colchicine (10^{-5}–10^{-4} M) leads to a significant accumulation of immunoreactivity of peptides in enteric neurons. For instance, in the myenteric plexus taken from freshly killed animals not injected with colchicine, the number of VIP immunoreactive nerve cell bodies in the intestine is only about 2% of the total number of myenteric neurons (Costa and Furness, 1983a; Fig. 8). After 24 h in culture with colchicine, the number of VIP immunoreactive cells increases to near half of the total number of myenteric neurons (Costa et al., 1985a; Fig. 10). The newly visualized cells have the shape of Dogiel Type I neurons (Figs. 2 and 10), while the rare VIP cells visible in freshly fixed preparations belong to the Type III of Dogiel (see Furness et al., 1986, for Dogiel's classification of cell shape). When double stained, many of the VIP Dogiel Type I cells also show immunoreactivity for ENK and DYN (Costa et al., 1985b) and indeed Type I cells containing ENK have been described previously (Furness et al., 1983c; Kobayashi et al., 1985). It is important to establish whether this effect of colchicine represents an enhancement of immunoreactivity already present in the cell or whether colchicine induces changes in phenotype. A number of observations suggest that colchicine increases the amount of immunoreactive material that is usually present at a level below detectability.

First, a few days after pathways within the enteric plexuses are interrupted in vivo, we see VIP immunoreactive nerve cell bodies of the type seen after in vitro colchicine treatment (Fig. 9). We know from projection studies of such neurons that

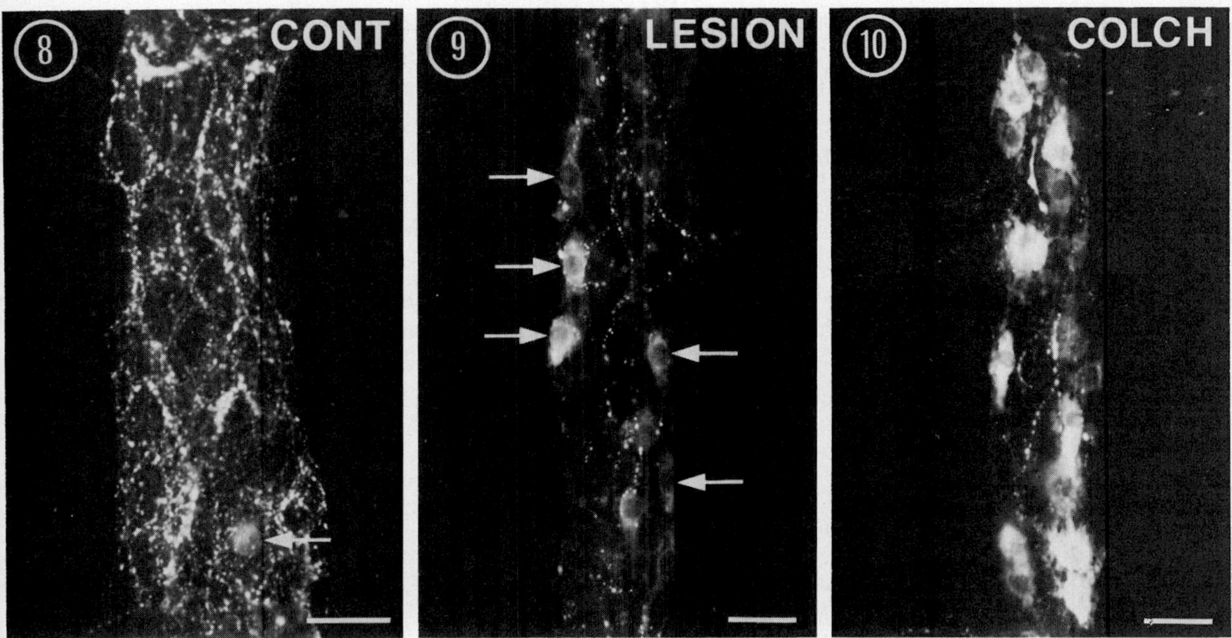

Figs. 8–10. Whole mount preparations of guinea-pig myenteric plexus, stained with VIP antibodies demonstrate the changes in the number of nerve cell bodies visible following an experimental lesion (Fig. 9) or after incubation with colchicine (Fig. 10) compared with a control preparation.

Fig. 8. From untreated control tissue (cont.) shows a large number of varicose nerve fibres within a myenteric ganglion. Only one nerve cell body is visible (arrow).

Fig. 9. A myenteric ganglion on the anal side of a surgical lesion which interrupted the myenteric plexus 5 days earlier; the number of varicose fibres is diminished because they originated from nerve cells located oral to the lesion, and the number of visible nerve cell bodies is increased (arrows).

Fig. 10. A myenteric ganglion following incubation in a culture medium with colchicine for 24 h; note the large number of very intense immunoreactive nerve cell bodies within the ganglion. Magnification bar: 50 μm.

they were not directly damaged by surgery, although their inputs were probably severed. Furthermore, maintaining a segment of intestine in culture medium for a few days without colchicine also results in the appearance of large numbers of VIP immunoreactive nerve cells. Finally, by using more sensitive immunohistochemical techniques such as the avidin-biotin method, these neurons are faintly but visibly stained even in freshly fixed preparations. Consequently, we think that colchicine treatment better defines the extent of a particular population of neurons by bringing to detectable levels peptides present in low concentrations within them.

Analysis of multiple overlap of staining

By using preparations incubated with colchicine, we have begun to study the multiple overlap of immunochemical staining and have found numerous examples of multiple coding of nerve cell bodies in the enteric plexuses with some neurons containing up to five substances in them (Table II; Fig. 29).

Since double staining techniques allow the study of only two substances at a time, the coexistence of multiple chemical messengers can only be deduced from indirect calculations. In the case of complete coexistence of more than two antigens it is easy to conclude that all the nerve cells contain all these substances. Thus in the submucous plexus of the guinea-pig ileum any pairing of antisera against choline acetyltransferase (ChAT), CCK, calcitonin gene-related peptide (CGRP) NPY and SOM shows complete overlap in nerve cell bodies (Furness et al., 1984, 1985). When there is not complete overlap of different immunoreactivities the analysis becomes more complex. For instance, in the submucous ganglia 55% of nerve cells contain ChAT immunoreactivity, but when double stained with antibodies against SP only a small proportion also stain for SP, whereas all SP submucous nerve cells show ChAT immunoreactivity. ChAT/SP cells represent 11% of the total submucous neurons. Similarly, double staining for ChAT and NPY indicates that not all ChAT neurons contain NPY but that all NPY neurons contain ChAT. The proportion of ChAT/NPY neurons is about 28% of the total submucous neurons (these neurons also contain CCK, CGRP and SOM). By adding up the population of ChAT/SP (11%) and the ChAT/CCK/CGRP/NPY/SOM neurons (28%), it follows that there must be a population of ChAT neurons without other markers which represents 55 − (11 + 28) = 16% of the total submucous neurons. With this

TABLE II

Proportions of subpopulations of enteric and sympathetic neurons

Coeliac ganglia	DBH/SOM	21%	Macrae et al., 1986
	DBH/NPY	52%	Macrae et al., 1986
	DBH/-	25%	Macrae et al., 1986
Myenteric ganglia	CCK/DYN/ENK/GRP/VIP	<1%	unpublished results
	ACh/(SP?)	unknown	
	ChAT/CCK/CGRP/NPY/SOM	5%	Furness et al., 1983b, 1985
	DYN/ENK/NPY/VIP	13%	unpublished results
	DYN/GRP/VIP	3%	unpublished results
Submucous ganglia	ChAT/CCK/CGRP/NPY/SOM	28%	Furness et al., 1984, 1985
	ChAT/SP	11%	Furness et al., 1984
	ChAT/-	16%	Furness et al., 1984
	DYN/VIP	45%	Costa et al., 1980b, 1985a

type of analysis it was possible to account for practically all submucous neurons in the guinea-pig ileum (Furness et al., 1984, 1985), and conclude that they fall into four immunochemical types (Table II).

The situation is made more complicated when all the overlaps between several pairs of double stained neurons are incomplete. For instance, in the myenteric plexus of the guinea-pig ileum not all VIP nerve cell bodies stain for ENK and, conversely not all ENK cells stain for VIP. Similarly, not all VIP cells stain for DYN (and vice versa) and not all DYN cells stain for ENK (and vice versa). If the degree of overlap between each pair of antigens is greater than 50% then it is possible to establish a minimum size of the population of cells with all three substances. Our results indicate that at least 30% of myenteric neurons in the guinea-pig small intestine contain all three peptides (i.e. VIP, ENK and DYN); they are Dogiel Type I neurons. Furthermore, there is a sizeable population of Dogiel Type I neurons with ENK and DYN but with no VIP (Costa et al., 1985a). The few VIP nerve cell bodies with Dogiel Type III morphology, referred to above, contain DYN but no ENK. Other large nerve cell bodies were found after colchicine treatment to contain VIP and DYN. Our recent studies show that the subclasses of myenteric neurons classified according to their shapes and to the combinations of peptides they contain are more numerous and varied than previously suspected. It is difficult to establish unequivocally the presence and the size of small populations. Combinations of other approaches are needed in such cases.

Quantitative analysis of dual localization of antigens in nerve fibres and terminals is difficult. When the varicosities of the terminals are crowded within the same nerve bundle it is often hard to establish the precise correspondence of particular varicosities when changing the filter blocks. Furthermore, within the same nerve fibres there may be significant variation of intensity of immunoreactive staining between varicosities. Because of the range of intensities, comparison of photographs taken with the two filters can be misleading since the fainter varicosities may have insufficient contrast to appear on the print. However, where there is incomplete overlap and the fibres are sparse it is possible to identify which nerve fibres contain the two antigens and which contain only one (Figs. 6 and 7).

When there is complete or almost complete overlap of immunoreactivity in double stained preparations, it can be easy to establish the multiple coexistence of peptides in the same nerve fibre terminals. The guinea-pig coeliac and inferior mesenteric ganglia receive nerve fibres from nerve cell bodies located in the enteric plexuses. Single staining experiments show that this projection contains VIP, GRP, CCK, DYN and ENK fibres (Dalsgaard et al., 1983a, b; Costa and Furness, 1983; Costa et al., 1984, 1985b). The double staining technique, using mixtures of antibodies against two of these peptides at a time, demonstrated that the vast majority of these terminals contain all five peptides (Figs. 11–18).

Unravelling the chemical codes and the projections of enteric neurons

The combination of experiments aimed at unravelling the projections of enteric neurons and of experiments aimed at establishing the chemical coding of the neurons has been very fruitful. The two approaches aid each other so that, if a projection of enteric neurons is worked out, then it becomes much easier to find which combination of peptides is present in these neurons. Conversely, if a combination of peptides is found in either nerve terminals or in some cell bodies, it is easier to search for the origin of the fibres or the termination of the cell bodies.

For example, we found, with single staining, that VIP fibres (Costa and Furness, 1983) and ENK fibres (Furness et al., 1983b) both projected in the anal direction within the myenteric plexus of guinea-pig ileum. This could be demonstrated by crushing the myenteric plexus in vivo to allow accumulation of immunoreactive material in the le-

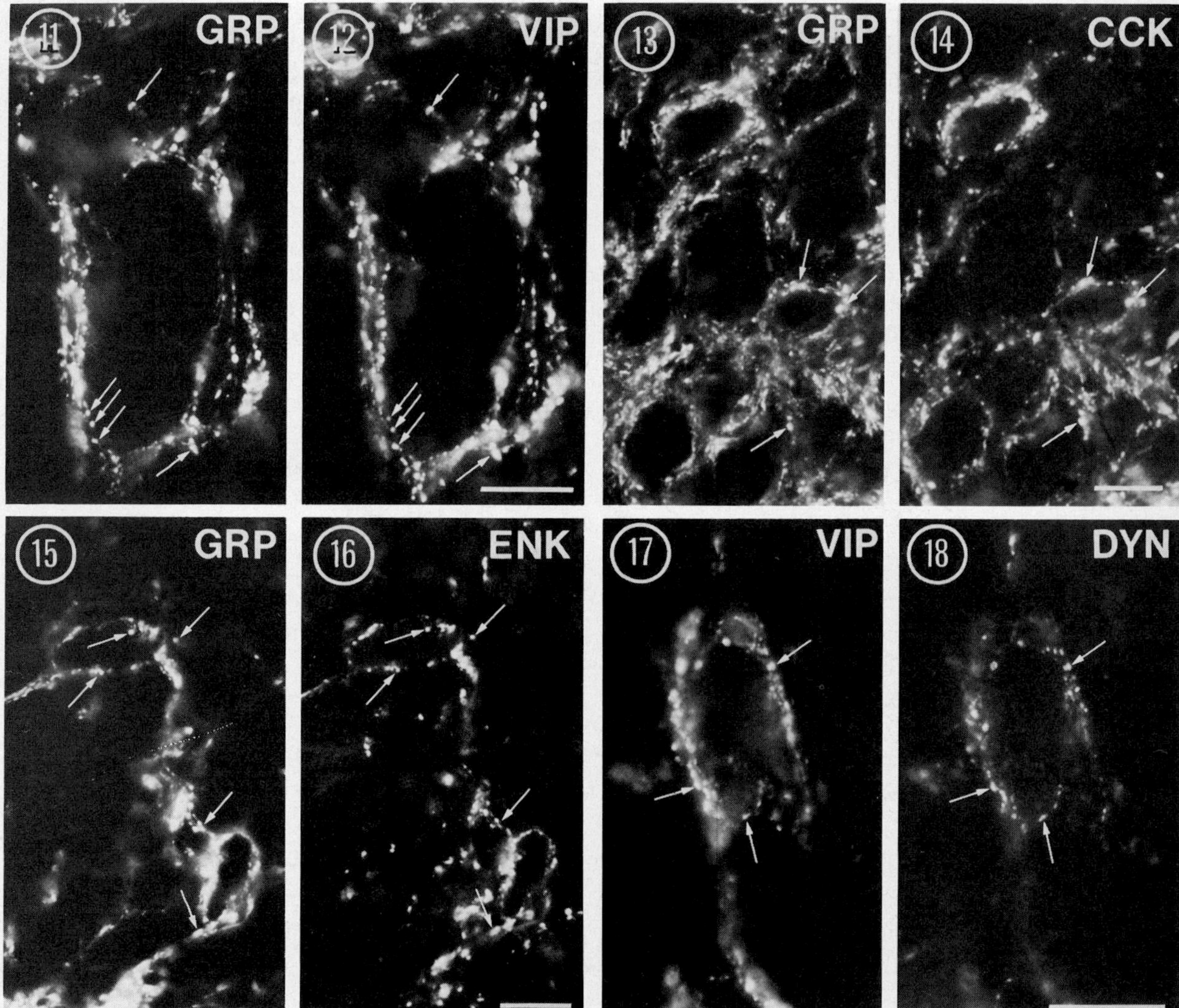

Figs. 11–18. Four pairs of photographs of double stained sections of guinea-pig coeliac ganglion showing fluorescence immunoreactivity for different neuropeptides: Figs. 11 and 12 (GRP and VIP), 13 and 14 (GRP and CCK), 15 and 16 (GRP and ENK), 17 and 18 (VIP and DYN). In each pair, corresponding arrows point to the same varicosities. Despite the difficulty in preparing adequate photographs (see text), the varicosities in each pair coincided and therefore there are fibres containing all these peptides, i.e. CCK, DYN, ENK, GRP and VIP. These fibres, which form pericellular endings around ganglion cells arise from myenteric neurons (see text). Magnification bar: 30 μm.

Figs. 19 and 20. Pair of pictures of the same field with double staining. Arrows with asterisks point to varicosities with both SOM and DBH immunoreactivity; arrows with no asterisk point to perivascular DBH fibres which do not stain for SOM and to a SOM varicosity in the ganglion not stained for DBH.

Figs. 21 and 22. Pair of pictures of the same submucous ganglion taken from an extrinsically denervated segment of intestine showing that all DBH (sympathetic noradrenaline) fibres degenerated while a large number of SOM fibres without DBH remain, indicating their intrinsic origin. Thus there are three populations of nerve fibres: (a) those with DBH/SOM supplying the central part of the submucous ganglia; (b) DBH perivascular fibres of sympathetic origin with no SOM; (c) SOM fibres without DBh of intrinsic origin supplying the submucous ganglia. Magnification bar: 20 μm.

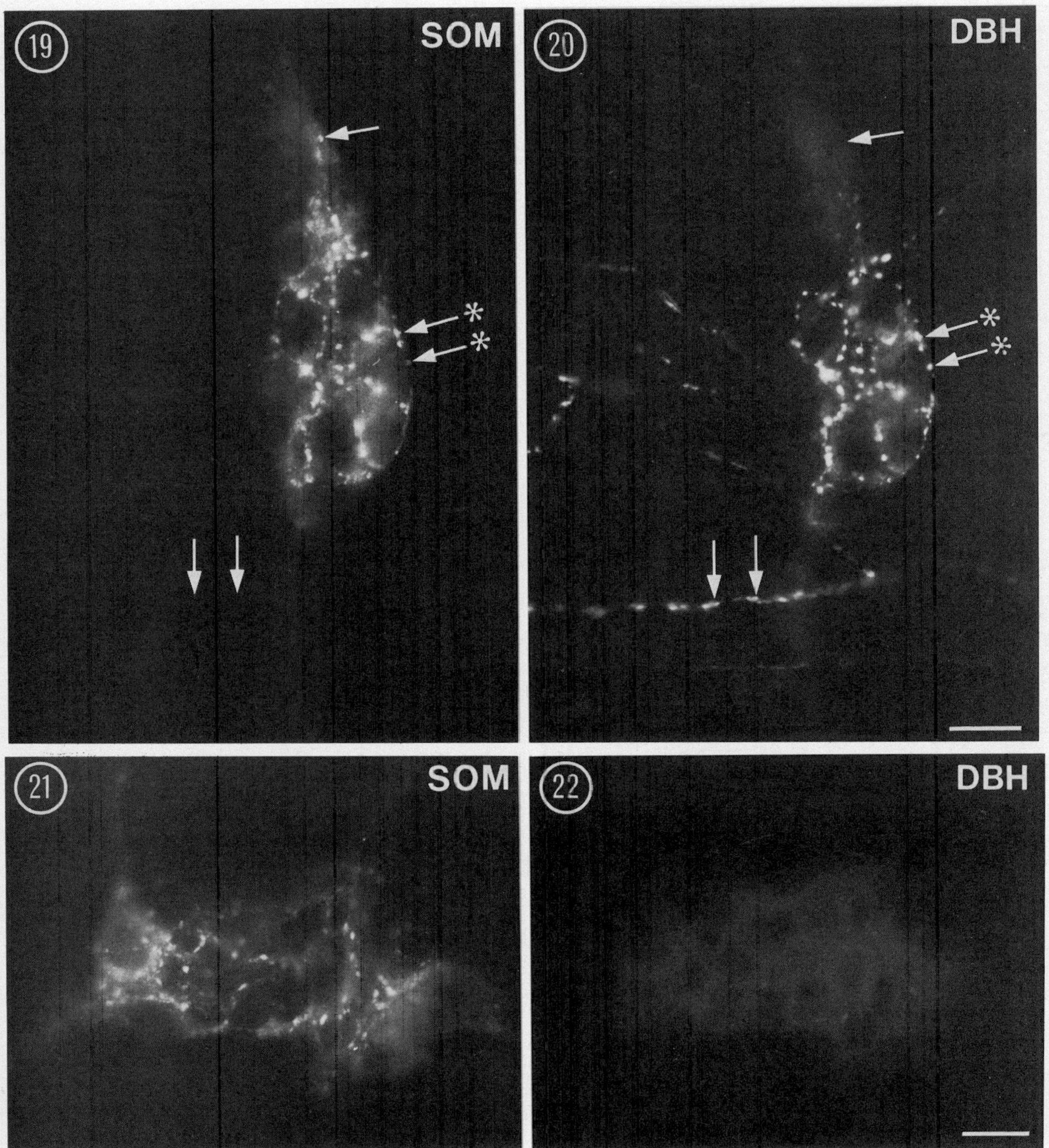

Figs. 19–22. Whole mount preparations of guinea-pig submucous ganglia showing the strategy to unravel the different types of SOM nerve fibres.

sioned axons. Repeating such experiments with the double staining technique for VIP and ENK shows that there are many more VIP fibres than ENK fibres and that all the ENK fibres also contain VIP

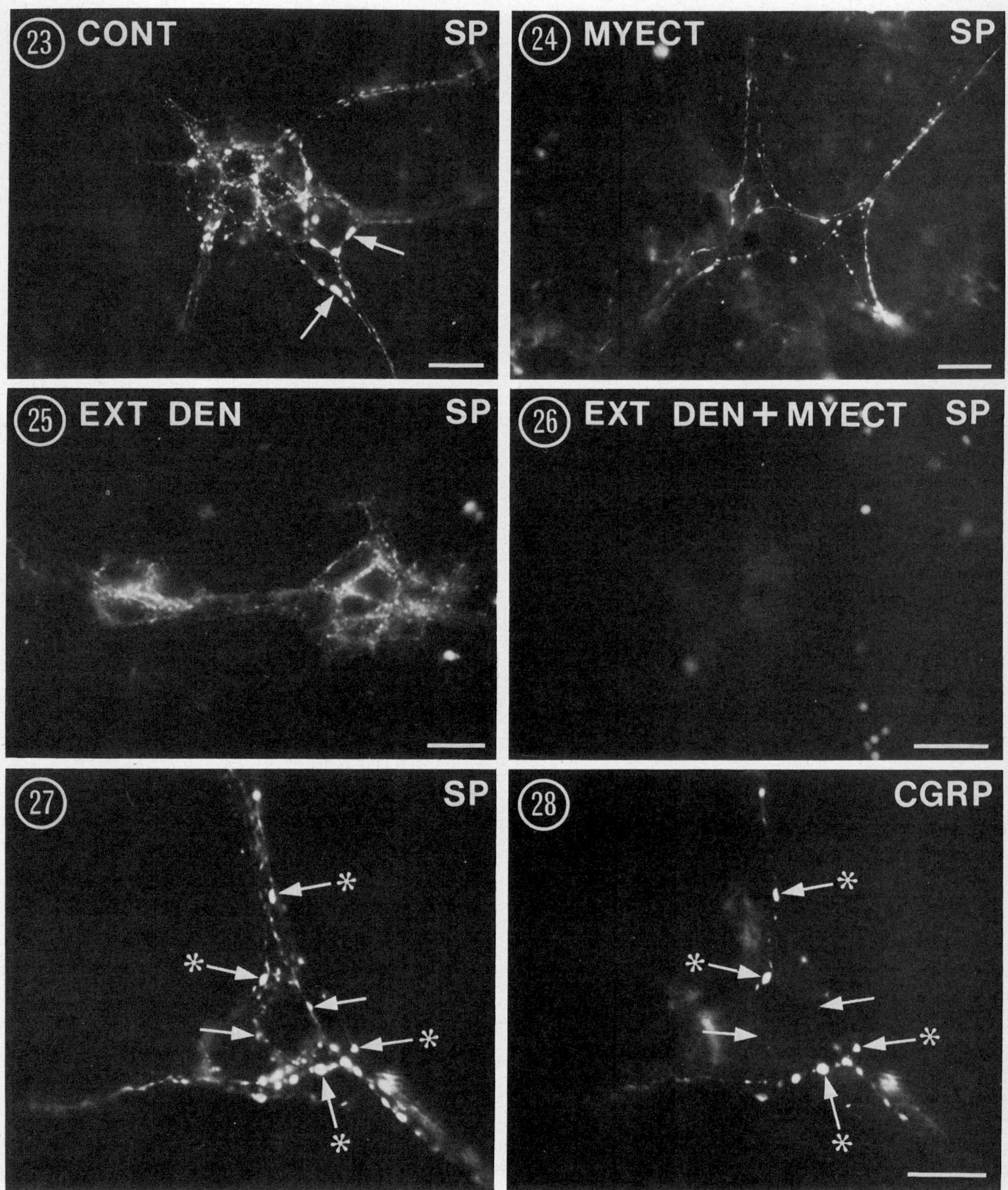

Figs. 23–28. Whole mount preparations of guinea-pig submucosa showing the strategy for establishing the existence of different populations of SP nerve fibres with different origin and chemistry.

(Figs. 4 and 5). Because there are no terminal fibres in the myenteric ganglia which contain both VIP and ENK but such fibres are numerous in the circular muscle it is suggested that the ENK/VIP fibres running anally in the myenteric plexus terminate in the circular muscle. Lesion studies confirm this projection. Furthermore, since the only types of nerve cell bodies in the myenteric ganglia with both ENK and VIP are Dogiel Type I, a fully characterized neuronal population and its projections could be deduced.

Another example of the fruitful combination of lesion and chemical coding studies to disclose a hidden projection is shown in Figs. 19 to 22. Hökfelt et al. (1977) reported that many nerve cell bodies in prevertebral sympathetic ganglia of the guinea-pig have SOM immunoreactivity. The gut is a likely target for such neurons and yet extrinsic denervation of the intestine did not reveal any obvious disappearance of SOM nerve terminals within the enteric plexus (Costa et al., 1980c). By using double staining for SOM and dopamine-β-hydroxylase (DBH) immunoreactivity we discovered that all the DBH fibres in the submucous ganglia, but not elsewhere, showed SOM immunoreactivity (Figs. 19 and 20; Costa and Furness, 1984). Since there are numerous SOM fibres of intrinsic origin in these ganglia even when the extrinsic ones are removed (Figs. 21 and 22), the presence of this population of SOM/DBH fibres, which arise from the coeliac ganglion, could only be distinghuished by its dual chemical coding.

In a study of the projections of SP nerve fibres in the guinea-pig small intestine, the presence of two sets of fibres with different origins in the submucous ganglia was established by lesion experiments (Costa et al., 1981; Figs. 23–26). There are two types of SP varicose fibres in the submucous ganglia, numerous fine varicose fibres and fewer fibres with larger varicosities (Fig. 23). After removal of the overlying myenteric plexus (myectomy) the fine fibres disappeared, leaving the larger ones intact (Fig. 24); following extrinsic denervation the large varicose fibres degenerated while the fine fibres remained intact (Fig. 25). Combining both operations resulted in the disappearance of all SP fibres (Fig. 26). These two sets of SP fibres were also found to be affected differently by capsaicin which depleted only the large varicose fibres of extrinsic origin suggesting that they are the peripheral processes of SP sensory neurons originating in the dorsal root ganglia (Furness et al., 1982b). Demonstration of a different neurochemical nature of these two types of SP fibres supplying the same ganglia came with a double staining study of the overlap of SP and CGRP (Gibbins et al., 1985). Only the large varicose SP fibres in these ganglia also show CGRP immunoreactivity (Figs. 27 and 28).

Fig. 23. Submucous ganglion from control tissue showing the full complement of SP fibres.

Fig. 24. Submucous ganglion underneath an area in which the myenteric plexus had been surgically removed 5 days earlier (myectomy) showing one set of fibres with large varicosities still present.

Fig. 25. Submucous ganglion from an extrinsically denervated segment of intestine showing a different set of finer fibres remaining.

Fig. 26. Submucous ganglion from a segment in which both extrinsic denervation and myectomy had been performed showing that both sets of SP nerve fibres have degenerated.

Figs. 27 and 28. Pair of pictures of the same field of a normal submucous ganglion double stained for SP and CGRP showing that the SP fibres with large varicosities (arrows with asterisks) (Fig. 27), also contain CGRP immunoreactivity (Fig. 28) while there are SP fibres which do not contain CGRP (single arrows). Magnification bars: Figs. 22–26, 30 μm; Figs. 27–28, 20 μm.

Multiple coding of neurons and connectivity

Some of these studies begin to indicate that subpopulations of enteric neurons are characterized by specific combinations of chemical messengers. Indeed, there is a remarkable correlation between this precise chemical coding of neurons and their connectivity. A striking example is the subgrouping of the sympathetic noradrenergic neurons supplying the intestine. In the coeliac ganglion of the guinea-pig there are three main types of noradrenergic neurons marked by the presence of DBH immunoreactivity, i.e. DBH/SOM neurons, DBH/NPY neurons and DBH/- neurons without other known peptides (Lundberg et al., 1982; Macrae et al., 1986). The DBH/SOM neurons, project to the submucous ganglia in the gut, the DBH/NPY neurons supply the blood vessels within the gut wall, and the DBH/- neurons project to myenteric ganglia (Furness et al., 1983a; Costa and Furness, 1984).

This principle of chemical coding of projections permits analysis of connectivity. For example, the nerve terminals of myenteric CCK/DYN/ENK/GRP/VIP neurons which project to prevertebral ganglia end specifically around two of the three main populations of sympathetic neurons, i.e. neurons with DBH/SOM or DBH alone, but not the vasomotor DBH/NPY neurons (Fig. 29).

This principle of organization of autonomic nerves may extend to the peptide-containing visceral and cutaneous sensory neurons in the dorsal root ganglia of guinea-pigs which form subpopulations with combinations of CGRP, CCK, DYN and SP according to their peripheral projections (Gibbins et al., 1985).

Figure 29 summarizes the subgroups of enteric neurons with well-established projections and with a known multiple chemical coding in the guinea-pig small intestine. Table II lists the relative sizes of these subgroups. there are many other chemical messengers in enteric neurons and many more specific projections but the definitive relationships between multiple chemical coding and projections remain to be determined.

Other authors have shown examples of coexistence of two substances in enteric neurons. Legay et al. (1984) showed that some SP neurons in the guinea-pig proximal colon also contained serotonin immunoreactivity. Ekblad et al. (1984) showed that in the mouse, pig and rat small intestine, VIP coexists with PHI and that some enteric neurons contained both VIP and NPY.

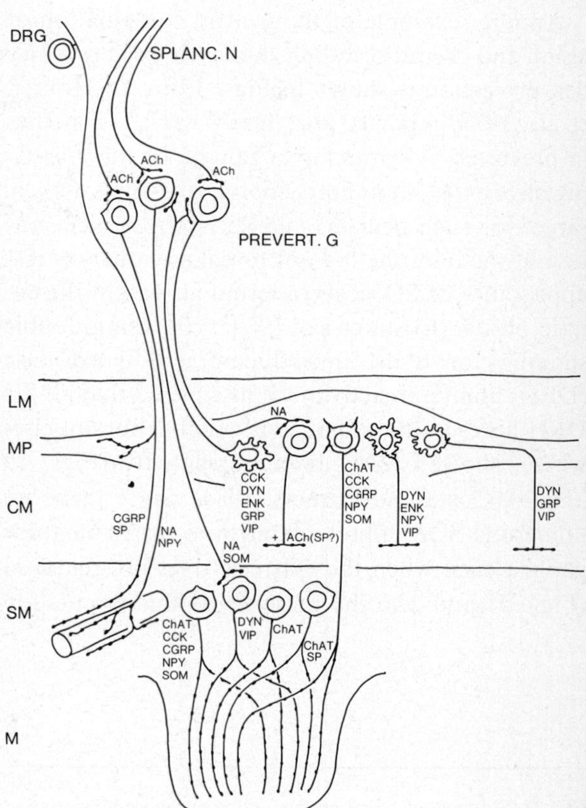

Fig. 29. Diagram showing the populations of enteric neurons and of extrinsic nerves with multiple coding and with established projections. Dorsal root ganglion (DRG); splanchnic nerve (SPLANC N); prevertebral ganglion (PREVERT G); longitudinal muscle (LM); myenteric plexus (MP); circular muscle (CM); submucosa (SM); mucosa (M); oral is on the left, anal on the right. The diagram shows that each group of neurons defined by a given combination of substances also has a specific projection and, conversely, neurons with a given projection have a well defined chemical coding. The possible functions of these populations of neurons are discussed in the text.

Correlation of chemical coding, shapes, and functional characteristics of intestinal neurons

It is now possible to attempt to correlate the histochemically identified populations of intrinsic and extrinsic intestinal neurons which contain multiple chemical messengers (Fig. 29) with the functional types of neurons described earlier in this chapter.

In some cases such correlations were made possible by combining intracellular electrophysiological recording with injections of fluorescent dye and immunohistochemistry (e.g. Bornstein et al., 1984). With this methodology, it was found that most of the ENK neurons, which all have Dogiel Type I shape, receive a fast cholinergic (nicotinic) synaptic input. A similar correlation has been recently reported by Katayama et al. (1985) who recorded fast cholinergic synaptic potentials from Dogiel Type I VIP neurons. We have shown immunohistochemically that there is a significant overlap between these two populations (Costa et al., 1985a). Although neurons with other shapes also may have fast cholinergic synaptic inputs, it is clear that the Dogiel Type II cells do not have fast synaptic potentials; electrophysiologically these neurons are defined as AH (after hyperpolarizing) neurons. Moreover, Dogiel Type II neurons are neurochemically different from Dogiel Type I neurons.

The two groups of neurons which project to the circular muscle and contain DYN and VIP (Fig. 29) are likely to correspond to the two groups of enteric inhibitory neurons which mediate fast, apamin-sensitive inhibitory junction potentials. Functional studies show one group to have a short projection and the other to have a long projection (Bornstein et al., 1985a). It is possible that the same two groups of neurons also mediate the slow apamin-insensitive inhibitory junction potential (Niel et al., 1983). Both these mechanisms of inhibition are effective in relaxing the muscle and are activated by reflex stimulation in the small intestine (Costa et al., 1986).

The chemical coding of the excitatory cholinergic motor neurons to the circular muscle has not been determined yet, but it is interesting that those SP neurons projecting to the muscle also mediate contraction and are also activated during the peristaltic reflex (Costa et al. 1985c; Bartho and Holzer, 1985). It is possible that both acetylcholine (ACh) and SP are released from the same neurons to mediate contraction via two different receptor mechanisms.

Of the histochemical identified populations of myenteric neurons the one that projects to the coeliac ganglion (CCK/DYN/ENK/GRP/VIP neurons) is likely to represent the afferent limb of the peripheral intestino-intestinal inhibitory reflex (Furness and Costa, 1974). If this is the case, these neurons are also cholinergic, since fast synaptic cholinergic (nicotinic) inputs from the intestine have been recorded from sympathetic neurons (Szurszewski, 1976).

The three subgroups of sympathetic postganglionic neurons which supply the intestine (Fig. 29) are likely to mediate different influences on intestinal functions. The noradrenergic fibres supplying the myenteric ganglia are involved in the sympathetic inhibition of intestinal motility, while the perivascular sympathetic nerves control blood flow, and it is likely that the sympathetic fibres to submucous ganglia control the activity of mucosal secretomotor neurons. This last group of nerve terminals, containing DBH and SOM, end around only one of the four classes of submucous neurons, the DYN/VIP neurons (see Table II and Fig. 29). This has a functional correlation; only the DYN/VIP neurons receive inhibitory inputs, at least some of which are noradrenergic (Bornstein et al., 1985b; North and Surprenant, 1985). The four populations of submucous neurons (Table II) all project to the mucosa and are likely to control its activity. There is functional evidence for both cholinergic and non-cholinergic secretomotor neurons (Cooke, 1984; Keast et al., 1985). If it is assumed that the different subgroups of the ChAT-containing neurons all mediate cholinergic responses it is likely that the DYN/VIP neurons mediate the non-cholinergic responses.

The CGRP/SP sensory neurons represent a subset of sensory neurons; they can be activated by excessive distension or irritative stimuli which elicit cardiovascular responses. Their antidromic activation can excite the intestine by stimulating intrinsic excitatory neurons (see Bartho and Holzer, 1985).

Significance and consequences of the coexistence of multiple chemical messengers

The widespread multiplicity of chemical messengers in enteric neurons, and in central neurons (see chapters by T. Hökfelt, L. Swanson and M. Brownstein, this volume), opens the obvious questions as to the roles of these substances in any one neuron. The chemical coding of each population of neurons distinguishes its location, its connections in neuronal circuits, and its functions. It is reasonable to expect that if a group of neurons in the same ganglion is subdivided by the presence or absence of one chemical marker, these two subgroups of neurons will have different projections. Their functions would also be expected to be different. Conversely, the discovery of neurons which have different projections from one source allows us to postulate that these neurons would also have differences in chemical coding. Finally, neurons with different functions in the same target tissue would also be expected to have distinct chemical codes. Even in the absence of any clue about the roles of particular chemical markers the chemical coding of neurons can be used fruitfully to unravel neuronal circuits.

Whether each peptide that contributes to the coding of a neuron mediates a message, i.e. acts as a neuronal transmitter or modulator, is not known yet, but it is interesting that all these peptides have potent actions on many biological tissues. Therefore, if they are released, they would have an effect on the target cells, and should be regarded as neurotransmitters.

The initial findings that peptides coexist with one of the amino acids or amine transmitters led to the development of the concept of cotransmission with a "classical" transmitter such as ACh, noradrenaline (NA), dopamine, serotonin or an amino acid aided by a coexisting peptide (see Burnstock, 1980; Cuello, 1982; Lundberg and Hökfelt, 1983; Hökfelt et al., 1984). There are, however, cases in which the classical transmitter substance may not have the principal role in neurotransmission, for example, in the vas deferens (Sneddon and Westfall, 1984). Furthermore, there are instances where no "classical" transmitter has yet been demonstrated, for example, peptide-containing sensory neurons.

A neuron cannot be defined by the suffix "ergic" (Trendelenberg, 1983) applied to just one of the substances it contains, if it utilizes more than one transmitter. The validity of preserving the terms cholinergic and adrenergic (or noradrenergic, dopaminergic, etc.) needs to be re-evaluated. Even more so, the use of the newly introduced term peptidergic should be seen with great suspicion. Each of these terms provides an incomplete description of a neuron or a synapse. It may be less misleading to simply speak of NA neurons, acetylcholine neurons, VIP neurons, etc., and, if the multiple chemical coding is known, to refer to a cell by listing in alphabetical order all the substances found in it (e.g. myenteric DYN/ENK/NPY/VIP neurons, sympathetic postganglionic NA/NPY neurons, etc.). Furthermore, it is often useful to distinguish neurons as not having an additional known marker, for example, DBH/- neurons referred to in Table II do not contain the other specified markers of DBH neurons, SOM and NPY, referred to in the Table.

It is not possible to attribute to a single substance, be it an amine, an amino acid or a peptide, a specific unique function. Thus the roles of SP in sensory nerves to the gut, in motor neurons to the gut muscle, and in mucosal neurons are likely to be different. No prediction can be made on the combination of chemical markers to be expected. The finding by Lundberg (Lundberg and Hökfelt, 1983) that VIP coexists with ACh in some of the neurons supplying the cat salivary glands led many workers to assume that VIP would always be in some ACh neurons. Yet as shown above, VIP is also found in the non-ACh enteric inhibitory neurons in the gut and VIP is present in enteric submucous neurons which lack ChAT.

The chemical coding of neurons is not rigidly established and there are many examples in which the levels of enzymes and chemical messengers change during development, in different functional states, or in experimentally altered conditions. A good example has been documented by Landis (1983) in sudomotor nerves in rats. These sympathetic neurons at early stages of development have the properties of NA neurons, but, as the animal matures, they acquire the characteristics of ACh/VIP neurons. The work of Sawchenko and Swanson (1985; and chapter in this volume) demonstrates functional variation of the chemical code of neurons. They found that adrenalectomy induced the expression of vasopressin in a subpopulation of CRF containing parvicellular neurons in the hypothalamus. Moreover, when the preganglionic input to the superior cervical ganglion of the rat is severed, the NA neurons show increased levels of SP which is not detectable in ganglia from normal rats (Kessler and Black, 1982). In the guinea-pig intestine, interruption of connections to some enteric neurons leads to an increase in the VIP-immunoreactive material in the nerve cells (Figs. 8 and 9).

It is important for the study of the neuronal functions by pharmacological means to consider that a neuron may release a cocktail of transmitters. These substances may have similar direct actions on effector cells, they may have facilitatory or inhibitory interactions on transmitter release, they may interact at release postjunctional receptors, or they may act on different targets. It is a primary challenge to neuroscientists to establish the extent of the multiple coding in neuronal circuits in different parts of the nervous system in different species.

Acknowledgements

This work was funded by the N.H. and M.R.C. of Australia and the Australian National Heart Foundation. We would like to thank Rae Tyler for typing the manuscript and Sue Graham and Pat Vilimas for helping in the preparation of the manuscript and figures.

Appendix

Procedures for validating double staining

Here we consider the situation in which two antigens (A and B) are to be located. We have available a first antibody raised against A in one species (1st AbA) and a first antibody raised against B in a different species (1st AbB). From the same species we have second antibodies against 1st AbA (designated 2nd AbA) and against 1st AbB (designated 2nd AbB). The procedure to be followed is that illustrated by Fig. 1.

(1) Test selectivity of the filters, i.e. adequacy of the filters to discriminate the two fluorophores:
  (a) stain tissue I which contains antigen A with 1st AbA and with 2nd AbA (Tritc).
  (b) stain another tissue II which contains antigen B with 1st AbB and with 2nd AbB (Fitc).
  (c) with filter block for Tritc, fluorescence should only be seen in tissue I and not in tissue II; with filter block for Fitc, fluorescence should only be seen in tissue II and not in tissue I.
  (d) if the wrong fluorophore is seen with one of the filter blocks, a more discriminating filter must be chosen.

(2) *Question:* Are the second antibodies species specific for the pairs of first antibodies used in double staining? i.e. does 2nd AbA bind to 1st AbB or does 2nd AbB bind to 1st AbA?
Test: Expose one sample of tissue to 1st AbA followed by 2nd AbB and expose another sample of the tissue to 1st AbB followed by 2nd AbA.
Outcome: If no inappropriate binding has occurred no staining should be observed. This test should be made on all pairs of first antibodies being used, since some second antibodies have variable cross-reactivity with different first antibodies raised in inappropriate species, e.g. some anti-rat 2nd Ab recognize some but not all 1st Ab raised in rabbits.

(3) *Question:* do 2nd Ab bind to each other?
Test: Expose one sample of tissue to 1st AbA followed by both 2nd AbA and 2nd AbB. Expose another sample of tissue to 1st AbB followed by both 2nd AbA and 2nd AbB.
Outcome: if in each case only single staining is observed, then 2nd AbA and 2nd AbB do not bind to each other.

(4) *Question:* do 1st Ab bind to each other?
Test: seek a tissue or create a model where only one of the two antigens under consideration is present and apply the double staining technique, using a pair of 2nd antibodies which have passed tests (2) and (3) above.
Outcome: only one fluorophore should be visible if there is no cross binding between the two first antibodies.

(5) Procedure for testing the validity of the double staining method in a new tissue using previously characterized antibodies:
(a) stain one set of new tissues with double staining procedure, i.e. 1st AbA + 1st AbB followed by 2nd AbA + 2nd AbB.
(b) stain another set of new tissues with the mixture of 1st AbA + 1st AbB which had been preincubated by either antigen A or antigen B followed by 2nd AbA + 2nd AbB.

If in test (5a) both fluorophores are visible and in test (5b) only one fluorophore is visible then there are no unwanted cross-reactivities (see Morris et al., 1985).

References

Auerbach, L. (1862) Ueber einen Plexus gangliosus myogastricus. 39er Jahr-Berich u Abh d Schlesischen Gesels f vaterland Cult, 103–104.

Bartho, L. and Holzer, P. (1985) Search for a physiological role of substance P in gastrointestinal motility. *Neuroscience,* 16: 1–32.

Bornstein, J. C., Costa, M., Furness, J. B. and Lees, G. M. (1984) Electrophysiology and enkephalin immunoreactivity of identified myenteric plexus neurones of guinea-pig small intestine. *J. Physiol. (Lond.),* 351: 313–325.

Bornstein, J. C., Costa, M., Furness, J. B. and Lang, R. J. (1985a) Electrophysiological analysis of projections of enteric inhibitory motor neurones in the guinea-pig small intestine. *J. Physiol (Lond.)* (in press).

Bornstein, J. C., Furness, J. B. and Costa, M. (1985b) An electrophysiological analysis of the synaptic input on to neurones immunoreactive for vasoactive intestinal peptide in the submucous plexus of the guinea-pig small intestine. *Proc. Aust. Physiol. Pharmacol. Soc.,* 16: 59P.

Burnstock, G. (1980) Do some nerve cells release more than one transmitter? In A. D. Smith, R. Llinas and P. G. Kostyuk (Eds.), *Commentaries in the Neurosciences,* Pergamon Press, Oxford, pp. 151–160.

Consolazione, A., Milstein, C., Wright, B. and Cuello, A. C. (1981) Immunocytochemical detection of serotonin with monoclonal antibodies. *J. Histochem. Cytochem.,* 29: 1425–1430.

Cooke, H. J. (1984) Influence of enteric cholinergic neurons on mucosal transport in guinea pig ileum. *Amer. J. Physiol.,* 248: G263–G267.

Coons, A. H. (1954) Fluorescent antibody methods. In J. F. Danielli (Ed.), *General Cytochemical Methods,* Academic Press, New York, pp. 399–422.

Costa, M. and Furness, J. B. (1982) Neuronal peptides in the intestine. *Brit. Med. Bull.,* 38: 247–252.

Costa, M. and Furness, J. B. (1983a) The origins, pathways and terminations of neurons with VIP-like immunoreactivity in the guinea-pig small intestine. *Neuroscience,* 8: 665–676.

Costa, M. and Furness, J. B. (1983b) Immunohistochemistry on whole mount preparations. In A. C. Cuello (Ed.), *Immunohistochemistry,* John Wiley & Sons, pp. 373–397.

Costa, M. and Furness, J. B. (1984) Somatostatin is present in a subpopulation of noradrenergic nerve fibres supplying the intestine. *Neuroscience,* 13: 911–920.

Costa, M., Buffa, R., Furness, J. B. and Solcia, E. L. (1980a) Immunohistochemical localization of polypeptides in peripheral autonomic nerves using whole mount preparations. *Histochemistry,* 65: 157–165.

Costa, M., Furness, J. B., Buffa, R. and Said, S. (1980b) Distribution of enteric neurons showing immunoreactivity for vasoactive intestinal polypeptide (VIP) in the guinea-pig intestine. *Neuroscience,* 5: 587–596.

Costa, M., Furness, J. B., Llewellyn-Smith, I. J., Davies, B. and Oliver, J. (1980c) An immunohistochemical study of the projections of somatostatin-containing neurons in the guinea-pig intestine. *Neuroscience,* 5: 841–852.

Costa, M., Furness, J. B., Llewellyn-Smith, I. J. and Cuello, A. C. (1981) Projections of substance P neurons within the guinea-pig small intestine. *Neuroscience,* 6: 411–424.

Costa, M., Furness, J. B., Cuello, A. C., Verhofstad, A. A. J., Steinbusch, H. W. M. and Elde, R. P. (1982) Neurons with 5-hydroxytryptamine-like immunoreactivity in the enteric nervous system: their visualization and reactions to drug treatment. *Neuroscience*, 7: 351–363.

Costa, M., Furness, J. B., Yanaihara, N., Yanaihara, C. and Moody, T. W. (1984) Distribution and projections of neurons with immunoreactivity for both gastrin-releasing peptide and bombesin in the guinea-pig small intestine. *Cell. Tiss. Res.*, 235: 285–293.

Costa, M., Furness, J. B. and Cuello, A. C. (1985a) Separate populations of opioid containing neurons in the guinea-pig intestine. *Neuropeptides*, 5: 445–448.

Costa, M., Furness, J. B., Gibbins, I. L. and Murphy, R. (1985b) Chemical coding and projections of opioid peptide containing neurons in the guinea-pig intestine. *Neurosci. Lett.*, Suppl. 19: S55.

Costa, M., Furness, J. B., Pullin, C. O. and Bornstein, J. (1985c) Substance P enteric neurons mediate non-cholinergic transmission to the circular muscle of the guinea-pig intestine. *Naunyn-Schmiedeberg's Arch. Pharmacol.*, 328: 446–453.

Costa, M., Furness, J. B. and Humphreys, C. M. S. (1986) Apamin distinguishes two types of relaxation mediated by enteric nerves in the guinea-pig gastrointestinal tract. *Naunyn-Schmiedeberg's Arch. Pharmacol.*, 332: 79–88.

Cuello, A. C. (Ed.) (1982) *Co-transmission*, Macmillan, London.

Dalsgaard, C.-J., Vincent, S. R., Hökfelt, T., Christensson, I. and Terenius, L. (1983a) Separate origins for the dynorphin and enkephalin immunoreactive fibres in the inferior mesenteric ganglion of the guinea-pig. *J. comp. Neurol.*, 221: 482–489.

Dalsgaard, C.-J., Hökfelt, T., Schultzberg, M., Lundberg, J. M., Terenius, L., Dockray, G. J. and Goldstein, M. (1983b) Origin of peptide-containing fibers in the inferior mesenteric ganglion of the guinea-pig: immunohistochemical studies with antisera to substance P, enkephalin, vasoactive intestinal polypeptide, cholecystokinin and bombesin. *Neuroscience*, 9: 191–211.

Dogiel, A. S. (1899) Uber den Bau der Ganglien in den Geflechten des Darmes and der Gallenblase des Menschen und der Saugetiere. *Arch. Anat. Physiol. Leipzig, Anat. Abtr.* (Jg. 1899): 130–158.

Ekblad, E., Ekman, R., Håkanson, R. and Sundler, F. (1984) GRP neurones in the rat small intestine issue long anal projections. *Regul. Peptides*, 9: 279–287.

Falck, B., Hillarp, N. A., Thieme, G. and Torp, A. (1962) Fluorescence of catecholamines and related compounds condensed with formaldehyde. *J. Histochem. Cytochem.*, 10: 348–354.

Furness, J. B. and Costa, M. (1974) The adrenergic innervation of the gastrointestinal tract. *Ergeb. Physiol.*, 69: 1–51.

Furness, J. B. and Costa, M. (1979) Projections of intestinal neurons showing immunoreactivity for vasoactive intestinal polypeptide are consistent with these neurons being the enteric inhibitory neurons. *Neurosci. Lett.*, 15: 199–204.

Furness, J. B. and Costa, M. (1980) Types of nerves in the enteric nervous system. *Neuroscience*, 5: 1–20.

Furness, J. B. and Costa, M. (1982a) Neurons with 5-hydroxytryptamine-like immunoreactivity in the enteric nervous system: their projections in the guinea-pig small intestine. *Neuroscience*, 7: 341–349.

Furness, J. B. and Costa, M. (1982b) Identification of gastrointestinal neurotransmitters. *Handbook of Exp. Pharmacol.*, 59: 383–460.

Furness, J. B., Costa, M. and Walsh, J. H. (1981) Evidence for and significance of the projection of VIP neurons from the myenteric plexus to the taenia coli in the guinea-pig. *Gastroenterology*, 80: 1557–1561.

Furness, J. B., Costa, M., Murphy, R., Beardsley, A. M., Oliver, J. R., Llewellyn-Smith, I. J., Eskay, R. L., Shulkes, A. A., Moody, R. W. and Meyer, D. K. (1982a) Detection and characterization of neurotransmitters, particularly peptides, in the gastrointestinal tract. *Scand. J. Gastroenterol.*, 17: 61–70.

Furness, J. B., Papka, R. E., Della, N. G., Costa, M. and Eskay, R. L. (1982b) Substance P-like immunoreactivity in nerves associated with the vascular system of guinea-pigs. *Neuroscience*, 7: 447–459.

Furness, J. B., Costa, M. and Eckstein, F. (1983a) Neurones localized with antibodies against choline acetyltransferase in the enteric nervous system. *Neurosci. Lett.*, 40: 105–109.

Furness, J. B., Costa, M., Emson, P. C., Hakanson, R., Moghimzadeh, E., Sundler, F., Taylor, I. L. and Chance, R. E. (1983b) Distribution, pathways and reactions to drug treatment of nerves with neuropeptide Y- and pancreatic polypeptide-like immunoreactivity in the guinea-pig digestive tract. *Cell Tiss. Res.*, 234: 71–92.

Furness, J. B., Costa, M. and Miller, R. J. (1983c) Distribution and projections of nerves with enkephalin-like immunoreactivity in the guinea-pig small intestine. *Neuroscience*, 8: 653–664.

Furness, J. B., Costa, M. and Keast, J. R. (1984) Choline acetyltransferase- and peptide immunoreactivity of submucous neurons in the small intestine of the guinea-pig. *Cell Tiss. Res.*, 237: 328–336.

Furness, J. B., Costa, M., Gibbins, I. L., Llewellyn-Smith, I. J. and Oliver, J. R. (1985) Neurochemically similar myenteric and submucous neurons directly traced to the mucosa of the small intestine. *Cell Tiss. Res.*, 241: 155–163.

Furness, J. B., Llewellyn-Smith, I. J., Bornstein, J. C. and Costa, M. (1986) Neuronal circuitry in the enteric nervous system. In C. Owman, A. Bjorklund and T. Hökfelt (Eds.), *Handbook of Chemical Neuroanatomy*, Elsevier, Amsterdam (in press).

Gabella, G. (1976) *Structure of the Autonomic Nervous System*, John Wiley & Sons, New York.

Gershon, M. D. (1981) The enteric nervous system. *Ann. Rev. Neurosci.*, 4: 227–272.

Gibbins, I. L., Furness, J. B., Costa, M., MacIntyre, I., Hillyard, C. J. and Girgis, S. (1985) Co-localization of calcitonin gene related peptide-like immunoreactivity with substance P in cutaneous, vascular and visceral sensory neurons of guinea-pigs. *Neurosci. Lett.*, 57: 125–130.

Griffith, S. G. and Burnstock, G. (1983) Serotoninergic neurons in human fetal intestine: An immunohistochemical study. *Gastroenterology*, 85: 929–937.

Haaijman, J. J. (1983) Labelling of proteins with fluorescent dyes: quantitative aspects of immunofluorescence microscopy. In A. C. Cuello (Ed.), *Immunohistochemistry*, John Wiley & Sons, pp. 47–85.

Hayashi, H., Ohsumi, K., Ueda, N., Fujiwara, M. and Mizuno, N. (1982) Effect of spinal ganglionectomy on substance P-like immunoreactivity in the gastroduodenal tract of cats. *Brain Res.*, 232: 227–230.

Hill, C. J. (1927) A contribution to our knowledge of the enteric plexuses. *Phil. Trans. roy. Soc. Lond. Ser. B*, 215: 355–387.

Hirst, G. D. S. (1979) Mechanisms of peristalsis. *Brit. Med. Bull.*, 35: 263–268.

Hirst, G. D. S. and McKirdy, H. C. (1975) Synaptic potentials recorded from neurones of the submucous plexus of guinea-pig small intestine. *J. Physiol. (Lond.)*, 249: 369–385.

Hökfelt, T., Johansson, O., Efendic, S., Luft, A. and Arimura, A. (1975) Are there somatostatin containing nerves in the rat gut? Immunohistochemical evidence for a new type of peripheral nerve. *Experientia*, 31: 852–854.

Hökfelt, T., Elfvin, L.-G., Elde, R., Schultzberg, M., Goldstein, M. and Luft, R. (1977) Occurrence of somatostatin-like immunoreactivity in some peripheral sympathetic noradrenergic neurons. *Proc. nat. Acad. Sci. USA*, 74: 3587–3591.

Hökfelt, T., Johansson, O., Ljungdahl, A., Lundberg, J. M. and Schultzberg, M. (1980) Peptidergic neurons. *Nature (Lond.)*, 284: 515–521.

Hökfelt, T., Johansson, O. and Goldstein, MM. (1984) Chemical anatomy of the brain. *Science*, 225: 1326–1334.

Jessen, K. R., Hills, J. M., Dennison, M. E. and Mirsky, R. (1983) γ-Aminobutyrate as an autonomic neurotransmitter: Release and uptake of ^{3}H γ-aminobutyrate in guinea pig large intestine and cultured enteric neurons using physiological methods and electron microscopic autoradiography. *Neuroscience*, 10: 1427–1442.

Katayama, Y., Lees, G. M. and Pearson, G. T. (1985) Electrophysiological and morphological characteristics of vasoactive intestinal peptide (VIP)-immunoreactive neurones in the guinea-pig myenteric plexus. *J. Physiol. (Lond.)* (in press).

Keast, J. R., Furness, J. B. and Costa, M. (1984) The origins of peptide and norepinephrine nerves in the mucosa of the guinea-pig small intestine. *Gastroenterology*, 86: 637–644.

Keast, J. R., Furness, J. B. and Costa, M. (1985) Investigations of nerve populations influencing ion transport that can be stimulated electrically, by serotonin, and by a nicotinic agonist. *Naunyn-Schmiedeberg's Arch. Pharmacol.* (in press).

Kessler, J. A. and Black, I. B. (1982) Regulation of substance P in adult rat sympathetic ganglia. *Brain Res.*, 234: 182–187.

Kobayashi, S., Suzuki, M. and Yanaihara, N. (1985) Enkephalin neurons in the guinea pig proximal colon: An immunocytochemical study using an antiserum to methionine-enkephalin-Arg^{6}-Gly^{7}-Leu^{8}. *Arch. Histol. Jap.*, 48: 27–44.

Kosterlitz, H. W. and Lees, G. M. (1964) Pharmacological analysis of intrinsic intestinal reflexes. *Pharmacol. Rev.*, 16: 301–339.

Krantis, A. and Kerr, D. I. B. (1981) Autoradiographic localization of ^{3}H-gamma aminobutyric acid in the myenteric plexus of the guinea-pig small intestine. *Neurosci. Lett.*, 23: 263–268.

Kuntz, A. (1953) *The Autonomic Nervous System*, Lea & Febiger, Philadelphia.

Landis, S. C. (1983) Development of cholinergic sympathetic neurons: evidence for transmitter activity in vivo. *Fed. Proc.*, 42: 1633–1638.

Lee, Y., Takami, K., Kawai, Y., Girgis, S., Hillyard, C. J., MacIntyre, I., Emson, P. C. and Tohyama, M. (1985) Distribution of calcitonin gene-related peptide in the rat peripheral nervous system with reference to its coexistence with substance P. *Neuroscience*, 15: 1227–1237.

Legay, C., Saffrey, M. J. and Burnstock, G. (1984) Co-existence of immunoreactive substance P and serotonin in neurons of the gut. *Brain Res.*, 302: 379–382.

Lindh, B., Dalsgaard, C.-J., Elfvin, L.-G., Hökfelt, T. and Cuello, A. C. (1983) Evidence of substance P immunoreactive neurons in dorsal root ganglia and vagal ganglia projecting to the guinea pig pylorus. *Brain Res.*, 269: 365–369.

Llewellyn-Smith, I. J., Furness, J. B., Wilson, A. J. and Costa, M. (1983) Organization and fine structure of enteric ganglia. In L.-G. Elfvin (Ed.), *Autonomic Ganglia*, John Wiley & Sons, pp. 145–182.

Lundberg, J. M. and Hökfelt, T. (1983) Co-existence of peptides and classical neurotransmitters. *Trends Neurosci.*, 6: 325–383.

Lundberg, J. M., Hökfelt, T., Ånggard, A., Terenius, L., Elde, R., Markey, K., Goldstein, M. and Kimmel, J. (1982) Organizational principles in the peripheral sympathetic nervous system: Subdivision by coexisting peptides (somatostatin-, avian pancreatic polypeptide-, and vasoactive intestinal polypeptide-like immunoreactive materials). *Proc. nat. Acad. Sci. USA*, 79: 1303–1307.

Macrae, I. M., Furness, J. B. and Costa, M. (1986) Distribution of subgroups of noradrenaline neurons in the coeliac ganglion of the guinea-pig. *Cell Tiss. Res.* (in press).

Meissner, G. (1857) Uber die Nerven der Darmwand. *Z. Ration. Med.*, 8: 364–366.

Morris, J. L., Gibbins, I. L., Furness, J. B., Costa, M. and Murphy, R. (1985) Co-localization of NPY, VIP and dynorphin in non-noradrenergic axons of the guinea-pig uterine artery. *Neurosci. Lett.*, 62: 31–37.

Niel, J. P., Bywater, R. A. R. and Taylor, G. S. (1983) Apamin--resistant poststimulus hyperpolarization in the circular muscle of the guinea-pig ileum. *J. Autonom. Nerv. Syst.*, 9: 565–569.

Norberg, K.-A. (1964) Adrenergic innervation of the intestinal wall studied by fluorescence microscopy. *Int. J. Neuropharmacol.*, 3: 379–382.

North, R. A. (1982) Electrophysiology of the enteric neurons. In G. Bertaccini (Ed.), *Mediators and Drugs in Gastrointestin-*

al Motility I, Springer, Verlag, Berlin, pp. 145–179.

North, R. A. and Surprenant, A. (1985) Inhibitory synaptic potentials resulting from α_2-adrenoceptor activation in guinea-pig submucous plexus neurones. *J. Physiol. (Lond.),* 358: 17–33.

Sawchenko, P. E. and Swanson, L. W. (1985) Localization, colocalization, and plasticity of corticotropin-releasing factor immunoreactivity in rat brain. *Fed. Proc.,* 44: 221–227.

Schabadasch, A. (1930) Intramurale Nervengeflechte des Darmrohrs. *Z. Zellforsch.,* 10: 320–385.

Schofield, G. C. (1968) Anatomy of muscular and neural tissues in the alimentary canal. In *Handbook of Physiology: Alimentary Canal,* American Physiol. Soc., Washington D.C., pp. 1579–1627.

Schultzberg, M. and Dalsgaard, C.-J. (1983) Enteric origin of bombesin immunoreactive fibres in the rat coeliac-superior mesenteric ganglion. *Brain Res.,* 269: 190–195.

Schultzberg, M., Hökfelt, T., Nilsson, G., Terenius, L., Rehfeld, J. F., Brown, M., Elde, R., Goldstein, M. and Said, S. (1980) Distribution of peptide and catecholamine neurons in the gastrointestinal tract of rat and guinea-pig: immunohistochemical studies with antisera to substance P, VIP, enkephalin, somatostatin, gastrin, neurotensin and dopamine-β-hydroxylase. *Neuroscience,* 5: 689–744.

Sharkey, K. A., Williams, R. G. and Dockray, G. J. (1984) Sensory substance P innervation of the stomach and pancreas. *Gastroenterology,* 87: 914–921.

Snedden, P. and Westfall, D. P. (1984) Pharmacological evidence that adenosine triphosphate and noradrenaline are cotransmitters in the guinea-pig vas deferens. *J. Physiol. (Lond.),* 347: 561–580.

Sternberger, L. A. (1974) *Immunocytochemistry,* Prentice-Hall, Englewood Cliffs, New Jersey.

Stöhr, P. (1930) Mikroskopische Studien zur Innervation des Magen-Darmkanales. *Z. Zellforsch. Mikroskop. Anat.,* 12: 66–154.

Stöhr, P. (1952) Zusammenfassende Ergebnisse uber die mikroskopiche Innervation des Magen-Darmkanals. *Ergebn. Anat. Entwick.,* 34: 250–401.

Sundler, F., Håkanson, R. and Leander, S. (1980) Peptidergic nervous systems in the gut. *Clin. Gastroenterol.,* 9: 517–543.

Surprenant, A. (1984) Slow excitatory synaptic potentials recorded from neurones of guinea-pig submucous plexus. *J. Physiol. (Lond.),* 351: 343–361.

Szurszewski, J. H. (1976) Towards a new view of prevertebral ganglion. In F. P. Brooks and P. W. Evers (Eds.), *Nerves and the Gut,* C. B. Black, Thorofore, N.J., pp. 244–260.

Trendelenberg, U. (1983) A plea for a uniform terminology for words ending with ergic. *Trends Pharmacol.,* 4: 49–50.

Walsh, J. H. (1981) Endocrine cells of the digestive system. In L. R. Johnson (Ed.), *Physiology of the Gastrointestinal Tract,* Raven Press, New York, pp. 59–144.

T. Hökfelt, K. Fuxe and B. Pernow (Eds.),
Progress in Brain Research, Vol. 68

CHAPTER 16

Multiple co-existence of peptides and classical transmitters in peripheral autonomic and sensory neurons—functional and pharmacological implications

Jan M. Lundberg[1] and Tomas Hökfelt[2]

Department of [1]Pharmacology and [2]Histology, Karolinska Institutet, S-104 01 Stockholm, Sweden

Introduction

Several biologically active polypeptides are present in autonomic motor and sensory neurons (see Lundberg and Hökfelt, 1983). Thus, the classical noradrenergic and cholinergic transmitter systems in the periphery seem to be subdivided into different populations of neurons on the basis of co-existence of specific peptides with noradrenaline (NA) or acetylcholine (ACh). Therefore, a concept of multiple synaptic messengers is emerging where the peptides can act together with and/or interact with the classical transmitters at the pre- and/or postsynaptic levels. Furthermore, autonomic transmission seems to be characterized by a frequency-dependent, chemical coding of multiple signals. Several pharmacological agents, which have been assumed to interfere specifically with classical transmitters, also influence peptide mechanisms, indicating that the interpretation of drug effects both in pharmacological experiments as well as in patient therapy should include aspects on co-existing peptides. In this chapter we will focus on some recent advances in studies on the co-existence of peptides with ACh and NA in certain autonomic nerves as well as on the occurrence of multiple peptides in sensory nerves.

Noradrenaline — NPY in sympathetic neurons

Noradrenaline has for long been known to be the primary transmitter of peripheral sympathetic neurons (von Euler, 1946) with minor exceptions, e.g. the sympathetic innervation of sweat glands, which is cholinergic. Immunohistochemical evidence has suggested that a member of the pancreatic polypeptide family, avian pancreatic polypeptide (APP) has a wide-spread neuronal localization in mammals. In fact, it could be established that APP-like immunoreactivity was present in a population of NA-containing, sympathetic ganglion cells (Lundberg et al., 1980). However, it could subsequently be shown that a structurally similar peptide with 36 amino-acid residues, neuropeptide Y (NPY) discovered by Tatemoto and Mutt (Tatemoto, 1982), was the endogenous peptide which is present in sympathetic neurons (Figs. 1A–C, 2A–D, and 3A) and with which the APP antiserum cross-reacts (Lundberg et al., 1982d,e; 1983c; 1984i). Only a proportion of sympathetic NA nerves seems to contain the NPY-like peptide and these neurons innervate target organs such as blood vessels, the muscle of the heart, spleen and vas deferens. Other populations of sympathetic neurons projecting to, for instance, exocrine elements in certain salivary glands or brown fat cells do not contain NPY, suggesting a chemical heterogeneity and a morphological basis for a functional differentiation of the sympathetic nerves (Fig. 1C,D). Thus, it may be of relevance to induce a sympathetic exocrine secretory response and lipolysis without a concomitant activation of vascular nerves and a reduction in blood flow. Furthermore, there are examples of considerably fewer NPY-immunoreactive (-IR) nerves than NA nerves on the venous side of the vascular tree. Examples are cerebral venules and venous sinusoids of the nasal mucosa (Fig. 1A,B). This indicates heterogeneity of sympathetic vascular nerves and possibly a separate control of blood flow (arterial nerves) and blood volume (venous nerves) (see Lundberg et al., 1982d). In the following we would like to summarize some of the recent findings in this research area, outlining where and how NPY and NA interact and cooperate in the sympathetic functional response.

Localization and storage

The presence of NPY-like immunoreactivity (-LI) in nerves has been established with immunohistochemical techniques both in sympathetic ganglia (Figs. 2A,B and 3) and in perivascular nerves in all investigated organs including brain, salivary glands, respiratory tract, intestine, urogenital tract, heart, spleen, skeletal muscle and skin (Figs. 1 and 2) as well as around non-vascular muscle cells in the myocardium of the heart, spleen and in vas deferens (see Lundberg et al., 1982e, 1983c, 1984i, 1985a; Edvinsson et al., 1983; Ekblad et al., 1984). NPY immunoreactivity (-IR) is closely related to the distribution of markers for NA neurons such as the catecholamine-synthesizing enzymes dopamine-β-hydroxylase (DBH) or tyrosine hydroxylase both in ganglion cells and in terminals. Co-existence of these enzymes with the NPY can directly be demonstrated in the same neuronal cell bodies of the ganglia. Additional evidence for co-existence of NPY and NA in the nerve endings are the pharmacological findings of (1) A concomitant disappearance of DBH- (or TH-) and NPY-LI after treatment with the neurotoxin 6-hydroxydopamine (6-OH-DA) (Lundberg et al., 1982e, 1985e); (2) a depletion of both NA and NPY-LI after reserpine (Lundberg et al., 1984h, 1985e) and (3) an inhibition of nerve stimulation-evoked release of NPY by the adrenergic neuron-blocking agent guanethidine (Lundberg et al., 1984a).

At the subcellular level, electron microscopic and fractionation studies from, for instance, the spleen and vas deferens have provided evidence that NA is stored in two types of organelles; small dense-cored vesicles (40–50 nm) and large dense-cored vesicles (80–90 nm) (see Fried, 1980). NPY, however, seems to be exclusively localized to the large dense-cored vesicles both in the cat spleen and rat vas deferens (Fried et al., 1985a,b). Being a peptide, NPY is after release most likely resupplied to nerve endings only by axonal transport after synthesis in the cell-body region (Fried et al., 1985a; Lundberg et al., 1985e). This characteristic property probably limits the amount of NPY being available for release compared to NA, which can be efficiently synthesized locally in the nerve endings. In accordance, the tissue content of NPY is several hundred times lower on a molar basis, as compared to NA. In the spleen, however, which has a higher proportion of large dense-cored vesicles in the sympathetic nerves (20% compared to 5% in the vas deferens), the NA/NPY ratio is somewhat lower (Lundberg et al., 1985e).

Release effects of sympatholytic drugs

Sympathetic nerve stimulation is accompanied not only by release of NA but also of NPY-LI. Thus, using the blood-perfused cat or pig spleen as experimental model, it has been demonstrated that nerve stimulation causes a co-release of NA and NPY-LI (Lundberg et al., 1984a,h, 1986b,d) (Fig. 4). Interestingly, intermittent stimulation with bursts of impulses at a high frequency enhances selectively the release of NPY-LI compared to NA (Fig. 4). Biochemical characterization of NPY-LI

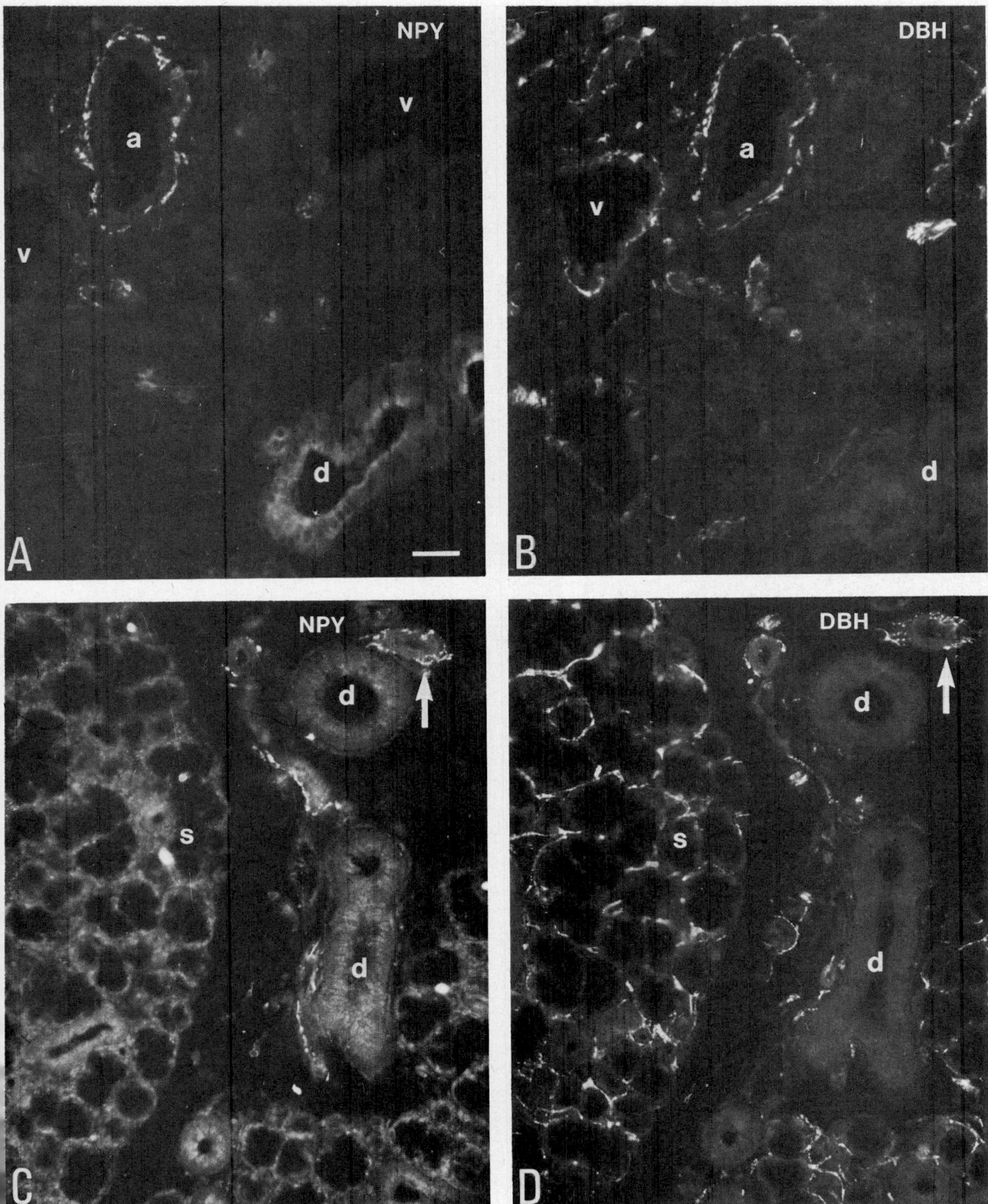

Fig. 1. Immunofluorescence micrographs of (A, B) cat nasal mucosa and (C, D) cat submandibular salivary gland after incubation with antiserum to NPY (A, C) and dopamine-β-hydroxylase, DBH (B, D). Note that NPY-immunoreactive terminals are confined to small arteries (a) and arterioles (arrows) both in the nasal mucosa (A) and submandibular gland (C), while DBH-positive (most likely NA-containing fibres) are also present around venous sinusoids (v) in the nasal mucosa (B) as well as close to exocrine elements, i.e. secretory accini (s) and ducts (d) in the submandibular gland (D). Bar in (A) indicates 50 μm. All micrographs have the same magnification.

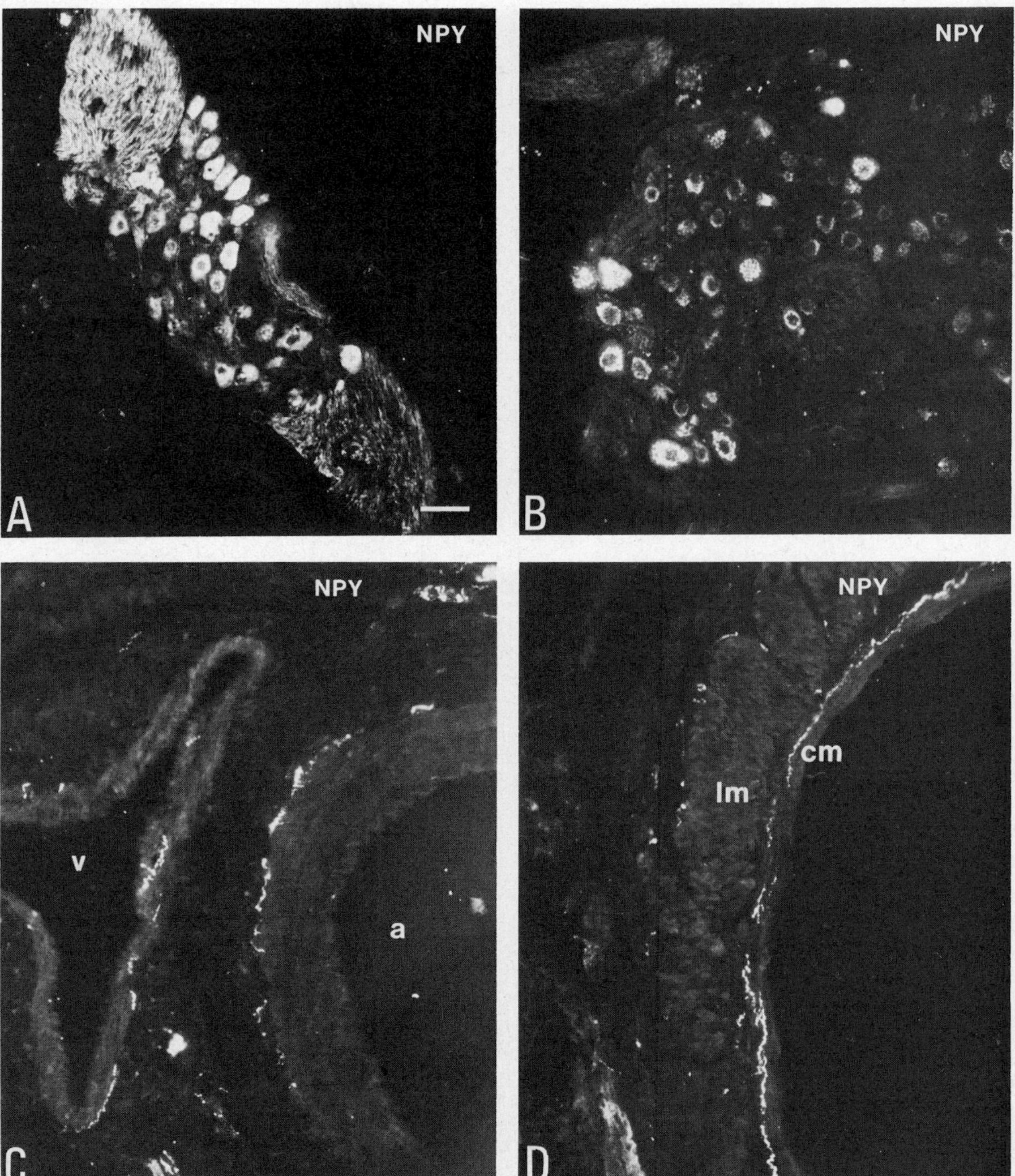

Fig. 2. Immunofluorescence micrographs of (A) L5-sympathetic ganglion, (B) coeliac ganglion, (C) femoral artery (a) and vein (v) and portal vein (D) of the rat after incubation with antiserum to NPY. Note numerous NPY-immunoreactive ganglion cells in (A) and (B), while terminals are seen at the adventitio-medial junction of the femoral vessels (C) and between the two muscle layers of the portal vein (longitudinal muscle layer, lm, and circular layer, cm) (D). Bar in (A) indicates 50 μm. All micrographs have the same magnification.

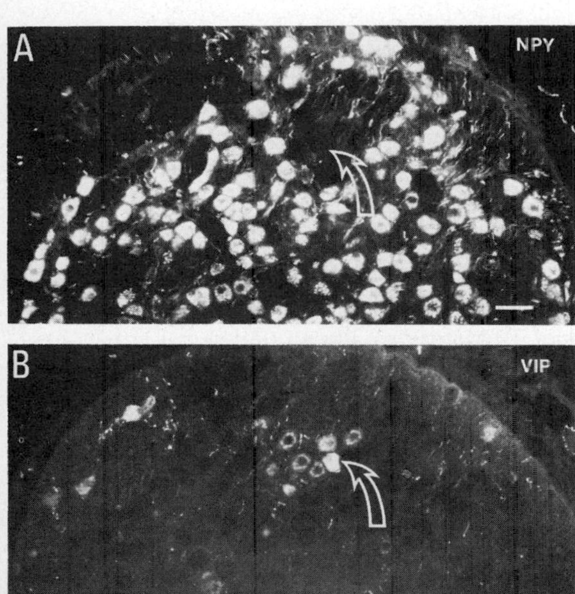

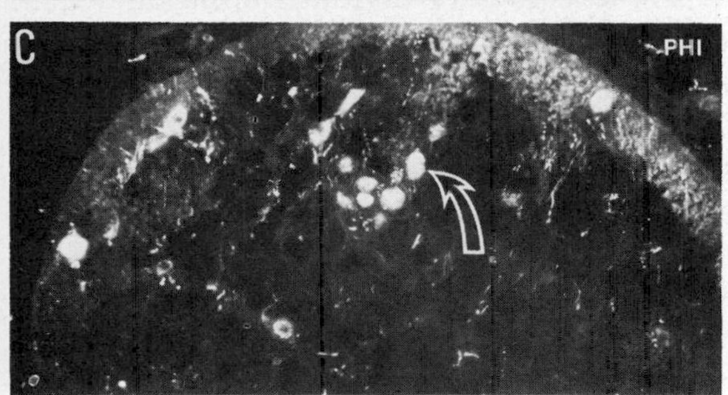

Fig. 3. Immunofluorescence micrographs of the L7-sympathetic ganglion in the cat after incubation with antiserum to (A) NPY, (B) VIP and (C) PHI. Note that VIP- (B) and PHI-immunoreactivity (C) co-exists in the same ganglion cells (arrow), while NPY is present in another population of sympathetic neurons. Bar in (A) indicates 50 μm. All micrographs have the same magnification.

in plasma from the splenic venous effluent collected during nerve stimulation and the spleen has revealed that the NPY-LI is similar to synthetic porcine NPY (Lundberg et al., 1984a, 1986d; Theodorsson-Norheim et al., 1985). The release of NPY-LI (as well as of NA) is markedly enhanced by α-adrenoceptor blockade, especially at low stimulation frequencies suggesting presynaptic inhibitory regulation of NPY release by NA via α-receptors (Fig. 4). Furthermore, stimulation-evoked NPY release is abolished by pretreatment with guanethidine. Guanethidine is known to be selectively taken

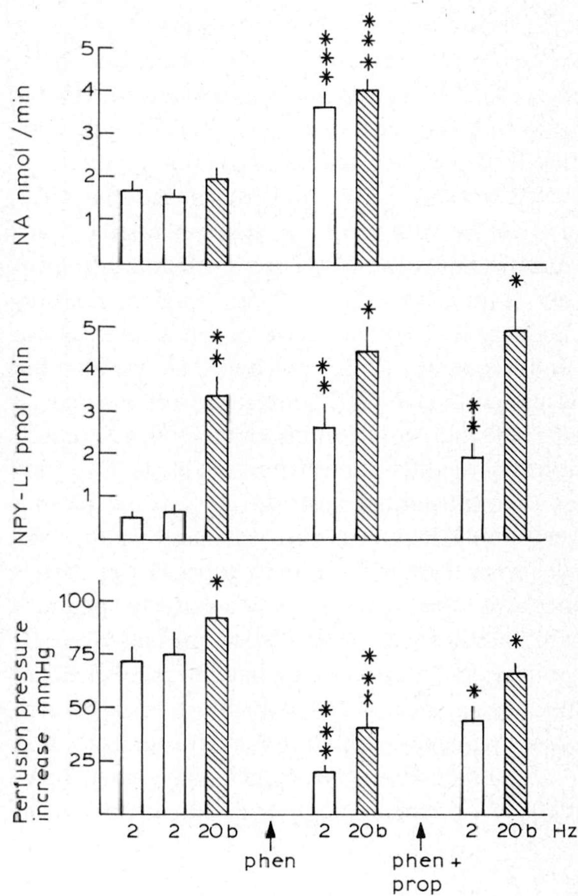

Fig. 4. Effects of splenic nerve stimulation for 2 min with a continuous low frequency at 2 Hz (2, open bars) or an intermittent high frequency stimulation at 20 Hz with 10-sec intervals (20b, hatched bars), giving the same total number of impulses (240) on perfusion pressure (mmHg) as well as the output of NPY-LI (pmol/min) or NA (nmol/min) from the pig spleen in vivo. Stimulations were performed with 15–20 min intervals. The responses during control conditions are compared with the effects 20 min after local infusion of phentolamine (Phen, estimated plasma concentration 5×10^{-5} M) or phentolamine plus propranolol (Prop, 10^{-5} M). Data are given as means ± S.E.M. and represent observations from five animals. Statistical significance between the second 2 Hz and the 20 Hz stimulations was calculated, using Student's t-test for paired observations, while Kruskal-Wallis analysis of variance with multiple comparisons was used to compare the responses of stimulations before and after adrenoceptor antagonists. (From Lundberg et al., 1986d.)

up into sympathetic nerve terminals, and after causing acute release of NA, it will then inhibit NA release (see Hertting et al., 1962a,b). It has often been considered that if guanethidine blocks a sympathetic response to nerve stimulation, the effect is mediated by NA. Since not only NA but also NPY has marked effects on the vasculature of various organs including the spleen (see below), guanethidine effects may also be related to inhibitory actions on NPY release. There is also evidence that NPY is co-released with NA upon reflex-sympathetic activation in man (Table I). Thus, both under surgical stress (Lundberg et al., 1985g), vaginal delivery (Lundberg et al., 1986c) as well as physical excercise (Lundberg et al., 1985c) not only NA but also the plasma levels of NPY-LI increase from around 20 pmol/l (during basal conditions) to 100–400 pmol/l (during sympathetic activation) (Table I). The findings that substantial increase in systemic plasma levels of NPY in man can be seen mainly upon maximal physical exercise tend to support our earlier hypothesis that release of co-existing peptides mainly occur at strong activation probably reflecting high impulse frequencies, in contrast to classical transmitters, such as NA, which are released also at low frequency stimulation (see Lundberg and Hökfelt, 1983). Hypoglycaemia in man, which rather activates preferentially the adrenal medulla, is in preliminary experiments not associated with any major increase in systemic plasma levels of NPY-LI (Table I). This suggests that the NPY content in the chromaffin cells of the adrenal medulla does not contribute to any major extent to plasma NPY-LI in man.

Reserpine is a monoamine-depleting drug which acts by interfering with vesicular storage mechanisms, thereby lowering the NA content in many peripheral tissues virtually to undetectable levels (see Carlsson, 1965). Recent evidence suggests that reserpine also depletes NPY-LI from certain sympathetic nerves, e.g. in the heart and some vascular beds such as skeletal muscle and spleen (Lundberg et al., 1984h, 1985e,f, 1986a,b). However, the content of NPY-LI in the vas deferens is not changed by reserpine in spite of a marked depletion of NA. The NPY levels in terminals of the heart and spleen are still reduced 5–10 days after a single reserpine injection, while apparently the cell-body content and axonal transport of NPY-LI slightly increase. The reserpine-induced changes in NPY levels are long-lasting (Lundberg et al., 1985e), and resupply via axonal transport of NPY from the cell bodies is not sufficient to maintain terminal levels of NPY.

The depletion of NPY-LI, but not of NA, after reserpine can be blocked by administration of the ganglionic-blocking agent chlorisondamine. This

TABLE I

Systemic plasma levels of NPY-LI (pmol/l), noradrenaline (NA, nmol/l) and adrenaline (ADR, nmol/l) in man during basal conditions compared to those during insulin-induced hypoglycaemia, thoracic surgery, graded physical exercise or in newborn infants after vaginal delivery (n = 4–12)

Condition	NPY-LI (pmol/l)	NA (nmol/l)	ADR (nmol/l)	References
Basal	29 ± 4	1.5 ± 0.2	0.16 ± 0.04	Lundberg et al., 1985g
Hypoglycaemia	39 ± 3	5.0 ± 1.0	11.30 ± 1.90	Unpublished
Thoracic surgery	59 ± 13	3.0 ± 0.6	0.30 ± 0.10	Lundberg et al., 1985g
Physical exercise:				
Mild	38 ± 2	3.0 ± 1.0	0.50 ± 0.10	Lundberg et al., 1985c
Moderate	45 ± 3	5.0 ± 0.5	0.70 ± 0.20	Lundberg et al., 1985c
Heavy	88 ± 7	29.0 ± 3.0	5.00 ± 1.20	Lundberg et al., 1985c
Vaginal delivery	161 ± 24	88.0 ± 17.0	8.70 ± 1.00	Lundberg et al., 1986c

supports the view that the depleting effect of reserpine on neuronal NPY stores is due to enhanced neuronal activity and/or release in excess of resupply of the peptide (Lundberg et al., 1985f, 1986a). An enhanced release of NPY-LI after reserpine is also most likely the basis of the chlorisondamine-sensitive raise in plasma levels of NPY-LI some hours after reserpine administration (Lundberg et al., 1986a). Nerve stimulation-evoked release of NPY-LI is markedly enhanced from the spleen in acutely reserpine-treated animals (Fig. 5) (Lundberg, 1986d). This may be related to lack of presynaptic inhibitory control on NPY release normally exerted by NA. Both the reserpine-induced depletion of NPY-LI in the heart and vascular nerves in skeletal muscle as well as the raise in plasma NPY can also be reduced by guanethidine (Lundberg et al., 1985f, 1986a), which inhibits the nerve stimulation-evoked release of NPY from sympathetic nerves (Lundberg et al., 1984a). Reserpine treatment combined with interruption of preganglionic nerve-impulse flow, using surgical decentralization, may create a situation where virtually no NA is present in sympathetic nerves, while the content of NPY is largely intact. Thus, in the cat spleen where the preganglionic fibres have been cut one week prior to reserpine treatment, NPY release evoked by postganglionic nerve stimulation is enhanced compared to control conditions (Fig. 6). A marked functional response then occurs in spite of a 96% depletion of NA content and adrenoceptor blockade (Lundberg et al., 1986b). Thus, this pharmacological model has provided strong evidence for the presence of a non-adrenergic transmitter in sympathetic splenic control.

In conclusion, the results obtained with reserpine treatment suggest different mechanisms for the subcellular storage of the co-existing classical transmitter and the peptide NPY in sympathetic nerves.

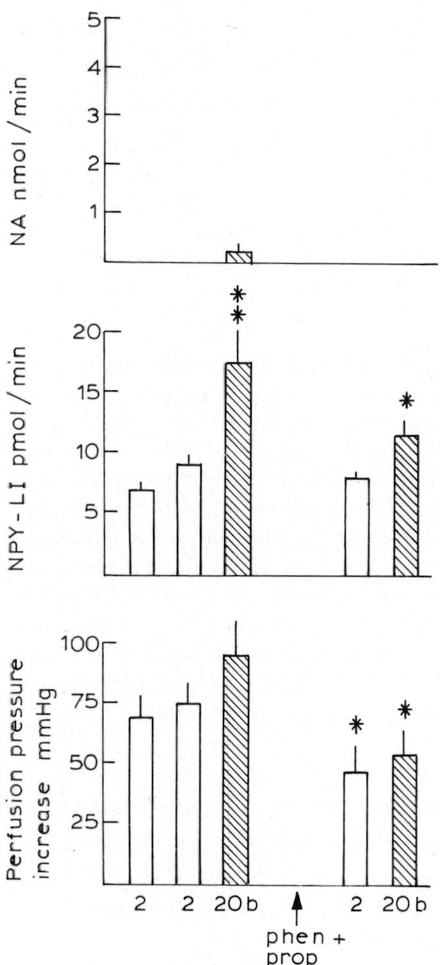

Fig. 5. Effects of splenic nerve stimulation for 2 min, using a continuous low frequency at 2 Hz (2, open bars) or an intermittent high frequency at 20 Hz (20b, hatched bars) on perfusion pressure (mmHg) as well as the output of NPY-LI (pmol/min) or NA (nmol/min) from the spleen of reserpinized pigs (1 mg/kg i.v., 12–14 h earlier). The responses after combined local infusion of phentolamine (Phen, estimated plasma concentration 5 × 10^{-5} M) and propranolol (Prop, 10^{-5} M) are also illustrated. Data are given as means ± S.E.M. and represent observations from five animals. * $p < 0.05$, ** $p < 0.01$, comparing the second 2 Hz and the 20 Hz stimulation with the corresponding response after phentolamine and propranolol treatment, using Student's *t*-test. (From Lundberg et al., 1986d.)

Postjunctional effects of NPY and NA

NPY exerts potent vasoconstrictor actions in vivo compared to NA (Lundberg and Tatemoto, 1982). Thus, NPY-induced vasoconstriction has been demonstrated as hypertensive reaction upon systemic administration (Lundberg and Tatemoto, 1982). Furthermore, local administration of NPY

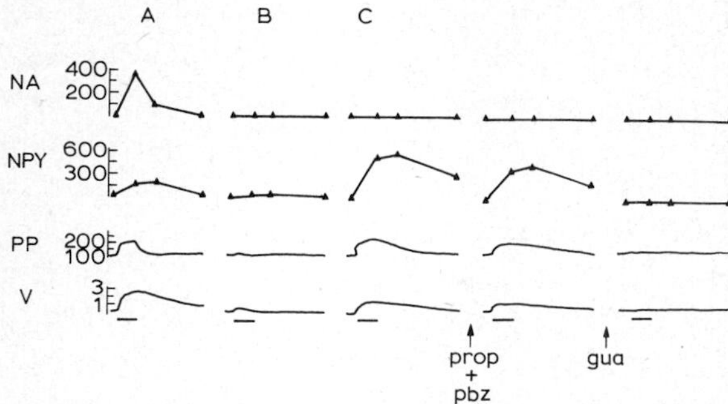

Fig. 6. Effects of postganglionic nerve stimulation (10 Hz, 10 V, 5 msec for 2 min) on volume (V, representing volume reduction, ml), perfusion pressure (PP, mmHg) as well as the output of NPY-LI (fmol/min) and NA (pmol/min) from the blood-perfused cat spleen from an untreated animal (A), 24 h after reserpine treatment (1 mg/kg s.c.) (B) or 24 h after reserpine treatment in an animal where the preganglionic nerves to the spleen had been cut one week earlier (C). Note that the long-lasting response to splenic nerve stimulation in (C) is largely resistant to pretreatment with phenoxybenzamine (pbz, 5 mg/kg i.v.) and propranolol (prop, 2 mg/kg i.v.) but is abolished by subsequent administration of guanethidine (gua, 3 mg/kg i.v.). (From Lundberg et al., 1986b.)

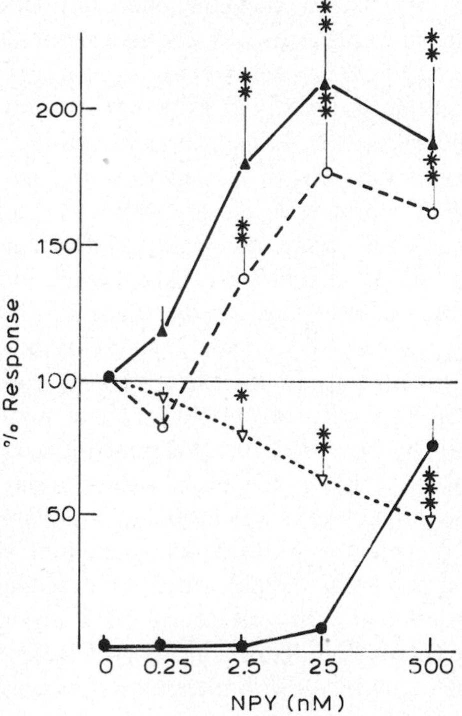

Fig. 7. Effects of increasing concentrations of NPY (nM) on (1) tension of the rat femoral artery (●—●) expressed as percentage of the response to transmural field stimulation at 6 Hz for 2 min. (2) NA (5×10^{-7} M) (▲—▲) and transmural field stimulation (TNS, 6 Hz for 2 min) (○---○)-evoked contractions as well as on TNS-evoked [^{3}H]NA efflux (▽---▽). Data are given as means ± S.E.M. and expressed as percentage of parallel control experiments in the absence of NPY. * $p < 0.05$, ** $p < 0.01$, *** $p < 0.001$ (n = 4-10). Note that NPY enhances both NA and TNS-evoked contractions in low concentrations, which do not cause any detectable contractions per se. The release of [^{3}H]NA is reduced by 50% at 500 nM NPY in spite of enhanced contraction to TNS. (From Pernow et al., 1986.)

causes vasoconstriction in the submandibular gland (Lundberg and Tatemoto, 1982), oral mucosa, dental pulp (Edwall et al., 1985), spleen (Lundberg et al., 1984a, 1986b,d) and intestine (Hellström et al., 1985). Topical application of NPY on small cerebral vessels causes vasoconstriction (i.e. caliber reduction) in vivo (Edvinsson et al., 1984b). NPY is also a vasoconstrictor agent in the coronary vascular bed shown in experiments using the whole perfused heart (Allen et al., 1983; Franco-Cereceda et al., 1985). The NPY effect on blood flow is slow in onset, long-lasting, resistant to α-adrenoceptor antagonists and present also in sympathectomized animals. Furthermore, blood flow (i.e. mainly reflecting arterial vascular tone) is relatively more affected by NPY than tissue volume (reflected by venous vascular tone) (Edvinsson et al., 1984b; Lundberg et al., 1984a). In isolated in vitro preparations of large blood vessels, NPY mostly exerts a rather weak contractile effect. Exceptions are cat cerebral arteries (Edvinsson et al., 1983) the femoral artery of the rat (Fig. 7) and the human submandibular artery where NPY is a potent vasoconstrictor (Lundberg et al., 1985d,g; Pernow et al., 1986). In the portal vein, NPY enhances the contractile force, but not the rate of the spontaneous contractions (Dahlöf et al., 1985b; Pernow et al., 1986).

In all vascular beds investigated in vivo and in vitro the contractile response to NPY seems unaffected by adrenoceptor antagonists in concentrations that totally abolish similar effects of exogenous NA (Lundberg and Tatemoto, 1982; Edvinsson et al., 1983; 1984a; Ekblad et al., 1984). This suggests that NPY has direct effects on vascular smooth muscle, which are independent of NA or adrenergic receptors. Specific binding sites for NPY with high affinity has been demonstrated with receptor-binding techniques on membrane preparations from the CNS (Saria et al., 1985b). It remains to be directly shown with similar techniques that vascular smooth muscle also possesses high affinity-binding sites for NPY.

The vasoconstrictor effects of NPY both in vitro (Edvinsson et al., 1983; Lundberg et al., 1985d; Pernow et al., 1986) as well as in vivo (Dahlöf et al., 1985a) can be antagonized by Ca^{2+}-entry blockers such as diltiazem or nifedipine (Fig. 8). Thus, the NPY-induced vascular smooth muscle spasm may be dependent on influx of extracellular calcium (see Andersson and Högestätt, 1984). This characteristic property of NPY seems to be partly different from the effects of NA, since NA-induced vasoconstriction of the α_1-type is to a major extent resistant to nifedipine, whereas α_2-mediated contractions are very sensitive to nifedipine (van Meel et al., 1981; Davero et al., 1982).

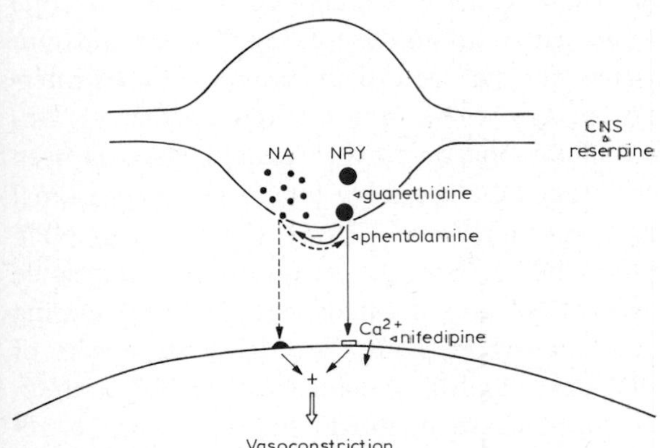

Fig. 8. Schematic illustration of a sympathetic varicosity close to a vascular smooth muscle cell. The differential storage of NA and NPY in small (NA) and large dense-cored vesicles (NPY plus NA) has been indicated. NA release already occurs at low-frequency stimulation via a guanethidine-sensitive mechanism. NA inhibits the release of NPY via α-receptors, an effect which is blocked by phentolamine. NPY seems to be released mainly at higher frequencies by a guanethidine-sensitive mechanism. NPY inhibits NA release via a presynaptic action, which is not dependent on Ca^{2+}-influx (nifedipine-resistant), while the NPY-induced vasoconstriction as well as the potentiation of NA contraction are inhibited by the calcium antagonist nifedipine. Reserpine depletes NA via interference with granular storage mechanisms, while the reserpine-induced NPY depletion seems to depend on increased release of the peptide in excess of resupply due to absence of local presynaptic NA control of release and/or CNS activation.

There is evidence that NPY has positive inotropic and chronotropic effects on the isolated right atrium of the guinea-pig in vitro (Lundberg et al., 1984; Franco-Cereceda et al., 1985). In the isolated preparations of the perfused whole heart, however, NPY reduces ventricular contractility in higher concentrations. This difference may at least partly be due to the simultaneous vasoconstriction in the perfusion experiments (Allen et al., 1983; Franco-Cereceda et al., 1985).

Another aspect of NPY in sympathetic vascular control is an enhancement of NA vasoconstriction both in vivo (Dahlöf et al., 1985a) and in vitro (Ekblad et al., 1984; Edvinsson et al., 1984a; Lundberg et al., 1985d; Pernow et al., 1986). This effect of NPY in vitro occurs at much lower concentrations (10^{-10} M to 10^{-9} M) than detectable contractile effects per se (Fig. 7). However, the potentiating effect of NPY on isolated vascular smooth muscle is not universal, since the NA response in, for instance, the femoral vein is not influenced compared to the femoral artery (Ekblad et al., 1984; Pernow et al., 1986). The vasoconstrictor response to adrenaline (Pernow et al., 1986) and histamine, but not to that to K^+ or $PGF_{\alpha 2}$, are also enhanced by NPY (Edvinsson et al., 1984a). The low concentrations of NPY necessary to enhance catecholamine-induced vasoconstriction are somewhat higher than the systemic plasma levels of the NPY-LI found during, for example, strong physical exercise in man or upon vaginal delivery of human infants (Lundberg et al., 1985c, 1986c) (see Table I). This suggests that NPY has mainly local effects, while the possible role of circulating NPY (originating from overflow after release from sympathetic terminals and/or adrenal medulla; Lundberg et al., 1983c) remains to be established.

The NPY-induced enhancement of NA contractions of vascular smooth muscle is blocked by nifedipine, suggesting that also this effect is related to changes in Ca^{2+} mechanisms (Lundberg et al., 1985d; Pernow et al., 1986). It has been reported that NPY increases the number of α_2- but not α_1-receptor-binding sites in membrane preparations from rat brain (Agnati et al., 1983). Similar mechanisms, however, do not seem to underly the NPY-induced potentiation of NA contractions of peripheral blood vessels. Thus, the α_1- and α_2-adrenoreceptor-binding in the femoral artery of the rat seems unaffected by NPY in concentrations that markedly enhance the functional response to NA (Pernow et al., 1986). Furthermore, the NA effect in this vessel is mainly mediated via α_1- and not by α_2-receptors.

Prejunctional effects of NPY

It was early observed that NPY inhibited the electrically induced twitch contractions of the vas deferens (Allen et al., 1982; Lundberg et al., 1982e). In some species the twitch response of the vas deferens, however, may not be due to NA but possibly to ATP (see Sneddon et al., 1982; Meldrum and Burnstock, 1983; Lundberg et al., 1984e; Stjärne and Åstrand, 1985). The second slow contractile phase of the transmural nerve stimulation (TNS) response of the vas deferens, which is likely to be NA-mediated, is also reduced by NPY (Lundberg et al., 1984e). Since the contractile effects of exogenous NA on the vas deferens are not inhibited by NPY, this suggests that NPY inhibits ATP and NA mechanisms via a prejunctional action. Direct evidence for this hypothesis was also obtained in release experiments where NPY was found to depress the TNS-induced secretion of [^{3}H]NA (Lundberg and Stjärne, 1984). Thus, three messenger signals in the vas deferens may be used by the same sympathetic nerves, (1) ATP as a rapid signal causing the twitch response; (2) NA causing the slow contraction and (3) NPY which principally regulates the release of the two "co-transmitters". The NPY-induced inhibition of NA release was also apparent in the presence of the α_2-antagonist yohimbine, suggesting that the effect was independent of presynaptic α_2-receptors (see also Pernow et al., 1986). Thereafter, NPY has been demonstrated to inhibit the TNS-evoked release of [^{3}H]NA from both perivascular (Dahlöf et al., 1985b; Lundberg et al., 1985d; Pernow et al., 1986) and cardiac nerves (Franco-Cereceda et al., 1985). The prejunctional effects of NPY occur at low concentrations (10^{-9}–10^{-8} M) in the femoral artery of the rat, where concentration-response relationships were studied (Fig. 7).

The prejunctional inhibitory effects of NPY on transmitter release can be correlated to a depression of the TNS-evoked contractile response in the vas deferens and the right atrium of the heart (Lundberg et al., 1984e). In the portal vein (Dahlöf et al., 1985b) and femoral artery (Lundberg et al., 1985d; Pernow et al., 1986), however, the TNS-induced contractile response is enhanced by NPY, in spite of a reduction in NA release (Fig. 7). This apparent discrepancy may be explained by a complex interplay between several factors taken together. (1) Only a minor portion of the released NA has been suggested to be necessary for an intact functional response (Ljung et al., 1976). (2) Although NPY reduces NA release, the postjunctional contractile effects of NA are simultaneously enhanced. During conditions where both the contractile effects of NPY per se and the enhancement of NA contractions are blocked by nifedipine, NPY seems to reduce the TNS response. In this situation the prejunctional inhibitory effects of NPY on NA release remains intact, since nifedipine does not influence this action of NPY (Pernow et al., 1986). Thus, interaction with calcium mechanisms seems to be a prerequisite for post- but not presynaptic actions of NPY in sympathetic vascular control.

Non-adrenergic sympathetic mechanisms — NPY?

In the literature, there is mainly pharmacological evidence that some functional effects of sympathetic nerve stimulation are not due only to NA. As mentioned above, there is ample evidence that the twitch component of the contractile response of the vas deferens is due to release of ATP from sympathetic nerves. Furthermore, electrophysiological studies have shown that a fast excitatory junction potential in smooth muscle cells obtained upon sympathetic nerve stimulation in both the vas deferens (see Stjärne and Åstrand, 1985) and arterioles (see Hirst and Neild, 1980) is non-adrenergic. With regard to sympathetic vascular control, Lundberg and Tatemoto (1982) noted that the secretory response of the submandibular gland induced by sympathetic nerve stimulation was more easily blocked by adrenoceptor antagonists than the simultaneous vasoconstriction. However, one major problem in many studies has been the use of only α-adrenoceptor antagonists, which leaves β-adrenergic vasodilation intact and possibly enhanced due to the simultaneous increase in NA release (see Fig. 4). Furthermore, many nerves that are electrically stimulated are mixed nerves with, for example, intermingled sensory or sympathetic vasoconstrictor and vasodilator fibres. In the isolated blood-vessel preparations in vitro, the situation is even more complex, since TNS is likely to induce the release of many types of nerve-stored, vasoactive principles from both vasoconstrictor and vasodilator fibres. When the combination of α- and β-adrenoceptor antagonists are used, several recent in vivo reports suggest that part of the sympathetic nervous vasoconstrictor response remains, while the effects of exogenous NA are totally blocked (cat submandibular gland, Lundberg and Tatemoto, 1982; cat or pig spleen, Lundberg et al., 1984a, i; cat intestine, Hellström et al., 1985; cat oral mucosa and dental pulp, Edvall et al., 1985). This "non-adrenergic" vasoconstriction induced by electrical nerve stimulation is abolished by guanethidine, suggesting that it is of sympathetic origin. Local infusion of NPY, but not of NA, mimics the adrenoceptor-antagonist resistant vasoconstriction, especially in the submandibular gland of the cat (Lundberg and Tatemoto, 1982). Thus, the vascular response to exogenous NA is short-lasting and followed by hyperemia. In contrast, the NPY effect is similar to the long-lasting, remaining response seen upon nerve stimulation after α- and β-adrenoceptor blockade.

Further evidence for non-adrenergic, sympathetic vasoconstriction has emanated from experiments using reserpine-pretreated animals. Already in 1962, Rosell and Sedvall reported that if the preganglionic pathways were interrupted prior to administration of reserpine, a nervously-mediated vasoconstriction partly remained in the skeletal muscle on the denervated side. This remaining response was subjected to fatigue upon repeated stimulation. Analysis of the NA content, however, revealed only a small difference in the NA depletion between the skeletal muscle of the intact and denervated side (Sedvall, 1964).

As discussed above, reserpine treatment depletes not only NA from skeletal muscle nerves but also NPY via a mechanism that is most likely dependent on intact ganglionic transmission (Lundberg et al., 1985f, 1986b). Preganglionic denervation was therefore combined with reserpine pretreatment in the cat-spleen model (Lundberg et al., 1986b). Interruption of ganglionic transmission did not influence the reserpine-induced NA depletion in the spleen 24 h later, which was 96% both after preganglionic sectioning and in control animals. Furthermore, no detectable endogenous NA release could be demonstrated upon nerve stimulations of the spleen in these reserpine-treated animals. However, sympathetic nerve stimulation of the spleen after such procedures caused a considerable functional response both with regard to vasoconstriction and volume reduction (Fig. 6). The functional effects declined upon repeated stimulation in parallel with a reduction in NPY release (Fig. 6). The "reserpine-resistant", sympathetic, vascular effects in the cat spleen also remained after administration of adrenoceptor antagonists (Fig. 6). These experiments give further evidence that other agents than NA, such as NPY, contribute to the sympathetic vascular control. However, since specific NPY antagonists are not yet available, the physiological role of NPY in sympathetic neurotransmission is still unclear, especially since both adrenoceptor blockers as well as reserpine enhance NPY release (Figs. 5 and 6). The development in the field of peripheral autonomic transmission is directed towards the discovery of several bioactive principles in the same nerves.

Therefore, it cannot be excluded that other not yet identified messengers than NPY may also be involved in these "non-adrenergic", sympathetic, vascular effects.

In conclusion, NPY is present together with NA in certain sympathetic nerves. Although the characteristics for NPY with regard to synthesis, storage, release and effects of sympatholytic drugs are partly different from those of NA, increasing evidence suggests that NPY is an important messenger in sympathetic neurotransmission both at the pre- and postsynaptic level.

VIP/PHI in cholinergic neurons

Postganglionic neurons to exocrine glands have been found to contain VIP-LI (see Lundberg et al., 1979; Lundberg, 1981). Several lines of evidence suggest that these VIP-immunoreactive neurons which project to, for instance, sweat glands, nasal mucosa and submandibular gland of the cat are cholinergic (see Lundberg, 1981). Another biologically active peptide designated PHI (PHI-27, the peptide (P) with NH_2-terminal histidine (H) and COOH-terminal isoleucine (I) amide and 27 amino-acid residues) with marked sequence homology to VIP has subsequently been isolated (Tatemoto and Mutt, 1980). PHI, which has a 50% amino-acid homology as compared to VIP, shares many of the biological activities of VIP, although PHI in most systems has a somewhat lower potency (Bataille et al., 1980; see Lundberg et al., 1984c). Interestingly, the VIP precursor gene besides VIP contains a coding sequence for a PHI-related peptide, which in man is designated PHM (the peptide (P) having NH_2-terminal histidine (H) and COOH-terminal methionine (M) amide) (Itoh et al., 1983). This finding suggests that VIP and PHI are co-synthesized in the same precursor molecule which is supported by immunohistochemical studies using specific antisera, showing that the same autonomic neurons to, for instance, exocrine glands contain both VIP- and PHI-IR (Lundberg et al., 1984c) (Fig. 3B, C).

Release of VIP, PHI and acetylcholine

Both VIP-LI (Lundberg, 1981; Edwards et al., 1982) and ACh (Lundberg et al., 1982b) are released upon parasympathetic stimulation of the submandibular gland of the cat. The release of VIP-LI increases characteristically with frequency, whereby fairly high stimulation frequencies are necessary to demonstrate significant VIP release. Having the parasympathetic vasodilatory response as a functional correlate to VIP and ACh release, it seems that ACh release is responsible for the increase in blood flow at low frequencies, since the response is potentiated by the cholinesterase inhibitor eserine and blocked by atropine (see Lundberg et al., 1982b). The vasodilatory response is atropine-resistant at higher stimulation frequencies and even prolonged (see Darke and Smaje, 1972), suggesting that a non-cholinergic mediator such as VIP is of importance upon strong activation (Lundberg, 1981; Lundberg et al., 1982b) (Fig. 9). Having the vasodilatory response in the submandibular salivary gland upon parasympathetic nerve stimulation as functional correlate, it seems that a frequency-dependent, chemical coding occurs in autonomic neurotransmission (Fig. 10). Thus, low-frequency stimulation causes perferential release of a classical transmitter (ACh, mainly stored in small vesicles), whereas high-frequency activation also induces the release of the peptide (VIP, from large dense-cored vesicles) (see Lundberg and Hökfelt, 1983). This difference has also beeen supported by directly analysing the overflow of these substances in the venous effluent of the gland (Lundberg et al., 1982b). A principally similar situation may exist for NA and NPY in sympathetic vascular control (see above).

Recent experiments have shown that parasympathetic nerve stimulation is also accompanied by increase in the output of PHI-LI (Lundberg et al., 1984d) (Fig. 9). VIP and PHI seem to be released in a 1:1 ratio from the salivary gland and the output of both peptides upon nerve stimulation increases in parallel after atropine (Fig. 9). The increase in

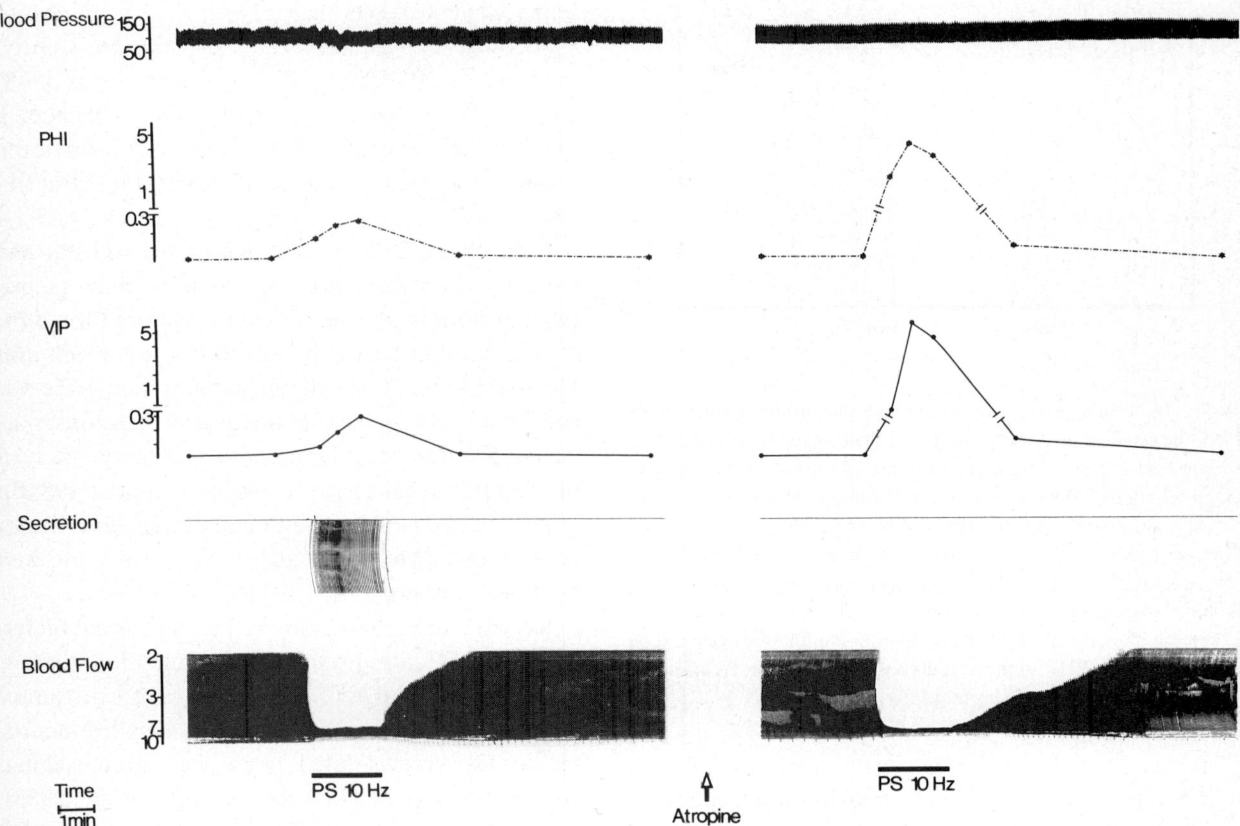

Fig. 9. Effects of parasympathetic nerve stimulation at 10 Hz for 2 min on blood flow (ml/min), salivary secretion recorded as drops of saliva and the output of VIP and PHI (pmol/min) from the submandibular salivary gland of the cat in vivo. Atropine treatment (1 mg/kg i.v.) abolishes salivary secretion, while the blood-flow response is enhanced and prolonged. Simultaneously, there is a marked parallel increase in the output of VIP and PHI from the venous outflow of the gland. (From Lundberg et al., 1984d.)

VIP and PHI output after atropine could either depend upon reduction of VIP metabolism in absence of a secretory response or indicate that VIP/PHI release is under an inhibitory influence by ACh via muscarinic, presynaptic receptors. Thus, a similar situation may exist in the parasympathetic system as in sympathetic nerves, where the classical transmitter (NA) has an inhibitory influence on the release of the co-existing peptide (NPY, see above).

Functional effects of VIP/PHI/ACh

Local infusions of ACh induce both vasodilation and salivary secretion in the submandibular gland of the cat. Although VIP causes vasodilation but no secretion per se, it enhances the secretory response to ACh. The VIP-induced potentiation of cholinergic salivary secretion may in part be due to the additional increase in blood flow, and also, to a direct effect of VIP on secretory elements (see Lundberg et al., 1982a, c). As mentioned above, porcine PHI in most species, such as rat, guinea-pig and cat, has been found to possess considerably less biological activity than VIP. However, this apparent poor activity of PHI may at least partly be due to variations in the endogenous PHI sequence between different species. Thus, when the human forms of VIP (which is identical to the porcine peptide) and PHI, i.e. PHM, have been tested with re-

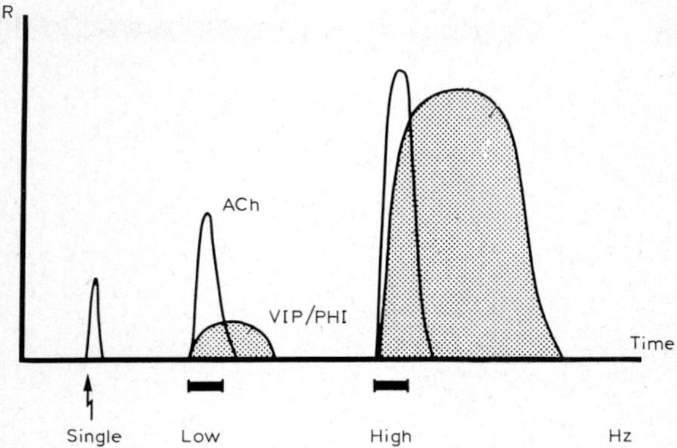

Fig. 10. Schematic illustration showing the putative contribution of the classical transmitter ACh and the co-existing peptides VIP and PHI to the vasodilatory response of the cat submandibular gland upon various degrees of activation induced by electrical nerve stimulation (single impulse, low and high frequencies, Hz). A single nerve impulse induces preferentially a response which is due to the release of the classical transmitter, as indicated by total blockade by atropine treatment. There seems to be an increasing functional effect caused by non-cholinergic agents, such as VIP and PHI upon stimulation with higher frequencies. (Modified from Lundberg and Hökfelt, 1983.)

gard to vasodilator activity in vitro on the submandibular artery of man, these two peptides were found to have a similar potency (Larsson et al., 1986).

In conclusion, the parasympathetic control of exocrine gland secretion and blood flow seem to depend on a multimessenger system, involving the classical transmitter ACh and at least two peptides, VIP and PHI.

Multiple peptides in capsaicin-sensitive sensory nerves

Substance P (SP) was the first biologically active peptide demonstrated in primary sensory neurons (see Hökfelt et al., 1975). SP-IR sensory neurons have peripheral branches in most peripheral organs, e.g. ureter, heart and lung, and seem to be of both parasympathetic (i.e. vagal), trigeminal and spinal origin. Acute exposure to capsaicin, the pungent agent in hot peppers, causes activation of chemosensitive nerves (see Nagy, 1982) and an initial release of SP-LI (Gamse et al., 1979). Subsequently, there is a depletion of SP-LI (Jessell et al., 1978) and, after exposure to high doses of capsaicin a functional desensitization and a degeneration of the sensory neurons (Jancso et al., 1981; Papka et al., 1984).

Endogenous release of SP (or related substances) from local sensory neurons seems to play an important role in the neurogenic inflammation syndrome upon chemical irritation (see Lembeck and Holzer, 1979). Thus, SP can largely mimic the vasodilator- and protein-extravasation responses as well as the non-vascular smooth muscle spasm seen in visceral organs (see Lundberg et al., 1984b). However, the capsaicin-induced excitation of heart contractility (Molnar et al., 1969) is not mimicked by SP (Lundberg et al., 1984f).

Recent studies have shown that additional tachykinins to SP are present in mammalian tissues. Thus, neurokinin A (NKA) (also called substance K) and neurokinin B (NKB) (also called neuromedin K) were isolated from the porcine spinal cord (Kangawa et al., 1983; Kimura et al., 1983). Simultaneously, it was demonstrated that one SP precursor gene contained both SP and NKA-like sequences (Nawa et al., 1983). Subsequently, Tatemoto et al. (1985) have found that an elongated form of SK named neuropeptide K (NPK) with 36 amino-acid residues is present in brain tissue. Thus, the SP precursor seems to produce three biologically active tachykinins, SP, NKA and NPK. Chromatographic characterization of ureter and lung extracts has shown that both SP- NKA- and NPK-LI seem to be sensitive to capsaicin pretreatment (Hua et al., 1985). Furthermore, immunohistochemical studies, using specific SP and NKA antisera, have demonstrated that cell bodies in spinal and vagal ganglia contain both SP- and NKA-LI (Hua et al., 1985). The pattern of the immunostaining of nerves in peripheral organs such as the ureter and lung is identical, using these two types of antisera. Capsaicin pretreatment of adult guinea-pigs leads to an almost total loss of both SP- and NKA-IR nerves in peripheral organs except in the intestine where most of the SP- and NKA-IR nerves are of intramural origin. No evidence was obtained that NKB-LI was present in capsaicin-sensitive sensory neurons (Hua et al., 1985).

Calcitonin-gene related peptide (CGRP) is a neuropeptide whose structure was deduced from a nucleotide sequence found on the calcitonin gene (Amara et al., 1982). CGRP-LI was also found to be present in primary sensory neurons, using immunohistochemical techniques (Rosenfeld et al., 1983). CGRP-LI nerves in peripheral organs like the heart were found to be sensitive to capsaicin pretreatment (Lundberg et al., 1985b). Correlation studies have shown that in many cases SP-LI and CGRP-LI co-exist in the same neurons in spinal ganglia (Wiesenfeld-Hallin et al., 1984; Lundberg et al., 1985b). The occurrence of CGRP-LI in capsaicin-sensitive, cardiac nerves (Lundberg et al., 1985b; Franco-Cereceda et al., 1986) is of interest, since CGRP, but not SP or other tachykinins mimics the cardio-excitatory effects of capsaicin (Lundberg et al., 1984f, 1985b; Tippins et al., 1984; Franco-Cereceda and Lundberg, 1985).

Capsaicin-induced release of SP, NKA, NPK and CGRP

Capsaicin exposure has been shown to release SP-LI from sensory branches in the spinal cord (Gamse et al., 1979) and ureter (Saria et al., 1983a). Furthermore, capsaicin releases NKA-LI from the perfused lung of the guinea-pig (Saria et al., 1985a). In addition, experiments from the spinal cord have shown that capsaicin releases CGRP-LI (Franco-Cereceda et al., 1986). Thus, there is evidence that activation of capsaicin-sensitive, sensory nerves is accompanied by release of several tachykinins and CGRP.

Functional effects of sensory peptides and capsaicin

Capsaicin exposure of mucosal membranes or the skin induces a series of events involving both local and central reflexes (Fig. 13). Reflex responses involve both perception of irritation, avoidance behaviour (e.g. sneezing) and sympathetic activation (increase in blood pressure) as well as parasympathetic activation (exocrine secretion). Therefore, the peptide containing capsaicin-sensitive sensory nerves seems to be connected in a reflex arc to autonomic sympathetic and parasympathetic motor fibres, which in turn contain other peptides (see Lundblad, 1984).

Local effects of capsaicin seem to be dependent on the release of mediators from sensory fibres in the tissues. Five types of principal responses have been linked to activation of capsaicin-sensitive nerves. (1) Vasodilation; this effect, which is expressed as fall in blood pressure upon systemic administration (Fig. 11) can be mimicked by all three tachykinins (SP, NKA and NPK). On a molar basis, however, CGRP seems to be the most potent vasodilating agent present in sensory nerves (Brain et al., 1984). (2) Extravasation of plasma proteins; this reaction takes place in postcapillary venules and all the tachykinins can induce this reaction, whereby SP has the most potent activity (Fig. 11). CGRP does not increase the vascular permeability

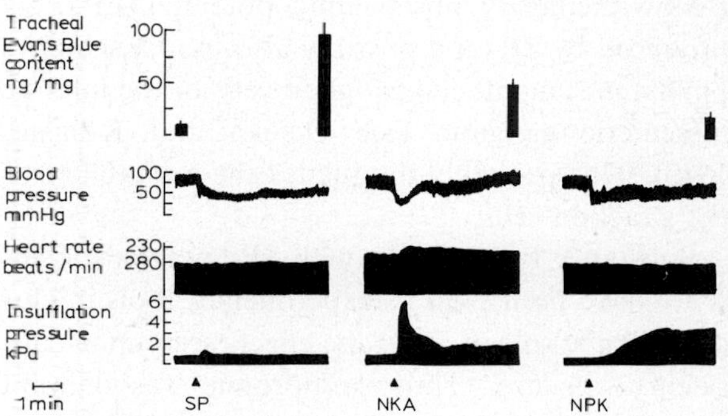

Fig. 11. Effects of i.v. administration (0.8 nmol/kg) of various tachykinins (substance P, SP; neurokinin A, NKA; neuropeptide K, NPK) on respiratory insufflation pressure, indicating bronchoconstriction, heart rate, systemic arterial blood pressure and tracheal Evans blue content, indicating protein extravasation. The content of Evans blue from control animals has been given as a bar before the SP effect. SP causes the largest protein-extravasation effect, while NKA induces a rapid and strong bronchoconstriction. NPK causes a slowly developing bronchoconstrictor effect.

of plasma proteins per se (Lundberg et al., 1985b). The capsaicin-induced extravasation response is most pronounced in mucosal membranes with sharp border lines to non-reactive areas such as in the gastrointestinal tract between the esophagus and anal mucosa (Lundberg et al., 1984b). (3) Non-vascular smooth muscle spasm in, for instance, the airways, intestine and urogenital tract (Molnar et al., 1969; see Lundberg et al., 1984b). Especially NKA and NPK have very potent contractile activity on the airway smooth muscle (Fig. 11) (Hua et al., 1984; Tatemoto et al., 1985). Thus, the two recently discovered tachykinins are more potent in this aspect compared to the well-known spasmogen SP. (4) Positive inotropic and chronotropic effects on the right atrium of the heart; this response is mimicked by CGRP (Tippins et al., 1984; Lundberg et al., 1985b), which exerts powerful cardio-excitatory effects (Fig. 12), but not by the tachykinins (Lundberg et al., 1984f). The capsaicin-induced stimulation of the heart is absent after CGRP tachyphylaxis, further suggesting the involvement of CGRP in this reaction (Fig. 12) (Franco-Cereceda and Lundberg, 1985). Thus, CGRP release by capsaicin from local sensory nerves within the myocardium may increase cardiac contractile activity. (5) A slow excitatory, postsynaptic potential (EPSP) is produced by SP (and possibly also by other tachykinins) in sympathetic ganglion cells of the inferior mesenteric ganglion (see Otsuka and Konishi, 1983). This probably modulates the excitability of the ganglion cells.

Substance P analogues with SP-antagonistic activity have been used as experimental tools in elucidating the role of SP in the effects seen upon capsaicin exposure. Thus, antidromic vasodilation (Rosell et al., 1981), extravasation of plasma proteins (Lembeck et al., 1982; Lundberg et al., 1983a, b), non-vascular smooth muscle spasm in, for instance, the airways (Lundberg et al., 1983b) or the slow EPSP in sympathetic ganglia induced by sensory nerve activation (see Otsuka and Konishi et al., 1983) have been found to be reduced after administration of SP antagonists. However, it seems clear that SP antagonists also block the response to

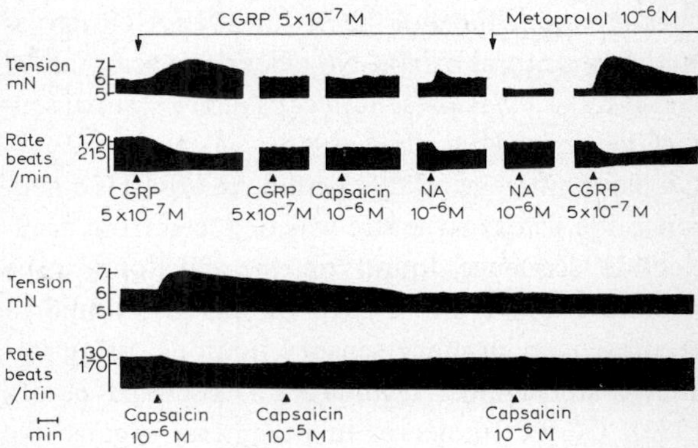

Fig. 12. Effects of CGRP (5×10^{-7} M), capsaicin (10^{-6} M or 10^{-5} M) or NA (10^{-6} M) on the spontaneously beating guinea-pig atrium. Metoprolol was added in upper panel, as indicated by arrow. After presence of CGRP for 20–30 min, addition of CGRP or capsaicin did not cause any response, while NA still stimulated the atrium. In the presence of metoprolol, which reduced basal tension per se, NA had no effect, while CGRP (60 min after CGRP washout) had a marked positive inotropic and chronotropic effect. Capsaicin caused a positive inotropic and chronotropic response, which also developed tachyphylaxis (lower panel). Bar indicates time scale for 1 min. (From Franco-Cereceda and Lundberg, 1985.)

other tachykinins (see Karlsson et al., 1984). Therefore, these analogues may be regarded as tachykinin antagonists rather than specific SP antagonists.

The capsaicin-pretreated animal — loss of chemogenic irritation

Pretreatment of animals either locally or systemically with high doses of capsaicin causes a depletion of sensory neuro-peptides and a degeneration of sensory nerve terminals (see Nagy, 1982). These animals show several typical deficiencies in reactions upon exposure to irritant chemicals. Thus, avoidance behaviour and protective reflexes as well as local tissue and smooth muscle reactions are absent or markedly reduced. One interesting example is the absence of irritation in the airways by cigarette-smoke exposure (Lundberg and Saria, 1983; Lundberg et al., 1983a). Furthermore, the oedema formation by histamine (Lundberg and Saria, 1983)

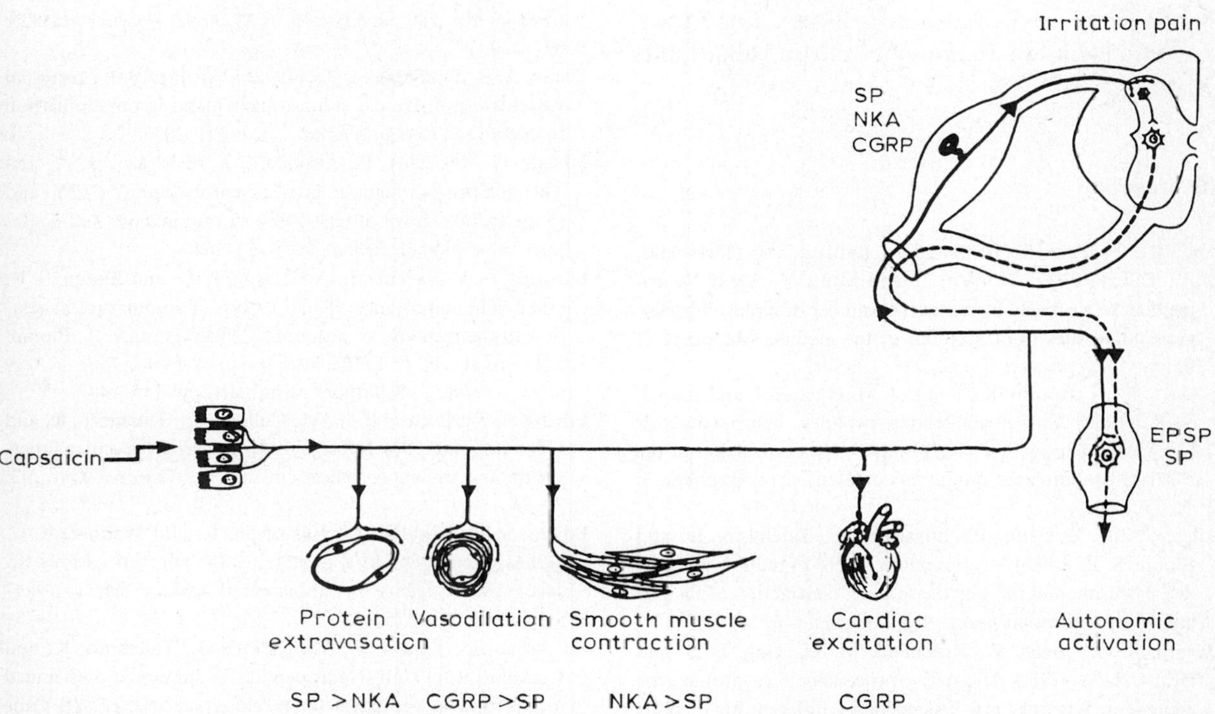

Fig. 13. Schematic illustration of the summary of events occurring upon capsaicin-induced activation of irritant receptors on C-fibre afferents in various organs. Capsaicin causes release of multiple co-existing peptides (substance P, SP; neurokinin A, NKA; calcitonin gene-related peptide, CGRP). Local release of these peptides from sensory nerve branches in various organs causes several biological effects with varying potencies; protein extravasation (SP > NKA), vasodilation (CGRP > SP > NKA), smooth muscle contraction, such as bronchoconstriction (NKA > SP), positive inotropic and chronotropic effects on heart contractility (CGRP), a slow EPSP in autonomic ganglia (SP) as well as central reflexes including sneezing, cough and autonomic activation leading to hypertension and exocrine secretion. Thus, peptides in sensory nerves seem to be linked with both sympathetic and parasympathetic vascular and secretory neurons containing other peptides such as NPY/ and VIP/PHI. (Modified from Lundberg et al., 1984b.)

or anaphylactic challenge in sensitized animals (Saria et al., 1983b) or man (Lundblad et al., 1985) are reduced after capsaicin pretreatment. This suggests a close relationship between mast cells and capsaicin-sensitive nerves. Activation of capsaicin-sensitive nerves also seems to contribute to the oedema formation in the skin upon heat exposure (Lundberg et al., 1984g). However, only certain deficiencies in sensory perception are obvious in the capsaicin-treated animals. Thus, mechanical sensitivity and reactions to certain chemicals including nicotine are to a large extent intact (see Lundblad, 1984).

In conclusion, multiple peptides with partly different biological activities are present in a population of sensory nerves which are sensitive to capsaicin. Activation of irritant receptors on these sensory nerves may initiate a cascade of both local reactions dependent on peptide release from sensory nerves as well as central reflexes, involving peptides in autonomic motor reflexes.

Acknowledgements

The present review has been based on studies supported by the Swedish Medical Research Council (14X-6554, 17X-5438), the American Council for Tobacco Research, the Swedish Tobacco Company, Petrus och Augusta Hedlunds Stiftelse and

Funds from the Karolinska Institute. For expert secretarial help we are grateful to Mrs Hilka Lindberg.

References

Agnati, L. F., Fuxe, K., Benfenati, F., Battistini, N., Härfstrand, A., Tatemoto, K., Hökfelt, T. and Mutt, V. (1983) Neuropeptide Y selectively increases the number of alpha$_2$-adrenergic binding sites in membranes of the medulla oblongata of the rat. *Acta physiol. Scand.*, 118: 293–295.

Allen, J. M., Tatemoto, K., Polak, J. M. Hughes, J. and Bloom, S. R. (1982) Two novel related peptides, neuropeptide Y (NPY) and peptide YY (PYY) inhibit the contraction of the electrically stimulated mouse vas deferens. *Neuropeptides*, 3: 71–77.

Allen, J. M., Bircham, P., Edwards, A., Tatemoto, K. and Bloom, S. R. (1983) Neuropeptide Y (NPY) reduces myocardial perfusion and inhibits the force of contraction of the isolated perfused rabbit heart. *Regul. Peptides*, 6: 247–252.

Amara, S. G., Jonas, V., Rosenfeld, M. G., Ong, E. S. and Evans, R. M. (1982) Alternative processing in calcitonin gene expression generates mRNAs encoding different polypeptide products. *Nature (Lond.)*, 198: 240–244.

Andersson, K. E. and Högestätt, E. D. (1984) On the mechanisms of action of calcium antagonists. *Acta med. Scand.*, Suppl. 681: 11–24.

Bataille, D., Gespach, D., Laburthe, M., Amiranoff, B., Tatemoto, K., Vauculin, N., Mutt, V. and Rosselin, G. (1980) Peptide having N-terminal histidine and C-terminal isolercineamide (PHI). Vasoactive intestinal peptide (VIP) and secretin-like effects in different tissues from the rat. *FEBS Lett.*, 114: 240–242.

Brain, S. D., Williams, T. J., Tippins, J. R. Moris, H. R. and Mac Intyre, I. (1984) Calcitonin gene-related peptide is a potent vasodilator. *Nature (Lond.)*, 313: 54–56.

Carlsson, A. (1965) Drugs which block the storage of 5-hydroxytryptamine and related amines. In V. Erspamer (Ed.), *Handbook Exp. Pharm., Vol. 19*, Springer-Verlag, Berlin–Heidelberg–New York, pp. 529–592.

Cavero, I., Shepperson, N., Lefeore-Bug, F. and Langer, S. Z. (1983) Differential inhibition of vascular smooth muscle responses to alpha$_1$- and alpha$_2$-adrenoceptor antagonists by diltiazem and verapamil. *Circulat. Res.*, Suppl. 1, 52: 69–76.

Dahlöf, C., Dahlöf, P. and Lundberg, J. M. (1985a) Neuropeptide Y (NPY): Enhancement of blood-pressure increase upon α-adrenoceptor activation and direct pressor effects in pithed rats. *Europ. J. Pharmacol.*, 109: 289–292.

Dahlöf, C., Dahlöf, P., Tatemoto, K. and Lundberg, J. M. (1985b) Neuropeptide Y (NPY) reduces field stimulation-evoked release of noradrenaline and enhances contractile force in the rat portal vein. *N.S. Arch. Pharmacol.*, 328: 327–330.

Darke, A. C. and Smaje, L. H. (1972) Dependence of functional vasodilation in the cat submaxillary gland upon stimulation frequency. *J. Physiol. (Lond.)*, 226: 191–203.

Edwall, B.,, Gazelius, B., Lundberg, J. M., Fazekas, A. and Theodorsson-Norheim, E. (1985) Neuropeptide Y (NPY) and sympathetic control of blood flow in oral mucosa and dental pulp. *Acta physiol. Scand.*, 125: 253–264.

Edwards, A. V., Järhult, J., Andersson, P.-O. and Bloom, S. R. (1982) The importance of the pattern of stimulation in relation to the response of autonomic effectors. in S. R. Bloom, J. M. Polak and E. Lindenlaub (Eds.), *Systemic Role of Regulatory Peptides*, Schattauer, Stuttgart, pp. 145–148.

Edvinsson, L., Emson, P. C., Mc Culloch, K., Tatemoto, K. and Uddman, R. (1983) Neuropeptide Y, cerebrovascular innervation and vasomotor effects in the cat. *Neurosci. Lett.*, 43: 79–84.

Edvinsson, L., Ekblad, E., Håkanson, R. and Wahlestedt, C. (1984a) Neuropeptide Y potentiates the effect of various vasoconstrictor agents on rabbit blood vessels. *Brit. J. Pharmacol.*, 83: 519–525.

Edvinsson, L., Emson, P., Mc Culloch, J., Tatemoto, K. and Uddman, R. (1984b) Neuropeptide Y: Immunocytochemical localization to and effect upon feline pial arteries and veins in vitro and in situ. *Acta physiol. Scand.*, 122: 155–163.

Ekblad, E., Edvinsson, L., Wahlestedt, C., Uddman, R., Håkanson, R. and Sundler, F. (1984) Neuropeptide Y co-exists and co-operates with noradrenaline in perivascular nerve fibres. *Regul. Peptides*, 8: 225–235.

Franco-Cereceda, A., Lundberg, J. M. and Dahlöf, C. (1985) Neuropeptide Y and sympathetic control of heart contractility and coronary vascular tone. *Acta physiol. Scand.*, 129: 361–370.

Franco-Cereceda, A. and Lundberg, J. M. (1986) Calcitonin gene-related peptide (CGRP) and capsaicin-induced stimulation of heart contractility. *N.S. Arch. Pharmacol.*, 331: 146–151.

Franco-Cereceda, A., Lundberg, J. M., Henke, H., Petermann, J. B., Hökfelt, T. and Fischer, J. A. (1986) Calcitonin gene-related peptide (CGRP) and substance P in capsaicin-sensitive sensory neurons: comparative distribution and CGRP release by capsaicin. *Regul. Peptides* (in press).

Fried, G. (1980) Small noradrenergic storage vesicles isolated from rat vas deferens — biochemical and morphological characterization. *Acta physiol. Scand.*, Suppl. 493: 1–28.

Fried, G., Lundberg, J. M. and Theodorsson-Norheim, E. (1985a) Subcellular storage and axonal transport of neuropeptide Y (NPY) in relation to catecholamines in the cat. *Acta physiol. Scand.*, 125: 145–154.

Fried, G., Terenius, L., Hökfelt, T. and Goldstein, M. (1985b) Evidence for differential localization of noradrenaline and neuropeptide Y (NPY) in neuronal storage vesicles isolated from rat vas deferens. *J. Neurosci.*, 5: 450–458.

Gamse, R., Molnar, A. and Lembeck, F. (1979) Substance P release from spinal cord slices by capsaicin. *Life Sci.*, 25: 629–636.

Hellström, P. M., Olerup, O. and Tatemoto, K. (1985) Neuropeptide Y may mediate effects of sympathetic nerve stimulation on colonic motility and blood flow in the cat. *Acta physiol. Scand.*, 124: 613–624.

Hertting, G., Axelrod, J. and Patrick, R. W. (1962a) Actions of bretylium and guanethidine on the uptake and release of ^{3}H-noradrenaline. *Brit. J. Pharmacol.*, 18: 161–166.

Hertting, G., Potter, L. and Axelrod, J. (1962b) Effects of decentralization and ganglionic-blocking agents on the spontaneous release of ^{3}H-norepinephrine. *J. Pharmacol.*, 136: 289–292.

Hirst, G. D. S. and Neild, T. O. (1980) Evidence for two populations of excitatory receptors for noradrenaline on arteriolar smooth muscle. *Nature (Lond.)*, 283: 767–768.

Hökfelt, T., Kellerth, J. O., Nilsson, G. and Pernow, B. (1975) Experimental immunohistochemical studies on the localization and distribution of substance P in cat primary sensory neurons. *Brain Res.*, 100: 235–252.

Hua, X., Lundberg, J. M., Theodorsson-Norheim, E. and Brodin, E. (1984) Comparison of cardiovascular and bronchoconstrictor effects of substance P, substance K and other tachykinins. *N.S. Arch. Pharmacol.*, 307: 196–201.

Hua, X., Theodorsson-Norheim, E., Brodin, E., Lundberg, J. M. and Hökfelt, T. (1985) Multiple tachykinins (neurokinin A, neuropeptide K and substance P) in capsaicin-sensitive sensory neurons in the guinea-pig. *Regul. Peptides*, 13: 1–19.

Itoh, W., Obata, K., Yanaihara, N. and Okamoto, H. (1983) Human mepro-vasoactive intestinal polypeptide (VIP) mRNA contains the coding sequence for a novel PHI-27 like peptide, PHM-27. *Nature (Lond.)*, 304: 547–549.

Jancsó, G., Hökfelt, T., Lundberg, J. M., Kiraly, E., Halász, N., Nilsson, G., Terenius, L., Rehfeld, J., Steinbusch, H., Vernofstad, A., Elde, R., Said, S. and Goldstein, M. (1981) Immunohistochemical studies on the effects of capsaicin on spinal and medullary peptide and monoamine neurons using antisera to substance P, gastrin/CCk, somatostatin, VIP, enkephalin, neurotensin and 5-hydroxytryptamine. *J. Neurocytol.*, 10: 963–980.

Jessell, T. M., Iversen, L. I. and Cuello, A. C. (1978) Capsaicin-induced depletion of substance P from primary sensory neurons. *Brain Res.*, 152: 183–188.

Kangawa, K., Minamino, N., Fukuda, A. and Matsuo, H. (1983) Neuromedin K: A novel mammalian tachykinin identified in porcine spinal cord. *Biochem. Biophys. Res. Commun.*, 114: 533–540.

Karlsson, J. A., Finney, M., Persson, C. G. and Post, C. (1984) Substance P antagonists and the role of tachykinins in noncholinergic bronchoconstriction. *Life Sci.*, 35: 2681–2691.

Kimura, S., Okada, M., Sugita, Y., Kanazawa, I. and Munekata, E. (1983) Novel neuropeptides, neurokinin α and β isolated from porcine spinal cord. *Proc. jap. Acad.*, 59B: 101–104.

Larsson, O., Dunér-Engström, M., Lundberg, J. M., Fredholm, B. B. and Änggård, A. (1986) Comparative effects of VIP, PHI and substance P on blood vessels and secretory elements of the human submandibular gland. *Regul. Peptides*, 13: 329–336.

Lembeck, F. and Holzer, P. (1979) Substance P as neurogenic mediator of antidromic vasodilatation and neurogenic plasma extravasation. *N.S. Arch. Pharmacol.*, 310: 175–183.

Lembeck, F., Donnerer, J.R. and Bartho, L. (1982) Inhibition of neurogenic vasodilatation and plasma extravasation by substance P antagonists, somatostatin and (D-met^{2}, Phe^{5})-enkephalinamide. *Europ. J. Pharmacol.*, 850: 171–179.

Ljung, B. (1976) Physiological patterns of neuroeffector control mechanisms: In J. A. Bevan et al. (Eds), *2nd Int. Symp. on Vascular Neuroeffector Mechanisms*, Karger, Basel, pp. 143–155.

Lundberg, J. M. (1981) Evidence for co-existence of vasoactive intestinal polypeptide (VIP) and acetylcholine in neurons of cat exocrine glands. Morphological, biochemical and functional studies. *Acta physiol. Scand.*, Suppl. 496, 112: 1–57.

Lundberg, J. M. and Hökfelt, T. (1983) Co-existence of peptides and classical neurotransmitters. *Trends Neurosci.*, 6: 325–333.

Lundberg, J. M. and Saria, A. (1983) Capsaicin-induced desensitization of the airway mucosa to cigarette smoke, mechanical and chemical irritants. *Nature (Lond.)*, 302: 251–253.

Lundberg, J. M. and Stjärne, L. (1984) Neuropeptide Y (NPY) depresses the secretion of ^{3}H-noradrenaline and the contractile response evoked by field stimulation in rat vas deferens. *Acta physiol. Scand.*, 120: 477–479.

Lundberg, J. M. and Tatemoto, K. (1982) Pancreatic polypeptide family (APP, BPP, NPY and PYY) in relation to α-adrenoceptor-resistant sympathetic vasoconstriction. *Acta physiol. Scand.*, 116: 393–402.

Lundberg, J. M., Hökfelt, T., Schultzberg, M., Uvnäs-Wallensten, K., Köhler, C. and Said, S. I. (1979) Occurrence of vasoactive intestinal polypeptide (VIP)-like immunoreactivity in certain cholinergic neurons of the cat: evidence from combined immunohistochemistry and acetylcholinesterase staining. *Neuroscience*, 4: 1539–1559.

Lundberg, J. M., Hökfelt, T., Änggård, A., Kimmel, J., Goldstein, M. and Markey, K. (1980) Co-existence of an avian pancreatic polypeptide (APP) immunoreactive substance and catecholamines in some peripheral and central neurons. *Acta physiol. Scand.*, 110: 107–109.

Lundberg, J. M., Änggård, A. and Fahrenkrug, J. (1982a) Complementary role of vasoactive intestinal polypeptide (VIP) and acetylcholine for cat submandibular blood flow and secretion. III. Effects of local infusions. *Acta physiol. Scand.*, 114: 329–338.

Lundberg, J. M., Änggård, A., Fahrenkrug, J., Lundgren, C. and Holmstedt, B. (1982b) Co-release of VIP and acetylcholine in relation to blood flow and salivary secretion in cat submandibular salivary gland. *Acta physiol. Scand.*, 115: 525–528.

Lundberg, J. M., Hedlund, B. and Bartfai, T. (1982c) Vasoactive intestinal polypeptide (VIP) enhances muscarinic ligand binding in the cat submandibular salivary gland. *Nature (Lond.)*, 295: 147–149.

Lundberg, J. M., Hökfelt, T., Änggård, A., Terenius, L., Elde, R., Markey, K. and Goldstein, M. (1982d) Organization principles in the peripheral sympathetic nervous system: Subdivision by co-existing peptides (somatostatin-, avian pancreatic polypeptide- and vasoactive intestinal polypeptide-like immunoreactive materials). *Proc. nat. Acad. Sci. USA*, 79: 1303–1307.

Lundberg, J. M., Terenius, L., Hökfelt, T., Martling, C. R., Tatemoto, K., Mutt, V., Polak, J., Bloom, S. R. and Goldstein, M. (1982e) Neuropeptide Y (NPY)-like immunoreactivity in peripheral noradrenergic neurons and effects of NPY on sympathetic function. *Acta physiol.Scand.*, 116: 477–480.

Lundberg, J. M., Martling, C. R., Saria, A., Folkers, K. and Rosell, S. (1983a) Cigarette smoke-induced oedema due to activation of capsaicin-sensitive vagal afferents and substance P release. *Neuroscience*, 10: 1361–1363.

Lundberg, J. M., Saria, A., Brodin, E., Rosell, S. and Folkers, K. (1983b) A substance P antagonist inhibits vagally induced inflammation and bronchial smooth muscle contraction in the guinea-pig. *Proc. nat. Acad. Sci. USA*, 80: 1120–1124.

Lundberg, J. M., Terenius, L., Hökfelt, L., Hökfelt, T. and Goldstein, M. (1983c) High levels of neuropeptide Y (NPY) in peripheral noradrenergic neurons in various mammals including man. *Neurosci. Lett.*, 42: 167–172.

Lundberg, J. M., Änggård, A., Theodorsson-Norheim, E. and Pernow, J. (1984a) Guanethidine-sensitive release of NPY-like immunoreactivity by sympathetic nerve stimulation. *Neurosci. Lett.*, 52: 175–180.

Lundberg, J. M., Brodin, E., Hua, X. and Saria, A. (1984b) Vascular permeability changes and smooth muscle contraction in relation to capsaicin-sensitive substance P afferents in the guinea-pig. *Acta physiol. Scand.*, 120: 217–227.

Lundberg, J. M., Fahrenkrug, J., Hökfelt, T., Martling, C.-R., Larsson, O., Tatemoto, K. and Änggård, A. (1984c) Co-existence of peptide HI (PHI) and VIP in nerves regulating blood flow and bronchial smooth muscle tone in various mammals including man. *Peptides*, 5: 593–605.

Lundberg, J. M., Fahrenkrug, J., Larsson, O. and Änggård, A. (1984d) Corelease of vasoactive intestinal polypeptide and peptide histidine isoleucine in relation to atropine-resistant vasodilation in cat submandibular salivary gland. *Neurosci. Lett.*, 52: 37–42.

Lundberg, J. M., Hua, X. Y. and Franco-Cereceda, A. (1984e) Effects of neuropeptide Y (NPY) on mechanical activity and neurotransmission in the heart, vas deferens and urinary bladder of the guinea-pig. *Acta physiol. Scand.*, 121: 325–332.

Lundberg, J. M., Hua, X. and Fredholm, B. (1984f) Capsaicin-induced stimulation of the guinea-pig atrium: Involvement of a novel sensory transmitter or a direct action on myocytes. *N.S. Arch. Pharmacol.*, 325: 176–182.

Lundberg, J. M., Saria, A., Rosell, S. and Folkers, K. (1984g) A substance P antagonist inhibits heat-induced oedema in the rat skin. *Acta physiol. Scand.*, 120: 145–146.

Lundberg, J. M., Saria, A., Änggård, A., Hökfelt, T., Terenius, L. (1984h) Neuropeptide Y and noradrenaline interaction in peripheral cardiovascular control. *Clin. exp. Theory Practice*, A6: 1961–1972.

Lundberg, J. M., Terenius, L., Hökfelt, T. and Tatemoto, K. (1984i) Comparative immunohistochemical and biochemical analysis of pancreatic polypeptide-like peptides with special reference to presence of neuropeptide Y in central and peripheral neurons. *J. Neurosci.*, 4: 2376–2386.

Lundberg, J. M., Änggård, A., Pernow, J. and Hökfelt, T. (1985a) Neuropeptide Y, substance P and VIP-immunoreactive nerves in cat spleen in relation to autonomic vascular and volume control. *Cell Tiss. Res.*, 239: 9–18.

Lundberg, J. M., Franco-Cereceda, A., Hua, X.-Y., Hökfelt, T. and Fischer, J. (1985b) Co-existence of substance P and calcitonin gene-related peptide immunoreactivities in substance P and calcitonin gene-related peptide immunoreactivities in sensory nerves in relation to cardiovascular and bronchoconstrictor effects of capsaicin. *Europ. J. Pharmacol.*, 108: 315–319.

Lundberg, J. M., Martinsson, A., Hemsén, A., Theodorsson-Norheim, E., Svedenhag, J., Ekblom, E. and Hjemdahl, P. (1985c) Co-release of neuropeptide Y and catecholamines during physical exercise in man. *Biochem. biophys. Res. Commun.*, 133: 30–36.

Lundberg, J. M., Pernow, J. and Dahlöf, C. (1985d) Pre- and postjunctional effects of NPY on sympathetic control of rat femoral artery. *Acta physiol. Scand.*, 123: 511–513.

Lundberg, J. M., Saria, A., Franco-Cereceda, Hökfelt, T., Terenius, L. and Goldstein, M. (1985e) Differential effects of reserpine and 6-hydroxydopamine on neuropeptide Y and noradrenaline in peripheral neurons. *N.S. Arch. Pharmacol.*, 328: 331–340.

Lundberg, J. M., Saria, A., Franco-Cereceda, A. and Theodorsson-Norheim, E. (1985f) Treatment with sympatholytic drugs changes tissue content of neuropeptide Y in cardiovascular nerves and adrenal gland. *Acta physiol. Scand.*, 124: 603–611.

Lundberg, J. M., Torsell, L., Sollevi, A., Theodorsson-Norheim, E., Pernow, J., Änggård, A. and Hamberger, B. (1985g) Neuropeptide Y and sympathetic vascular control in man. *Regul. Peptides*, 13: 41–52.

Lundberg, J. M., Al-Saffar, A., Saria, A. and Theodorsson-Norheim, E. (1986a) Reserpine-induced depletion of neuropeptide Y from cardiovascular nerves and adrenal gland due to neurogenic activation. *N.S. Arch. Pharmacol.*, 332: 163–168.

Lundberg, J. M., Fried, G., Pernow, J., Theodorsson-Norheim, E. And Änggård, A. (1986b) NPY — a mediator of reserpine-resistant, non-adrenergic vasoconstriction in cat spleen after preganglionic denervation? *Acta physiol. Scand.*, 126: 151–152.

Lundberg, J. M., Hemsén, A., Fried, G., Theodorsson-Norheim, E. and Lagercrantz, H. (1986c) High plasma levels of neuropeptide Y (NPY)-like immunoreactivity and catecholamines in newborn infants. *Acta physiol. Scand.*, 126: 471–473.

Lundberg, J. M., Rudehill, A., Sollevi, A., Theordorsson-Norheim, E. and Hamberger, B. (1986d) Frequency and reserpine-dependent chemical coding of sympathetic transmission: Differential release of noradrenaline and neuropeptide Y from pig spleen. *Neurosci. Lett.*, 63: 96–100.

Lundblad, L. (1984) Protective reflexes and vascular effects in the nasal mucosa elicited by activation of capsaicin-sensitive substance P-immunoreactive trigeminal neurons. *Acta physiol. Scand.*, Suppl. 529: 1–42.

Lundblad, L., Lundberg, J. M., Änggård, A. and Zetterström, O. (1985) Capsaicin pretreatment inhibits the flare component of the cutaneous allergic reaction in man. *Europ. J. Pharmacol.*, 113: 461–462.

Meldrum, L. A. and Burnstock, G. (1983) Evidence that ATP acts as a co-transmitter with noradrenaline in sympathetic nerves supplying the guinea-pig vas deferens. *Europ. J. Pharmacol.*, 92: 161–163.

Molnar, J. G., György, L., Unyi, G. and Kenyeres, J. (1969) The effect of capsaicin on the isolated guinea-pig ileum and auricle. *Acta physiol. Acad. Sci. Hung.*, 35: 369–374.

Nagy, J. (1982) Capsaicin's action on the nervous system. *Trends Neurosci.*, 5: 62–65.

Nawa, H., Hirose, T., Takashima, H., Inayama, S. and Nakanishi, S. (1983) Nucleotide sequences of cloned cDNAs for two types of bovine brain substance P precursor. *Nature (Lond.)*, 306: 32–36.

Otsuka, M. and Monishi, S. (1983) Substance P — the first peptide neurotransmitter? *Trends Neurosci.*, 6: 317–320.

Papka, R., Furness, J. B., Della, N. G., Murphy, R. and Costa, M. (1984) Time course effect of capsaicin on ultrastructure and histochemistry of substance P-immunoreactive nerves associated with the cardiovascular system of the guinea-pig. *Neuroscience*, 12: 1277–1292.

Pernow, J., Saria, A. and Lundberg, J. M. (1986) Mechanisms underlying pre- and postjunctional effects of neuropeptide Y in sympathetic vascular control. *Acta physiol. Scand.*, 126: 239–249.

Rosell, S. and Sedvall, G. (1962) The rate of disappearance of vascoconstrictor responses to sympathetic chain stimulation after reserpine treatment. *Acta physiol. Scand.*, 56: 306–314.

Rosell, S., Olgart, L., Gazelius, B., Panopoulos, P., Folkers, K. and Hong, J. (1981) Inhibition of antidromic and substance P-induced vasodilatation by a substance P antagonist. *Acta physiol. Scand.*, 111: 381–382.

Rosenfeld, M. G., Mermod, J. J., Amara, S. G., Swanson, W., Sawchenko, P., Rivier, J., Vale, W. and Evans, R. (1983) Production of a novel neuropeptide by the calcitonin gene via tissue-specific RNA processing. *Nature (Lond.)*, 304: 129–132.

Saria, A., Lundberg, J. M., Hua, X. and Lembeck, F. (1983a) Capsaicin-induced substance P release and sensory control of vascular permeability in the guinea-pig ureter. *Neurosci. Lett.*, 41: 167–172.

Saria, A., Lundberg, J. M., Skofitsch and Lembeck, F. (1983a) Vascular protein leakage in various tissues induced by substance P, capsaicin, bradykinin, serotonin, histamine and by antigen challenge. *N.S. Arch. Pharmacol.*, 324: 212–218.

Saria, A., Theodorsson-Norheim, E., Gamse, R. and Lundberg, J. M. (1985a) Release of substance P- and substance K-like immunoreactivities from the isolated perfused guinea-pig lung. *Europ. J. Pharmacol.*, 106: 207–208.

Saria, A., Theodorsson-Norheim, E. and Lundberg, J. M. (1985b) Evidence for specific neuropeptide Y-binding sites in rat brain synaptosomes. *Europ. J. Pharmacol.*, 107: 105–107.

Sedvall, G. (1964) Short-term effects of reserpine on noradrenaline levels in skeletal muscle. *Acta Physiol. Scand.*, 62: 101–108.

Sneddon, P., Westfall, D. F. and Fedan, J. S. (1982) Co-transmitters in the motor nerves of the guinea-pig vas deferens: Electrophysiological evidence. *Science N.Y.*, 218: 693–695.

Stjärne, L. and Åstrand, P. (1985) Relative pre- and postjunctional roles of noradrenaline and adenosine 5'triphosphate as neurotransmitters of the sympathetic nerves of guinea-pig and mouse vas deferens. *Neuroscience*, 3: 929–946.

Tatemoto, K. (1982) Neuropeptide Y: the complete amino-acid sequence of the brain peptide. *Proc. nat. Acad. Sci. USA*, 79: 5485–5489.

Tatemoto, K. and Mutt, V. (1981) Isolation and characterization of the intestinal peptide porcine PHI (PHI-27) a new member of the glucagon secretion family. *Proc. nat. Sci. USA*, 28: 6603–6607.

Tatemoto, K., Lundberg, J. M., Jörnvall, M. and Mutt, V. (1985) Neuropeptide K: Isolation, structure and biological activities of a novel brain tachykinin. *Biochem. biophys. Res. Commun.*, 128: 947–953.

Tippins, J. R., Morris, H. R., Panico, M., Etienne, T., Bevis, P., Girgis, S., MacIntyre, I., Pazria, M. and Attinger, M. (1984) The myotropic and plasma calcitonin modulating effects of calcitonin gene-related peptide. *Neuropeptides*, 4: 425–434.

Theodorsson-Norheim, E., Hemsén, A. and Lundberg, J. M. (1985) Radioimmunoassay for neuropeptide Y (NPY): chromatographic characterization of immunoreactivity in plasma and tissue extracts. *Scand. J. Lab. Invest.*, 45: 355–365.

Van Meel, J., De Jonger, A., Kalkman, H. H., Wilffert, B., Timmermans, P. and Van Zwielen, P. (1981) Organic and inorganic calcium antagonists reduce vasoconstriction in vivo mediated by postsynaptic $alpha_2$-adrenoceptors. *N.S. Arch. Pharmacol.*, 316: 288–293.

Von Euler, U. S. (1946) A specific sympathomimetic ergone in adrenergic nerve fibres (sympathin) and its relations to adrenaline and noradrenaline. *Acta physiol. Scand.*, 12: 73–97.

Wisenfeld-Hallin, Z., Hökfelt, T., Lundberg, J. M., Forssmann, W., Reinecke, M., Tschopp, F. and Fischer, J. (1984) Immunoreactive calcitonin gene-related peptide and substance P co-exist in sensory neurons and interact in spinal behavioural responses of the rat. *Neurosci. Lett.*, 52: 199–204.

T. Hökfelt, K. Fuxe and B. Pernow (Eds.),
Progress in Brain Research, Vol. 68

CHAPTER 17

On the possible roles of noradrenaline, adenosine 5′-triphosphate and neuropeptide Y as sympathetic cotransmitters in the mouse vas deferens

Lennart Stjärne[1] and Jan M. Lundberg[2]

Department of [1]Physiology and [2]Pharmacology, Karolinska Institutet, S-104 01 Stockholm, Sweden

Introduction

The vasa deferentia in various rodent species (guinea-pig, mouse, rat) have a uniquely high content of noradrenaline (NA; Sjöstrand, 1962), contained in postganglionic sympathetic fibres forming a dense network around the smooth muscle cells (Falck, 1962). Further, the electrical and mechanical responses to electrical nerve stimulation are depressed or abolished by the sympathetic neurotoxin 6-hydroxydopamine, as well as by the known blockers of sympathetic transmitter secretion, bretylium and guanethidine (Burnstock and Holman, 1964; Ambache and Zar, 1971; Swedin, 1971; McGrath, 1978; Sjöstrand, 1981). Hence the motor innervation of the smooth muscle has been regarded as purely sympathetic and neuro-muscular transmission as exclusively "noradrenergic", i.e. mediated by NA (Huković, 1961). However, the role of NA as the only mediator of all responses to sympathetic nerve stimulation in these tissues has been questioned (Ambache and Zar, 1971). As shown most clearly in the guinea-pig vas deferens, the excitatory junction potentials (EJPs) in smooth muscle cells, or the twitch ("phase I") contractile response to nerve stimulation, cannot be mimicked by exogenous NA, abolished by reserpine-induced depletion of the NA stores, or blocked by NA antagonists (Burnstock and Holman, 1964; Ambache and Zar, 1971; Fedan et al., 1981; Sneddon et al., 1982; Meldrum and Burnstock, 1983; Sneddon and Burnstock, 1984; Sneddon and Westfall, 1984). In contrast, these responses can be mimicked by adenosine 5′-triphosphate (ATP), a known constituent of all NA storage vesicles in sympathetic nerves (Schümann, 1958; von Euler et al., 1963; Fried, 1981; Lagercrantz and Fried, 1982), and abolished by pharmacological agents blocking or desensitizing ATP receptors (Fedan et al., 1981; Sneddon et al., 1982; Meldrum and Burnstock, 1983; Sneddon and Burnstock, 1984; Sneddon and Westfall, 1984). In view of these findings, a cotransmission hypothesis (Burnstock, 1976) has been proposed for sympathetic motor control, according to which the EJP and twitch ("phase I") contraction of the smooth muscle in rodent vas deferens are triggered by ATP, and the delayed ("phase II") contraction by NA, co-secreted with ATP, possibly from the same vesicle of the sympathetic nerve varicosities (Sneddon et al., 1982; Meldrum and Burnstock, 1983; Sneddon and Burnstock, 1984; Sneddon and Westfall, 1984).

In general agreement with this hypothesis, we have found that the electrical and mechanical responses to nerve stimulation in the guinea-pig and the mouse vas deferens do not seem to be mediated by NA alone, but at least in part also by ATP (Stjärne and Åstrand, 1984, 1985). However, our results suggest that ATP may not be the exclusive mediator of all electrical responses of the smooth muscle cells (Stjärne and Åstrand, 1984) and that the twitch ("phase I") contraction is not caused by ATP alone, nor the delayed ("phase II") contraction by NA alone. Our evidence rather indicates that both contractile responses are caused by the summed effects of NA and ATP (NA being relatively more important in the mouse and ATP relatively more important in the guinea-pig vas deferens). Further, our results indicate that a third, unknown transmitter substance may be also involved in generation of the contractile responses to nerve stimulation, in both species (Stjärne and Åstrand, 1985).

A likely candidate would be neuropeptide Y (NPY), a substance known to occur in relatively high concentration in sympathetically innervated tissues, including the vas deferens in various species (Lundberg et al., 1982b, 1983, 1984a). NPY seems to be stored in sympathetic nerves in "large dense cored" vesicles (Fried et al., 1985a,b), together with NA and ATP (Fried, 1981). As shown in cat spleen, on electrical nerve stimulation NPY may be secreted along with NA; the secretion of both substances is blocked by guanethidine, showing that both are released from sympathetic nerves (Lundberg et al., 1984b). In pig spleen it has been found that the relative proportions of secreted NA:NPY vary with the stimulation parameters; bursts at high frequency increased the secretion of NPY relatively more than that of NA (Lundberg et al., 1986). Exogenous NPY has a number of marked direct and indirect pre- and postjunctional effects, which vary in intensity with the individual sympathetically innervated tissue. Thus in some tissues and species NPY is a potent vasoconstrictor per se (Lundberg and Tatemoto, 1982), but it induces only a weak contraction of the (mouse) vas deferens (Stjärne et al., 1985). In several tissues NPY strongly enhances the smooth muscle contractile response to exogenous NA (Ekblad et al., 1984; Lundberg et al., 1985) as well as to ATP (Stjärne et al., 1985). Therefore it has been proposed that co-secretion of endogenous NPY with NA and ATP may result in amplification of the contractile response of smooth muscle to sympathetic nerve stimulation. This is not the only effect of NPY, however. Exogenous NPY has been found to also depress transmitter secretion; in the vas deferens the net effect of exogenous NPY is depression of sympathetic neuromuscular transmission (Lundberg and Stjärne, 1984; Dahlöf et al., 1985; Lundberg et al., 1985; Stjärne et al., 1985).

Evidence is thus accumulating that sympathetic neuroeffector transmission in a tissue is often mediated by more than one transmitter substance; the relative role of each transmitter seems to vary with the tissue and/or species (Stjärne and Åstrand,

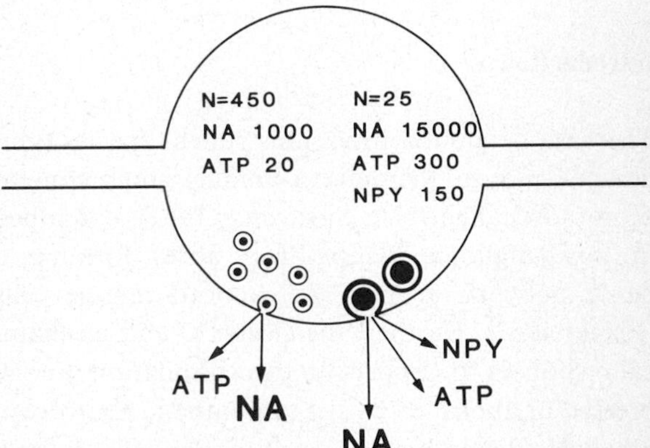

Fig. 1. Proposed model of the storage, and the possibly selective secretion, of sympathetic co-transmitters in a varicosity of the sympathetic nerves of the mouse vas deferens. The available evidence indicates that the average varicosity contains some 450 "small dense cored" vesicles, each with approximately 1000 molecules of NA and 20 molecules of ATP, and 25 "large dense cored" vesicles, each with up to 15,000 molecules of NA, 300 molecules of ATP and 150 molecules of NPY (Dahlström et al., 1966; Hökfelt, 1969; Fried, 1981; Lagercrantz and Fried, 1982; Thuresson-Klein, 1982; Fried et al., 1985a, b; Stjärne et al., 1985). The stimulus parameters may determine the proportions of the different co-transmitters secreted: at low frequency a nerve impulse may trigger (exocytotic: Smith and Winkler, 1972; Fried, 1981; Thuresson-Klein, 1983) secretion of transmitter (NA and ATP) from a "small" vesicle, while during bursts at high frequency the probability is increased that the nerve impulse will release transmitter (NA, ATP and NPY) from a "large" vesicle (Lundberg et al., 1986). It should be noted that bursts of nerve impulses at a high frequency have been observed to occur under physiological conditions in vivo, in many sympathetic nerves (Hallin and Thorebjörk, 1974). (Reproduced with permission from Stjärne et al., 1985.)

1985). In this chapter, we concentrate therefore on one tissue: the mouse vas deferens. Our aim is to discuss in some detail results indicating that sympathetic neuromuscular transmission in this tissue is not mediated by NA alone, but also by ATP and, perhaps, NPY, and to present a working hypothesis concerning the possible pre- and postjunctional roles of these three putative co-mediators of the electrical and mechanical responses to sympathetic nerve stimulation (Fig. 1).

Experimental procedures

Preparations used. Male C57 mice (15–25 g) were stunned and bled, and the vasa deferentia dissected out and mounted in perspex chambers (volume: 2 ml) perfused at 36°C at 1 ml/min with Tyrode's solution of the following composition (mM): NaCl 136.9, KCl 2.7, $CaCl_2$ 1.8, $MgCl_2$ 0.5, $NaHCO_3$ 11.9, NaH_2PO_4 0.4, glucose 5.6. The solution was gassed with 93.5% O_2 and 6.5% CO_2, giving a final pH of 7.0.

Estimation of the secretion of [^{3}H]NA. In "overflow" experiments to study the secretion of [^{3}H]NA (see Alberts et al., 1981), the vasa deferentia were preincubated at 37°C for 30 min with 2×10^{-6} M [^{3}H]NA (5 Ci/mol, New England Nuclear Co.), in Tyrode's solution containing 0.11×10^{-6} M ascorbic acid, washed and mounted in perspex chambers at a resting tension of 5 mN, in 2 ml baths perfused with [^{3}H]NA-free Tyrode's solution, at a rate of 1 ml/min. The nerves were excited by field stimulation (90 V, 0.3 msec) at various frequencies and train lengths (see figure legends), using a Grass S44 stimulator and a pair of platinum ring electrodes, either around the prostatic end of the vas deferens (electrode separation: 3 mm) or at the top and bottom of the preparation (see figure legends). The effluent was divided into 4 ml fractions and used for analysis of [^{3}H]NA. After adding 2.5 ml Instagel (Packard Instruments) to 1 ml aliquots of the effluent and of extracts of the tissue, the ^{3}H activity was counted in a Packard liquid scintillation spectrometer. In earlier work it has been shown by chromatography on alumina and Dowex 50-X4 (Graefe et al., 1973) that intact [^{3}H]NA accounts for more than 90% of the ^{3}H remaining in the tissue (Stjärne and Åstrand, 1984). Therefore, the stimulus evoked increase in efflux of ^{3}H, divided by the (calculated) ^{3}H in the tissue at the time of stimulation, was used as an approximation of the evoked secretion of [^{3}H]NA (see Alberts et al., 1981).

Measurement of the contractile responses to nerve stimulation, or to exogenous agonists. The vas deferens was mounted vertically at 5 mN resting tension in a 4 ml organ bath, during resting periods perfused at 1 ml/min with Tyrode's solution gassed with 93.5% O_2 and 6.5% CO_2, as described above. Substances to be tested were added to the bath under stop flow conditions. For nerve stimulation the perspex bath was equipped with two platinum ring electrodes (3 mm apart) close to the bottom of the bath. The prostatic end of the vas deferens was pulled just through the upper ring. The nerves were excited by field stimulation (90 V, 0.3 msec) at various frequencies and train lengths (see figure legends), using a Grass S44 stimulator. The longitudinal tension was recorded isometrically, by force displacement transducers and amplifiers (Hottinger Baldwin Messtechnik GmbH, Q 11/5 and KWS 3072, respectively) and Omniscribe recorders (Houston instrument).

Electrophysiological recordings. The right vas deferens was transferred to a 2 ml perspex chamber perfused continuously (1 ml/min) with Tyrode's solution of the composition mentioned above, gassed in the reservoir with 93.5% O_2, 6.5% CO_2. The temperature was maintained at 35–36°C. The membrane potential of smooth muscle cells on or near the surface of the preparation was recorded intracellularly (Blakeley and Cunnane, 1979; Cunnane and Stjärne, 1982, 1984a) using glass microelectrodes filled with 5 M potassium acetate (resistances 30–60 Mohms). The stimulating electrodes (chlorided Ag rings, diameter 3 mm, separation 2 mm, enclosed in an insulating teflon tube) were placed around the prostatic end of the vas deferens. Stimulation was applied in the form of trains of rectangular pulses at 0.4–1 Hz. The stimulus intensity was varied in each experiment by altering either the duration (0.05–0.4 msec) or the voltage (2–10 V) of the applied pulses (stimulators: Square One Instruments, Stimulus Isolator; or Somedic AB). Spontaneous and evoked EJPs ("sEJPs", "eEJPs") and the electrically derived dV/dt of their rising phases, "discrete events" (Blakeley and Cunnane, 1979), were recorded on magnetic tape and displayed on a Tektronix 5116 digital storage oscilloscope. Figures 2 and 10 in the present paper are slightly retouched Polaroid photographs of records displayed on the oscilloscope screen.

Assay of NPY-like immunoreactivity, and of endogenous NA. The content of NPY-like immunoreactivity (NPY-LI) was determined by radioimmunoassay (RIA). Briefly, six mice were killed by an overdose of Nembutal. Then the vas deferens (from the epididymis to the prostate) was dissected out on one side, weighed and frozen on dry ice. After heating at 95°C for 10 min in 1 M acetic acid the tissues were homogenized. Following centrifugation, the supernatant was collected and lyophilized. RIA was performed using NPY antiserum N1 which does not cross-react with peptide YY or bovine pancreatic polypeptide. The detection limit of the assay for NPY is 2 fmol/tube (Theodorsson-Norheim et al., 1985).

In a few cases, at the end of electrophysiological experiments the vasa deferentia were homogenized and extracted in 0.4 M perchloric acid. The extracts were purified and concentrated by adsorption on alumina, and the NA content measured electrochemically after separation by high pressure liquid chromatography (Hjemdahl et al., 1979).

Immunohistochemistry. Vasa deferentia from Nembutal-anaesthetized mice were dissected out, immersion-fixed in a mixture of formalin and parabenzoquinone and processed for immunohistochemistry (see Lundberg et al., 1982a). Antiserum 102D was raised against natural porcine NPY (see Lundberg et al., 1984a). To find out whether NPY-immunoreactivity co-existed with catecholamines, antisera raised against the catecholamine synthesising enzyme, tyrosine hydroxylase (TH) was used. Control sections were incubated with

Fig. 2A. Effects of pharmacological "elimination" of ATP- or NA- mediated transmission, on the spontaneous electrical activity in cells of the mouse vas deferens; representative recordings of spontaneous EJPs ("sEJPs") and their first time differentials (spontaneous discrete events, "sDEs") in different cells, under three different conditions. Top: In controls; Middle: During continuous exposure to "mATP" (α,β-methylene ATP, 10^{-5} M, added to desensitize ATP receptors, Meldrum and Burnstock, 1983); Bottom: In a preparation depleted of more than 93% of its NA content (by pretreatment with reserpine). While sEJPs and sDEs could be normal in amplitude (although depressed in frequency of occurrence) in NA-depleted preparations, these responses were lacking completely when ATP receptors were desensitized, i.e. for as long as mATP was present in the medium. (Modified and reproduced with permission from Stjärne and Åstrand, 1984.) (B) Lack of radical effects of NA depletion (by pretreatment with reserpine) on stimulus-evoked "fast" and "slow" EJPs ("eEJPs") and discrete events ("DEs"), in mouse vas deferens. Trains of stimuli of submaximal intensity at 1 Hz. Top: Control preparation (stimulus intensity: 6.5 V, 0.1 msec). Bottom: Reserpine treated preparation (stimulus intensity: 5 V, 0.1 msec). (Modified and reproduced with permission from Stjärne and Åstrand, 1984.) (C) Effects of pharmacological "elimination" of ATP-mediated transmission, on stimulus-evoked EJPs ("eEJPs") in the mouse vas deferens: representative examples of eEJPs under control conditions and during continuous exposure to "mATP" (α,β-methylene ATP, 10^{-5} M). Continuous nerve stimulation at 1 Hz, with stimuli of submaximal strength (10 V, 0.07 msec). The records were taken after completion of the initial facilitation during the first 5–10 stimuli of a train. Top: Recording in a cell under control conditions. "Fast" eEJPs of variable amplitudes occurred intermittently, superimposed on non-intermittent "slow" eEJPs of relatively constant amplitudes. Bottom: Recording in a different cell, in the presence of mATP. "Fast" eEJPs did not occur for as long (up to 1 h) as mATP was present in the medium; "slow" eEJPs were incompletely suppressed, and could be increased in amplitude by increasing the stimulus intensity (this never caused the appearance of "fast" eEJPs; not shown here but see reference below). (Modified and reproduced with permission from Stjärne and Åstrand, 1984.)

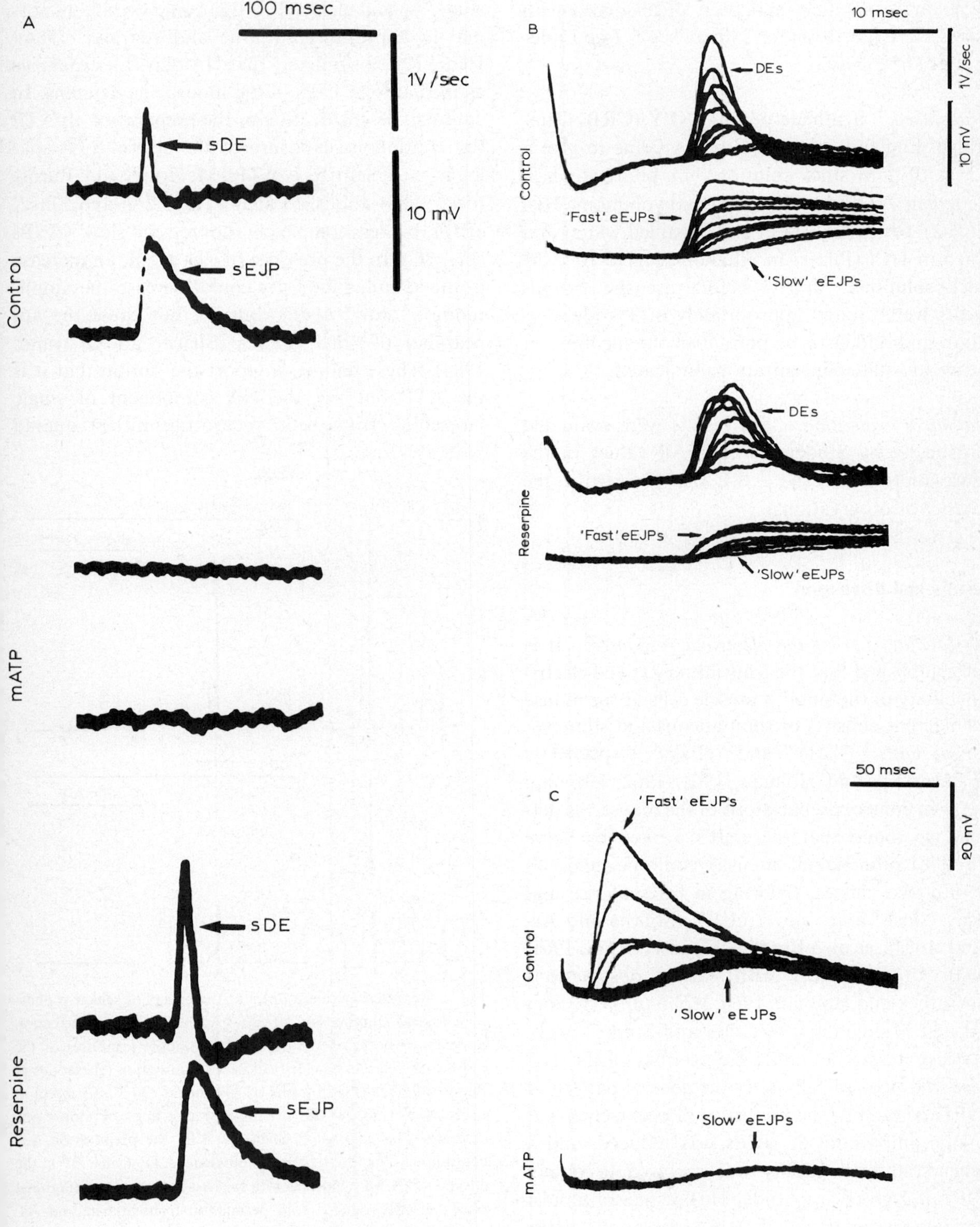
A
100 msec
1V/sec
10 mV
sDE
sEJP
Control
mATP
sDE
sEJP
Reserpine
B
10 msec
1V/sec
10 mV
DEs
Control
'Fast' eEJPs
'Slow' eEJPs
DEs
Reserpine
'Fast' eEJPs
'Slow' eEJPs
C
50 msec
20 mV
'Fast' eEJPs
Control
'Slow' eEJPs
'Slow' eEJPs
mATP

NPY antiserum that had been preabsorbed with excess NPY (10^{-5} M) for 24 h at +4°C (see Lundberg et al., 1984a).

Drugs used. Synthetic porcine NPY (CRB, Cambridge, England) was dissolved in saline to give a 2.3×10^{-4} M stock solution. NA bitartrate, α,β-methylene ATP, clonidine HCl and yohimbine HCl (Sigma) were dissolved in glass distilled water, and prazosin HCl (Pfizer) in ethanol, to give 10^{-2} M stock solutions. Shortly before use the various agents were diluted appropriately in Tyrode's solution and added to be present in the medium, at the steady state concentrations indicated.

Statistical evaluation. The results were evaluated statistically by Student's *t*-test. All values in the figures represent means ± S.E. of mean (*n* gives the number of observations).

Results and discussion

(A) *Mediator(s) of the electrical responses.* It is well established that the transmitter-evoked electrical activity of the smooth muscle cells of the mouse vas deferens consists of spontaneous and stimulus-evoked EJPs ("sEJPs" and "eEJPs" respectively; cf. Burnstock and Holman, 1961, 1962; Holman, 1970). In control preparations of the mouse vas deferens we found that the eEJPs evoked by nerve stimuli of submaximal intensity could be subdivided into two classes, differing in rates of rise and decay: "fast" and "slow" eEJPs (Stjärne and Åstrand, 1984; see also Burnstock and Holman, 1961, 1962). In agreement with earlier observations (Burnstock and Holman, 1964; Holman, 1970; Bennett and Middleton, 1975; Illés and Starke, 1983), extensive reserpine-induced depletion of the NA stores did not radically alter the general pattern of sEJPs and eEJPs. The frequency of occurrence (but not the amplitude) of sEJPs was reduced, and a higher stimulus intensity was required to obtain eEJPs of a given amplitude, but in spite of almost complete (more than 93%) NA depletion, sEJPs (Fig. 2A) and eEJPs (Fig. 2B) could be largely normal in appearance (Stjärne and Åstrand, 1984). Hence it seems unlikely that NA plays a crucial role as mediator of EJPs in the mouse vas deferens. In contrast, desensitization of the preparation to ATP (by continuous exposure to the stable ATP analogue, α,β-methylene ATP; Meldrum and Burnstock, 1983) abolished sEJPs (Fig. 2A) and "fast" eEJPs, but less completely suppressed "slow" eEJPs (Fig. 2C). In the presence of this agent, an increase in the stimulus intensity could increase the amplitude of "slow" eEJPs, but did not cause the appearance of "fast" eEJPs (Stjärne and Åstrand, 1984). These findings support the notion that it is the ATP but not the NA component of single "mixed" sympathetic neurotransmitter quanta

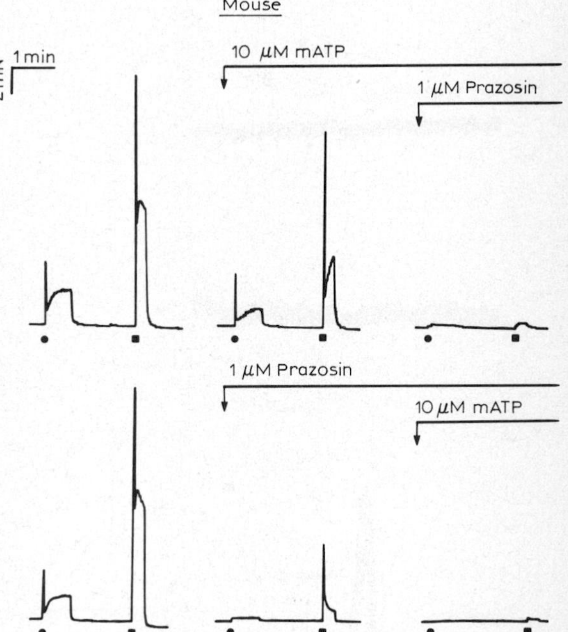

Fig. 3. Representative examples of the effects of selective pharmacological "elimination" of either ATP- or NA-mediated components, or both, on the diphasic contractile responses of the mouse vas deferens to electrical nerve stimulation (electrodes at the prostatic end) with trains of 300 shocks (90 V, 0.3 msec) at 8 Hz (●) or 20 Hz (■) in single preparations of mouse vas deferens. To "eliminate" effects of ATP the preparation was continuously exposed to α,β-methylene ATP ("mATP"); the effects of NA were blocked with the α_1-adrenoceptor antagonist prazosin. (Reproduced with permission from Stjärne and Åstrand, 1985.)

which mediates sEPJs and "fast" eEJPs; the genesis of "slow" eEJPs is unclear (Stjärne and Åstrand, 1984). It should be noted that although NA did not seem to play a crucial role as trigger of the electrical responses, this transmitter may still indirectly influence EJPs by amplifying the effects of ATP (Stjärne and Åstrand, 1984). The smooth muscle membrane was not distinctly depolarized by bath application of NPY in concentrations up to 10^{-6} M (not shown). It seems unlikely therefore that endogenous NPY plays a major role as trigger of EJPs (Stjärne et al., 1985).

(B) *Mediators of the mechanical responses.* Nerve stimulation with single shocks does not contract the mouse vas deferens, which responds typically to trains of stimuli at frequencies above 4 Hz, with a diphasic contraction (Fig. 3). Both "phase I" and "phase II" of the contractile responses were depressed (but not abolished) by "elimination" of NA-mediated effects (by reserpine-induced NA depletion, or by addition of the α_1-adrenoceptor blocking agent prazosin), or of ATP-mediated effects (by continuous exposure to α,β-methylene ATP). A combination of both procedures depressed both responses by more than 95% (Fig. 3; Stjärne and Åstrand, 1985). The effects on "phase I" contractions are shown in more detail in Fig. 4, which also illustrates several characteristic features of "autoinhibition" of transmitter secretion mediated by prejunctional α_2-adrenoceptors (an item discussed below, under C).

A reasonable conclusion from these results would be that the electrical and mechanical effects of sympathetic nerve stimulation in this preparation are caused almost exclusively by the combined pre- and postjunctional effects of NA and ATP (Fig. 5). However, as shown in Fig. 6, it seems difficult to explain all aspects of the contractile responses to nerve stimulation purely in terms of the calculated concentrations of NA and ATP at the smooth muscle receptors. Thus the strikingly sigmoid shape of the curves describing the twitch contractions as functions of the train length and/or frequency of nerve stimulation (see also Fig. 4) contrasts sharply with the smooth, upward concave curve showing the calculated "instant" concentration of NA (and presumably, also of co-secreted ATP) at the receptors (Fig. 6). The sudden, sharp increase in the contractile response when the stimulus frequency or

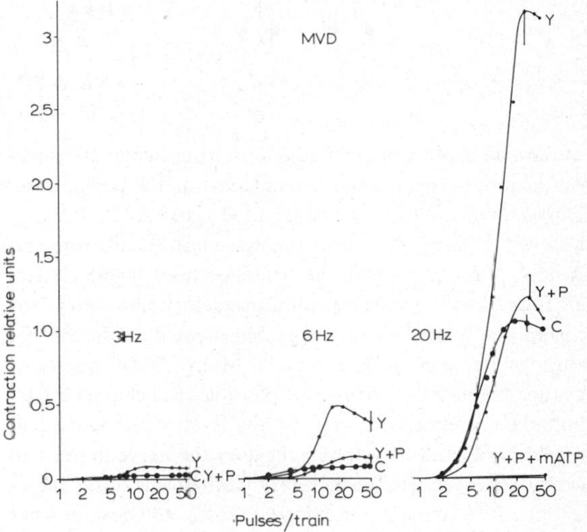

Fig. 4. Effects of pharmacological "elimination" of NA- and ATP-mediated transmission, on the contractile response of the mouse vas deferens to electrical nerve stimulation (electrodes at the prostatic end) at 3, 6 or 20 Hz, as a function of train length. C: Controls, in the absence of pharmacological agents; Y: in the presence of the α_2-adrenoceptor antagonist yohimbine (10^{-6} M), added to block NA-mediated "autoinhibition"; Y + P: in the presence of yohimbine + the α_1-adrenoceptor antagonist prazosin (10^{-6} M); Y + P + mATP: in the presence of yohimbine + prazosin + α,β-methylene ATP ("mATP", 10^{-5} M). Note the strikingly sigmoid form of all curves: a minimum of 3 shocks/train was required to trigger a twitch contraction; above this threshold there was a sharp increase in contractile amplitude with increasing train length. Yohimbine did not enhance contractions in NA-depleted preparations; hence presumably the up to 4-fold yohimbine-induced increase in twitch contractions in preparations with a normal NA content was due to blockade of α_2-adrenoceptor mediated "autoinhibition" of transmitter secretion (Stjärne and Åstrand, 1985). Note that the effect of yohimbine became apparent only when the train length exceeded 6 shocks (for comments, see text). Addition of prazosin reduced contractions by about 2/3, and further addition of mATP (shown only at 20 Hz, but the effect was similar at the other frequencies) almost completely suppressed the remaining contraction. Thus apparently NA mediated about 2/3 and ATP 1/3 of the twitch contractions under these conditions. All points are the means of 8–10 observations. The vertical bars show typical examples of the S.E.

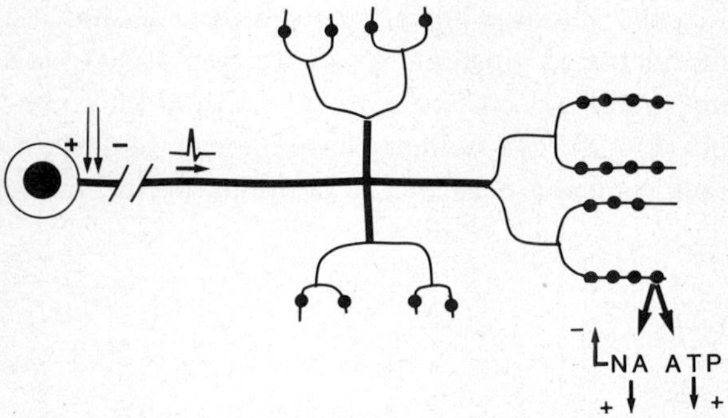

Fig. 5. Can all aspects of sympathetic neuromuscular transmission in the mouse vas deferens be explained on the basis of pre- and postjunctional effects of quanta of NA and ATP? The diagram shows an "idealized" sympathetic neuron (Dahlström and Häggendal, 1966) in rodent vas deferens: total length of terminals 10 cm, about 20,000 potentially secretory varicosities (for their supply of "small" and "large dense cored" vesicles, and their transmitter content, see Fig. 1). Many crucial questions remain unanswered, concerning the physiological characteristics of "stimulus-secretion coupling" at the level of the individual varicosity. How, and to what extent does the nerve impulse in the parent axon activate the secretory mechanisms of the individual varicosity (Cunnane and Stjärne, 1984b), and how (at what site? by what mechanism? to what extent?) do the transmitter substances secreted from a varicosity "autoinhibit" the secretory mechanisms? Based on combined electrophysiological (Cunnane and Stjärne, 1982, 1984a; Cunnane, 1984) and biochemical analysis (Stjärne, 1985), a working hypothesis has been proposed, according to which the total population of varicosities behaves in part as a "digital" system (but see below concerning the influence of stimulation frequency); the secretory mechanisms of the individual varicosity are only rarely activated (by 1–3 out of 100 stimuli; "p" 0.01–0.03), and then respond in a "one-or-none" manner, secreting only a single transmitter quantum (Cunnane and Stjärne, 1982, 1984a), presumably the NA and ATP contained in a "small dense cored" vesicle (Stjärne and Åstrand, 1984). ATP acts almost exclusively postjunctionally, while NA in addition to stimulating the smooth muscle also "autoinhibits" the secretory mechanisms (Stjärne, 1985; Stjärne and Åstrand, 1985).

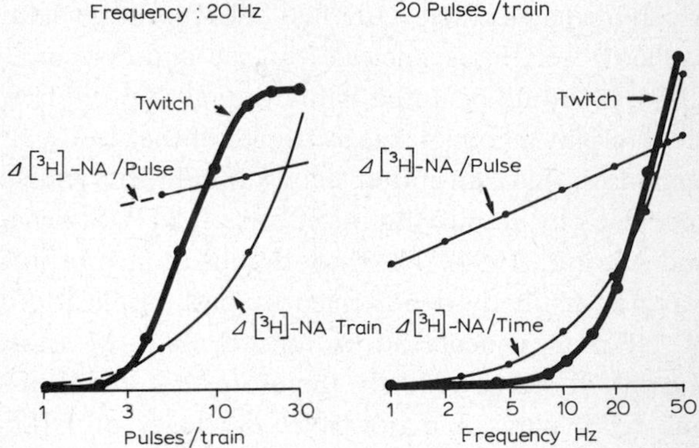

Fig. 6. An attempt to correlate the measured amplitude of the nerve stimulation-induced contractile response of the mouse vas deferens with the calculated "instant" concentration of transmitters (endogenous NA and co-secreted ATP, as inferred from measurement of the secretion of [^{3}H]NA). The diagram shows the amplitudes of "phase I" (twitch) contractions, and the fractional secretion of [^{3}H]NA (expressed per pulse, per train or per time; see Methods, p. 265), evoked by nerve stimulation at 20 Hz with trains of increasing length, or with 20-shock trains at increasing frequency (stimulating electrodes at prostatic end). Vertical scales are linear (relative units); horizontal scales logarithmic. For calculation of the secretion of [^{3}H]NA as a function of the length of stimulus trains, the preparations were stimulated at 20 Hz with 300 shocks, either in one sequence, or in repeated trains of 5, 15 or 50 shocks, separated by 10 sec stimulus-free intervals. For determination of the frequency dependence of the secretion of [^{3}H]NA they were stimulated with 300 shocks at various frequencies from 1 to 50 Hz. All points represent the mean values of four observations. The sudden steep increase in tension as the threshold in train length or frequency was exceeded is not obviously related to the secretion of NA (or of ATP, presumably), either expressed per train or per unit time, and hence probably not to the concentration of these transmitters at the smooth muscle receptors. For further comments see text.

train length were increased above certain threshold levels seems to require additional explanation. The sigmoid form suggests that some kind of "co-operative" mechanism may be involved, acting either postjunctionally, e.g. by increasing lateral interaction between neighbouring activated sites on the smooth muscle, or prejunctionally, e.g. by increasing secretion of a third, unknown transmitter, amplifying the effects of co-secreted NA and ATP (the amplifying transmitter would have to be essentially devoid of a contractile effect of its own, since as mentioned above blockade or desensitization of NA and ATP receptors almost completely inhibited the contractile responses of the mouse vas deferens to nerve stimulation; Stjärne and Åstrand, 1985).

Our results are compatible with the possibility that "prejunctional co-operativity", mediated by increasing co-secretion of NPY along with NA and

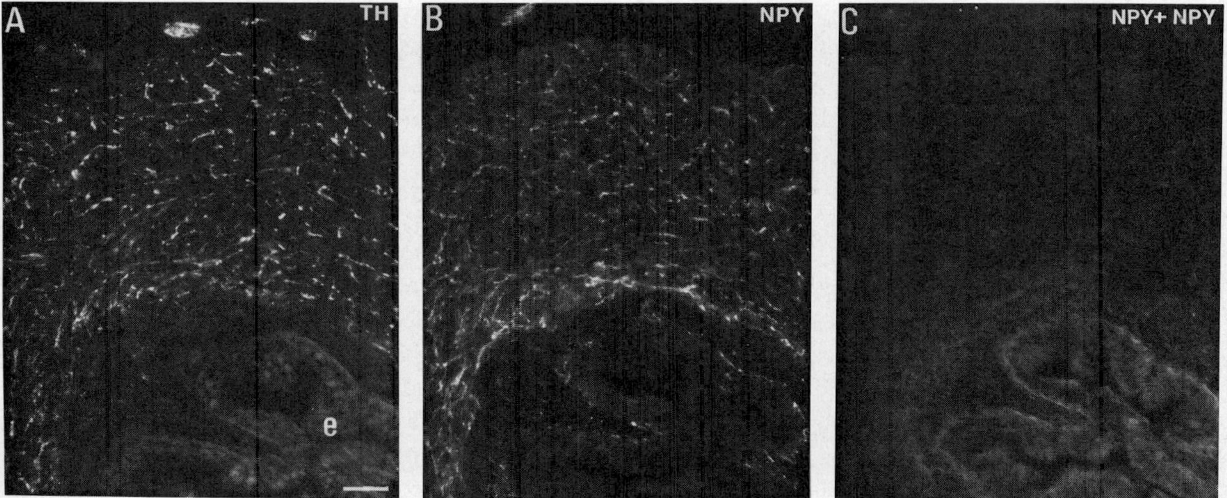

Fig. 7. Immunofluorescence micrographs of the prostatic portion of the mouse vas deferens after incubation with antiserum, (A) to tyrosine hydroxylase (TH) and (B) to NPY, or (C) with NPY antiserum which had been preabsorbed with an excess of NPY. Note the similar distribution of TH- and NPY-immunoreactive nerve fibres in the smooth muscle layers while NPY-immunoreactive nerves close to the luminal epithelium (e) seem to lack corresponding TH-immunoreactivity. No NPY-immunoreactive fibres can be seen after incubation with antiserum that was preabsorbed with NPY (C). Bar in (A) indicates 50 μm. All micrographs have the same magnification.

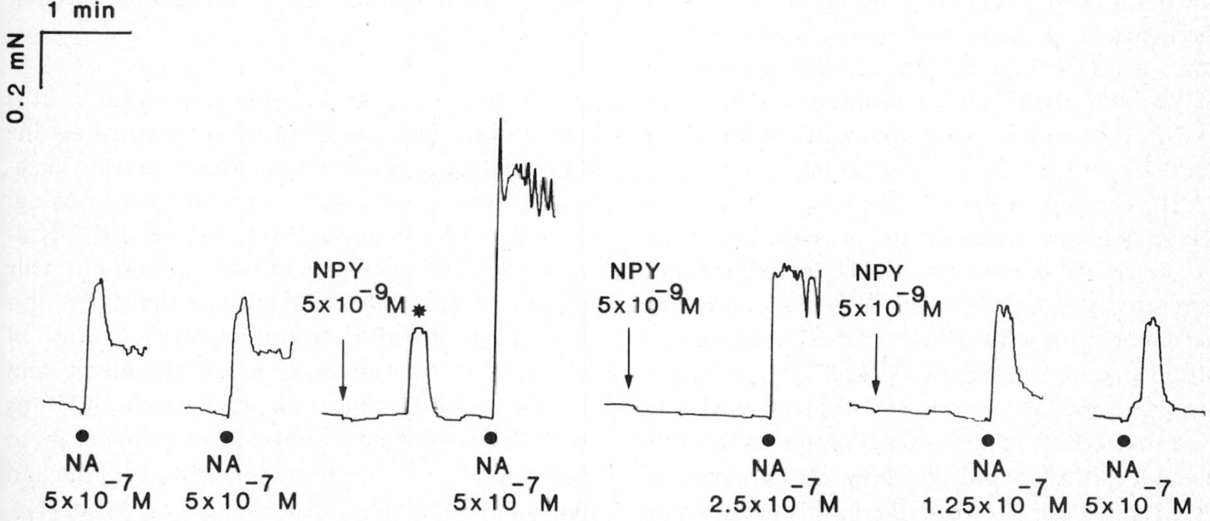

Fig. 8. Examples of the enhancing effect of NPY on the mechanical contractions caused by submaximal concentrations of noradrenaline (NA). In this preparation which was unusually sensitive, NPY per se could induce phasic contractions (*, the more consistent effect of higher concentrations of NPY in all preparations was a small long-lasting tonic contraction; see Fig. 11), and from 5×10^{-10} M dose-dependently increased the contractile response to NA (added 1.5 min later). Shown is the 5-fold increase in the response to NA, by 5×10^{-9} M NPY. Dots denote additions of NA to the final concentrations indicated. NPY potentiated the contractile response to exogenous NA even when the two substances were added simultaneously to the bath (not shown). (Reproduced with permission from Stjärne et al., 1985.)

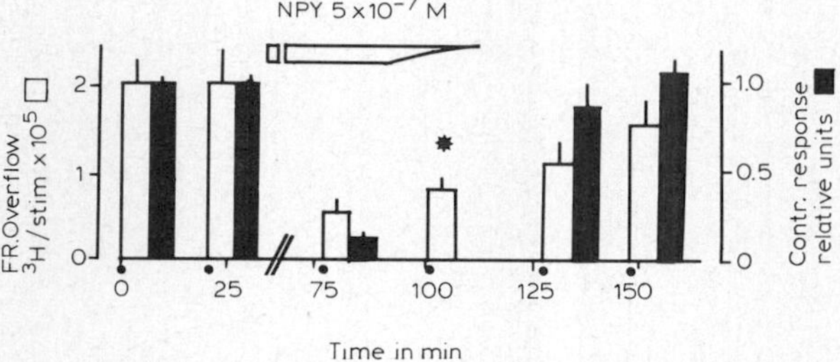

Fig. 9. Comparison of the inhibitory effects of exogenous NPY on the secretion of [³H]NA and on the contractile response to nerve stimulation, in the mouse vas deferens. NPY (5×10^{-7} M) was present in the medium for 20 min before, and during the 3rd stimulation period (wash with NPY-free Tyrode's solution started before the 4th stimulation period). Field stimulation (electrodes at top and bottom of the preparation) at 10 Hz, with 5×20 pulses with 10-sec intervals, or with one pulse train of 100 shocks (*). Vertical bars indicate S.E. ($n = 4$). Note similarities and differences in the extent and time course of the inhibitory effects of NPY on the secretory and contractile responses. (Reproduced with permission from Stjärne et al., 1985.)

ATP, may be one factor responsible for the steep increase in tension on nerve stimulation with increasing frequency (and train length?). The reasons are the following: (1) NPY occurs in the sympathetic nerves of the mouse vas deferens: the tissue has a relatively high content of NPY (molar ratio of NA:NPY about 300:1; Stjärne et al., 1985), most of which according to immunohistochemical evidence is located in NA-containing nerves (Fig. 7A,B). Thus the majority of the nerve cell bodies of the sympathetic nerves (at the prostatic end of the vas deferens) showed both TH and NPY-immunoreactivity, and TH- and NPY-immunoreactive nerve fibres formed a closely similar, dense network in the smooth muscle layers (Fig. 7A), as well as around local blood vessels. It should be noted however that NPY-immunoreactive fibres close to the luminal epithelium did not show TH-immunoreactivity; hence some of the NPY in this tissue occurs in "non-adrenergic" nerve fibres (cf. Figs. 7A,B; Fried et al., 1986). (2) Judging from findings in pig spleen (Lundberg et al., 1985) the secretion of NPY from the sympathetic nerves in the mouse vas deferens, and hence the concentration of NPY at the smooth muscle receptors, may similarly to the contraction increase steeply with the stimulation frequency (whether or not this is the case remains to be determined experimentally). (3) Exogenous NPY (at concentrations from 10^{-9} M) "instantly" increased the contractile effects of submaximal concentrations of exogenous NA or ATP in the mouse vas deferens, by 2 to 4-fold (shown for NA, in Fig. 8). Hence if the secretion of endogenous NPY is preferentially increased at high nerve impulse frequency, the effect may well be an increase in the evoked contraction, due to potentiation of the contractile effects of co-secreted NA and ATP. (4) NPY was found to have the required property mentioned above, to be almost devoid of a contractile effect of its own, in the mouse vas deferens (see Fig. 11). Therefore, the finding that pharmacological "elimination" of the transmitter effects of NA and ATP almost completely abolished the contractile responses to nerve stimulation does not exclude that endogenous NPY plays a quantitatively important role as an amplifier of the contractile response to nerve stimulation (Stjärne et al., 1985). Whether or not this is actually the case remains to be determined when specific NPY antagonists become available.

(C) *Mediators of prejunctional "autocontrol".* It is well known that endogenous NA may depress the secretory mechanisms of sympathetic nerves via activation of prejunctional α_2-adrenoceptors (see e.g. Gillespie, 1980; Langer, 1981; Starke, 1981; Kalsner, 1984 and references in that symposium). Our results in the vas deferens indicate that NPY also may exert powerful "autoinhibitory" control of sympathetic transmitter secretion (Lundberg and Stjärne, 1984; Stjärne et al., 1985), while ATP (as such or after degradation to adenosine) appears to be less potent (or inert) in this regard (Stjärne and Åstrand, 1985). Thus exogenous α_2-agonists (NA or clonidine, from 10^{-8} M; cf. Cunnane, 1984) or NPY (from 10^{-9} M) dose-dependently and reversibly depressed the secretion of [³H]NA (shown for NPY in Fig. 9) and (in most but not all cells) depressed or abolished the stimulus-evoked, but not the spontaneous EJPs (Fig. 10A,B). The selective

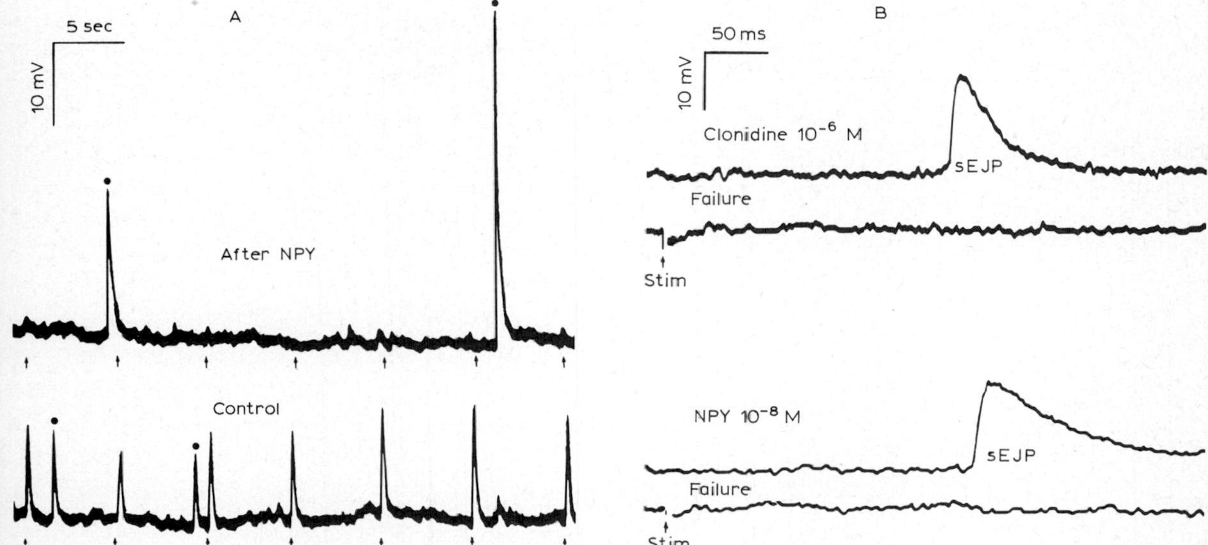

Fig. 10A. Differential effect of NPY on stimulus-evoked EJPs ("eEJPs") and on spontaneously occurring EJPs ("sEJPs") in a smooth muscle cell of the mouse vas deferens. Continuous stimulation at 0.4 Hz (4 V, 0.1 msec). NPY was added directly to the 2 ml bath (0.1 nmol NPY in 200 μl, stop flow conditions; final average concentration: 5×10^{-8} M; 3 min later perfusion with NPY-free medium was resumed). Starting about 1 min after addition of NPY, eEJPs became increasingly depressed in amplitude, then started to fail intermittently and after 2.5 min were abolished completely, while sEJPs were unchanged (or increased) in frequency of occurrence and in amplitude. The effect on eEJPs persisted for a long time (up to 30 min) during wash. Lower trace: During the control period before NPY all stimuli evoked an eEJP. Shown are 7 eEJPs (no failures) and 2 sEJPs (dots). Top trace: In this cell NPY abolished eEJPs but did not depress sEJPs; the effect persisted for 30 min during wash. Representative record 4 min after starting wash. At higher sweep speed it could be seen that none of the EJPs during this period occurred within 150 msec after the stimulus artifact; hence both EJPs in the top trace were "spontaneous" ("sEJPs"); they were normal or increased in amplitude. The membrane potential showed some drift, but remained in the range −60–70 mV under both conditions. Arrows denote nerve stimuli. Dots represents sEJPs. (Reproduced with permission from Stjärne et al., 1985.) (B) Examples of the selective inhibitory effect of clonidine (upper panel) and of NPY (lower panel) on evoked electrical responses, but not on spontaneous activity (two different preparations). Continuous field stimulation at 0.4 Hz (4 V, 0.3 msec). Under control conditions every stimulus evoked an eEJP in all cells of these preparations. In the cells shown, 5–10 min after addition of clonidine or NPY, all stimuli failed to evoked an eEJP, while sEJPs were not depressed. In each panel the upper trace shows an sEJP, and the lower trace failure of a stimulus to evoke an eEJP. Membrane potential: About −60 mV. (Clonidine effect reproduced with permission from Stjärne et al., 1985.)

blockade of evoked responses shows that the inhibitory effect of these agents is not directed towards the secretory step as such, but towards the mechanisms whereby this step is normally activated by nerve impulses. Clonidine and NPY also strongly depressed (mainly "phase I" of) the contractile responses to nerve stimulation (shown for NPY in Fig. 11; note the considerable latency of this effect).

The results shown in Fig. 4 illustrate two important features of the "autoinhibition" exerted by endogenous NA, via prejunctional α_2-adrenoceptors: (1) Its *scope*: since yohimbine did not increase the contractile response to nerve stimulation in NA-depleted preparations (Stjärne and Åstrand, 1985), presumably the magnitude of the yohimbine-induced (maximally 4-fold, at 6 Hz) increase in twitch contractions in controls, reflects the extent to which neuro-muscular transmission in this tissue is "normally" depressed by endogenous NA. (2) Its *trigger mechanisms*: yohimbine did not enhance the contractile response to trains shorter than 6 shocks (cf. Rand et al., 1982). This shows that the NA concentration and/or distribution under the resting conditions in vitro was insufficient to inhibit tonically the secretory mechanisms. The finding that approximately the same number of shocks was required to

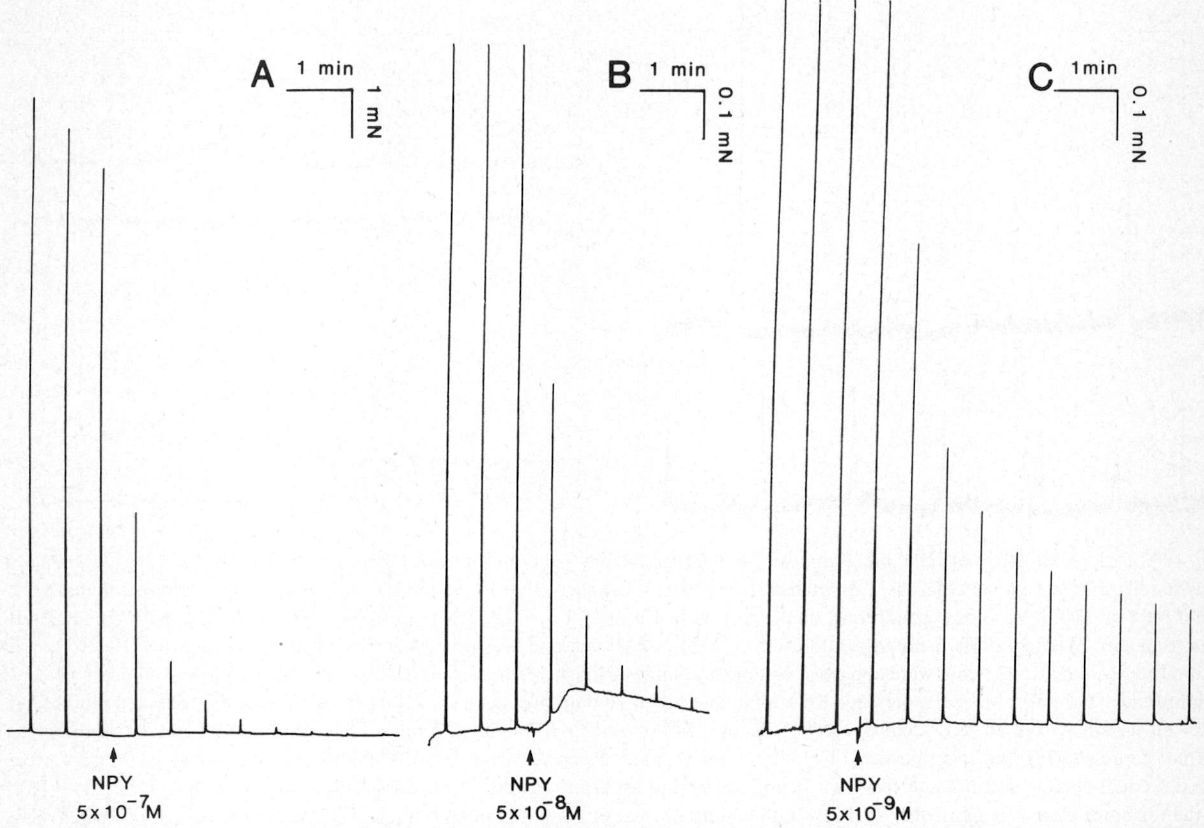

Fig. 11. Examples of two mechanical effects of NPY: (1) the dose-dependent NPY-induced rise in resting tension (threshold concentration: 5×10^{-9} M NPY; time to peak: 1–2 min), and (2) the depression of the twitch response to field stimulation with trains of 20 shocks at 10 Hz, with 1 min intervals (threshold concentration: less than 5×10^{-9} M NPY; after maximal effect, about 4 min). Yohimbine 10^{-6} M present; this agent increased twitch amplitudes by about 2-fold, and "exaggerated" the inhibitory effect of NPY on twitch contractions, when compared to controls in the absence of yohimbine. Three different concentrations of NPY were tested on the same preparation. Note the increased gain in B and C (for better visibility of direct contractile effects of NPY); here twitch peaks before NPY are off scale. NPY caused a small increase in the resting tension, but strongly depressed the twitch response to nerve stimulation. (Modified and reproduced with permission from Stjärne et al., 1985.)

begin to trigger "α-autoinhibition", independently of the stimulation frequency, shows that the threshold for this mechanism is not related to *latency in time* (cf. Gillespie, 1980; Starke, 1981; Rand et al., 1982; in our experiments at 3 Hz the minimum latency was 2 sec; at 20 Hz it was 0.3 sec). Nor is it related to a certain *minimum concentration of NA* at the receptors (since due to frequency dependent facilitation, presumably the *average* NA concentration extraneuronally after 6 shocks was at least 10-fold higher at 20 Hz than at 3 Hz). The threshold may rather be related somehow to a *minimum number of activated release sites* (each responding presumably to only 1% of the stimuli and then releasing only a single quantum; cf. Cunnane and Stjärne, 1982, 1984a). The time course of possible "autoinhibition" of transmitter secretion by endogenous NPY is not known. The brief latency of development of the "autoinhibitory" effect of *endogenous* NA (Fig. 4: latency for beginning and maximal effect at 3 Hz, 2 and 3 sec; at 20 Hz, 0.3 and 1.5 sec, respectively) contrasts sharply with the slowness of onset and development of the inhibitory effect of *exogenous* α_2-agonist (or of exogenous NPY; see

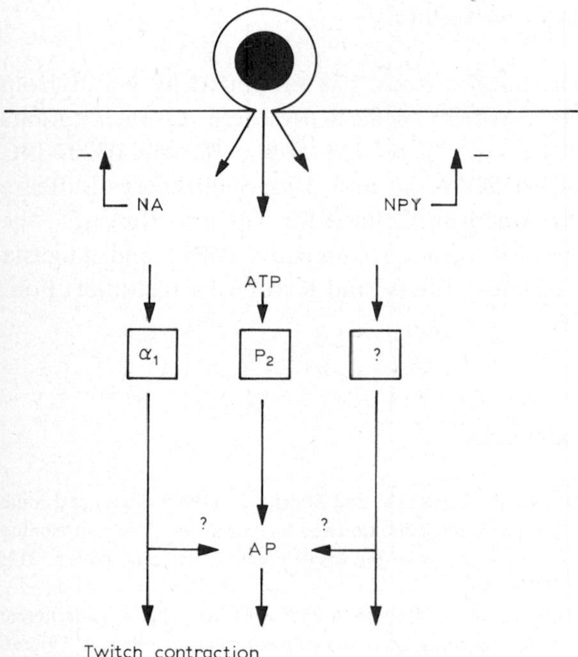

Fig. 12. Diagram to illustrate our working hypothesis concerning the possible roles of NA, ATP and NPY as putative co-transmitters mediating neuro-muscular control in the mouse vas deferens by pre- and postjunctional effects: (a) The stimulus parameters determine (cf. Fig. 1) whether transmitter will be secreted (A) from "small" (NA + ATP) or (B) from "large" vesicles (NA + ATP + NPY); high frequency bursts increase the probability for (B). (b) ATP is the main "electrogenic" transmitter, i.e. the main mediator of the EJP and the muscle action potential ("AP"). The relative importance of ATP as a motor transmitter may be limited to "close" neuromuscular junctions (Stjärne and Åstrand, 1984). (c) NA is both important as an excitatory (on the smooth muscle) and inhibitory (on the nerve terminals) transmitter. NA may stimulate the muscle without changing the membrane potential, but may also indirectly affect EJPs and muscle APs by increasing the sensitivity of the smooth muscle to ATP (Stjärne and Åstrand, 1984). Local "autoinhibition" of transmitter secretion by NA may provide a mechanism for negative feedback control (i.e. stabilization) of the *extrajunctional* concentration of NA; this parameter may be important for regulation of the excitability of the tissue to transmitter quanta (Schipper, 1979; Stjärne and Åstrand, 1984; Stjärne, 1985). (d) NPY has little effect per se on the smooth muscle of mouse vas deferens, but with increasing nerve impulse frequency NPY may be an increasingly important "instant amplifier" of the effects of its co-transmitters, NA and ATP ("booster" effect of NPY). Presumably with some delay, NPY may locally "turn off" transmitter secretion in active regions of the nerve endings. The function may be to prevent local secretory overload ("economy" effect of NPY; Stjärne et al., 1985).

Fig. 11). The latency difference may be due in part to differences in diffusion delay, but as discussed elsewhere (Stjärne, 1982), they may also reflect more fundamental differences between the modes of inhibition of transmitter secretion by exogenous and endogenous agonist.

(D) *A working hypothesis for the relative roles of NA, ATP and NPY in sympathetic neuro-muscular transmission in the mouse vas deferens.* In our opinion the simplest assumption to explain the results presented above is that NA, ATP and NPY are co-mediators of sympathetic neuro-muscular transmission in this tissue. The evidence is strong for NA and ATP; as yet, due to lack of specific pharmacological blocking agents, it is weaker for NPY. The main features of our current working hypothesis concerning the relative roles of these three putative co-transmitters in this junction are the following (Fig. 12, and legend): (a) NA exerts potent pre- and postjunctional effects, but is not the exclusive mediator of the nerve signal across this junction. (b) ATP, which seems to act almost exclusively postjunctionally, plays an important role as sympathetic co-transmitter with NA (Fedan et al., 1981; Sneddon, Westfall and Fedan, 1982; Meldrum and Burnstock, 1983; Sneddon and Burnstock, 1984; Sneddon and Westfall, 1984), but is not the exclusive mediator of EJPs (apparently "slow" eEJPs are not triggered by ATP alone; Stjärne and Åstrand, 1984), or of "phase I" contractions (both "phase I" and "phase II" contractions in this tissue seem to be caused by co-operative interaction between NA and ATP, possibly aided by NPY; Stjärne and Åstrand, 1985; Stjärne et al., 1985). (c) NPY may play an increasingly important dual role as co-transmitter with NA and ATP, with increasing nerve impulse frequency. Postjunctionally in this tissue its effects would be expressed almost exclusively through the co-transmitters, NPY acting as "instant" amplifier of the effects of NA and ATP on the smooth muscle. Prejunctionally NPY may act as a delayed local inhibitor of transmitter secretion (Stjärne et al., 1985). (d) The "autoinhibitory" prejunctional effects are "digital", i.e. involve further reduction of the (intrinsically low; cf. Cunnane and Stjärne, 1982, 1984a) proportion of "monoquantal" varicosities activated by a nerve impulse (Stjärne, 1985). The prejunctional effects of NA and NPY do not coincide in *time* (they seem to be delayed; Stjärne et al., 1985) and/or in *space* (they may be exerted extra- rather than intrajunctionally; cf. Stjärne 1978, 1982) with their excitatory postjunctional effects on the smooth muscle cells.

A corollary to this working hypothesis is that it is inappropriate to continue to characterize sympathetic nerve fibres as "noradrenergic" (or, worse, as "adrenergic"), purely on the basis of their high NA content (since they seem to be in part also "ATP-ergic", and possibly "NPY-ergic"). More generally, as long as each neurone was thought to act through a single transmitter substance the terms "adrenergic" or "cholinergic", for fibres in the autonomic system and their effects (Dale, 1934), have been useful. However, it seems wrong to apply this nomenclature to nerves known to utilize multiple transmitters (e.g. "X", "Y" and "Z"). Here it may be meaningful to describe results of stimulation in terms of "X-", "Y-" or "Z-ergic" *effects,* but it appears inappropriate and potentially misleading to label the *nerve fibres* themselves as either "X-", "Y-" or "Z-ergic".

Conclusions

In our opinion the most reasonable hypothesis to satisfy the available experimental evidence is that sympathetic neuro-muscular transmission in the mouse vas deferens involves complex pre- and post-junctional interactions between three transmitter substances: NA, ATP and NPY. The validity of the hypothesis for the mouse vas deferens, and its applicability to other sympathetic neuro-effector junctions, remain to be established in future work.

Acknowledgements

The present study was supported by grants from the Swedish Medical Research Council (grants B84-85-14X-03027-15A-16B, B8304X-03207-14C 14X-6554), Knut and Alice Wallenbergs Stiftelse, the American Council for Tobacco Research, the Swedish Tobacco Company, Petrus and Augusta Hedlunds Stiftelse and Karolinska Institutets Fonder.

References

Alberts, P., Bartfai, T. and Stjärne, L. (1981) Site(s) and ionic basis of α-autoinhibition and facilitation of ^{3}H-noradrenaline secretion in guinea-pig vas deferens. *J. Physiol. (Lond.)*, 312: 297–334.

Ambache, N. and Zar, M. A. (1971) Evidence against adrenergic motor transmission in the guinea-pig vas deferens. *J. Physiol. (Lond.)*, 216: 359–389.

Bennett, M. R. and Middleton, J. (1975) An electrophysiological analysis of the effects of reserpine on adrenergic neuromuscular transmission. *Brit. J. Pharmacol.*, 55: 79–85.

Blakeley, A. G. H. and Cunnane, T. C. (1979) The packeted release of transmitter from the sympathetic nerves of the guinea-pig vas deferens: An electrophysiological study. *J. Physiol. (Lond.)*, 296: 85–96.

Burnstock, G. (1976) Do some nerve cells release more than one transmitter? *Neuroscience*, 1: 239–248.

Burnstock, G. and Holman, M. E. (1961) The transmission of excitation from autonomic nerve to smooth muscle. *J. Physiol. (Lond.)*, 155: 115–133.

Burnstock, G. and Holman, M. E. (1962) Spontaneous potentials at sympathetic nerve endings in smooth muscle. *J. Physiol. (Lond.)*, 160: 446–460.

Burnstock, G. and Holman, M. E. (1964) Effect of denervation and reserpine treatment on transmission at sympathetic nerve endings. *J. Physiol. (Lond.)*, 160: 461–469.

Cunnane, T. C. (1984) The mechanisms of neurotransmitter release from sympathetic nerves. *Trends Neurosci.*, 7: 248–253.

Cunnane, T. C. and Stjärne, L. (1982) Secretion of transmitter from individual varicosities of guinea-pig and mouse vas deferens: All-or-none and extremely intermittent. *Neuroscience*, 7: 2565–2576.

Cunnane, T. C. and Stjärne, L. (1984a) Transmitter secretion from individual varicosities of guinea-pig and mouse vas deferens: Highly intermittent and monoquantal. *Neuroscience,* 13: 1–20.

Cunnane, T. C. and Stjärne, L. (1984b) Frequency dependent intermittency and ionic basis of impulse conduction in postganglionic sympathetic fibres of guinea-pig vas deferens. *Neuroscience,* 11: 211–229.

Dahlöf, C., Dahlöf, P., Tatemoto, U. and Lundberg, J. M. (1985) Neuropeptide Y (NPY) reduces field stimulation-evoked release of noradrenaline and enhances force of contraction in the rat portal vein. *N.S. Arch. Pharmacol.,* 328: 327–330.

Dahlström, A. and Häggendal, J. (1966) Some quantitative studies on the noradrenaline content in the cell bodies and terminals of a sympathetic adrenergic neuron system. *Acta physiol. Scand.,* 67: 271–177.

Dahlström, A. Häggendal, J. and Hökfelt, T. (1966) The noradrenaline content of the varicosities of sympathetic adrenergic nerve terminals in the rat. *Acta physiol. Scand.,* 67: 289–294.

Dale, H. H. (1934) Nomenclature of fibres in the autonomic system and their effects. *J. Physiol. (Lond.),* 80: 10–11.

Ekblad, E., Edvinsson, L., Wahlestedt, C., Uddman, R., Håkanson, R. and Sundler, F. (1984) Neuropeptide Y co-exists and co-operates with noradrenaline in perivascular nerve fibres. *Regul. Peptides,* 8: 225–235.

Falck, B. (1962) Observations on the possibilities of the cellular localization of monoamines by a fluorescence method. *Acta physiol. Scand.,* 56: Suppl., 197.

Fedan, J. S., Hogaboom, G. K., O'Donnell, J. P., Colby, J. and Westfall, D. (1981) Contribution by purines to the neurogenic response of the vas deferens of the guinea-pig. *Europ. J. Pharmacol.,* 69: 41–53.

Fried, G. (1981) Small noradrenergic vesicles isolated from rat vas deferens — biochemical and morphological characterization. *Acta physiol. Scand.,* 11: Suppl., 493.

Fried, G., Terenius, L., Hökfelt, T. and Goldstein, M. (1985) Evidence for differential localization of noradrenaline and neuropeptide Y (NPY) in neuronal storage vesicles isolated from rat vas deferens. *J. Neurosci.,* 5: 450–458.

Fried, G., Lundberg, J. M. and Theodorsson-Norheim, E. (1986) Subcellular storage and axonal transport of neuropeptide Y (NPY) in relation to catecholamines in the cat. *Acta physiol. Scand.,* 125: 145–154.

Gillespie, J. S. (1980) Presynaptic receptors in the autonomic nervous system. In L. Szekeres (Ed.), *Adrenergic Activators and Inhibitors, Handbook of Experimental Pharmacology, Vol. 44.* Springer Verlag, Berlin, pp. 353–425.

Graefe, K. H., Stefano, F. J. and Langer, S. Z. (1973) Preferential metabolism of (-)-^{3}H-norepinephrine through the deaminated glycol in the rat deferens. *Biochem. Pharmacol.,* 22: 1147–1160.

Hallin, R. G. and Thorebjörk, H. E. (1974) Single unit sympathetic activity in human skin nerves during rest and various manoeuvers. *Acta physiol. Scand.,* 92: 303–317.

Hjemdahl, P., Daleskog, M. and Kahan, T. (1979) Determination of plasma catecholamines by high performance liquid chromatography with electrochemical detection: comparison with a radioenzymatic method. *Life Sci.,* 25: 131–138.

Hökfelt, T. (1969) Distribution of noradrenaline storing particles in peripheral adrenergic neurons as revealed by electron microscopy. *Acta physiol. Scand.,* 76: 427–440.

Holman, M. E. (1970) Junction potentials in smooth muscle. In E. Bülbring, A. F. Brading, A. W. Jones and T. Tomita (Eds.), *Smooth Muscle,* Edward Arnold, London, pp. 244–288.

Huković, S. (1961) Responses of the isolated sympathetic nerve — ductus deferens preparation of the guinea-pig. *Brit. J. Pharmacol.,* 16: 188–194.

Illés, P. and Starke, K. (1983) An electrophysiological study of presynaptic-adrenoceptors in the vas deferens of the mouse. *Brit. J. Pharmacol.,* 78: 365–373.

Kalsner, S. (1984) Symposium on "The noradrenergic presynaptic controversy". *Fed. Proc.,* 43: 1351–1389.

Lagercrantz, H. and Fried, G. (1982) Chemical composition of the small noradrenergic vesicles. In R. L. Klein, H. Lagercrantz and H. Zimmermann (Eds.) *Neurotransmitter Vesicles,* Academic Press, London, pp. 174–188.

Langer, S. Z. (1981) Presynaptic regulation of the release of catecholamines. *Pharmacol. Rev.,* 32: 337–362.

Lundberg, J. M. and Stjärne, L. (1984) Neuropeptide Y (NPY) depresses the secretion of ^{3}H-noradrenaline and the contractile response evoked by field stimulation in rat vas deferens. *Acta physiol. Scand.,* 120: 477–479.

Lundberg, J. M. and Tatemoto, K. (1982) Pancreatic polypeptide family (APP, BPP, NPY and PYY) in relation to sympathetic vasoconstriction resistant to alpha-adrenoceptor blockade. *Acta physiol. Scand.,* 116: 393–402.

Lundberg, J. M., Hökfelt, T., Änggård, A., Terenius, L., Elde, R., Markey, K. and Goldstein, M. (1982a) Organization principles in the peripheral sympathetic nervous system: subdivision by coexisting peptides (somatostatin-, avian pancreatic polypeptide- and vasoactive intestinal polypeptide-like immunoreactive materials). *Proc. nat. Acad. Sci. USA,* 79: 1303–1307.

Lundberg, J. M., Terenius, L., Hökfelt, T., Martling, C.-R., Tatemoto, K., Mutt, V., Polak, J. M., Bloom, S. R. and Goldstein, M. (1982b) Neuropeptide Y (NPY)-like immunoreactivity in peripheral non-adrenergic neurons and the effects of NPY on sympathetic function. *Acta physiol. Scand.,* 116: 477–480.

Lundberg, J. M., Terenius, L., Hökfelt, T. and Goldstein, M. (1983) High levels of neuropeptide Y (NPY) in peripheral noradrenergic neurons in various mammals including man. *Neurosci. Lett.,* 42: 167–172.

Lundberg, J. M., Terenius, L., Hökfelt, T. and Tatemoto, K. (1984a) Comparative immunohistochemical and biochemical analysis of pancreatic polypeptide-like peptides with special reference to presence of neuropeptide Y in central and peripheral neurons. *J. Neurosci.,* 4: 2376–2386.

Lundberg, J. M., Änggård, A., Theodorsson-Norheim, E. and Pernow, J. (1984b) Guanethidine-sensitive release of neuropeptide Y-like immunoreactivity in the cat spleen by sympathetic nerve stimulation. *Neurosci. Lett.*, 52: 175–180.

Lundberg, J. M., Pernow, J., Dahlöf, C. and Tatemoto, K. (1985) Pre- and postjunctional effects of neuropeptide Y (NPY) on sympathetic control of rat femoral artery. *Acta physiol. Scand.*, 125: 511–513.

Lundberg, J. M., Rudehill, A., Sollevi, A., Theodorsson-Norheim, E. and Hamberger, B. (1986) Frequency- and reserpine-dependent chemical coding of sympathetic transmission: differential release of noradrenaline and neuropeptide Y from pig spleen. *Neurosci. Lett.*, 63: 96–100.

McGrath, J. C. (1978) Adrenergic and "non-adrenergic" components of the contractile response of the vas deferens to a single indirect stimulus. *J. Physiol. (Lond.)*, 283: 23–39.

Meldrum, L. A. and Burnstock, G. (1983) Evidence that ATP acts as a co-transmitter with noradrenaline in sympathetic nerves supplying the guinea-pig vas deferens. *Europ. J. Pharmacol.*, 92: 161–163.

Rand, M. J., McCulloch, M. W., Standford-Starr, C., Story, D. F. and Yang, C. (1982) The time course of the development and persistence of the autoinhibitory effect in noradrenergic transmission. In H. Yoshida, Y. Hagihara and S. Ebashii (Eds.), *Neurotransmitter Receptors; Advances in Pharmacology and Therapeutics II, Vol. 2,* Pergamon Press, Oxford and New York, pp. 121–130.

Schipper, J. (1979) A scanning microfluorimetric study on noradrenergic neurotransmission. Thesis. Rodopi, Amsterdam.

Schümann, H. (1958) Über den Noradrenalin und ATP-Gehalt sympathischer Nerven. *Arch. exp. Pathol. Pharmak.*, 233: 296–300.

Sjöstrand, N. O. (1962) Effect of reserpine and hypogastric denervation on the noradrenaline content of the vas deferens of the guinea-pig. *Acta physiol. Scand.*, 56: 376–380.

Sjöstrand, N. O. (1981) Smooth muscles of vas deferens and other organs in the male reproductive tract. In E. Bülbring, A. F. Brading, A. W. Jones and T. Tomita (Eds.), *Smooth Muscle,* Edward Arnold, London, pp. 367–376.

Smith, A. D. and Winkler, H. (1972) Fundamental mechanisms in the release of catecholamines. In H. Blaschko and E. Muscholl (Eds.), *Catecholamines: Handbook of Experimental Pharmacology, Vol. XXX,* Springer Verlag, Berlin, pp. 538–617.

Sneddon, P. and Burnstock, G. (1984) Inhibition of excitatory junction potentials in guinea-pig vas deferens by α,β-methylase-ATP: further evidence for ATP and noradrenaline as cotransmitters.*Europ J. Pharmac.*, 100: 85–90.

Sneddon, P. and Westfall, D. P. (1984) Pharmacological evidence that adenosine triphosphate and noradrenaline are co-transmitters in the guinea-pig vas deferens. *J. Physiol. (Lond.)*, 347: 561–580.

Sneddon, P., Westfall, D. P. and Fedan, J. S. (1982) Cotransmitters in the motor nerves of the guinea-pig vas deferens: Electrophysiological evidence. *Science,* 218: 693–695.

Starke, K. (1981) Presynaptic receptors. *Ann. Rev. Pharmacol. Toxicol.*, 21: 7–30.

Stjärne, L. (1978) Facilitation and receptor mediated regulation of noradrenaline secretion by control of recruitment of varicosities as well as by control of electro-secretory coupling. *Neuroscience,* 3: 1147–1155.

Stjärne, L. (1982) Site(s) and ionic mechanisms in facilitation and α-autoinhibition of ^{3}H-noradrenaline secretion in guinea-pig vas deferens. In H. Yoshida, Y. Hagihara and S. Ebashii (Eds.), *Neurotransmitter Receptors: Advances in Pharmacology and Therapeutics II. Vol. 2,* Pergamon Press, Oxford and New York, pp. 111–120.

Stjärne, L. (1985) Scope and mechanisms of control of stimulus-secretion coupling in single varicosities of sympathetic nerves. *Clin. Sci.*, 68, Suppl. 10: 77s–81s.

Stjärne, L. and Åstrand, P. (1984) Discrete events measure single quanta of adenosine 5′-triphosphate secreted from sympathetic nerves of guinea-pig and mouse vas deferens. *Neuroscience,* 13: 21–28.

Stjärne, L. and Åstrand, P. (1984) Relative pre- and postjunctional roles of noradrenaline and adenosine 5′-triphosphate as neurotransmitters of the sympathetic nerves of guinea-pig and mouse vas deferens. *Neuroscience,* 14: 929–946.

Stjärne, L., Lundberg, J. M. and Åstrand, P. (1986) Neuropeptide Y — a cotransmitter with noradrenaline and adenosine 5′triphosphate in the sympathetic nerves of the mouse vas deferens? A biochemical, physiological and electropharmacological study. *Neuroscience,* 18: 151–166.

Swedin, G. (1971) Studies on neurotransmission mechanisms in the rat and guinea-pig vas deferens. *Acta physiol. Scand.*, 83, Suppl., 369.

Theodorsson-Norheim, E., Hemsén, A. and Lundberg, J. M. (1985) Radioimmunoassay for NPY: Chromatographic characterization of immunoreactivity in plasma and tissue extracts. *Scand. J. Clin. Invest.*, 45: 355–365.

Thuresson-Klein, Å. (1982) Fine structure of the isolated noradrenergic vesicles. In R. L. Klein, H. Lagercrantz and H. Zimmermann (Eds), *Neurotransmitter Vesicles,* Academic Press, London, pp. 119–132.

Thuresson-Klein, Å. (1983) Exocytosis from large and small dense cored vesicles in noradrenergic nerve terminals. *Neuroscience,* 10: 245–252.

Von Euler, U. S., Lishajko, F. and Stjärne, L. (1963) Catecholamines and adenosine triphosphate in isolated adrenergic nerve granules. *Acta physiol. Scand.*, 59: 495–496.

T. Hökfelt, K. Fuxe and B. Pernow (Eds.),
Progress in Brain Research, Vol. 68

CHAPTER 18

Neuropeptide Y: coexistence with noradrenaline. Functional implications

R. Håkanson, C. Wahlestedt, E. Ekblad, L. Edvinsson and F. Sundler

Departments of Pharmacology, Clinical Pharmacology and Histology, University of Lund, Lund, Sweden

Introduction

Neuropeptide Y (NPY) and peptide YY (PYY) are structurally similar 36-amino acid peptides, belonging to the pancreatic polypeptide (PP) family (Tatemoto, 1982a,b). By immunocytochemistry NPY has been shown to have a wide distribution in a variety of central and peripheral neurones and to coexist with noradrenaline (NA) in sympathetic (Lundberg et al., 1982a; Ekblad et al., 1984; Uddman et al., 1985) and certain brain-stem neurones (Everitt et al., 1984). PYY, on the other hand, occurs predominantly in endocrine cells in the gut (Lundberg et al., 1982b; El-Salhy et al., 1983; Böttcher et al., 1984). NPY has been attributed with various functional roles. A vasoconstrictor effect, which seems to be exerted directly on the smooth muscle, has been demonstrated in vivo (Lundberg and Tatemoto, 1982; Lundberg et al., 1982a; Edvinsson et al., 1984a) and in vitro (Edvinsson et al., 1983, 1984a,b; Ekblad et al., 1984; Lundberg et al., 1985). In addition, NPY affects the sympathetic neuro-effector junction by potentiating NA-evoked vasoconstriction post-junctionally (Edvinsson et al., 1984b; Ekblad et al., 1984; Lundberg et al., 1985; Wahlestedt et al., 1985). Pre-junctionally, NPY inhibits the release of NA (Allen et al., 1982; Lundberg et al., 1982a, 1985; Lundberg and Stjärne, 1984). In addition to these three actions (direct, and pre- and post-junctional modulatory effects), which have been observed in the periphery, NPY has been claimed to upregulate α_2-adrenoceptors in the rat medulla oblongata (Agnati et al., 1983). Despite the many diverse actions of NPY, the functional significance of the coexistence — and possible cosecretion — of NPY and NA is still far from fully understood.

The finding that NPY is present in a large population of nerve cell bodies in the sympathetic ganglia was the first indication that NPY and NA might coexist (Lundberg et al., 1982a, 1983). The following observations support this view: surgical or chemical (6-hydroxydopamine) sympathectomy eliminates both NA and NPY from sympathetic targets including blood vessels (Ekblad et al., 1984; Edvinsson et al., 1984a; Uddman et al., 1985). Double-staining immunocytochemical techniques have suggested the coexistence of NPY and the NA-forming enzyme, dopamine-β-hydroxylase, in perivascular fibres, and, finally, such techniques have established beyond any doubt the coexistence of NPY and NA in cell bodies of post-ganglionic sympathetic neurones (Ekblad et al., 1984; Uddman et al., 1985; cf. Sundler et al., 1986).

Effects of NPY

NPY-evoked vasoconstriction

The first effect of NPY to be observed was a direct constrictor effect on local blood flow (Lundberg et

TABLE I

Contractile effect of NPY on isolated blood vessel segments from guinea-pigs, rats and humans

	Neuropeptide Y (molar contraction)				
	2×10^{-11} M	2×10^{-10} M	2×10^{-9} M	2×10^{-8} M	2×10^{-7} M
Guinea-pig (n = 7)					
Femoral artery (10.1 ± 3.4 mN)	0	0	0	1.0 ± 1.0	3.1 ± 2.0
Femoral vein (3.4 ± 1.4 mN)	0	0.7 ± 0.7	1.1 ± 1.1	9.0 ± 5.0	26.1 ± 13.0
Rat (n = 7)					
Femoral artery (10.8 ± 2.1 mN)	0	0	0	1.4 ± 1.3	5.7 ± 4.1
Femoral vein (4.3 ± 0.8 mN)	0	0	0	9.3 ± 5.4	23.3 ± 15.8
Human (n = 3)					
Mesenteric artery (16.1 ± 2.4 mN)	0	0	0	0	0
Mesenteric vein (11.1 ± 4.3 mN)	0	0	0	1.2 ± 0.2	n.d.

Mean ± S.E.M.; the maximum contraction elicited by 124 mM K^+ (within parentheses) was set as 100 and the effects of NPY are given as a percentage. n.d. = Not determined.

al., 1982a; see also Edvinsson et al., 1983; Hellström et al., 1985; Tuor et al., 1985). On the whole, however, NPY up to 10^{-6} M has been found to have a poor contractile effect on most isolated peripheral blood vessels (Table I) (cf. Edvinsson et al., 1984a,b) but for certain cerebral arteries (Fig. 1). The guinea-pig femoral vein and iliac vein and rat femoral vein were also exceptions in that they responded fairly well. Moreover, vasoconstriction required medium to high concentrations of the peptide. The responses were markedly reduced in Ca^{2+}-free medium and could be blocked by Ca^{2+} entry blockers, such as nifedipine and verapamil, but not by adrenergic or serotonergic blockers (Edvinsson et al., 1983).

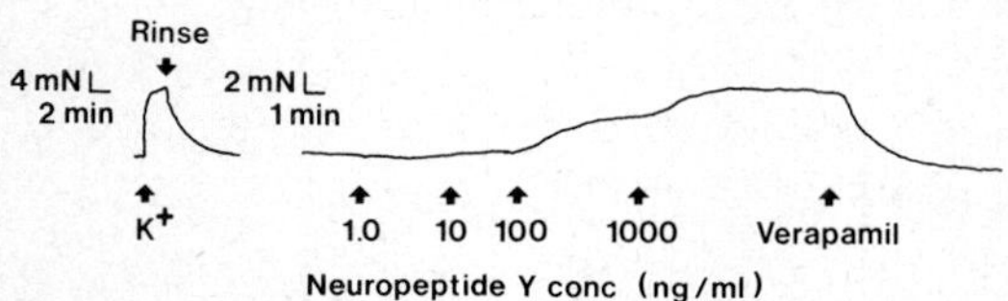

Fig. 1. Contractile response of feline middle cerebral artery to the cumulative applications of neuropeptide Y. The Ca^{2+} entry blocker verapamil (10^{-5} M) rapidly relaxes the neuropeptide Y-contracted blood vessel. Calibration bars are inserted.

NPY-evoked enhancement of NA-evoked vasoconstriction

Several isolated rabbit arteries respond to electrical stimulation with a contraction that is probably mediated by NA since it can be blocked by guanethidine or by the α_1-adrenoceptor blocker prazosine (Ekblad et al., 1984; Wahlestedt et al., unpublished). NPY greatly enhanced the response to electrical stimulation (Fig. 2) (Ekblad et al., 1984). Also the contractile responses to NA (and adrenaline) were enhanced in the presence of NPY (Fig. 3). Studies on several isolated arteries from the rabbit showed that the NA concentration-response curve was shifted to the left in the presence of NPY (Fig. 3); veins did not respond to NPY with enhanced NA-evoked contraction (Table II) (Edvinsson et al., 1984b). The potentiating effect was, however, not restricted to NA but included also histamine (both arteries and veins were sensitized to histamine) and in one instance prostaglandin $F_2\alpha$. Vasoconstrictions evoked by 5-HT or K^+ were not affected by NPY. The potentiating effect of NPY on NA-evoked vasoconstriction was observed at low concentrations of NPY (beginning at approxi-

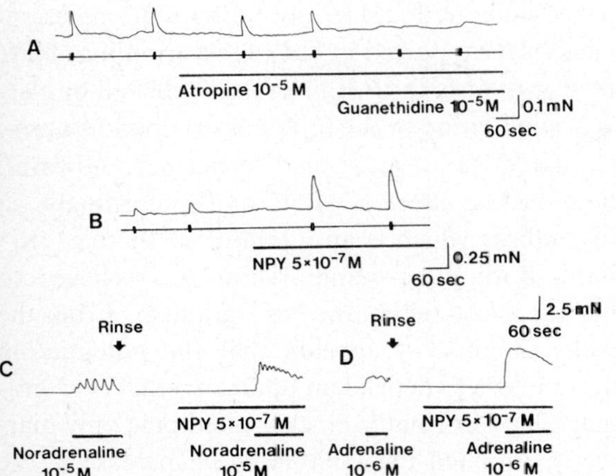

Fig. 2. Typical registrations of electrically induced constriction of isolated rabbit gastro-epiploic artery. Stimulation (5–10 Hz, 5–15 V over the electrodes, 0.3 msec duration) was maintained for 3–5 sec (■). Exposure to drugs is indicated by a straight line. (A) Electrical stimulation evoked a vasomotor response that was unaffected by atropine but inhibited by guanethidine and by tetrodotoxin (not shown). (B) The electrically induced vasomotor response was greatly potentiated by NPY. (C, D) Also the vasomotor responses evoked by noradrenaline and adrenaline were potentiated by NPY.

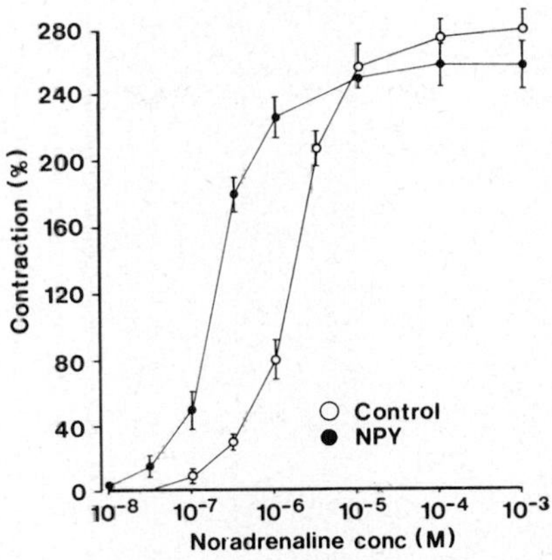

Fig. 3. Concentration-response curves for noradrenaline (rabbit femoral artery) in the absence or presence of NPY (3×10^{-8} M). Mean values of ten separate runs on paired specimens. Vertical bars give S.E.M.

mately 10^{-10} M) (Fig. 4) (Edvinsson et al., 1984b). A potentiating effect of NPY on NA-evoked responses has also been observed in isolated arteries from man (Edvinsson et al., 1985) and rat (Lundberg et al., 1985).

TABLE II

pD_2-values for various vasoconstrictors in the absence and presence of NPY (30 nM)

Agonist	Vessel	pD_2 control	pD_2 NPY	Significance level
Noradrenaline	Central ear artery	6.12 ± 0.12	6.26 ± 0.15	NS
	Gastro-epiploic artery	5.14 ± 0.10	5.76 ± 0.07	$p < 0.001$
	vein	5.33 ± 0.19	5.52 ± 0.20	NS
	Femoral artery	5.80 ± 0.07	6.56 ± 0.04	$p < 0.001$
	vein	6.16 ± 0.08	6.20 ± 0.16	NS
Histamine	Basilar artery	5.72 ± 0.11	6.02 ± 0.06	$p < 0.05$
	Central ear artery	5.79 ± 0.14	5.97 ± 0.09	NS
	Gastro-epiploic artery	5.22 ± 0.07	5.63 ± 0.07	$p < 0.005$
	vein	5.25 ± 0.15	6.06 ± 0.30	$p < 0.05$
	Femoral artery	5.68 ± 0.04	6.74 ± 0.11	$p < 0.001$
	vein	5.56 ± 0.05	6.31 ± 0.03	$p < 0.001$
Prostaglandin $F_{2\alpha}$	Gastro-epiploic artery	5.26 ± 0.24	5.73 ± 0.11	NS
	vein	4.76 ± 0.04	6.09 ± 0.12	$p < 0.001$
	Femoral artery	5.31 ± 0.06	5.32 ± 0.008	NS
	vein	5.72 ± 0.33	5.83 ± 0.10	NS

Values are given as means ± S.E.M., 6–10 experiments in each group. NS = Not significant.

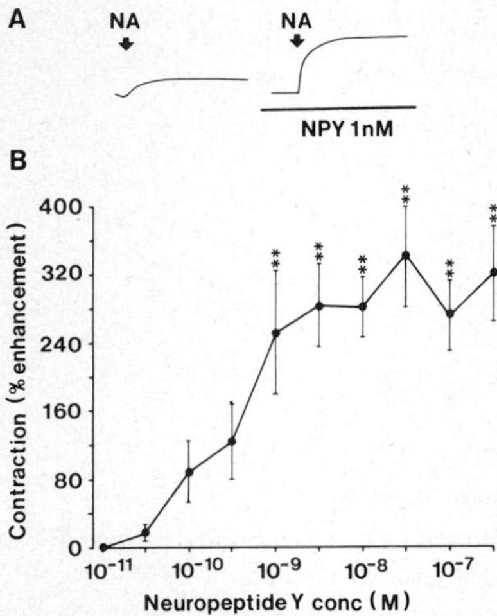

Fig. 4. (A) Tracings of the contraction of a rabbit gastro-epiploic artery after addition of 1 μM noradrenaline (NA) and 20 min later of the same concentration of NA in the presence of 1 nM NPY. (B) Enhancement of the responses of the gastro-epiploic artery to 1 μM NA by different concentrations of NPY. The contractions were measured before and after addition of NPY to the bath, and the enhancement is expressed as the percentage of the response before addition of NPY. Mean values of 8–10 runs. Vertical bars give S.E.M. Significance level: ** $p < 0.01$, *** $p < 0.001$, using paired Student's t-test.

NPY-induced potentiation: mode of action

The potentiating effect of NPY is reflected in an increased pD_2 value (i.e. the negative logarithm of the ED_{50} value) for the NA concentration-response curve (Edvinsson et al., 1984b). A series of experiments employing the rabbit femoral artery was carried out in an attempt to throw light on the mechanism behind the NPY-induced potentiation (Wahlestedt et al., 1985). Paired experiments were performed in which control specimens were compared with matched specimens that had been pre-treated in various ways (Table III). The control specimens invariably displayed the anticipated increase in the pD_2 value for the NA concentration-response curve under the influence of NPY. Cocaine was found not to affect the NPY-induced change in pD_2 value, suggesting that NPY acts to potentiate the response to NA regardless of the efficiency of the amine re-uptake mechanism. The notion that the NPY-evoked potentiation does not reflect a pre-junctional action is supported by the observation that NPY failed to modify the [^{3}H]NA release elicited by electrical stimulation of the rabbit gastroepiploic artery (Ekblad et al., 1984). Na^+ deficiency, however, abolished the effect of NPY, and interestingly, so did ouabain which is an inhibitor of the Na^+/K^+ pump. Both these manipulations are believed to alter the trans-membrane Na^+ gradient. From the results obtained it appears that the potentiating effect of NPY is dependent upon an intact Na^+ gradient. The Ca^{2+} entry blocker nifedipine only marginally inhibited the NPY-induced increase in the pD_2 value. Also, keeping the specimens in a Ca^{2+}-deficient medium for about 4 min did not inhibit the increase in pD_2. However, if the specimens were kept in Ca^{2+}-deficient medium fortified with EGTA for 30 min the result was a marked reduction of NA-evoked contractions and a complete inhibition of the NPY-induced increase in pD_2. Based on the results with nifedipine and assuming that exposure to Ca^{2+}-deficient medium for 4 min removes most extracellular Ca^{2+} it may be suggested that an influx of extracellular Ca^{2+} is not absolutely essential for the NPY-induced potentiation. From the results with exposure to Ca^{2+}-deficient medium for 30 min, when NPY failed to alter the pD_2 value, it may be concluded that even though Ca^{2+} influx is probably not essential for the NPY-evoked potentiation, a facilitated mobilization of an intracellular sequestered Ca^{2+} pool may be required.

The potentiating effect of NPY-related peptides

The potentiation of the response to NA is produced not only by NPY but also by other chemically related peptides (Table IV). This is the case with PYY, which displays great structural similarities with NPY, particularly in the C-terminal part. Out of 36 positions 28 are identical in the two peptides. PP, another NPY-related peptide, differs from NPY and PYY by potentiating the NA response only at very high concentrations. Peptides, chemically unrelated to NPY, such as calcitonin gene-re-

TABLE III

pD_2-values for the contractile effect of NA or NPY + NA in rabbit isolated femoral artery following a variety of pretreatments

Pretreatment	pD_2(NA)	pD_2(NPY + NA)	Statistical level
Cocaine (10^{-5} M)	5.87 ± 0.05	6.48 ± 0.10	$p < 0.001$
None	5.78 ± 0.07	6.40 ± 0.09	$p < 0.001$
Na^+-deficiency[a]	5.92 ± 0.08	6.03 ± 0.11	n.s.
None	5.65 ± 0.06	6.43 ± 0.08	$p < 0.001$
Ouabain (10^{-7} M)	5.85 ± 0.09	6.19 ± 0.10	n.s.
None	5.58 ± 0.07	6.38 ± 0.11	$p < 0.001$
Nifedipine	5.84 ± 0.05	6.28 ± 0.008	$p < 0.01$
None	5.89 ± 0.10	6.45 ± 0.05	$p < 0.001$
Ca^{2+}-free (4 min)[b]	5.71 ± 0.09	6.16 ± 0.07	$p < 0.01$
None	5.76 ± 0.06	6.30 ± 0.09	$p < 0.001$
Ca^{2+}-free (30 min) + EGTA[c]	5.57 ± 0.21	5.50 ± 0.19	n.s.
None	5.67 ± 0.04	6.31 ± 0.07	$p < 0.001$

Means ± S.E.M., n = 7–12. NPY was applied 2 min before NA.
[a] The Na^+ content of the medium was lowered from 150 to 80 mM.
[b] The preparations were exposed to a medium without Ca^{2+} for 4 min before application of NA.
[c] The preparations were exposed to a medium without Ca^{2+} and enriched with 1 mM EGTA for 30 min before application of NA.

lated peptide and LPLRFamide, were without effect (Wahlestedt et al., 1985a).

Effect of NPY on NA release

In several sympathetically controlled smooth muscle preparations, such as the vas deferens and certain blood vessels (rat femoral artery and portal vein), it has been possible to show that NPY inhibits the release of NA evoked by electrical stimulation (Allen et al., 1982; Lundberg et al., 1982a, 1985; Dahlöf et al., 1984; Lundberg and Stjärne, 1984). This does not seem to be the case everywhere, however. Thus, in studies of the isolated rab-

TABLE IV

pD_2-values for the contractile effect of NA in rabbit isolated femoral artery in the absence or presence of various peptides (for details, see text)

Peptide	Concentration	pD_2(NA)	pD_2(peptide + NA)	Statistical level
NPY	3×10^{-8} M	5.70 ± 0.02	6.39 ± 0.02	$p < 0.001$
PYY	10^{-7} M	5.91 ± 0.06	6.53 ± 0.09	$p < 0.001$
BPP	10^{-7} M	5.64 ± 0.08	5.75 ± 0.10	n.s.
HPP	10^{-6} M	5.85 ± 0.08	6.33 ± 0.13	$p < 0.01$
CGRP	10^{-6} M	5.86 ± 0.04	5.90 ± 0.05	n.s.
LPLRFamide	10^{-6} M	6.09 ± 0.09	6.02 ± 0.08	n.s.

Means ± S.E.M., n = 6–10. The peptides were applied 2 min before NA. n.s. = Not significant.

TABLE V

	1 2 3 4 5 6 7 8 9 10 11 12 13 14 15 16 17 18
NPY 1-36	Tyr-Pro-Ser-Lys-Pro-Asp-Asn-Pro-Gly-Glu-Asp-Ala-Pro-Ala-Glu-Asp-Met-Ala
Desamido-NPY 1-36	Tyr-Pro-Ser-Lys-Pro-Asp-Asn-Pro-Gly-Glu-Asp-Ala-Pro-Ala-Glu-Asp-Met-Ala
PYY 1-36	Tyr-Pro-Ala-Lys-Pro-Glu-Ala-Pro-Gly-Glu-Asp-Ala-Ser-Pro-Glu-Glu-Leu-Ser
PYY 13-36	Ser-Pro-Glu-Glu-Leu-Ser
	19 20 21 22 23 24 25 26 27 28 29 30 31 32 33 34 35 36
NPY 1-36	Arg-Tyr-Tyr-Ser-Ala-Leu-Arg-His-Tyr-Ile- Asn-Leu-Ile- Thr-Arg-Gln-Arg-Tyr-NH_2
Desamido-NPY 1-36	Arg-Tyr-Tyr-Ser-Ala-Leu-Arg-His-Tyr-Ile- Asn-Leu-Ile- Thr-Arg-Gln-Arg-Tyr
PYY 1-36	Arg-Tyr-Tyr-Ala-Ser-Leu-Arg-His-Tyr-Leu-Asn-Leu-Val-Thr-Arg-Gln-Arg-Tyr-NH_2
PYY 13-36	Arg-Tyr-Tyr-Ala-Ser-Leu-Arg-His-Tyr-Leu-Asn-Leu-Val-Thr-Arg-Gln-Arg-Tyr-NH_2
NPY 19-36	Arg-Tyr-Tyr-Ser-Ala-Leu-Arg-His-Tyr- Ile-Asn-Leu-Ile- Thr-Arg-Gln-Arg-Tyr-NH_2
NPY 24-36	Leu-Arg-His-Tyr-Ile- Asn-Leu-Ile- Thr-Arg-Gln-Arg-Tyr-NH_2
PYY 24-36	Leu-Arg-His-Tyr-Leu-Asn-Leu-Val-Thr-Arg-Gln-Arg-Tyr-NH_2
PYY 27-36	Tyr-Leu-Asn-Leu-Val-Thr-Arg-Gln-Arg-Tyr-NH_2

Amino acid sequences of NPY, PYY and the fragments employed in the study.
Abbreviations: NPY = neuropeptide Y; PYY = peptide YY.

bit gastro-epiploic artery, it has not been possible to demonstrate suppression of NA release by NPY (Ekblad et al., 1984).

What part of NPY carries the activating signal?

The question arose whether the whole NPY sequence was needed to produce the biological effects or whether fragments of NPY would be sufficient. A series of C-terminal fragments of NPY and PYY was synthesized (Dr. N. Yanaihara, Shizouka, Japan) (Table V). None of the fragments produced any direct vasoconstriction, nor did they cause potentiation of the NA- or histamine-evoked vasoconstriction, even at very high concentrations (Wahlestedt et al., 1986). Interestingly, however, PYY 13-36 turned out to be almost equipotent with NPY and PYY in suppressing electrically evoked contractions in the rat vas deferens, presumably reflecting inhibition of NA release (Fig. 5). None of the other fragments displayed this effect. The finding that desamido-NPY was inactive stresses the importance of the amidated C-terminus. The results of the studies on the bioactivities of the NPY/PYY fragments are summarized in Table VI. From these data it is tempting to speculate that pre-junctional

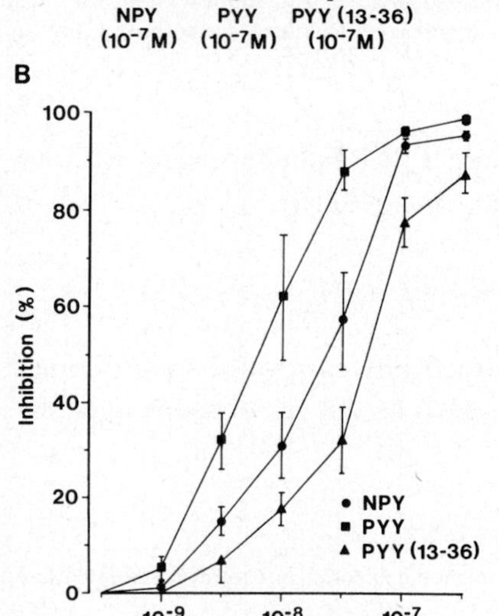

Fig. 5. Suppression by NPY, PYY and PYY (13–36) of the motor response of the rat vas deferens (prostatic part) to continuous electrical stimulation at low frequency. (A) Typical tracings following application of NPY, PYY or PYY 13–36 (10^{-7} M of either). (B) Concentration-response curves illustrating the suppressive effects of various peptides on the electrically induced twitches expressed as percentage of the twitch amplitude before application of peptide: NPY (●), PYY (■) or PYY 13–36 (▲). Each value is the mean of 4–8 observations; bars give S.E.M.

TABLE VI

Effects of NPY, PYY and PYY 13-36 on the sympathetic neuro-effector junction

	Direct post-junctional effect (vasoconstriction)	Post-junctional modulatory effect (potentiated NA and histamine response)		Pre-junctional modulatory effect (suppressed NA-release)
	Guinea-pig iliac vein	Rabbit femoral artery	Rabbit femoral vein	Rat vas deferens
NPY	+	+	+	+
PYY	+	+	+	+
PYY 13-36	0	0	0	+
Desamido-NPY	0	0	0	0

All other peptide fragments tested were without effect.
+ = Effectiveness; 0 = lack of effect.

NPY receptors recognize a part of NPY that is different from that recognized by post-junctional NPY receptors (Table VII). It must be pointed out, however, that since PYY seems to react as readily as NPY with the binding sites, we may not be justified in referring to them as NPY receptors. By the use of this term we are implicitly — and perhaps incorrectly — suggesting that NPY is the physiological ligand.

Physiological significance of NPY/NA coexistence

NPY seems to have at least three effects on the sympathetic neuro-effector junction. There is a pre-junctional effect, expressed as suppression of stimulated NA release, and two post-junctional effects, a direct response, which is not mediated via adrenoceptors, and a potentiation of the NA-evoked response. The possible end result of these diverse actions may be an improvement in the "economy" at the sympathetic neuro-effector junction, reflected in a reduced NA demand and a suppression or shortening of the NA release process after nerve stimulation (Table VIII). However, most of the results obtained so far are from in vitro studies and it is unclear to what extent they apply in vivo. It is important also to keep in mind that NPY does not seem to evoke all three effects at every sympathetic neuro-effect junction. One of the effects may be manifested in one target, other effects in another one, possibly reflecting differences in the distribution of receptor subtypes. Secondly, the potentiating effect of NPY is not limited to NA, since the effects of e.g. histamine are also enhanced. Finally,

TABLE VII

Evidence for NPY/PYY receptor subpopulations

Pre-junctional binding sites recognize PYY 13-36
Post-junctional binding sites require the whole NPY or PYY sequence

TABLE VIII

Effects of NPY on the sympathetic neuro-effector junction

Pre-junctional:	Suppression of NA release
Post-junctional:	(a) Direct response (e.g. vasoconstriction, (b) Potentiation of the NA-evoked response

Possible consequences
Improvement in NA "economy"
(reduced NA demand, suppressed NA release).

TABLE IX

NPY-evoked effects at the sympathetic neuro-effector junction

Suggested rank-order of physiological importance based on pD_2 values:
(1) Post-junctional modulation of NA response (rabbit femoral artery, pD_2 8.82) (Edvinsson et al., 1984b; Wahlestedt et al., 1986)
(2) Pre-junctional suppression of NA release (rat vas deferens, pD_2 8.16) (Wahlestedt et al., 1986)
(3) Direct vasoconstriction (guinea-pig iliac vein, pD_2 7.47; cat cerebral arteries, pD_2 7.89) (Edvinsson et al., 1984a; Wahlestedt et al., 1986)

NPY is not the only peptide that is capable of exerting the three actions at the sympathetic neuro-effector junction. Its chemical relative PYY, and to some extent PP, are also capable of inducing the same effects and it is therefore still difficult to define a physiological role for NPY as such at the sympathetic neuro-effector junction. Certainly, the effects produced by NPY and PYY are manifested at concentrations which makes it tempting to speculate on their physiological significance. If we were to rank the three actions of NPY (and PYY) based on the concentrations needed to bring about the action, the post-junctional potentiation of the NA response would be at the top (because very low concentrations of peptides are needed), the pre-junctional suppression of stimulated NA release (in the rat vas deferens) would be second, and the direct vasoconstriction would be third (even though the results presented are from a blood vessel that was very sensitive to NPY) (Table IX). It is possible that the ranking order will have to be altered when more detailed information becomes available.

In conclusion, there is mounting evidence that the coexistence of NPY and NA in sympathetic neurones is of physiological importance, although the nature of their cooperation is only partly understood. It must be emphasized that the functional role of NPY in the periphery is probably not related exclusively to noradrenergic neurotransmission. NPY seems to have effects on vascular smooth muscle that are unrelated to adrenergic receptors. Furthermore, NPY has been demonstrated by immunocytochemistry in other neuronal systems apart from the sympathetic one. Thus, NPY coexists with VIP in certain non-adrenergic enteric neurones (Sundler et al., 1983; Ekblad et al., 1985) and in non-adrenergic neurones in pelvic ganglia (Inyama et al., 1985). In addition, NPY has been demonstrated in non-adrenergic nerve fibres in the heart (Hassall and Burnstock, 1984). The functional significance of NPY in non-adrenergic neurones is even more enigmatic than in the sympathetic neurons.

Acknowledgement

The study was supported by grants from the Swedish Medical Research Council (1007, 5958).

References

Agnati, L. F.,Fuxe, K., Benfenati, F., Battistini, N., Härfstrand, A., Tatemoto, K., Hökfelt, T. and Mutt, V. (1983) Neuropeptide Y in vitro selectively increases the number of α_2-adrenergic binding sites in membranes of the medulla oblongata of the rat. *Acta physiol. Scand.*, 118: 293–295.

Allen, J. M., Adrian, T. E., Tatemoto, K., Polak, J. M., Hughes, J. and Bloom, S. R. (1982) Two novel related peptides, neuropeptide Y (NPY) and peptide YY (PYY) inhibit the contraction of the electrically stimulated mouse vas deferens. *Neuropeptides*, 3: 71–77.

Böttcher, G., Sjölund, K., Ekblad, E., Håkanson, R., Schwartz, T. W. and Sundler, F. (1984) Coexistence of peptide YY and glicentin immunoreactivity in endocrine cells of the gut. *Regul. Peptides*, 8: 261–266.

Dahlöf, C., Dahlöf, P., Tatemoto, K. and Lundberg, J. M. (1984) Neuropeptide Y (NPY) reduces field stimulation-evoked release of noradrenaline and enhances contractile force in the rat portal vein. *Naunyn-Schmiedebergs Arch. Pharmacol.*, 328: 327–330.

Edvinsson, L., Emson, P., McCulloch, J., Tatemoto, K. and Uddman, R. (1983) Neuropeptide Y: Cerebrovascular innervation and vasomotor effect in the cat. *Neurosci. Lett.*, 43: 79–84.

Edvinsson, L., Ekblad, E., Håkanson, R. and Wahlestedt, C. (1984b) Neuropeptide Y potentiates the effect of various vasoconstrictor agents on rabbit blood vessels. *Brit. J. Pharmacol.*, 83: 519–525.

Edvinsson, L., Emson, P., McCulloch, J., Tatemoto, K. and Uddman, R. (1984a) Neuropeptide Y: Immunocytochemical localization to and effect upon feline pial arteries and veins in vitro and in situ. *Acta physiol. Scand.*, 122: 155–163.

Edvinsson, L., Håkanson, R., Steen, S., Uddman,R. and Wahlestedt, C. (1985) Innervation of human omental arteries and veins and vasomotor responses to noradrenaline, neuropeptide Y, substance P and vasoactive intestinal peptide. *Regul. Peptides*, 12: 67–79.

Ekblad, E., Edvinsson, L., Wahlestedt, C., Uddman, R., Håkanson, R. and Sundler, F. (1984) Neuropeptide Y co-exists and co-operates with noradrenaline in perivascular nerve fibers. *Regul. Peptides*, 8: 225–235.

Ekblad, E., Ekelund, M., Graffner, H., Håkanson, R. and Sundler, F. (1985) Peptide-containing nerve fibers in the stomach wall of rat and mouse. *Gastroenterology*, 89: 73–85.

El-Salhy, M., Wilander, E., Huntti-Berggren, L. and Grimelius, L. (1983) The distribution and ontogeny of polypeptide YY (PYY)- and pancreatic polypeptide (PP)-immunoreactive cells in the gastrointestinal tract of rat. *Histochemistry*, 78: 53–60.

Everitt, B. J., Hökfelt, T., Terenius, L., Tatemoto, K., Mutt, V. and Goldstein, M. (1984) Differential co-existence of neuropeptide Y (NPY)-like immunoreactivity with catecholamines in the central nervous system of the rat. *Neuroscience*, 11: 443–462.

Hassall, C. J. S. and Burnstock, G. (1984) Neuropeptide Y-like immunoreactivity in cultured intrinsic neurones of the heart. *Neurosci. Lett.*, 52: 111–115.

Hellström, P. M., Olerup, O. and Tatemoto, K. (1985) Neuropeptide Y may mediate effects of sympathetic nerve stimulations on colonic motility and blood flow in the cat. *Acta physiol. Scand.*, 124: 613–624.

Inyama, C. O., Hacker, G. W., Gu, J., Dahl, D., Bloom, S. R. and Polak, J. M. (1985) Cytochemical relationships in the paracervical ganglion (Frankenhäuser) of rat studied by immunocytochemistry. *Neurosci. Lett.*, 55: 311–316.

Lundberg, J. M., Terenius, L., Hökfelt, T., Martling, C. R., Tatemoto, K., Mutt, V., Polak, J. M., Bloom, S. R. and Goldstein, M. (1982a) Neuropeptide Y (NPY)-like immunoreactivity in peripheral noradrenergic neurons and effects of NPY on sympathetic function. *Acta physiol. Scand.*, 116: 477–480.

Lundberg, J. M. and Tatemoto, K. (1982) Pancreatic polypeptide family (APP, BPP, NPY and PYY) in relation to sympathetic vasoconstriction resistant to alpha-adrenoceptor blockade. *Acta physiol. Scand.*, 116: 393–402.

Lundberg, J. M., Tatemoto, K., Terenius, L., Hellström, P. M., Mutt, V., Hökfelt, T. and Hamberger, B. (1982b) Localization of peptide YY (PYY) in gastrointestinal endocrine cells and effects on intestinal blood flow and motility. *Proc. nat. Acad. Sci. USA*, 79: 4471–4475.

Lundberg, J. M., Terenius, L., Hökfelt, T. and Goldstein, M. (1983) High levels of neuropeptide Y in peripheral noradrenergic neurons in various mammals including man. *Neurosci. Lett.*, 42: 167–172.

Lundberg, J. M. and Stjärne, L. (1984) Neuropeptide Y (NPY) depresses the secretion of ^{3}H-noradrenaline and the contractile response evoked by field stimulation in rat vas deferens. *Acta physiol. Scand.*, 120: 477–479.

Lundberg, J. M., Pernow, J., Tatemoto, K. and Dahlöf, C. (1985) Pre- and postjunctional effects of NPY on sympathetic control of rat femoral artery. *Acta physiol. Scand.*, 123: 511–513.

Sundler, F., Moghimzadeh, E., Håkanson, R., Ekelund, M. and Emson, P. (1983) Nerve fibers in the gut and pancreas of the rat displaying neuropeptide Y immunoreactivity. Intrinsic and eneteric nervous origin. *Cell Tissue Res.*, 230: 487–493.

Sundler, F., Håkanson, R., Ekblad, E., Uddman, R. and Wahlestedt, C. (1986) Neuropeptide Y in peripheral adrenergic and enteric nervous systems. *Ann. Rev. Cytol*, 102: 243–269.

Tatemoto, K. (1982a) Neuropeptide Y. Complete amino acid sequence of the brain peptide. *Proc. nat. Acad.Sci. USA*, 79: 5485–5489.

Tatemoto, K. (1982b) Isolation and characterization of peptide YY (PYY), a candidate gut hormone that inhibits pancreatic exocrine secretion. *Proc. nat. Acad. Sci. USA*, 79: 2514–2518.

Tuor, U. I., Edvinsson, L. and McCulloch, J. (1985) Neuropeptide Y and cerebral blood flow. *Lancet*, i: 1271.

Uddman, R., Ekblad, E., Edvinsson, L., Håkanson, R. and Sundler, F. (1985) Neuropeptide Y-like immunoreactivity in perivascular nerve fibers of the guinea-pig. *Regul. Peptides*, 10: 243–257.

Wahlestedt, C., Edvinsson, L., Ekblad, E. and Håkanson, R. (1985) Neuropeptide Y potentiates noradrenaline-evoked vasoconstriction:Modeofaction.*J.Pharmacol.exp.Ther.*,234:735–741.

Wahlestedt, C., Yanaihara, N. and Håkanson, R. (1986) Evidence for different pre- and postjunctional receptors for neuropeptide Y and related peptides. *Regul. Peptides*, 13: 317–328.

SECTION VI

Central Systems

T. Hökfelt, K. Fuxe and B. Pernow (Eds.),
Progress in Brain Research, Vol. 68

CHAPTER 19

Aspects on the information handling by the central nervous system: focus on cotransmission in the aged rat brain

L. F. Agnati[1], K. Fuxe[2], M. Zoli[1], E. Merlo Pich[1], F. Benfenati[1], I. Zini[1] and M. Goldstein[3]

[1]*Department of Human Physiology, University of Modena, Via Campi 287, 41100 Modena, Italy,* [2]*Department of Histology, Karolinska Institutet, Stockholm, Sweden, and* [3]*Department of Psychiatry, New York University Medical Center, N.Y., U.S.A.*

Introduction

In order to evaluate the possible functional meaning of cotransmission we have studied a particular animal model, the aged brain of the rat (Giacobini et al., 1982; Agnoli et al., 1983). Aging is a progressive change in the morphological and biochemical features of the organism which takes place after the adult life. According to Finch (1973), senescence is the last quarter of expected life, when body functions become deteriorated and organs start to show pathological changes.

In this chapter we will report regional data on the effects of aging on two basic parameters of neural function, namely Na^+/K^+ ATPase, which is involved in the maintenance of membrane polarization, and protein phosphorylation, which is a biochemical system related to the intracellular decoding of extracellular signals (Nestler and Greengard, 1984). It was also of interest to evaluate a recently discovered feature of synaptic transmission, the coexistence of more putative transmitters in the same neuron (see Hökfelt et al., 1984), in adult versus aged rats. Until now only limited information on this subject is available (Agnati et al., 1984b, 1985a,b) and such knowledge may help to discover the morphofunctional basis for the failure of the old brain to perform its integrative tasks.

Finally, one possible functional meaning of cotransmission (the receptor-receptor interactions) will be illustrated (see Agnati et al., 1984d; Fuxe and Agnati 1985) and discussed in the large context of the electro-metabolic integrative capabilities of the CNS.

On this basis the age-induced changes in Na^+/K^+ATPase, in protein phosphorylation and in cotransmission will be discussed in the frame of a general view of the information handling in the CNS.

A general pattern of changes will be demonstrated for the two first mentioned biochemical parameters, while it has not been possible to draw any general rules for the effects of aging on costored putative transmitters.

Material and methods

Three-month-old and 24-month-old Sprague-Dawley rats have been used. The rats were kept under standardized humidity, temperature and lighting conditions (lights on at 8.00 a.m., lights off at 8.00 p.m.) and they had free access to water and food.

[^{3}H]Ouabain binding was used to evaluate Na^+/K^+ATPase binding sites in tissue sections and in cellular subfractions prepared from parieto-frontal cerebral cortex (dorsal cortex) and spinal cord (see Fig. 1). [^{3}H]Ouabain binding was performed

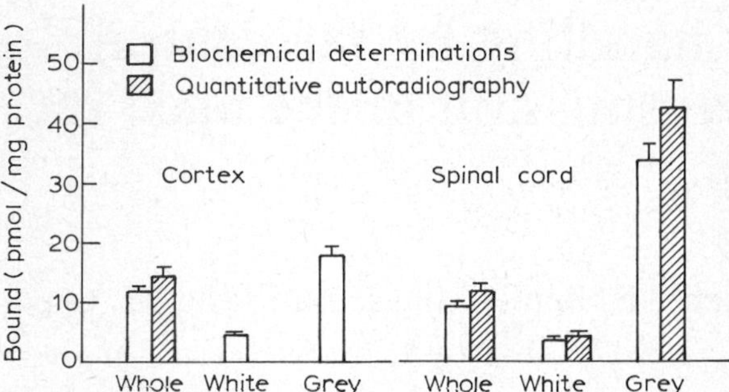

Fig. 1. [^{3}H]Ouabain binding in the parieto-frontal cerebral cortex and thoracic spinal cord. The binding has been performed on homogenates and in sections (autoradiographic procedure). For technical details, see text. B_{max} values are shown on the y-axis; means (out of 8 rats) ± S.E.M. Whole = white plus grey matter; white = white matter; grey = grey matter. The agreement between biochemical and autoradiographic determinations should be noted as well as the low binding in the white matter.

according to Swann et al. (1982). The results have been obtained by using either increasing ligand concentrations (1–500 nM) in saturation experiments or by a fixed concentration close to the K_D value (25–30 nM).

The cAMP and Ca^{2+}-induced protein phosphorylation was carried out according to Nestler and Greengard (1984) (see Agnati et al., 1985c). The studies were performed on crude mitochondrial membrane preparations obtained from dorsal cortex, striatum, limbic system (mainly tuberculum olfactorium and nuc. accumbens), hippocampal formation and spinal cord.

Protein phosphorylation was carried out following the procedures described by Nestler and Greengard (1984) both in basal conditions and after maximal stimulation with 2nd messengers, namely cyclic AMP (10 μM) and calcium (1 mM). The whole membrane preparation was diluted to a protein concentration of 1 mg/ml and lysed in Hepes buffer (50 mM pH 7.4) containing $MgCl_2$ 10 mM, EGTA 0.1 mM, IBMX 0.5 mM and DTT 1 mM. After preincubation for 2 min at 30°C, the phosphorylation assay was started by the addition of 0.5 pmoles of (γ^{32}P)-ATP to 100 μl samples and blocked after 10 sec at 30°C with 100 μl stopping solution, containing 2% SDS, followed by boiling for 2 min. Proteins were then separated by polyacrylamide gel electrophoresis (10% acrylamide/Bis in the separating gel) (Laemmli, 1970) and autoradiographed. Differences in the phosphorylation pattern of substrate proteins were analyzed by scanning microdensitometry and expressed in optical density units. In all experiments at least three replications (four animals for each replication) were used for both adult (3 month) and old (24 month) groups of animals (Fig. 2).

The immunochemical procedure (PAP technique) in combination with image analysis was carried out as reported by Agnati et al. (1984a). The morphometrical and microdensitometrical analysis as well as the quantitative method to evaluate coexistence at cell body level (occlusion method), was principally performed as described by Agnati et al. (1984a), while the method to evaluate coexistence in terminals was performed as described by Fuxe et al. (1985).

The biochemical findings on NT/DA receptor interaction in nuc. accumbens (Agnati et al., 1983c, 1985d) have been correlated to behavioral experiments. The locomotor activity of rats has been evaluated in photocell activity cages after intra-accumbens injections of DA and DA plus NT dissolved in 0.5 μl saline. Two groups of rats have been chronically implanted with 26 gauge stainless steel guide cannulas 2 mm over the nuc. accumbens: intact rats and rats with bilateral 6OH-DA-induced lesions of the DA terminals in nuc. accumbens (see Fig. 3). The experiments were performed at least one week after the intra-accumbens injection of 6OH-DA (3 μg/2 μl).

Also the NT receptor binding characteristics in these two groups of rats were tested by measurements of [^{3}H]NT binding to synaptic membranes from the nuc. accumbens area. The binding assay was carried out according to Quirion et al. (1982) by using a fixed concentration of NT close to the K_D value (2.3 nM). The evaluation of the overall

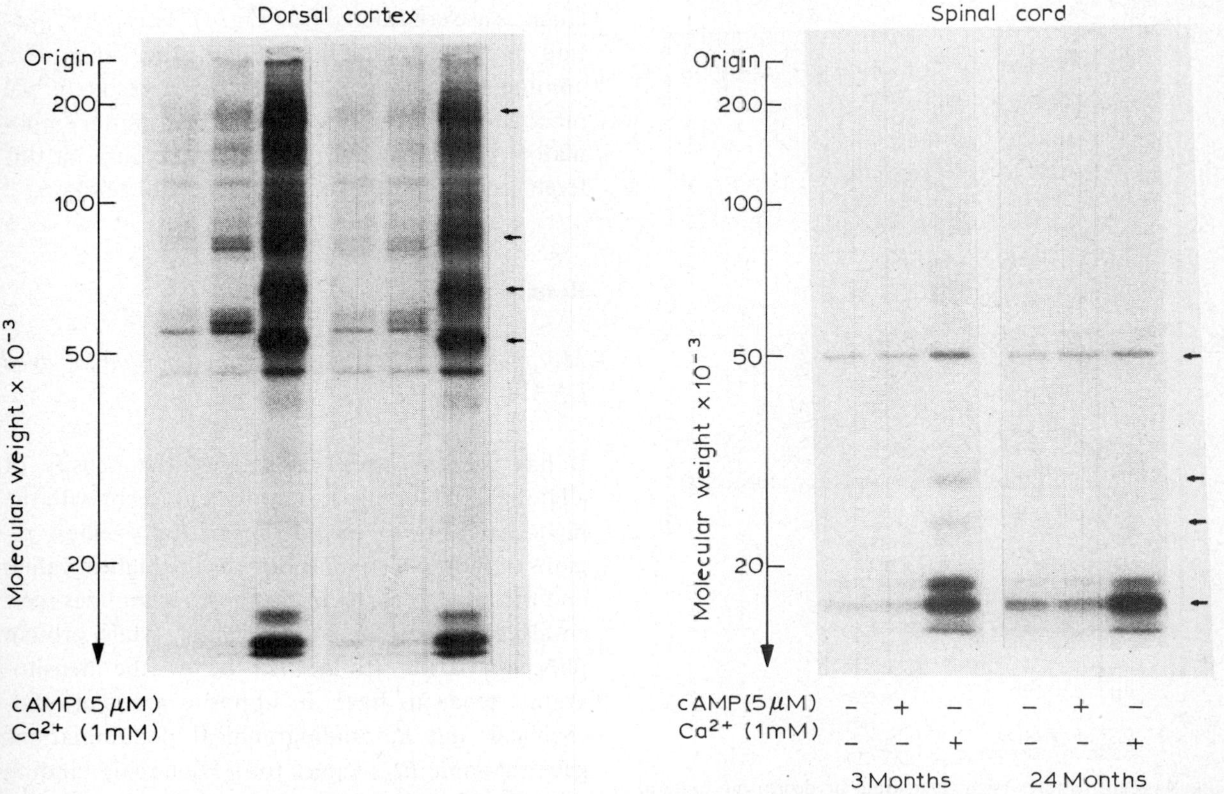

Fig. 2. Autoradiography of basal, cyclic AMP and calcium-stimulated phosphorylation in P2 fractions from dorsal cortex (left panel) and spinal cord (right panel) of 3- and 24-month-old rats. Phosphoproteins have been separated by means of SDS polyacrylamide gel electrophoresis. The arrows show the 140, 80–86, 64 and 55 kDa proteins from dorsal cortex and the 46, 28, 23 and 14 kDa proteins from the spinal cord.

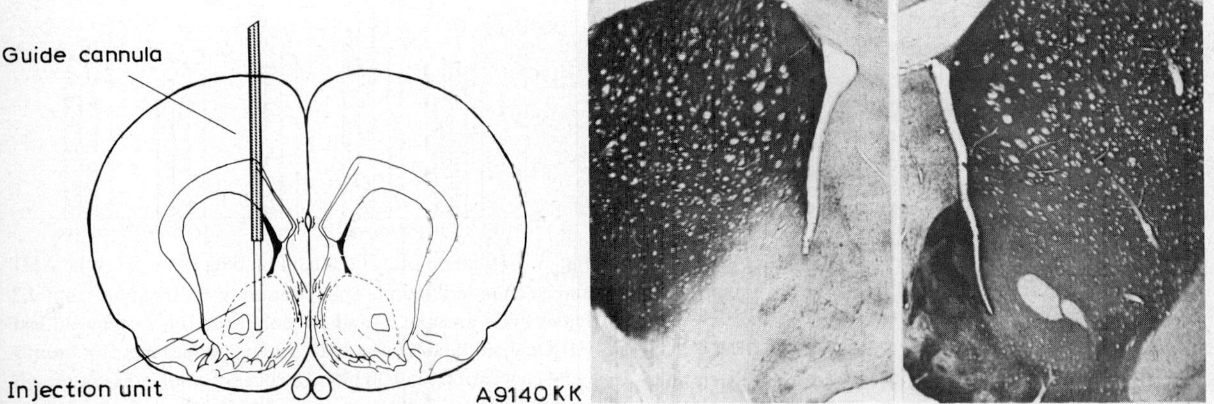

Fig. 3. The left panel shows a schematic view of the procedure used to cause degeneration of the TH-positive terminals in the nuc. accumbens. For further details, see text. The right panel presents immunocytochemical evidence for the selective disappearance of the TH-positive terminals in nuc. accumbens versus striatum. The staining was performed by the PAP procedure (see section on Material and methods in the text). TH antibody dilution: 1:1000.

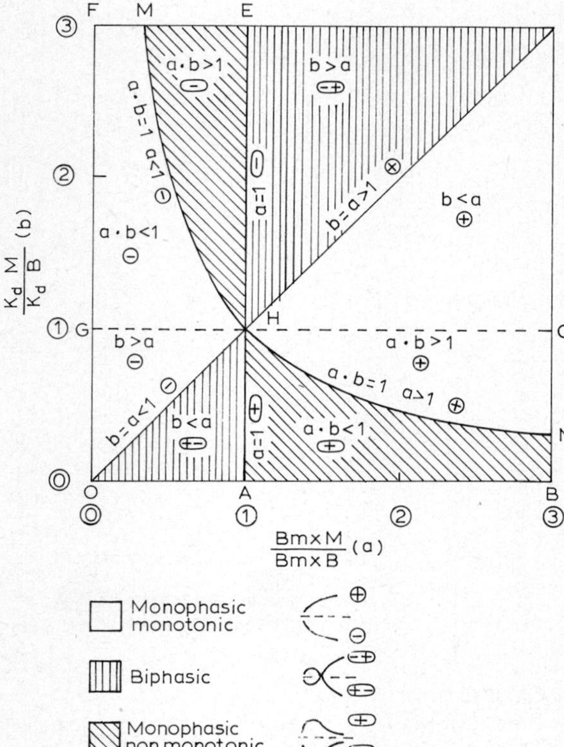

Fig. 4. Main features (sign, increasing or decreasing pattern, presence of min or max values) of equation Y = (aMx/bK + x) − (Mx/K + x), where M = B_{max} and K = K_D, x = free ligand concentration and Y = the change in ligand bound to the receptor as a function of simultaneous changes in "a" (modulated Bmx/basal Bmx) and "b" (modulated K_d/basal K_d) coefficients, which are reported on the *x*- and *y*-axis, respectively. The white areas represent a monophasic and monotonic pattern of the function (no *X*-axis crosses, no MIN or MAX values) whereas the dashed areas indicate the presence of a MIN or MAX value with (vertical hatching) or without (diagonal hatching) a sign change. In the various areas of the plot, the sign of the function is also displayed inside circles (monotonic pattern) or ellypses (occurrence of MIN or MAX values). (For further details, see text.)

effects of peptide modulation on monoamine receptors has been carried out by means of a new developed mathematical approach (Benfenati, Fuxe, Agnati, submitted). Through this approach one can get an overall evaluation of the modulatory effects of e.g. a neuropeptide on monoamine receptor binding characteristics, since both the K_D and B_{max} changes are considered (see Fig. 4). Thus, the equation presented in Fig. 4 gives the differential amount of radioligand bound, as a result of the modulatory effects of a putative transmitter (modulator) present in the incubation medium, at different concentrations of the free radioligand.

Results

Morphometrical and biochemical studies on the aged CNS

It has been shown (Fig. 5) that the density of [^{3}H]ouabain binding sites shows a gradient with the highest density in the phylogenetically oldest regions of the CNS (spinal cord has the highest value) and the lowest density in the most recent ones (cerebral cortex has the lowest value), while protein phosphorylation (total area below the densitograms) tends to have an opposite gradient. Biochemical and autoradiographical determinations gave the same B_{max} values for [^{3}H]ouabain binding sites (Fig. 1).

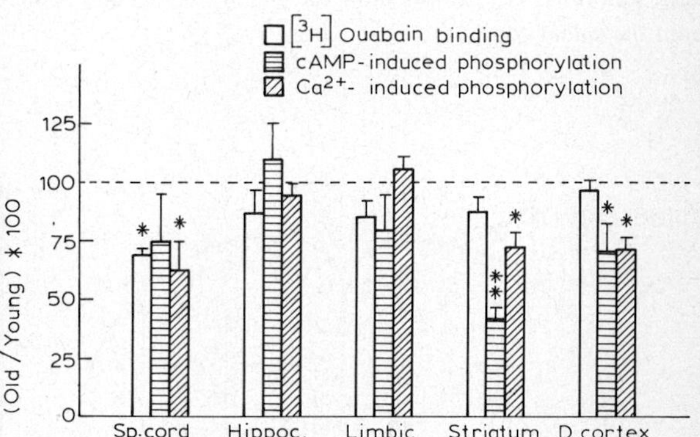

Fig. 5. Evaluation of [^{3}H]ouabain binding (n = 5), cyclic AMP and calcium-induced phosphorylation in P2 fractions from different brain areas of 3- and 24-month-old rats (3 replications). [^{3}H]Ouabain binding was evaluated as pmoles/mg prot. at a ligand concentration of 30 nM. The overall stimulation of protein phosphorylation induced by cyclic AMP and calcium was evaluated measuring the optical density of the labelled areas. All the data are expressed as mean percentages of the ratio (old/young) ± S.E.M.; Student's *t*-test for independent samples. * = $p < 0.05$; ** = $p < 0.01$.

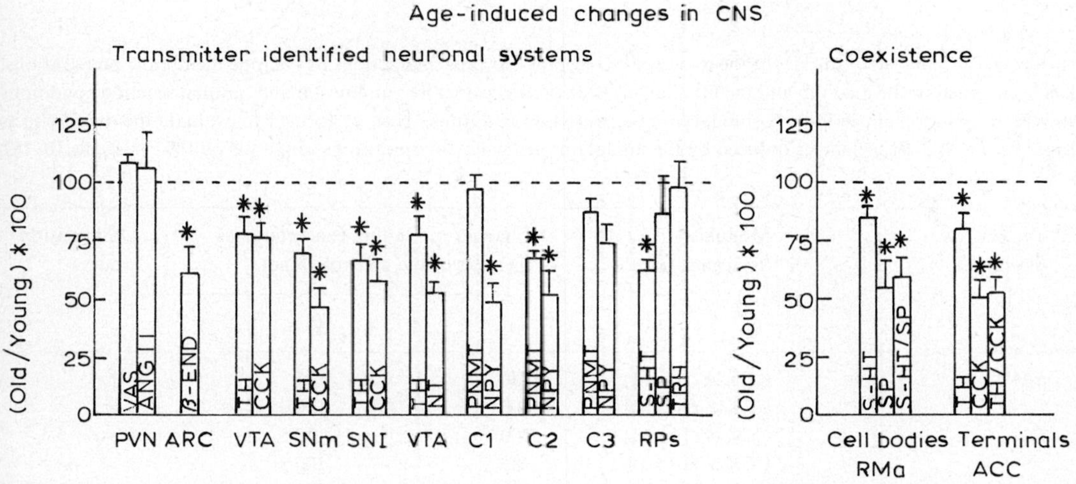

Fig. 6. Codistribution or coexistence of putative transmitters and transmitter biosynthetic enzymes in cell bodies and terminals of the CNS of young and old rats. All the data (number of cells on the left panel and entity of coexistence on the right panel) are expressed as mean percentages of the ratio (old/young) ± S.E.M. Student's *t*-test for independent samples (n = 5). Abbreviations: PVN = nuc. paraventricularis; ARC = nuc. arcuatus; VTA = ventral tegmental area; SNm = substantia nigra medial part; SNl = substantia nigra lateral part; RPa = nuc. raphe pallidus; RMa = nuc. raphe magnus; ACC = nuc. accumbens.

The [³H]ouabain binding shows a well-defined pattern in the aged brain with changes only in the phylogenetically oldest regions. Thus, a significant reduction in the density of binding sites was observed in the spinal cord. However, protein phosphorylation is not as resistant to the aging processes as [³H]ouabain binding sites and is affected especially in the phylogenetically recent regions (striatum and cerebral cortex) (Fig. 5).

When we analyze the age-induced changes either in coexistence (presence of two or more putative transmitters in the same neuron) or more broadly in codistribution (presence of two or more putative transmitters in the same nerve cell cluster or local circuit) it seems as if neuropeptides are often more affected than the enzymes involved in the monoamine synthesis and the monoamines themselves (Fig. 6).

Receptor-receptor interaction: the NT/DA receptor interaction in the limbic area (mainly nuc. accumbens and tuberculum olfactorium)

Starting from 1980 to 1981 (Agnati et al., 1980; Fuxe et al., 1981) we have demonstrated that receptors once activated by their transmitter can modulate recognition sites for other transmitters. Some of these results are summarized in Table I.

It has also been discovered that receptor-receptor interactions can be altered in pathological states such as genetic hypertension (Agnati et al., 1983b), in animal models of human pathology such as the 6OH-DA denervated striatum (model for Parkinson's disease) (Fuxe et al., 1985b) and the aged rat (Agnati et al., 1984c).

It has been observed that the CCK/DA2 receptor interaction in striatum is changed in the old animal (Agnati et al., 1984c). As a matter of fact by means of a computer simulation it is possible to assess that there is a switch from a reduction in the binding of [³H]spiperone (D2 radioligand) in presence of CCK-8 towards an increase in the binding of [³H]spiperone (Table I). We have also further characterized the interactions between NT and DA receptors in the subcortical limbic structures. In fact, our previous data demonstrated that while NT can decrease ³H-*N*-propyl-norapomorphine (NPA) binding (agonist radioligand) to limbic synaptic

TABLE I

Summary of the evidence from our laboratories for the existence of receptor-receptor interactions in synaptic membrane preparations. The modulator has been added to the medium and the binding has been performed under equilibrium and optimal reaction conditions (Fuxe and Agnati, 1985; Agnati et al., 1984d). A simulation procedure (see Fig. 4) has been performed to evaluate the oveall effects on the binding based on K_D and B_{max} changes induced by the modulator at ligand concentrations ranging from $10^{-1} \cdot K_D$ to $10 \cdot K_D$

Ligand (brain region)	Type of receptor	Modulator (concentration)	Changes in binding characteristics (percent of the control value)		Simulation curve
			K_d	B_{max}	
[3H]SPI	5-HT_2	CCK-4 (10 nM)	130	125	↓↑
(cortex)		CCK-8 (10 nM)	100	100	=
[3H]SPI	D_2	CCK-4 (10 nM)	100	100	=
(striatum)		CCK-8 (10 nM)	83	100	↓
	Old rats	CCK-8 (10 nM)	100	108	↑
[3H]NPA	D_2-D_3	CCK-4 (10 nM)	121	100	↓
(striatum)		CCK-8 (10 nM)	119	109	↓↑
[3H]NT	NT	DA (10 nM)	126	117	↑
(striatum)	6OH-DA denervation	DA (10 nM)	283	210	↓↑
[3H]NPA (striatum)	D_2-D_3	GLU (1 μM)	123	100	↓
[3H]NPA (limbic)	D_2-D_3	NT (10 nM)	160	100	↓
[3H]NT (limbic)	NT	DA (500 nM)	182	140	↓↑
[3H]NPA (limbic)	D_2-D_3	CCK-8 (10 nM)	140	110	↓↑
[3H]SPI (limbic)	D_2	NT (10 nM)	100	100	=
[3H]PAC		NPY (10 nM)	130	135	↓↑
(med. obl.)	SHR rats	NPY (10 nM)	100	100	=
[3H]5-HT (spinal cord)	5-HT_1	SP (10 nM)	134	125	↓↑

membranes (Agnati et al., 1983c), DA has the opposite effect on [^{3}H]NT binding in the same region, pointing to the possible existence of intramembrane negative feedback loops controlling the sensitivity of receptors (Agnati et al., 1985d). In view of above, behavioral experiments have been carried out evaluating the locomotor activity of intact rats and of rats with bilateral 6OH-DA induced degeneration of the DA terminals of nuc. accumbens, after a DA or DA plus NT injection into the nuc. accumbens.

There is a supersensitive response to DA in the lesioned rats, and more surprisingly, NT (0.3 μg) can reduce this response, while the same dose of NT is not effective in inhibiting DA-induced locomotor activity in intact rats (Fig. 7). Thus, it seems as if 6OH-DA also causes development of NT receptor supersensitivity. This view is supported by the biochemical experiments, which, at the [^{3}H]NT concentration used, demonstrate an increase in [^{3}H]NT binding to synaptic membranes of the nuc. accumbens of denervated rats (Fig. 8).

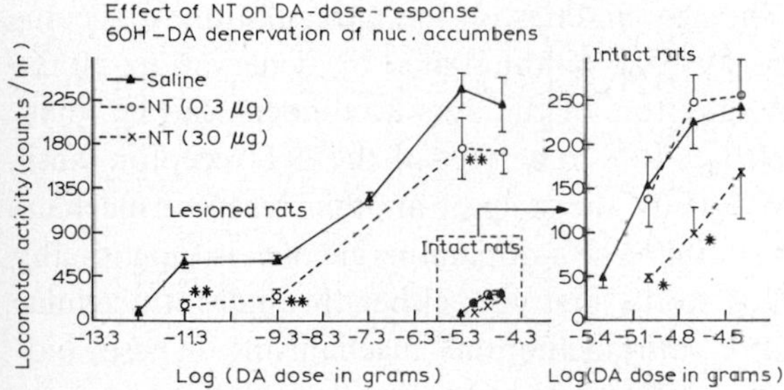

Fig. 7. Effects of bilateral intra-accumbens administration of NT (0.3 and 3.0 μg/0.5 μl saline) on DA-induced locomotor activity in intact rats (right panel) and in rats after bilateral DA denervation of the nuc. accumbens by 6OH-DA (left panel). The small insert shows the right panel in the same scale of that used for the left panel. Dunnet's test for multiple comparisons (n = 8–10); * = $\alpha < 0.05$; ** $\alpha = < 0.01$.

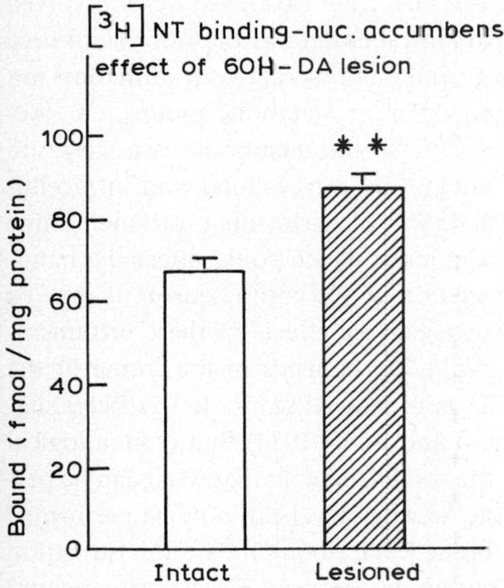

Fig. 8. [^{3}H]NT binding (2.3 nM) to synaptic membranes from nuc. accumbens of intact rats and of rats with a 6OH-DA denervated nuc. accumbens. Student's paired t-test (n = 8); ** = $p < 0.01$.

Discussion

The aging processes modify in a differential way two basic biochemical parameters of the neural tissue: the NA^+/K^+ATPase activity and the protein phosphorylation, the latter being preferentially affected. Both parameters mainly reflect functional features of the nerve cells rather than of the glial component (Swann et al., 1982; Nestler and Greengard, 1984). It is worthwhile noting that only the phylogenetically most recent brain areas show a profound alteration in protein phosphorylation. It can be surmised that the postsynaptic metabolic responses are changed especially in these areas during aging. Thus, the plastic changes, which can take place mainly through the former type of nerve cell response, are decreased in the aged brain.

Changes in the contents of putative transmitters or of transmitter biosynthetic enzymes have also been demonstrated at various levels of the neuraxis during aging. It is not possible to state a general rule for the aging of transmitters in the brain, since each transmitter or transmitter biosynthetic enzyme shows its own pattern of changes during aging within different cell groups having the same transmitter (see e.g. changes in CCK/TH coexistence in the A10 vs. A9 DA cell group; Agnati et al., 1985b), and sometimes even within different parts of the same cell group (see e.g. changes in CCK/TH coexistence in the lateral and medial parts of the A9 DA cell group).

We have previously discussed the possible functional meaning of coexistence (Agnati et al., 1984d) based on the discovery of the receptor-receptor interactions; decrease or increase of the efficiency of the main transmission line, isoreceptor interconversion, multiple interrelated postsynaptic responses, increase the number of possible messages. Thus, these functional aspects may be altered in aging. Furthermore, the most recent evidence obtained in studies on receptor-receptor interactions and on age-induced changes in the entity of coexistence (Fig. 9) suggests that the miniaturization of the neural network as well as the intramembrane feedback loops can be affected in the aged brain.

The discovery of receptor-receptor interactions opens up new aspects on the integrative capabilities of the neural networks. In fact, these interactions stress the view of the existence at the synaptic level of multiple transmission lines, which can interact at the presynaptic level, the postsynaptic membrane

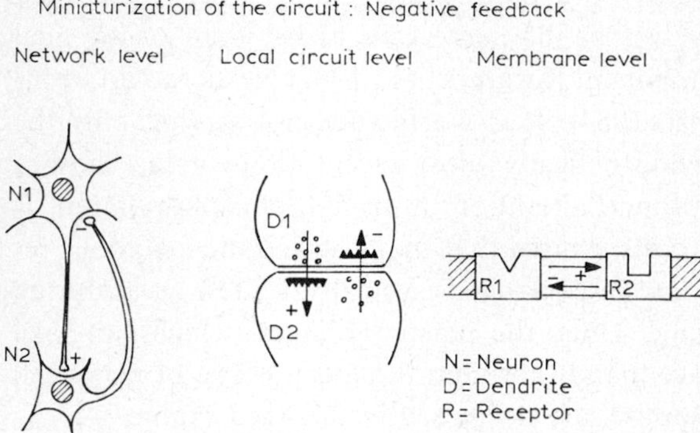

Fig. 9. The concept of miniaturization of the circuit.

level and the postsynaptic transduction system (Fig. 10). Furthermore, at the level of the local circuit (Rakic, 1979) this phenomenon suggests that the local circuit should be considered as an electrometabolic integrative unit (see Fig. 10).

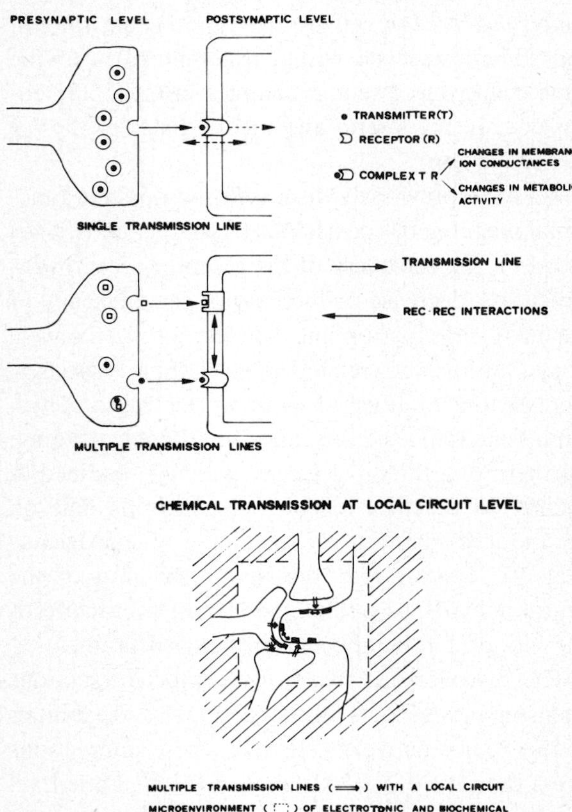

Fig. 10. The local circuit as an electrometabolic unit.

The new findings on the upregulation of accumbens [^{3}H]NT binding sites by denervation of the DA receptors of the nuc. accumbens can be interpreted as due to a reset of the NT receptor sensitivity. Thus, the state of another receptor mechanism, in this case a dopaminergic one, is functionally linked to the first one, either through intracellular and/or intramembrane mechanisms. These biochemical data may at least in part explain the more effective inhibitory action of NT- on DA-induced locomotor activity when injected into the nuc. accumbens in rats with a bilateral 6OH-DA-induced degeneration of DA terminals of the nuc. accumbens compared with intact rats.

The receptor-receptor interactions are only one example of the many types of regulatory mechanisms which can affect the various systems involved in the information handling at the intramembrane level, as e.g. interactions between different ion channels, and different metabolic pumps, etc. According to this view, the membrane is a structure capable of integrating extracellular and intracellular signals as well as of performing intramembrane regulatory responses, which could affect the handling of information by the entire neuron. It may be relevant to consider the effects of these intramembrane integrative mechanisms in the frame of the wiring of the neuronal network. It has been suggested (Agnati and Fuxe, 1984) that from a logical standpoint the results indicate that what can be performed at the network level can now be performed at the membrane level, obtaining a miniaturization of the computing devices (see Fig. 9), which could have been of importance for the appearance of the higher brain functions during evolution. This aspect should be considered when we are discussing the functional role of cotransmission and, as pointed out above, receptor interactions at the local circuit level. A general view of the relevance of the receptor-receptor interaction (either at the synaptic or at the local circuit level) is schematically presented in Fig. 11, where, in parenthesis, the possible functional meaning of the experimental observations are reported. In conclusion, moving from the synapse to the neural network we put forward the

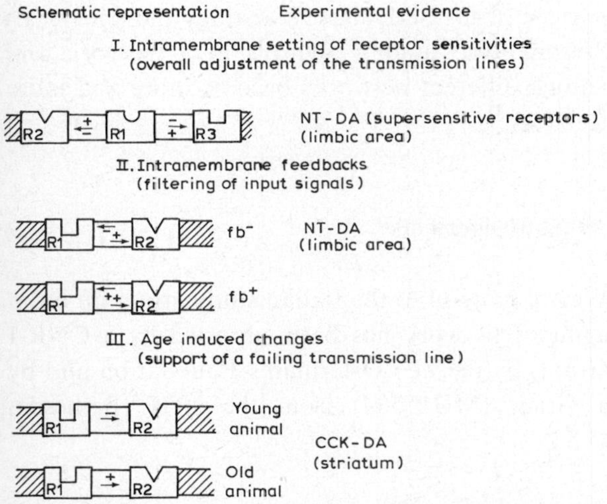

Schematic representation Experimental evidence

I. Intramembrane setting of receptor sensitivities (overall adjustment of the transmission lines)

R2 R1 R3 NT-DA (supersensitive receptors) (limbic area)

II. Intramembrane feedbacks (filtering of input signals)

R1 R2 fb^- NT-DA (limbic area)

R1 R2 fb^+

III. Age induced changes (support of a failing transmission line)

R1 R2 Young animal

CCK-DA (striatum)

R1 R2 Old animal

Fig. 11. Possible functional meaning of coexistence and more generally of integration of electrochemical signals at the membrane level.

idea that the synaptic transmission should be considered as made up by multiple transmission lines which can interact with each other in the same or adjacent synapses, making possible also intersynaptic integrations (level of the local circuit). Finally, it should be considered that the neural network, thanks also to the non-synaptic transmission (Vizi, 1984) is controlled by signals in the medium surrounding the network (volume of transmission). Thus, the neural network operates in a medium, through which electrical and chemical (paracrine, endocrine) messages can reach any element of the system. Thus, besides the focal sites of information handling, i.e. the synaptic contacts, we must consider the volume of transmission as taking part in the integrative processes of the neural network.

In this way the information handling of the CNS relies upon two different types of transmission (see Table II): "the neuron linked electrochemical transmission" and the "volume of transmission' (signals of the network medium). Through the latter type the neural network is liberated from the constraints of the neuroanatomical wiring, since now the electrical and the chemical signals can theoretically reach in any order, any part of the various nerve cells, making possible large numbers of informational networks. We believe that the suggested identification of these two types of transmission may be considered highly complementary to the concept of ionotropic and metabotropic transmission (McGeer et al., 1978). In agreement with our view is the experimental evidence (see e.g. Agnati et al., 1984; Fuxe et al., this volume; Kuhar, 1985) that the transmitter receptors often cover substantially larger areas than the nerve terminal networks containing the corresponding transmitter. This discrepancy is so large that it is unlikely that it is only

TABLE II

Schematic summary of our hypothesis on the existence of two principal types of electrochemical transmission at network and local circuit level

Kind of transmission	Speed of transmission	Degree of divergence	Segregation ("safety" of the transmission)	Plasticity	Preferential information processing
"*Wiring*" neuron linked electrochemical transmission	High	Low to moderate	High	Low	Elementary elaboration short-term action
"*Volume of transmission*" humoral ("open") electrochemical transmission	Low	High to very high	Low	High	Holistic elaboration long-term action

caused by the fact that the receptors are localized not only in the postsynaptic membrane but also in the cell body, axon and terminals of the neuron. Thus, our concepts underline the view of Changeux (1983) that the chemical transmission has added a new dimension to the integrative capabilities of the neural networks.

A fascinating analogy of the capabilities of neural networks to affect each other as far as the higher brain functions are concerned, is offered by Dennis Diderot (1713–1784) who wrote:

"Mais les cordes vibrantes ont encore une autre propriété, c'est d'en faire frémir d'autres; et c'est ainsi qu'une première idée en rappelle une seconde, ces deux-la une troisième, toutes les trois une quatrième, et ainsi de suite, sans qu'on puisse fixer la limite des idées réveillées, enchaînées, du philosophe qui médite ou qui s'écoute dans le silence et l'obscurite. Cet instrument a des sauts étonnants, et une idée réveillée va faire quelquefois frémir une harmonique qui en est à un intervalle incompréhensible."

During aging neural systems degenerate (Finch, 1973; Agnati et al., 1984b, 1985a,b). Thus, the "neuron linked electrochemical transmission" is affected. However, in view of the redundancy of the CNS no clearcut deficits may appear (see Granit, 1977). But the "volume of transmission" type of electrochemical communication is also affected and this alteration may have profound effects on the higher functions of the CNS.

We can now discuss in this new frame our findings on the changes in Na^+/K^+ATPase binding sites and protein phosphorylation in the aged brain, which well match the observations of a decrease of brain glucose utilization with age (Smith et al., 1980). It is apparent that the metabolic responses in the aged brain are altered and above all in the phylogenetically most recent regions, where they have the highest level of activity. These types of responses are basic for the proper decoding of chemical signals (such as peptides, amines, etc.) which can reach a neuron also through the "volume of transmission" and thus are important, as discussed above, to free the neural network from the constraints of the neuroanatomical wiring. Thus, in the aged CNS, the new dimension opened up by the chemical transmission is getting more and more narrow or to use Diderot's analogy the (chemical) "resonances" among neurons in a network and among different networks become more and more feeble.

Acknowledgements

We are grateful to the Italian study group on brain aging. This work has been suported by a CNR-I Grant, by the Leo Osterman's Foundation and by a Grant (MH25504) from the NIH (Bethesda, U.S.A.).

References

Agnati, L. F. and Fuxe, K. (1984) New concepts on the structure of the neural networks: the miniaturization and hierarchical organization of the central nervous system. *Biosci. Rep.*, 4: 93–94.

Agnati, L. F., Fuxe, K., Zini, I. Lenzi, P. and Hökfelt, T. (1980) Aspects on receptor regulation and isoreceptor identification. *Med. Biol.*, 58: 182–187.

Agnati, L. F., Fuxe, K., Benfenati, F., Battistini, N., Härfstrand, A., Tatemoto, K., Hökfelt, T. and Mutt, V. (1983a) Neuropeptide Y in vitro selectively increases the number of α2-adrenergic binding sites in membranes of the medulla oblongata of the rat. *Acta physiol. Scand.*, 118: 293–295.

Agnati, L. F., Fuxe, K., Benfenati, F., Battistini, N., Härfstrand, A., Hökfelt, T., Cavicchioli, L., Tatemoto, K. and Mutt, V. (1983b) Failure of neuropeptide Y in vitro to increase the number of α2-adrenergic binding sites in membranes of medulla oblongata of the spontaneous hypertensive rats. *Acta physiol. Scand.*, 119: 309–312.

Agnati, L. F., Fuxe, K., Benfenati, F. and Battistini, N. (1983c) Neurotensin in vitro markedly reduces the affinity in subcortical limbic ^{3}H-N-propylnorapomorphine binding sites. *Acta physiol. Scand.*, 119: 459–461.

Agnati, L. F., Fuxe, K., Benfenati, F., Zini, I., Zoli, M., Fabbri, L. and Härfstrand, A. (1984a) Computer assisted morphometry and microdensitometry of transmitter identified neurons with special reference to the mesostriatal dopamine pathway. I. Methodological aspects. *Acta physiol. Scand.*, Suppl. 532: 5–36.

Agnati, L. F., Fuxe, K., Benfenati, F., Toffano, G., Cimino, M., Battistini, N., Calza, L. and Merlo Pich, E. (1984b) Computer assisted morphometry and microdensitometry of transmitter identified neurons with special reference to the mesostriatal dopamine pathway. III. Studies on aging processes. *Acta physiol. Scand.*, Suppl. 532: 45–61.

Agnati, L. F., Fuxe, K., Battistini, N. and Benfenati, F. (1984c) Aging brain and dopamine receptors: Abnormal regulation by CCK-8 of ^{3}H-spiperone labelled dopamine receptors in striatal membranes. *Acta physiol. Scand.*, 120: 465–467.

Agnati, L. F., Fuxe, K., Benfenati, F., Battistini, N., Zini, I., Camurri, M. and Hökfelt, T. (1984d) Postsynaptic effects of neuropeptide comodulators at central monoamine synapses. In E. Usdin, A. Carlsson, A. Dahlström and J. Engel (Eds.), *Neurology and Neurobiology, Vol. 8B,* Alan R. Liss Inc., New York, pp. 191–198.

Agnati, L. F., Fuxe, K., Calza, L., Giardino, L., Zini, I., Toffano, G., Goldstein, M., Marrama, P., Gustafsson, J.-Å., Yu, Z.-Y., Cuello, C., Terenius, L., Lang, R. and Ganten, D. (1985a) Morphometrical and microdensitometrical studies on monoaminergic and peptidergic neurons in the aging brain. In L. F. Agnati and K. Fuxe (Eds.), *Quantitative Neuroanatomy in Transmitter Research,* MacMillan Press, London, pp. 91–112.

Agnati, L. F., Fuxe, K., Giardino, L., Calza, L., Zoli, M., Battistini, N., Benfenati, F., Vanderhaegen, J. J., Guidolin, D., Ruggeri, M. and Goldstein, M. (1985b) Evidence for cholecystokinin-dopamine receptor interactions in the central nervous system of the adult and old rat. Studies on their functional meaning. In J. J. Vanderhaeghen (Ed.), *Neuronal Cholecystokinin,* Ann. N.Y. Acad. Sci., 448: 315–333.

Agnati, L. F., Fuxe, K., Benfenati, F., Zoli, M., Owman, C., Diemer, N. H. Kåhrström, J., Toffano, G. and Cimino, M. (1985c) Effects of ganglioside GM1 treatment on striatal glucose metabolism, blood flow and protein phosphorylation of the rat. *Acta physiol. Scand.*, 125: 43–53.

Agnati, L. F., Fuxe, K., Battistini, N., Giardino, L., Benfenati, F., Martire, M. and Ruggeri, M. (1985d) Further evidence for the existence of interactions between neurotensin and dopamine receptors. Dopamine reduces the affinity and increases the number of ^{3}H-neurotensin binding sites in the subcortical limbic forebrain of the rat. *Acta physiol. Scand.*, 124: 125–128.

Agnoli, A., Crepaldi, G., Spano, P. F. and Trabucchi, M. (1983) *Aging Brain and Ergot Alkaloids,* Raven Press, New York.

Benfenati, F., Agnati, L. F., Fuxe, K., Cimino, M., Battistini, N., Merlo Pich, E., Farabegoli, C. and Zini, I. (1985) Quantitative autoradiography as a tool to study receptors in neural tissue. Studies on 3H-Ouabain binding sites and correlation with synaptic protein phosphorylation in different brain areas. In L. F. Agnati and K. Fuxe (Eds.), *Quantitative Neuroanatomy in Transmitter Research,* MacMillan Press, London, pp. 381–396.

Changeux, J.-P. (1983) *L'Homme Neuronal,* Librairie Arthème Fayard, Paris.

Diderot, D. (1965) *Entretien entre d'Alembert et Diderot,* Garnier-Flammarion, Paris.

Finch, C. B. (1973) Catecholamine metabolism in the brains of aging male mice. *Brain Res.*, 52: 261–276.

Fuxe, K. and Agnati, L. F. (1985) Receptor-receptor interactions in the central nervous system. A new integrative mechanism in synapses. Medicinal Research Reviews, John Wiley & Sons, Inc., USA (in press).

Fuxe, K., Agnati, L. F., Benfenati, F., Cimino, M., Algeri, S., Hökfelt, T. and Mutt, V. (1981) Modulation of cholecystokinins of ^{3}H-spiroperidol binding in rat striatum: evidence for increased affinity and reduction in the number of binding sites. *Acta physiol. Scand.*, 113: 567–569.

Fuxe, K., Agnati, L. F., Zoli, M., Härfstrand, A., Grimaldi, R., Bernardi, P., Camurri, M. and Goldstein, M. (1985a) Development of quantitative methods for the evaluation of the entity of coexistence of neuroactive substances in nerve terminal populations in discrete areas of the central nervous system: Evidence for hormonal regulation of cotransmission. In L. F. Agnati and K. Fuxe (Eds.), *Quantitative Neuroanatomy in Transmitter Research,* MacMillan Press, London, pp. 157–174.

Fuxe, K., Agnati, L. F., Martire, M., Neumeyer, A., Benfenati, F. and Frey, P. (1985b) Studies of neurotensin-dopamine receptor interactions in striatal membranes of the male rat. The influence of 6-hydroxydopamine induced dopamine receptor supersensitivity. *Acta physiol. Scand.* (submitted).

Giacobini, E., Filogamo, G., Giacobini, G. and Vernadakis, A. (1982) *The Aging Brain: Cellular and Molecular Mechanisms of Aging in the Nervous System,* Raven Press, New York.

Granit, R. (1977) *The Purposive Brain,* The MIT Press, Cambridge Mass.

Hökfelt, T., Johansson, O. and Goldstein, M. (1984) Chemical Anatomy of the brain. *Science,* 225: 1326–1334.

Kuhar, M. J. (1985) The mismatch problem in receptor mapping studies. *Trends Neurosci.,* 27: 190–191.

Laemmli, U. K. (1970) Cleavage of structural proteins during the assembly of the head of bacteriophage T4. *Nature (Lond.),* 227: 680–685.

McGeer, P. Z., Eccles, J. C. and McGeer, E. G. (1978) *Molecular Neurobiology of the Mammalian Brain,* Plenum Press, New York.

Nestler, E. J. and Greengard, P. (1984) *Protein Phosphorylation in the Nervous System,* John Wiley, New York.

Quirion, R., Gaudreau, P., StPierre, S., Rioux, F. and Pert, C. B. (1982) Autoradiographic distribution of ^{3}H-neurotensin receptors in rat brain: visualization by tritium sensitive film. *Peptides,* 3: 757–766.

Rakic, P. (1979) Genetic and epigenetic determinants of local neuronal circuits in the mammalian central nervous system. In F. O. Schmitt and F. G. Worden (Eds.), *The Neurosciences, 4th Study Program,* The MIT Press, Cambridge, Mass.

Smith, D. O., Goochee, C., Rapaport, S. I. and Sokoloff, L. (1980) Effects of aging on local rates of cerebral glucose utilization in the rat. *Brain,* 103: 351–365.

Swann, A. C., Grant, S. C. and Maas, J. W. (1982) Brain Na^+/K^+ATPase and noradrenergic activity: effects of hyperinnervation and denervation on high affinity ouabain binding. *J. Neurochem.,* 38: 836–839.

Vizi, E. S. (1984) *Non-Synaptic Interactions between Neurons: Modulation of Chemical Transmission,* John Wiley, New York.

T. Hökfelt, K. Fuxe and B. Pernow (Eds.),
Progress in Brain Research, Vol. 68

CHAPTER 20

Morphofunctional studies on the neuropeptide Y/adrenaline costoring terminal systems in the dorsal cardiovascular region of the medulla oblongata. Focus on receptor-receptor interactions in cotransmission

K. Fuxe[1], L. F. Agnati[2], A. Härfstrand[1], A. M. Janson[1], A. Neumeyer[1], K. Andersson[1], M. Ruggeri[2], M. Zoli[2] and M. Goldstein[3]

[1]*Department of Histology, Karolinska Institutet, Stockholm, Sweden,* [2]*Department of Human Physiology, University of Modena, Modena, Italy, and* [3]*Department of Psychiatry, New York University Medical Center, N.Y., U.S.A.*

Introduction

We have for many years analyzed the anatomy and function of the central adrenaline neurons in the rat (Hökfelt et al., 1974, 1980, 1984a; Goldstein et al., 1978; Fuxe et al., 1980a,b,c, 1981a, 1982a,b, 1983; Agnati et al., 1985a). The morphological studies have also been performed by means of computer assisted morphometry and microdensitometry (See Agnati et al., 1984b, 1985b,c) to give an objective representation of the central adrenaline (A) nerve cell groups in the medulla oblongata (Agnati et al., 1985c; Kalia et al., 1985). The functional and biochemical studies of the A neurons within the medulla oblongata, especially within the dorsal cardiovascular region (nuc. tractus solitarius and dorsal motor nuc. of the vagus), have given evidence that the adrenergic neurons have an important vasodepressor function in the central nervous system (see Fuxe et al., 1980a,b,c, 1981a, 1982a,b). Hökfelt and colleagues (1984a) have demonstrated the existence of neuropeptide Y like immunoreactivity in the A cell groups C1, C2 and C3 in the medulla oblongata. Based on these observations, we have the last few years analyzed the effects of centrally administered neuropeptide Y (NPY) on cardiovascular and respiratory parameters and on pre- and postsynaptic mechanisms in central A nerve terminal networks in the dorsal cardiovascular region of the medulla oblongata of the rat. These studies have shown that NPY gives i.c. in the α-chloralose anaesthetized rat can reduce arterial blood pressure and heart rate and that these actions are observed also in the presence of α-adrenergic receptor blockade (see Fuxe et al., 1983b; Härfstrand et al., 1984). Furthermore, in membrane preparations from the medulla oblongata NPY (10 nM) was found to, selectively, modulate the binding characteristics of α_2-adrenergic agonists and antagonist binding sites using *p*-[^{3}H]aminoclonidine ([^{3}H]PAC), [^{3}H]Rauwolscine and [^{3}H]Rx 781094 as radioligands (Agnati et al., 1983c; Fuxe et al., 1984a). It was found that under equilibrium conditions NPY could induce an increase in B_{max} values and an increase in the K_D values for both the [^{3}H]adrenergic agonist and antagonist binding sites. These results indicate the existence of interactions between NPY and α_2-adrenergic receptors in the medulla oblongata, which may take place at the level of the coupling device as well as at the level of the recognition site (Agnati et al., 1984a; Fuxe et al., 1984a; 1984b).

In this chapter we have further analyzed the role

of receptor-receptor interactions in cotransmission via a more detailed morphofunctional analysis of the NPY/A costoring neurons of the medulla oblongata. The results give evidence that receptor-receptor interactions in costoring synapses make possible a miniaturization of neuronal circuits and a heterostatic regulation of the synapse, since the α_2-adrenergic transduction mechanisms in the membrane can be altered without any associated change in A levels and utilization (see Fuxe et al., 1984a; Agnati et al., 1985a).

Quantitative evaluation of neuropeptide Y/PNMT coexistence in dorsal cardiovascular region of the medulla oblongata by means of the occlusion method

Of fundamental importance for the understanding of the functional significance of coexistence of neuronal messengers has been the development of quantitative methods to evaluate the entity of coexistence in nerve cell bodies and nerve terminals (Agnati et al., 1984b, 1985b; Fuxe et al., 1985a). Thus, the so-called occlusion method has been used to quantitate coexistence in nerve terminal networks. The principle of this technique is shown in Fig. 1. Three adjacent vibratome sections have been stained for PNMT immunoreactivity, NPY immunoreactivity and for NPY/PNMT immunoreactivity as shown in the lower part of Fig. 1. In all three sections, coexisting profiles are shown and therefore the sum of the immunoreactive profiles shown in sections 1 and 2 minus those demonstrated in section 3 will give the number of NPY/PNMT costoring profiles. The determination of the immunoreactive profiles has been made by means of image analysis using an IBAS image analyzer (Zeiss Kontron). The analysis has been performed on binary images which have been obtained by the discrimination procedure indicated in Fig. 1. The gray tone histogram of the background has been obtained and the mean gray tone minus two standard deviations has been used in the discrimination procedure. An overall evaluation of the amount of the immunoreactive nerve terminals present was obtained by

The occlusion for the quantitative determination of coexistence in terminals

1. Background definition: Graytone histogram ($\bar{X}$: SD)
2. Discrimination by using the graytone level ($\bar{X}$-2. SD)
3. Assessment of the specific area for NPY(SA_{NPY})
4. Assessment of the specific area for PNMT(SA_{PNMT})
5. Assessment of the specific area for NPY + PNMT($SA_{NPY+PNMT}$)
6. Evaluation of the specific area of distribution of the single objects: The minimum value is the area of the single terminal (SA_T)

$SA_{NPY} + SA_{PNMT} - SA_{NPY+PNMT} = SA_{NPY/PNMT}$

$(SA_{NPY/PNMT})/(SA_T) = N_{NPY/PNMT}$ = Number of terminals with coexistence

$(SA_{PNMT})/(SA_T) = N_{PNMT}$ = Number of PNMT positive terminals

$((N_{NPY/PNM})/(N_{PNMT}))\cdot 100$ = Percent of coexistence

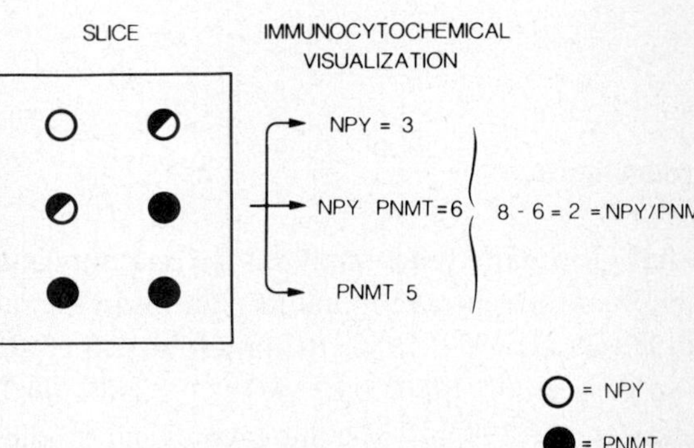

Fig. 1. Schematic illustration of the procedures used to determine the coexistence in nerve terminal networks present in sections by means of the occlusion method. SA = the size of the specific area evaluated by means of the IBAS Image Analyzer. The specific area has been obtained for PNMT, NPY and NPY + PNMT-like immunoreactivity. A_T = area of the single terminal obtained by means of the histogram of the single objects present in the image. The principles of the occlusion method are indicated in the lower part of the figure.

measuring the total specific area of immunoreactive profiles as indicated in Fig. 1. Thus, by means of the occlusion principle, the coexisting immunoreactive area is obtained and by dividing this area with the area of the single profile an estimation of the number of terminals showing coexistence can be obtained.

In the present study, coexistence of PNMT and

TABLE I

Studies on coexistence in the NPY and PNMT immunoreactive nerve terminals in the medial subnucleus of NTS and in the dorsal motor nucleus of the vagus using the occlusion principle WKY rats (16 weeks old). Formula for coexistence (%)

$$\frac{FA(NPY) + FA(PNMT) - FA(NPY\ and\ PNMT)}{FA(NPY)} \times 100$$

Animal group	NPY terminals		PNMT terminals		NPY and PNMT terminals		Coexistence (see formula above) (%)
	Mean area $\bar{A}$ (μ^2)	Field area FA(NPY) (μ^2)	Mean area $\bar{A}$ (μ^2)	Field area FA(PNMT) (μ^2)	Mean area $\bar{A}$ (μ^2)	Field area FA(NPY+PNMT) (μ^2)	
WKY	4.40 ±0.07	2160 ±399	4.52 ±0.03	1220 ±239	4.44 ±0.01	1660 ±429	82 ±5

Mean ± S.E.M. are shown above.

NPY immunoreactivity has been analyzed in nerve terminals of the dorsal motor nucleus of the vagus and of the medial subnucleus of the nuc. tractus solitarius at the level of the area postrema of the normotensive Wistar-Kyoto rat. This region is part of the dorsal cardiovascular center of the medulla oblongata of the rat (see Kalia et al., 1985). The results of the analysis are shown in Table I. The NPY and PNMT immunoreactive nerve terminals have been demonstrated by the use of 30 μm thick vibratome sections in combination with indirect peroxidase procedure of Sternberger (1979), for details see Agnati et al., 1984b. As seen in Table I, we can now for the first time show that NPY and PNMT immunoreactivity are costored in the vast majority of the NPY immunoreactive nerve terminals (82%). Thus, it seems likely that the interactions between NPY and A demonstrated in functional and biochemical experiments partly reflect processes which may take place during cotransmission in the NPY/A costoring synapses of the dorsal cardiovascular centers of the medulla oblongata (see below).

Functional meaning of NPY/adrenaline coexistence in the cardiovascular centers of the medulla oblongata of the rat

In previous studies, intracisternal administration of NPY has been shown to produce dose-related reduction of arterial blood pressure in the α-chloralose anesthetized male rat (Fuxe et al., 1983b; Härfstrand et al., 1984). In this chapter we demonstrate that NPY given into the lateral ventricle of conscious unrestrained male rats can also produce a marked lowering of arterial blood pressure, of heart rate and of respiration rate underlining an important role of NPY in central cardiovascular control (Fig. 2). The total duration of action observed for a maximal dose of NPY is in the order of 2 h, similar to that seen after central clonidine administration. As seen in Fig. 3, the prevention experiments in the α-chloralose anesthetized rats with the α_2-adrenergic antagonist Rx 781094 (208 nmol, i.c.) show that the α_2-adrenergic antagonist can prevent the hypotensive action of clonidine (0.37 nmol, i.c.) but not the hypotensive action of

EFFECTS OF NPY(1.25 nmol i.v.t.) ON CONSCIOUS UNRESTRAINED MALE RATS.

CSF
NPY

BASAL VALUES	LEVEL OF SIGNIFICANCE
CSF 107±2mmHg n=5	0-30' p<0.002
NPY 103±3mmHg n=5	0-60' p<0.002
CSF 425±17 beats/min	0-30' 0.05<p<0.1
NPY 408±21 beats/min	0-60' 0.05<p<0.1
CSF 98±3 breaths/min	0-30' 0.05<p<0.1
NPY 103±3 breaths/min	0-60' 0.05<p<0.1

Fig. 2. Effects of i.v.t. injections of NPY (1.25 nmol/30 μl mock CSF) on mean arterial blood pressure (MAP), heart rate (HR) and respiratory rate (RR) in the awake unrestrained male rat. Means ± S.E.M. (n = 5) are shown in per cent of respective basal value at the time of NPY or CSF injections. The areas of hypotensive, bradycardic and bradypneuic activity observed in each animal during the period analysed (1 h) were evaluated. These values have been used to test a significant effect of NPY on cardiovascular and respiratory parameters (see table in the figure; Mann-Whitney U-test).

Prevention experiments with Rx 781094 (208nmol) ic.

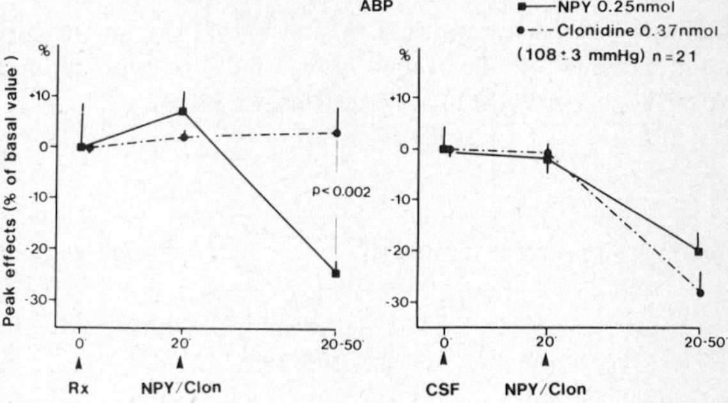

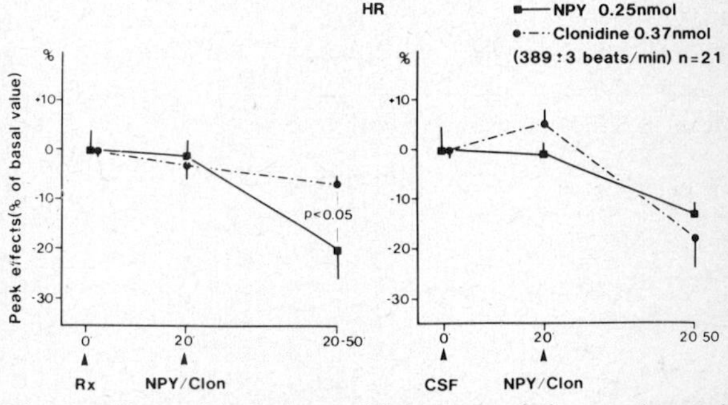

Fig. 3. Effects of intracisternal injections of the α_2-adrenergic receptor antagonist Rx 781094 on the hypotensive and bradycardiac actions of intracisternal injections of clonidine and NPY in the α-chloralose anesthetized rat. Rx 781094 was administered 20 min prior to the injection of NPY or clonidine. The peak effects of NPY and clonidine are shown in per cent of respective basal value (means ± S.E.M.). In the statistical analysis, Mann Whitney U-test was performed.

NPY (0.25 nmoles, i.c.). These results give evidence that NPY can exert its cardiovascular actions in the presence of α_2-adrenergic receptor blockade (see also Härfstrand et al., 1984). However, the α_2-adrenergic and NPY receptors probably interact, since when NPY and clonidine are administered together no additional effect is seen as illustrated in Fig. 4. Thus, combined intracisternal administration of maximal or submaximal doses of NPY and clonidine in the α-chloralose anesthetized rat does not lead to any significant increase of the hypotensive action observed after the respective single drug administration and the same has also been found to be true when using threshold doses of NPY and clonidine.

Based on these observations, the hypothesis has been introduced that the NPY and α_2-adrenergic receptors probably located in the postsynaptic membrane of the NPY/adrenaline costoring synapses of the dorsal cardiovascular region of the medulla oblongata can interact with each other at least at the level of the coupling device (Fig. 5). As

Combined i.c. administration of submaximal doses of NPY and Clonidine in α-chloralose anaesthetized rats

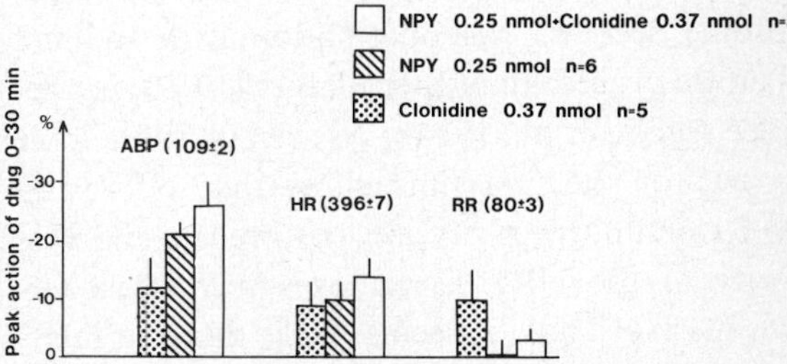

Fig. 4. Effects of combined intracisternal administration of submaximal doses of NPY and clonidine on arterial blood pressure, heart rate and respiratory rate in the α-chloralose anesthetized male rat. The peak effects of the drugs are shown during the first 30 min time interval following injection and are expressed in per cent of respective basal mean value. The drugs were dissolved in artificial CSF and the effects shown represent the effects seen after subtracting the slight effects produced by artificial CSF alone.

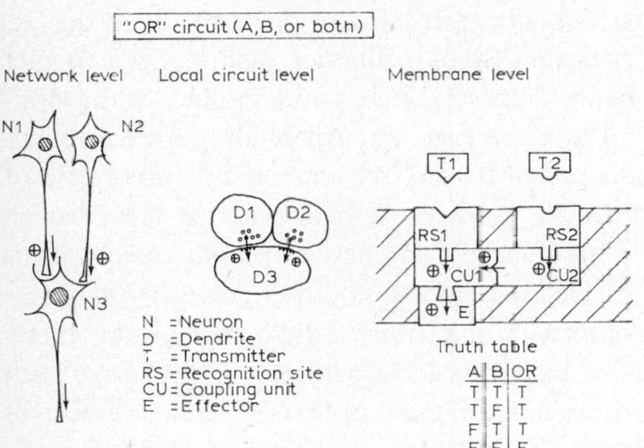

Fig. 5. Schematic representation of the possible logic model underlying the receptor-receptor interaction as exemplified for NPY receptors and α_2-adrenergic receptors. It should be observed that this mechanism in the present case works as an "OR" circuit, since the hypotensive action can be obtained after NPY or clonidine but combined treatment cannot cause a clearcut increase of the hypotensive actions of NPY and clonidine alone. Furthermore, NPY causes hypotension also after α_2-receptor blockade with Rx 781094, (see Fig. 3). By means of receptor-receptor interactions a miniaturization of the circuit (Agnati and Fuxe, 1984) can be achieved (note the successive steps in miniaturization from the left to the right of neural circuits capable of an "OR" operation). The truth table gives the logical value for the output (T = true = active; F = false = inactive), when the inputs (A,B) take different logical values.

indicated in the figure, such an interaction makes possible the performance of an "or" logical operation at membrane level. The performance of such a logical function can also take place at network level and at local circuit level. However, the receptor-receptor interaction may also be envisaged as a miniaturization of neuronal circuits of the brain (see Agnati and Fuxe, 1984). Current evidence indicates that the α_2-adrenergic receptor controls in an inhibitory way adenylate cyclase via a guanylate-regulated protein (Gi protein). It is therefore possible that the interaction between the NPY and α_2-adrenergic receptors partly represents an interaction at the Gi protein. It has been shown by Undén and Bartfai (1984) that the GTP-regulated proteins probably are involved in the control of NPY recognition sites, since GTP can produce in vitro a reduction in the B_{max} value of the NPY binding sites. Recently, we have also observed that GTP given intracisternally in the α-chloralose anesthetized rat can delay the onset of the hypotensive action of NPY but not that of clonidine (Härfstrand et al., 1985).

Biochemical and receptor autoradiographical evidence for an interaction between NPY and α_2-adrenergic receptors in the dorsal cardiovascular center of the medulla oblongata of the rat

As stated in the Introduction, we have previously demonstrated that in vitro NPY (10 nM) produces an increase in the number of [^{3}H]PAC and α_2-[^{3}H]adrenergic antagonist binding sites as well as a small reduction in the affinity of these binding sites when performing the binding under optimal and equilibrium conditions (Agnati et al., 1983c; Fuxe et al., 1984b). Bovine serum albumin (BSA) (0.5%) and bacitracin (10^{-5} M) were also present to prevent a breakdown of NPY. In these experiments, Tris HCl buffer (50 mM) was used as described in the original procedure of Rouot and Snyder (1979).

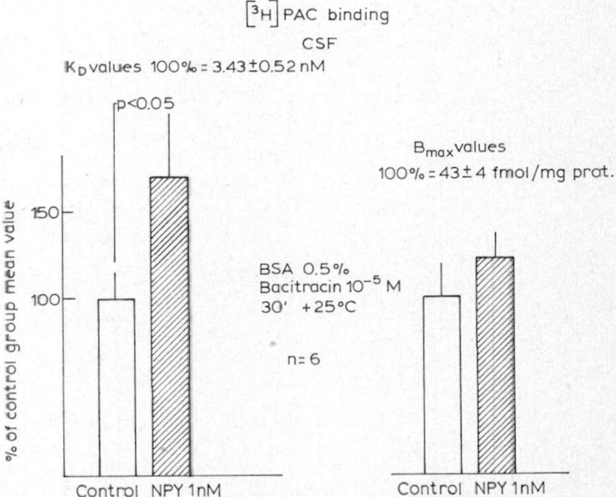

Fig. 6. Effects of NPY (1 nM) in vitro on the binding characteristics of *p*-[^{3}H]aminoclonidine (PAC) in membrane preparations of the male rat medulla oblongata using artificial CSF as incubation medium. Bovine serum albumin and bacitracin were also present in order to prevent breakdown of NPY. The experiment was performed under equilibrium conditions with an incubation time of 30 min at room temperature (see Rouot and Snyder, 1979). Means ± S.E.M. are shown (n = 6 experiments). Student's paired t-test was used.

In order to perform these experiments under more physiological conditions the Tris HCl buffer has been replaced by artificial cerebrospinal fluid (CSF), which by itself increases the K_D value by about 300% and reduced the B_{max} value by about 30% in the [^{3}H]PAC binding sites. Also lower concentrations of NPY have been evaluated (down to 0.1 nM) in view of the demonstration that the K_D value of the NPY binding sites range from 0.5 to 1 nM (Undén et al., 1984; Goldstein et al., this volume). Under these equilibrium conditions (30 min, 37°C) NPY was found to produce a substantial increase in the K_D value but no significant increase in the B_{max} value in membrane preparations of the medulla oblongata of the normotensive male rat using a concentration of 1 nM of NPY (Fig. 6). When using a higher concentration of NPY (10 nM) and CSF as incubation medium, a significant increase in the B_{max} value of the [^{3}H]PAC binding sites was observed as described previously in the experiments with Tris HCl buffer (see Fig. 7). A nonsignificant increase in the K_D value was now observed. These in vitro studies, involving the use of artificial CSF as incubation medium, give further evidence that NPY receptor can influence the affinity of α_2-adrenergic agonist binding sites in membrane preparations from the medulla oblongata of the rat. In order to establish whether NPY can in vivo modulate α_2-adrenergic receptor mechanisms in the medulla oblongata, experiments involving intraventricular injections of NPY into awake unrestrained male rats for a period of 8 days have been performed (see Fig. 8). NPY was given in a dose of 1.25 nmoles once daily and the last dose was given 1 h before decapitation. As shown above, this dose of NPY produces a marked lowering of arterial blood pressure and heart rate lasting for about 2 h. However, it is likely that the activation of NPY receptors takes place during a significantly longer time period, since the lowering of arterial blood pressure is always associated with compensatory activation of other types of neuronal mechanisms aiming to restore normal arterial blood pressures. As control animals we have used cannulated rats which were treated once daily with artificial CSF. The [^{3}H]PAC binding procedure was performed as originally described by Rouot and Snyder (1979),

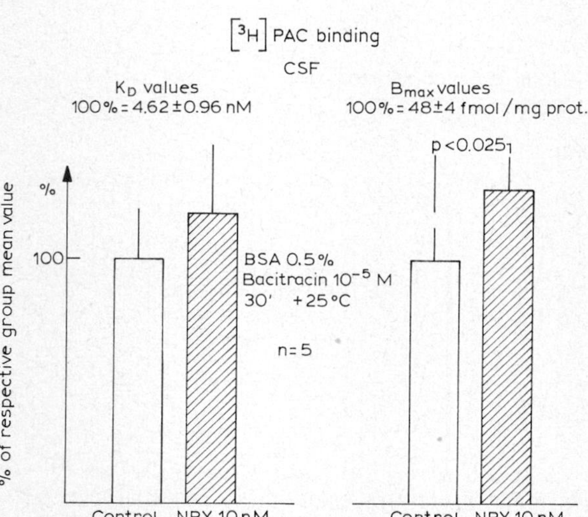

Fig. 7. Effects of NPY (10 nM) in vitro on the binding characteristics of p-[^{3}H]aminoclonidine binding in membrane preparations from the rat male medulla oblongata using artificial CSF as incubation medium. For further details see text to Fig. 6. Means ± S.E.M. (n = 5) are shown and the values are expressed in per cent of respective group mean value (CSF alone). Student's paired t-test was used in the statistical analysis.

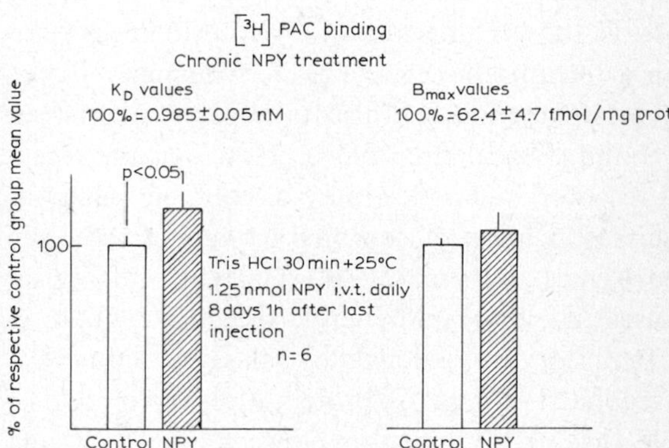

Fig. 8. Effects of daily intraventricular injections of NPY for a period of 8 days on the binding characteristics of p-[^{3}H]aminoclonidine in membrane preparations of rat male medulla oblongata using Tris-HCl buffer (50 mM) as incubation medium. The binding assay was performed as described by Rouot and Snyder (1979). Means ± S.E.M. (n = 6) are shown in per cent of respective control group mean value (Tris-HCl alone). Student's paired t-test was used in the statistical analysis.

that is, 30 min at 25°C using a Tris HCl buffer. The results are summarized in Fig. 8. It is shown that the in vivo intermittent treatment with NPY produces a small but significant increase in the K_D value of the [^{3}H]PAC binding sites compared with the group of animals treated with the artificial CSF alone. Six experiments were performed and in each experiment five rats were used per group. Thus, the results obtained in these in vivo experiments are similar to those obtained in vitro using artificial CSF and NPY in a concentration of 10^{-9} M. The molecular mechanism underlying the NPY-induced changes in the binding characteristics of [^{3}H]PAC binding sites is presently unknown, but the results are compatible with an interaction occurring both at the level of the coupling device as well as at the level of the recognition sites.

At this stage of the analysis it became of importance to demonstrate the presence of high densities of [^{125}I]NPY binding sites in the dorsal cardiovascular region of the medulla oblongata, and that these binding sites in fact overlap with the [^{3}H]PAC binding sites. For this purpose receptor autoradiographical studies were started. In the experiments we followed the biochemical procedure for NPY binding of Goldstein and colleagues (this volume). For details on the receptor autoradiography see Fuxe et al., (1983c), Agnati et al. (1984b) and Benfenati et al. (1985). The concentrations of iodinated NPY ranged from 0.5 to 2 nM. The Tris HCl buffer used contained 5 mM $MgCl_2$ and 5 mM $CaCl_2$ as well as 0.5% BSA and 10^{-5} M of bacitracin. The unfixed cryostate sections were incubated for 90

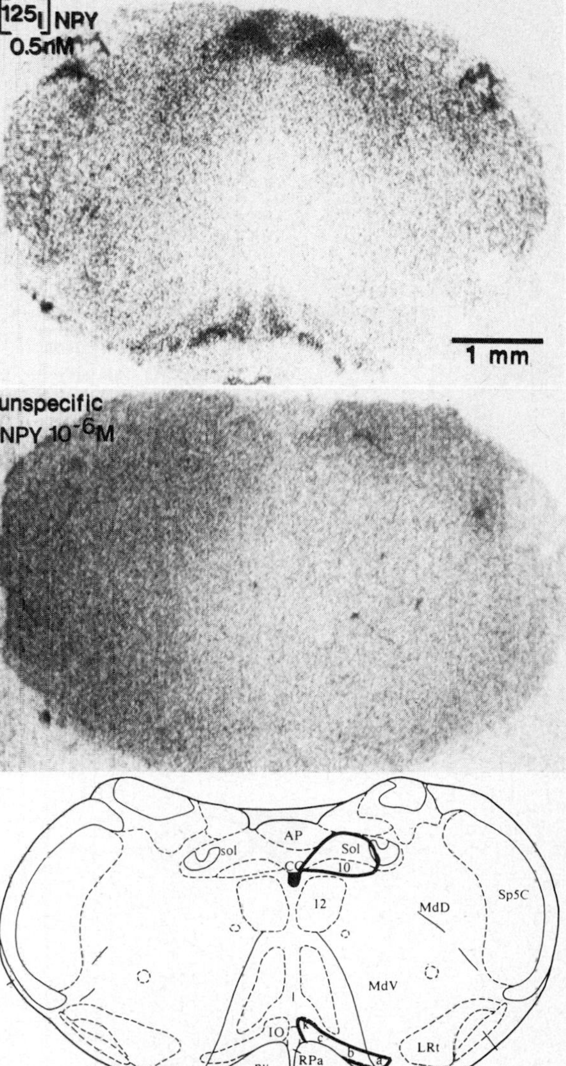

Fig. 9. Autoradiographic localization of [^{125}I]NPY binding sites in a coronal section of the rat medulla oblongata using tritium sensitive sheet film. The concentration used was 0.5 nM and the iodinated NPY was obtained from Amersham, England (above 2000 Ci/mmol). The reaction conditions were similar to those described by Goldstein et al., for biochemical experiments (this volume). 50 mM Tris-HCl buffer (pH 7.6) was used, containing 5 mM $MgCl_2$ and $CaCl_2$ as well as 0.1 mM bacitracin. The binding was studied under equilibrium conditions (incubation time 90 min at room temperature). The unspecific binding was defined as the binding in the presence of NPY in a concentration of 1 μM (middle panel). In the lower panel the neuroanatomical landmarks are shown based on a coronal section from the Atlas of Paxinos and Watson (1982). The binding was measured by quantitative autoradiography in the areas outlined by the solid lines. As seen the measurements in the nuc. tractus solitarius (Sol) are includes besides Sol also the dorsal motor nucleus of the vagus (10). The bregma level is −13.8 mm. The following abbreviations have been used: sol = nuc. tractus solitarius; IO = inferior olive; RPa = nuc. raphe pallidus; py = pyramidal tract; XII = nuc. hypoglossus; MdV = ventral reticular nuc. of the medulla oblongata; MdD = dorsal reticular nuc. of the medulla oblongata; LRt = lateral reticular nuc.; AP = area postrema; Sp5 = spinal nuc. of the trigeminal nerve.

min at 25°C to ensure the presence of equilibrium conditions. In Figs. 9 and 10, receptor autoradiograms are shown demonstrating in coronal sections regions in the medulla oblongata having a high density of NPY binding sites. Low concentrations of NPY were used (0.5 nM around the K_D value) in order to obtain a high signal to noise ratio and to have a "conservative" approach to the evaluations of the areas of overlap between NPY and α_2-binding sites (see Fig. 13). At the levels analyzed (Bregma −14.3 mm to −12.3 mm) the highest density of NPY binding sites is shown to exist within the nuc. tractus solitarius, nuc. paratrigeminalis, the medial nuclei of the inferior olive and the substantia gelatinosa of the caudal part of the spinal trigeminal nucleus. Somewhat lower densities were observed in the dorsal motor nuc. of the vagus and in the parasolitary area.

High densities of NPY binding sites can also be observed within the outer layers (I–III) of the entire cerebral cortex, especially in the occipital cortex and within the somatosensory cortex the layer IV is outlined while layer III here is less labelled (Figs. 11 and 12). A high density of NPY binding sites is also found within islands of the olfactory tubercle, which may correspond to the islands of Calleja, within claustrum, within several thalamic nuclei (laterodorsal and lateroposterior thalamic nuclei), within the outer layers of the superior collicle, within the anterior olfactory nuclei and in the deeper layers of the frontal lobe and of the occipital cortex.

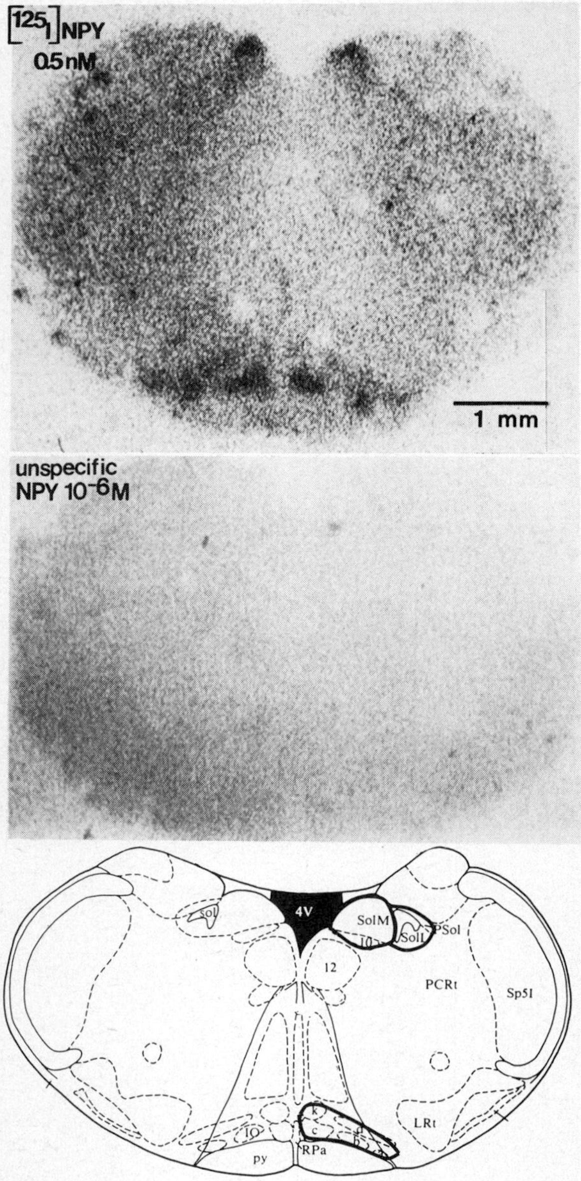

Fig. 10. Autoradiographic localization of [^{125}I]NPY binding sites in a coronal section of the rat medulla oblongata using tritium sensitive sheet film. The highest binding was observed in the dorsal strip region of the nuc. tractus solitarius and within the medial nuc. of the inferior olive. For details on the binding procedure, see text to previous figure. The middle panel shows the unspecific binding (binding in the presence of NPY (1 μM)). In the lower panel the neuroanatomical landmarks are shown according to Paxinos and Watson Atlas (1982) (Bregma −13.3 mm). Abbreviations used: see text to previous figure; SolM = medial nuc. of tractus solitarius; SolL = lateral nuc. of the tractus solitarius; PSol = parasolitary nucleus; PCRt = parvocellular reticular nuc. of the medulla oblongata. The binding was measured by quantitative receptor autoradiography in the areas outlined by the solid lines. As seen the NTS area includes the medial nuc. of the tractus solitarius and the dorsal motor nuc. of the vagus. The parasolitary area includes the lateral nuc. of the tractus solitarius as well as the parasolitary nuc. The area in the inferior olive includes all the medial nuclei as well as the dorsal nucleus.

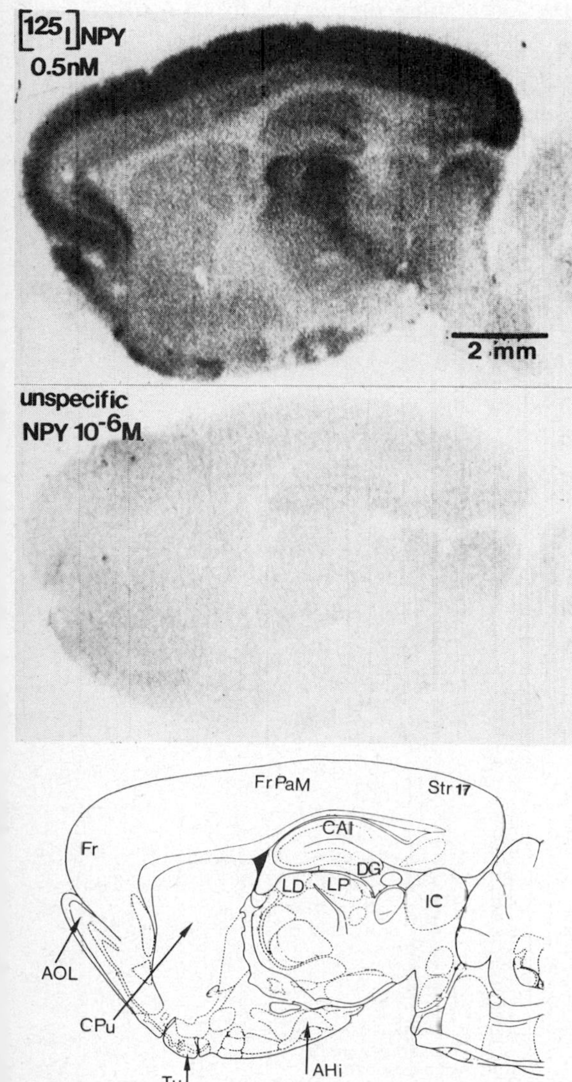

Fig. 11. Autoradiographic localization of [^{125}I]NPY binding sites in a saggital section of rat brain using tritium sensitive sheet film (lateral 2.9 mm, Paxinos and Watson, 1982). For details on incubation procedures, see text to previous figure legends. In the middle panel the unspecific binding is shown (binding in the presence of NPY (1 μM)). In the lower panel the neuroanatomical areas are shown in section taken from the sagital plane located laterally of the midline by 2.9 mm (see Paxinos and Watson, 1982). Abbreviations used: AOl = anterior olfactory nuc., lateral part; CPu = nuc. caudatus putamen; Tu = tuberculum olfactorium; AHi = amygdala-hippocampal area; FR = frontal cortex; FrPaM = frontoparietal cortex, motor area; Str17 = striatal cortex, area 17; CA1 = subfield Ca1 of Ammon's horn; DG = dentate gyrus; LD = laterodorsal thalamic nucleus; LP = lateroposterior thalamic nucleus; IC = inferior collicle.

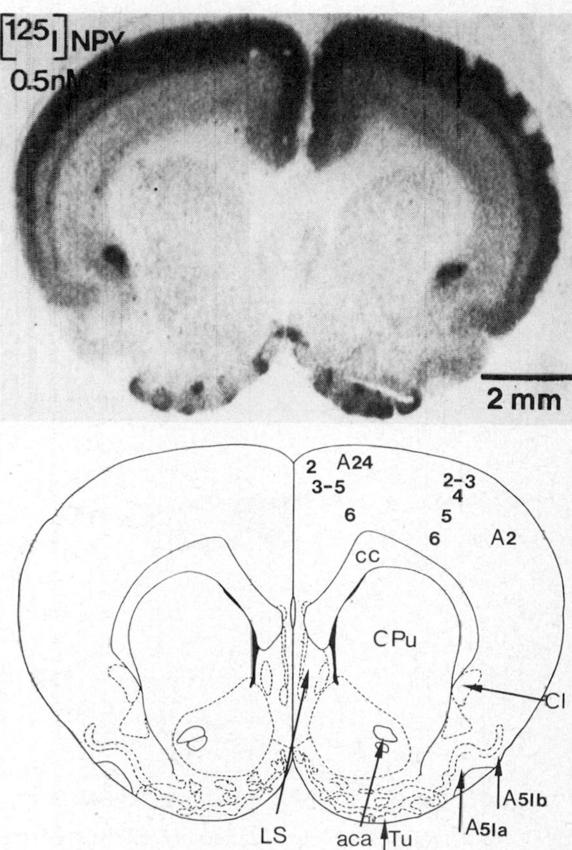

Fig. 12. Autoradiographical localization of [^{125}I]NPY binding sites in a coronal section of the rat brain using a tritium sensitive sheet film (Bregma −1.7 mm according to Paxinos and Watson Atlas, 1982). For details on the binding procedure, see text to Fig. 9. The neuroanatomical details are indicated in the lower part of the figure. Abbreviations used: LS = lateral septal nucleus; aca = anterial limb of the anterior commissure; To = tuberculum olfactorium; A51a, A51b represent areas of the pyriform cortex; Cl = claustrum; CP = nucl. caudatus putamen; cc = corpus callosum; A24 = ventral anterior area; A2 = caudal postcentral area (see Krieg, 1947).

In Fig. 13, a high density of [^{3}H]PAC binding sites in the nuc. tractus solitarius region and in the parasolitary region is illustrated. The concentration used of [^{3}H]PAC was 10 nM. In the lower part of the figure, the overlap areas between the [^{3}H]PAC and iodinated NPY binding sites are shown in the dorsal cardiovascular region. The concentration used of iodinated NPY was 0.5 nM, which will not label all the iodinated NPY binding sites. It must

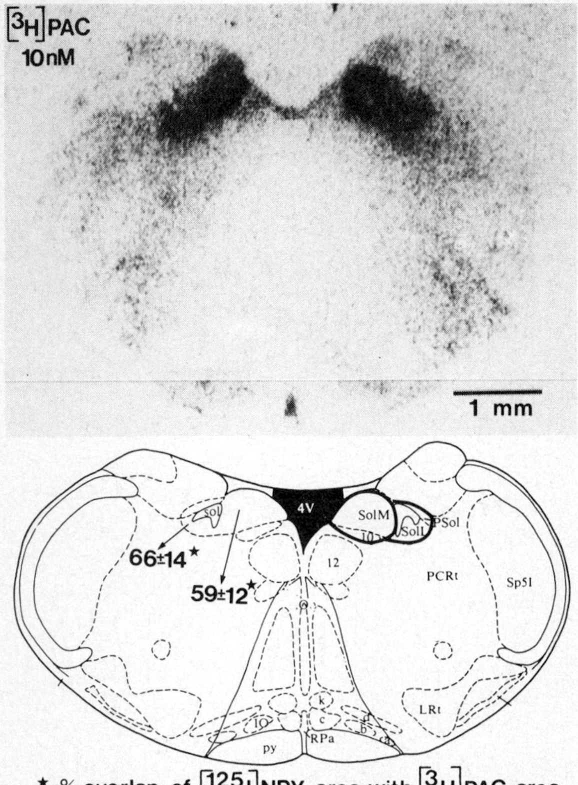

Fig. 13. Autoradiographical localization of [^{3}H]PAC (PAC 10 nM) binding sites in a coronal section of the rat medulla oblongata using tritium sensitive sheet film (Bregma −13.3 mm, according to Paxinos and Watson Atlas, 1982). In the lower part of the figure the neuroanatomical landmarks are shown as well as the per cent overlap of the [^{125}I]NPY area with the [^{3}H]PAC area. The regions analyzed for overlap are indicated by the solid lines in the lower panel of the figure. Nuc. tractus solitarius area includes the medial nucleus of the nuc. tractus solitarius (SolM) and the dorsal motor nucleus of the vagus and the parasolitary area includes the lateral nucleus of the tractus solitarius and the parasolitary nuc. (SolL) and PSol). For other abbreviations used, see text to Fig. 10.

be realized, however, that with high concentrations of iodinated NPY, unspecific binding is increased in sections of the medulla oblongata. Therefore, the signal to noise ratio is reduced and the high density regions can then not be as clearly delineated as with the somewhat lower concentrations. Under all conditions the results clearly demonstrated a marked overlap (about 60%) between the [^{125}I]NPY and [^{3}H]PAC binding sites in the dorsal cardiovascular area of the medulla oblongata. As seen in the figures, the peak labelling with iodinated NPY is observed in the most dorsal and medial parts of the nuc. tractus solitarius.

When it had been established that the high den-

Modulation of [3H] PAC binding in sections of medulla oblongata as studied by receptor autoradiography

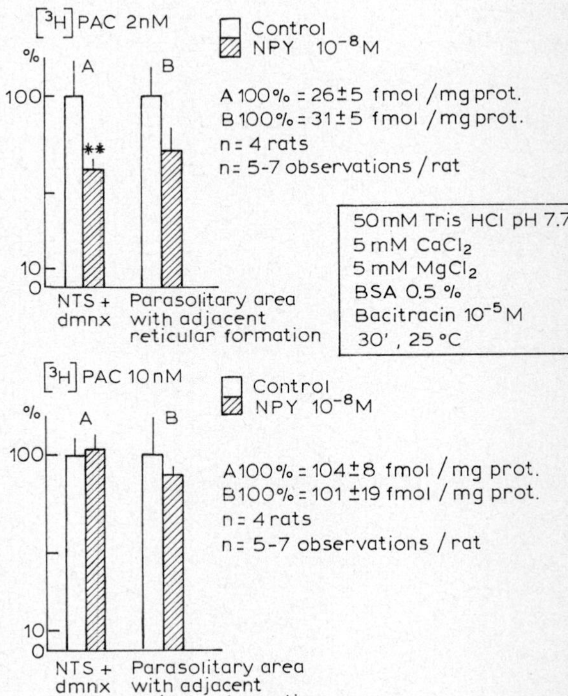

Fig. 14. Effects of NPY (10 nM) on the binding of [^{3}H]PAC to coronal sections of the medulla oblongata of the rat using quantitative receptor autoradiography (see Fuxe et al., 1983; Benfenati et al., 1985). Two concentrations of [^{3}H]PAC were used, 2 nM and 10 nM. The incubation procedure is indicated in the figure and is based on the procedure of Rouot and Snyder (1979) with the addition of $CaCl_2$ and $MgCl_2$ to improve NPY binding to its receptor and of bovine serum albumin and bacitracin in the concentrations indicated to prevent breakdown of NPY. Coronal sections of the medulla oblongata have been analyzed from 0.5 mm caudal to obex up to 1 mm rostral to obex. Means ± S.E.M. (n = 4) are shown and the values are expressed in per cent of the solvent mean group value. Student's paired t-test ** = $p < 0.01$. The areas analyzed are neuroanatomically shown in Figs. 9 and 10.

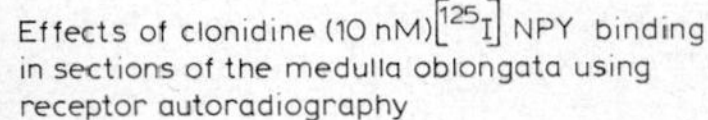

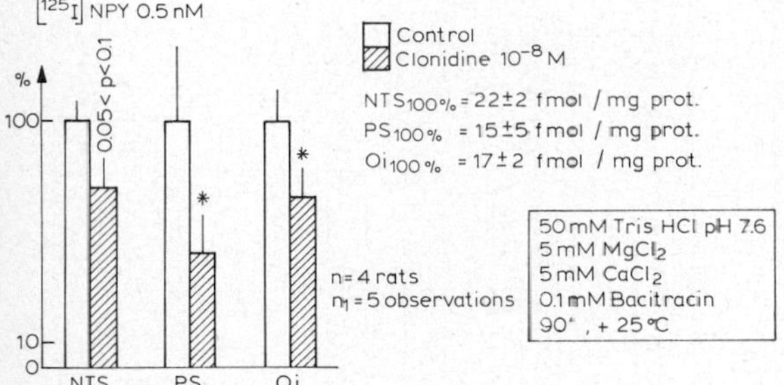

Fig. 15. Effects of clonidine (10 nM) on [^{125}I]NPY binding in coronal sections of the medulla oblongata using quantitative receptor autoradiography. Coronal sections were analyzed from a level 0.5 mm caudal to obex to a level 1 mm rostral to obex. The concentration used was 0.5 nM of iodinated NPY. The incubation procedure was based on that of Goldstein et al. (this volume). Means ± S.E.M. are shown. n = 4 rats with a total of 5 observations per rat. In the statistical analysis Student's paired t-test was used. * = $p < 0.05$. NTS = nuc. tractus solitarius area which includes also the dorsal motor nucleus of the vagus; PS = parasolitary area which includes the lateral solitary nucleus and the parasolitary nucleus; Oi = inferior olive.

sities of NPY and PAC binding sites overlapped in the dorsal cardiovascular region of the medulla oblongata, it became of importance to study if it was possible by means of quantitative receptor autoradiography to show if NPY in vitro could modulate the binding of PAC to the dorsal cardiovascular region of the medulla oblongata, and also if clonidine in turn could modulate NPY binding to this region. The results are summarized in Fig. 14. When analyzing the effects of NPY on [^{3}H]PAC binding in the section the original procedure (see Rouot and Snyder, 1979) has been modified adding into the incubation medium also 5 mM of $CaCl_2$ and $MgCl_2$. These ions appear to play an important role for the binding of NPY to its binding sites (see Goldstein et al., this volume). The results show that NPY (10 nM) can significantly reduce binding of [^{3}H]PAC in the nuc. tractus solitarius using a concentration of 2 nM but not a concentration of 10 nM of this radioligand. No significant reduction was observed in the parasolitary area with 2 nM of [^{3}H]PAC. These results are compatible with the view that NPY can increase the K_D value of the [^{3}H]PAC binding sites in the nuc. tractus solitarius without modulating the B_{max} values in the nuc. tractus solitarius (no effects when the high concentration of [^{3}H]PAC was used). These results are highly complementary to those obtained in the biochemical experiments reported above. In fact, they indicate that NPY receptors can regulate the affinity of the α_2-adrenergic receptors in the nuc. tractus solitarus and in the dorsal motor nuc. of the vagus.

In Fig. 15, it is shown that clonidine (10 nM) can significantly reduce the binding of 0.5 nM of iodinated NPY to the parasolitary area, to the inferior olive and produce a trend for a reduction of the binding in the nuc. tractus solitarius region, which also includes the dorsal motor nuc. of the vagus. These results give evidence that α_2-adrenergic receptors in turn can regulate the binding characteristics of the iodinated NPY binding sites via receptor-receptor interactions. Thus, reciprocal interactions may exist between the α_2-adrenergic receptors and NPY receptors in the dorsal cardiovascular region, where NPY/adrenaline costoring synapses are present. However, it must be underlined that clonidine also modulates iodinated NPY binding sites in the inferior olive where no coexistence between NPY and CA takes place. Thus, α_2-adrenergic and NPY receptors probably also interact at the local circuit level by means of receptor-receptor interaction. The importance of receptor-receptor interactions at the local circuit level has been demonstrated in our laboratories, also for other recognition sites such as glutamate/DA, cholecystokinin/DA and neurotensin/DA binding sites (see Fuxe et al., 1981b, 1984a; Agnati et al., 1983b; Fuxe and Agnati, 1985). Thus, receptors belonging to neighbouring terminals can via receptor-receptor interactions provide a heteroregulation of receptors (see Agnati et al., 1980). Such a heteroregulation is also possible by means of receptors for paracrine and endocrine signals which can regulate transmitter receptors, inter alia, via receptor-receptor interaction. The results obtained in the physiological experiments indicate that this type of interaction takes place at least in part at the level of the coupling device. It is therefore possible that the reduced K_D value observed in the α_2-[^{3}H]adrenergic agonist binding sites under the influence of NPY (1 nM) is a part of an intramembrane feedback response, caused by a NPY-induced increase in transduction to the common biological effector. It must be emphasized, however, that a number of findings indicate that interactions also take place between the receptor proteins carrying the recognition sites (see Agnati et al., 1984a; Fuxe et al., 1984a; Fuxe and Agnati, 1985).

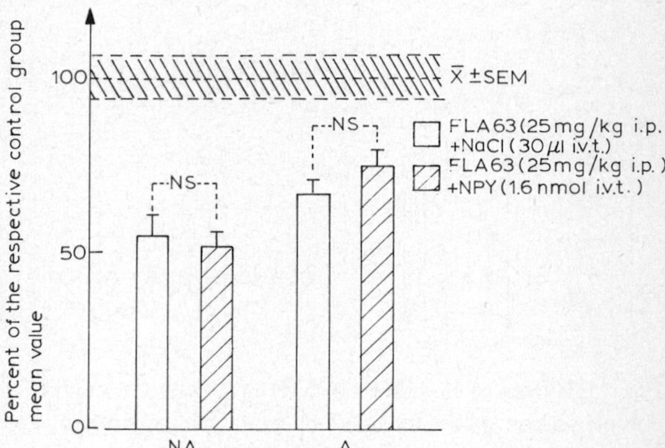

Fig. 16. Effects of intraventricular injections of NPY (1.6 nmol/rat) on noradrenaline (NA) and (A) utilization in the nTS area of the rat, using the DA-β-hydroxylase inhibitor FLA 63 (25 mg/kg, i.p., 2 h before killing). NPY was given immediately before FLA 63 injection. The area sampled was the mediodorsal and caudal part of the medulla oblongata. HPLC in combination with electrochemical detection was used. The results are given as means ± S.E.M. (n = 10). Statistical analysis according to Mann Whitney U-test. In the control group the absolute levels of NA and A were 1629 ± 29 (NA) and 41 ± 7 ng/g (A).

Evidence for a heterostatic regulation of the synapse: involvement of intrasynaptic, intersynaptic and extrasynaptic signals

In order to understand the functional meaning of coexistence and of the receptor-receptor interactions, it has been of importance to study the effects of the peptide comodulators in the monoamine neurons also on the presynaptic monoaminergic mechanisms in vivo and in vitro. In this study, it has consistently been found that the peptide comodulators upon in vivo administration fail to modulate the level and utilization of its costoring monoamine (Fuxe et al., 1980, 1984b, 1985c; Agnati et al., 1984a; Fuxe and Agnati, 1985). Thus, intraventricular injections of CCK peptides in the awake unrestrained rat failed to influence DA utilization and levels in the CCK/DA costoring synapses of the tuberculum olfactorium and the nuc. accumbens (Fuxe et al., 1980d). Furthermore, neurotensin and GRF given centrally and systemically fail to modulate DA levels and utilization in the external layer of the median eminence, where they are partly costored with DA in some of the tubero-infundibular DA neurons (Fuxe et al., 1984c, 1985c).

In agreement with the previous results (see Fig. 16) it has been found in the present study that intraventricular injections of NPY into the unrestrained awake male rat do not modulate noradrenaline and A levels and utilization within the overall dorsal cardiovascular area of the medulla oblongata (dorsomedial and caudal part of the medulla oblongata). Thus, it seems possible that in the NPY/adrenaline costoring synapses of the medulla oblongata NPY predominantly acts via postsynaptic actions as indicated above, affecting the α_2-adrenergic receptor sensitivity by means of the receptor-receptor interactions without inducing any compensatory change in the A storage and release. In this way, a heterostatic regulation of the synapse becomes possible as illustrated in Fig. 17. Thus, the α_2-adrenergic transmission line can be modulated by NPY without interfering with the homeostatis of the A mechanism, that is without inducing compensatory changes in A synthesis and release. The new concept of "heterostatic" regulation is shown in detail in the figure. The message reaching the intracellular machinery of the cell is above all dependent upon the release and synthesis of the transmitter, of the binding of the transmitter to its recognition site and to the efficiency of the transduc-

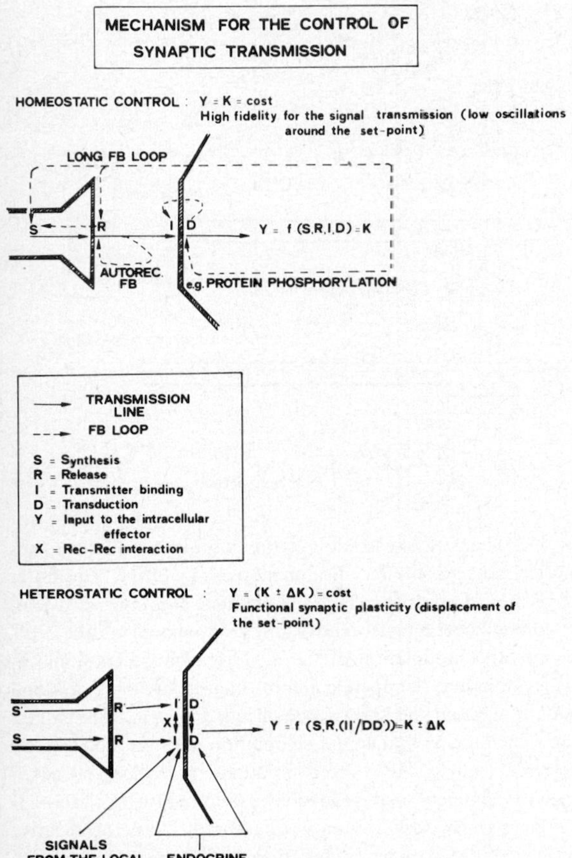

Fig. 17. Schematic representation of the mechanisms which may contribute to two types of basic behaviors of synapses: the constancy of the efficacy of the transmission line (synaptic homeostasis) and the change of the level, at which this constancy is maintained (synaptic heterostasis).

tion mechanism. In the upper part of the figure the homeostatic regulation of the synapse is shown and a large number of the feedbacks are indicated, which maintain the constancy of the transmission (K). The feedbacks involve inter alia the long feedback, reaching the nerve cell bodies and regulating the frequency of nerve impulses, the autoreceptor feedback, controlling the synthesis and release of the transmitter, and the feedbacks from intracytoplasmatic second messengers regulating the receptor mechanisms via protein phosphorylation. Via the various feedbacks, a high fidelity of the transmission line is maintained (low oscillations around the K value). By means of the receptor-receptor interactions the receptor sensitivity can be changed as well as the message reaching the intracellular machinery without any associated changes in the presynaptic features of the transmission line. This regulation has been defined as a "heterostatic" regulation of the synaptic transmission. In fact, as stated in the figure, it allows to change the level at which the synapse works. Thus, it can be envisaged as a change of the set-point of the synapse ($K \pm \Delta \bar{K}$). We suggest that synaptic heterostasis has an important role in functional synaptic plasticity.

Although the participation of the costoring messengers in the heterostatic regulation of the synapse appears to dominate in many in vivo situations, it must be realized that the costoring messengers probably interact also at the presynaptic level (see also Burnstock, and Bartfai, this volume). Martire and colleagues (Martire, Cerrito, Härfstrand, Agnati and Fuxe, unpublished data) have recently shown in vitro that 1 nM of NPY can enhance the inhibitory effects of clonidine (0.1 μM) on CA release from synaptosomal preparations from the dorsal cardiovascular centers of the medulla oblongata. Thus, the coexisting messenger can change the sensitivity of the autoreceptor feedback, in this case presented by the presynaptic α_2-adrenergic receptors located on A and NA nerve terminals. In other experiments in vivo it has also been possible to show that clonidine acutely (5 min following an intracisternal injection) in a dose of 3.75 nmoles can produce a trend for a reduction of NPY immunoreactivity within the rostral part of the dorsomedial and caudal part of the medulla oblongata (dorsal cardiovascular center) (Härfstrand, Fuxe, Agnati, Lang and Ganten, unpublished data). These results indicate that α_2-adrenergic receptors in the NPY/adrenaline costoring synapses, located presynaptically may control NPY synthesis and/or release. The significance of these putative presynaptic interactions between the cotransmission lines are presently unclear but may represent part of the integrative activity of the synapses. The relative importance of the postsynaptic receptor-receptor interactions and the presynaptic interactions between the costoring messengers may obviously vary from one synapse to the other. The important factor remains, however, that in several neuronal systems analyzed in vivo the costoring messenger appears to make possible the heterostatic regulation of the synapse and may in this way increase synaptic plasticity. It must be emphasized, however, that such types of heterostatic mechanisms are also made possible by receptor-receptor interactions occurring between neighboring synapses at the local circuit level and by means of paracrine and hormonal signals, which can alter receptor sensitivity without inducing changes in the presynaptic mechanisms (see Fuxe et al., 1984a). Thyroidectomy can, e.g. change DA-receptor sensitivity in the striatum without causing any compensatory changes in striatal DA utilization and levels (Fuxe et al., 1984a).

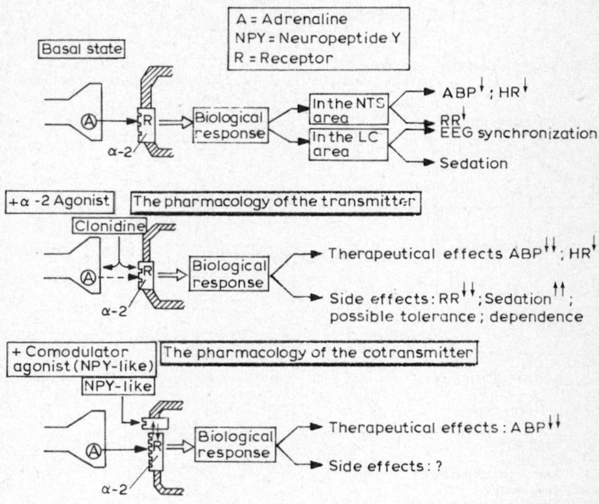

Fig. 18. Schematic illustration of the modulation of the α_2-adrenergic transmission line. The pharmacology of the transmitter and of the cotransmitter (NPY) is outlined. It is suggested that, e.g. comodulator agonists (NPY-like compounds) via the NPY receptor and modulation of the α_2-adrenergic receptor mechanism can induce therapeutic actions, that is, lowering of blood pressure, without the known side effects due to α_2-stimulation. Thus, since the α_2-adrenergic recognition sites are not directly interfered with by NPY-like compounds, tolerance and abstinence development as seen following treatment with the α_2-adrenergic agonist clonidine should be absent. Also the sedative effects of NPY-like compounds may be less pronounced than those seen after clonidine treatment (Zini et al., 1984).

Possible therapeutic implications of the heterostatic mechanisms. Focus on NPY/adrenaline coexistence within the cardiovascular region of the medulla oblongata

By the demonstration that the A comodulator NPY exerts powerful vasodepressor actions when injected intracisternally and intraventricularly new possibilities open up for the treatment of hypertension, especially since NPY can reduce arterial blood pressure via an action beyond the α_2-adrenergic recognition site without clearly interfering with the A homeostasis. One way to modulate the control of arterial blood pressure could obviously be to change the coexistence of NPY and A. We have recently discovered that there exist a hormonal regulation of coexistence of neuronal messengers (see also Swanson, this volume). Thus, via two color immunohistochemistry using the PAP technique, it has been possible to demonstrate the existence of glucocorticoid receptor immunoreactivity in the nuclei of the PNMT/NPY nerve cell bodies of the medulla oblongata, especially in the C1 group (Härfstrand et al., 1986). Furthermore, adrenalectomy markedly increases the entity of NPY/PNMT coexistence in hypothalamic nerve terminals from 29 to 89.5%. Corticosterone treatment of the adrenalectomized rats markedly reduces the coexistence of NPY and PNMT in the nerve terminals of the hypothalamus (see Fuxe et al., 1985). These results indicate that glucocorticoid receptor activation inhibits the transcription of RNA in the A cell bodies responsible for the synthesis of NPY. Thus, following the removal of the adrenal gland, NPY synthesis will be enhanced in the A neurons, which may mainly be responsible for the increased degree of coexistence of NPY and PNMT immunoreactivity in the A nerve terminals of the hypothalamus. It seems possible that actions of this type by glucocorticoids on the synthesis of peptide comodulators in the central nervous system can contribute to their ability to favor development of hypertension.

In Fig. 18, the pharmacology of the comodulator is illustrated in comparison with the pharmacology of the transmitter (e.g. α_2-agonist clonidine used in antihypertensive treatments). Both the transmitter adrenaline and the α_2-agonist clonidine as well as NPY have been shown in the present and previous studies to reduce blood pressure, heart rate and respiratory frequency. However, the α_2-adrenergic agonist clonidine produces side-effects such as sedation, which are at least partly caused by an inhibition of the activity in the noradrenergic locus coeruleus system, which is of importance for tonic arousal. It seems possible that NPY-like molecules can be devoid of such side-effects, since in the spontaneously hypertensive rat NPY lowers arterial blood pressure but at the same time causes an increase in arousal (see Zini et al., 1984). It will, therefore, be of substantial interest to develop a therapy based on NPY-like peptides, which can penetrate into the central nervous system and be devoid of the vasoconstrictor activity observed after systemic injection of NPY. It seems possible that there could exist a subtype of NPY receptor in the central nervous system, which may be preferentially activated by certain types of NPY fragments. This is, e.g. true for the central CCK receptors which have a substantial affinity also for CCK-4 unlike the peripheral CCK receptors (Innis and Snyder, 1980). Of primary importance for the development of this type of therapy are recent demonstrations that no tolerance develops to the cardiovascular actions of NPY following an 8-day treatment with intraventricular injections of NPY given once daily (see Fig. 19). Thus, following treatment which involves daily injections of NPY for a period of 8 days, the NPY receptors involved in cardiovascular control are still capable of producing a lowering of arterial blood pressure upon activation of NPY. To evaluate the possible importance of NPY therapy it also becomes necessary to test whether withdrawal from chronic treatment with NPY leads to the development of withdrawal hypertension as is the case after abrupt interruption of chronic clonidine treatment.

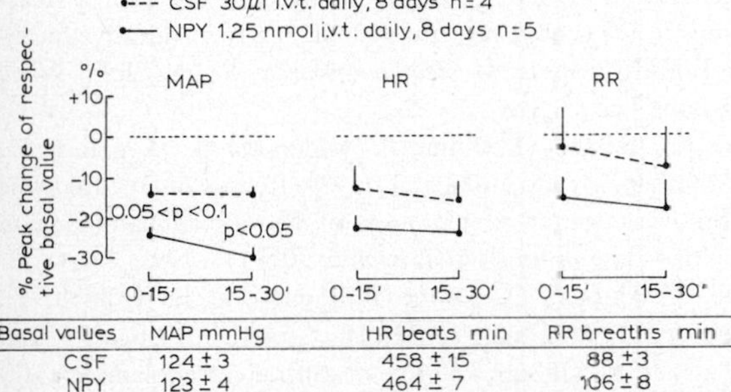

Basal values	MAP mmHg	HR beats min	RR breaths min
CSF	124 ± 3	458 ± 15	88 ± 3
NPY	123 ± 4	464 ± 7	106 ± 8

Fig. 19. Acute effects of an intraventricular injection of NPY in awake unrestrained rats, which have been treated previously with NPY (0.5 nmoles in 30 µl artificial CSF, i.v.t., once daily for 8 days). The effects on mean arterial blood pressure, heart rate and respiratory rate are shown and expressed as peak change of respective basal value. Means ± S.E.M. (n = 5) are shown. Statistical analysis was performed by means of Mann-Whitney *U*-test when comparing the effects of artificial CSF alone and NPY.

In order to further understand the possible therapeutic effects of NPY-related peptides in the treatment of spontaneous hypertension, we are presently mapping out possible changes in the NPY and A costoring neurons during the development of spontaneous hypertension. A number of alterations have already been observed, such as a trend for a disappearance of the PNMT immunoreactivity in neurons of the dorsal strip of the nuc. tractus solitarius, which may have an important cardiovascular vasodepressor function. However, no deficiency in NPY stores has been demonstrated in the dorsal cardiovascular region of the medulla oblongata in spontaneously hypertensive (SH) rats versus the normotensive control rat as determined by radioimmunoassay (Härfstrand et al., unpublished data). Furthermore, in view of the results observed when studying the dose-response curves for the cardiovascular actions of NPY given intracisternally into the α-chloralose anesthetized spontaneously hypertensive rat, it becomes important when performing NPY-like therapy, to use sufficiently high doses to overcome the reduced affinity in the NPY receptor mechanism in the SH rat (Härfstrand et al., 1984).

Acknowledgements

This work has been supported by a Grant from the Swedish Medical Research Council (04X-715), by a Grant from the Magnus Bergvall's Stiftelse, by a Grant from Knut and Alice Wallenberg's Foundation and by a CNR-I Grant. We are grateful for the excellent technical assistance of Ms. Birgitta Nyberg, Ms. Ulla-Britt Finnman, Ms. Barbro Tinner, Ms. Lotta Frösell, Mr. Lars Rosén, Ms. Beth Hagman. We are also grateful for the excellent secretarial assistance of Ms. Anne Edgren.

References

Agnati, L. F. and Fuxe, K. (1983) Subcortical limbic ^{3}H-N-propylnorapomorphine binding sites are marked modulated by cholecystokinin-8 in vitro. *B iosci. Rep.*, 3: 1101–1105.

Agnati, L. F. and Fuxe, K. (1984) New concepts on the structure of the neuronal networks: The miniaturization and hierarchical organization of the central nervous system. *Biosci. Rep.*, 4: 93–98.

Agnati, L. F., Fuxe, K., Zini, I., Lenzi, P. and Hökfelt, T. (1980) Aspects on receptor regulation and isoreceptor identification. *Med. Biol.*, 58: 182–187.

Agnati, L. F., Fuxe, K., Benfenati, F., Battistini, N., Härfstrand, A., Hökfelt, T., Caviccioli, L., Tatemoto, K. and Mutt, V. (1983a) Failure of neuropeptide Y in vitro to increase the number of α_2-adrenergic binding sites in membranes of medulla oblongata of the spontaneous hypertensive rat. *Acta physiol. Scand.*, 119: 309–312.

Agnati, L. F., Fuxe, K., Benfenati, F. and Battistini, N. (1983b) Neurotensin in vitro markedly recuces the affinity in subcortical limbic ^{3}H-N-propylnorapomorphine binding sites. *Acta physiol. Scand.*, 119: 459–461.

Agnati, L. F., Fuxe, K., Benfenati, F., Battistini, N., Härfstrand, A., Tatemoto, K., Hökfelt, T. and Mutt, V. (1983c) Neuropeptide Y in vitro selectively increases the number of adrenergic binding sites in membranes of the medulla oblongata of the rat. *Acta physiol. Scand.*, 118: 293–295.

Agnati, L. F., Fuxe, K., Benfenati, F., Battistini, N., Zini, I., Camurri, M. and Hökfelt, T. (1984a) Postsynaptic effects of neuropeptide comodulators at central monoamine synapses. In E. Usdin, A. Carlsson, A. Dahlström and J. Engel (Eds.), *Neurology and Neurobiology, Vol. 8b,* Alan R. Liss Inc., New York, pp. 191–198.

Agnati, L. F., Fuxe, K., Benefenati, F., Zini, I., Zoli, M., Fabbri, L. and Härfstrand, A. (1984b) Computer assisted morphometry and microdensitometry of transmitter identified neurons with special reference to the mesostriatal dopamine pathway. I. Methodological aspects. *Acta physiol. Scand.*, Suppl. 532: 5–36.

Agnati, L. F., Fuxe, K., Grimaldi, R., Härfstrand, A., Zoli, M., Zini, I., Ganten, D. and Bernardi, P. (1985a) Aspects on the role of neuropeptide Y and atrial peptides in control of vascular resistance. In W. Osswald, D. Reis and P. Vanhoutte (Eds.), *The Molecular Basis for the Central and Peripheral Regulation of Vascular Resistance,* Plenum Press (in press).

Agnati, L. F., Fuxe, K., Calza, L., Giardino, L., Zini, I., Toffano, G., Goldstein, M., Marrama, P., Gustafsson, J.-Å., Yu, Z.-Y., Cuello, A. C., Terenius, L., Lang, R. and Ganten, D. (1985b) Morphometrical and microdensitometrical studies on monoaminergic and peptidergic neurons in the aging brain. In L. F. Agnati and K. Fuxe (Eds.), *Wenner-Gren Symposium on Quantitative Neuroanatomy in Transmitter Research, Stockholm, Sweden, May 3–4, 1984,* Macmillan Press, London, pp. 91–113.

Agnati, L. F., Fuxe, K., Jansson, A.-M., Zoli, M., Härfstrand, A., Zini, I. and Goldstein, M. (1985c) Morphofunctional studies on the central nervous system by means of image analysis. *Eric K. Fernström Symposium on Neural Regulation of Brain Circulation: Effects of Neurotransmitters and Neuromodulators, Lund, Sweden, June 21–23* (in press).

Benfenati, F., Agnati, L.F., Fuxe, K., Cimino, M., Battistini, N., Merlo Pich, E., Farabegoli, C. and Zini, I. (1985) Quantitative autoradiography as a tool to study receptors in neural tissue. Studies on 3H-Ouabain binding sites and correlation with synaptic protein phosphorylation in different brain areas. In L. F. Agnati and K. Fuxe (Eds.), *Wenner-Gren Symposium on Quantitative Neuroanatomy in Transmitter Research, Stockholm, Sweden, May 3–4, 1984,* Macmillan Press, London, pp. 381–397.

Fuxe, K. and Agnati, L. F. (1985) Receptor-receptor interactions in the central nervous system. A new integrative mechanism in synapses. *Medicinal Research Reviews,* John Wiley & Sons, Inc., USA.

Fuxe, K., Jonsson, G., Bolme, P., Andersson, K., Agnati, L. F., Goldstein, M. and Hökfelt, T. (1979) Reduction of adrenaline turnover in cardiovascular areas of the rat medulla oblongata by clonidine. *Acta physiol. Scand.*, 107: 177–179.

Fuxe, K., Ganten, D., Bolme, P., Agnati, L. F., Hökfelt, T., Andersson, L., Goldstein, M., Härfstrand, A., Unger, T. and Rascher, W. (1980a) The role of central catecholamine pathways in spontaneous and renal hypertension in rats. In K. Fuxe, M. Goldstein, B. Hökfelt and T. Hökfelt (Eds.), *Central Adrenaline Neurons: Basic Aspects and Their Role in Cardiovascular Functions,* Pergamon Press, Oxford and New York, pp. 259–276.

Fuxe, K., Agnati, L. F., Ganten, D., Jonsson, G., Hökfelt, T., Bolme, P., Andersson, K., Goldstein, M., Unger, T. and Rascher, W. (1980b) Studies on the cardiovascular functions of the central catecholamine pathways. Evidence for a vasodepressor function of the central adrenaline neurons. *Les*

Neuromédiateurs du Tronc Cérébral (Lyon, October, 26–27, 1979), Sandoz Editions, pp. 13–35.

Fuxe, K., Bolme, P., Agnati, L. F., Jonsson, G., Andersson, K., Köhler, C. and Hökfelt, T. (1980c) On the role of central adrenaline neurons in central cardiovascular regulation. In K. Fuxe, M. Goldstein, B. Hökfelt and T. Hökfelt (Eds.), *Central Adrenaline Neurons: Basic Aspects and Their Role in Cardiovascular Functions*, Pergamon Press, Oxford and New York, pp. 161–182.

Fuxe, K., Andersson, K., Locatelli, V., Agnati, L. F., Hökfelt, T., Skirboll, L. and Mutt, V. (1980d) Cholecystokinin peptides produce marked reduction of dopamine turnover in discrete areas in the rat in following intraventricular injection. *Europ. J. Pharmacol.*, 67: 329–331.

Fuxe, K., Agnati, L. F., Ganten, D., Goldstein, M., Yukimura, T., Jonsson, G., Bolme, P., Hökfelt, T., Andersson, K., Härfstrand, A., Unger, T. and Rascher, W. (1981a) The role of noradrenaline and adrenaline neuron systems and substance P in the control of central cardiovascular functions. In J. P. Buckley and C. M. Ferrario (Eds.), *Central Nervous System Mechanisms in Hypertension*, Raven Press, New York, pp. 89–113.

Fuxe, K., Agnati, L. F., Benfenati, F., Cimmino, M., Algeri, S., Hökfelt, T. and Mutt, V. (1981b) Modulation by cholecystokinins of ^{3}H-spiroperidol binding in rat striatum: Evidence for increased affinity and reduction in the number of binding sites. *Acta physiol. Scand.*, 113: 567–569.

Fuxe, K., Vincent, M., Andersson, K., Härfstrand, A., Agnati, L. F., Sassard, J., Benfenati, F., Hökfelt, T. (1982a) Selective reduction of adrenaline turnover in the dorsal midline area of the caudal medulla oblongata and increase of hypothalamic adrenaline levels in the lyon strain of genetically hypertensive rats. *Europ. J. Pharmacol.*, 77: 187–191.

Fuxe, K., Agnati, L. F., Ganten, D., Andersson, K., Calza, L., Vincent, M., Sassard, J., Yukimura, T., Eneroth, P., Goldstein, M., Hökfelt, T., Rosell, S., Härfstrand, A., Vale, W., Brown, M. and Rivier, J. (1982b) Central and peripheral hormones and peptides: Focus on the involvement of noradrenaline and adrenaline neurons, opioid peptides, substance P and somatostatin in central cardiovascular regulation of the rat. In W. Rascher, C. Clough and D. Ganten (Eds.), *Hypertensive Mechanisms. The Spontaneously Hypertensive Rat as a Model of Study Human Hypertension*, Schattauer-Verlag, Stuttgart and Berlin, pp. 417–441.

Fuxe, K., Agnati, L. F., Benfenati, F., Celani, M. F., Zini, I., Zoli, M. and Mutt, V. (1983a) Evidence for the existence of receptor-receptor interactions in the central nervous system. Studies on the regulation of monoamine receptors by neuroleptics. *J. Neuronal Trans.*, 18: 165–179.

Fuxe, K., Agnati, L. F., Härfstrand, A., Zini, I., Tatemoto, K., Merlo Pich, E., Hökfelt, T., Mutt, V. and Terenius, L. (1983b) Central administration of neuropeptide Y induces hypotension bradypnea and EEG synchronization in the rat. *Acta physiol. Scand.*, 118: 189–192.

Fuxe, K., Calza, L., Benfenati, F., Zini, I. and Agnati, L. F. (1983c) Quantitative autoradiographic localization of (^{3}H) imipramine binding sites in the brain of the rat: Relationship to ascending 5-hydroxytryptamine neuron systems. *Proc. nat. Acad. Sci. USA*, 80: 3836–3840.

Fuxe, K., Agnati, L. F., Andersson, K., Martire, M., Ögren, S.-O., Giardino, L., Battistini, N., Grimaldi, R., Farabergoli, C., Härfstrand, A. and Toffano, G. (1984a) Receptor-receptor interactions in the central nervous system. Evidence for the existence of heterostatic synaptic mechanisms. In E. S. Vizi and K. Magyar (Eds.), *Regulation of Transmitter Function: Basic and Clinical Aspects: Developments in Neuroscience Series, Vol. 17*, Elsevier Science Publ., pp. 129–140.

Fuxe, K., Agnati, L. F., Härfstrand, A., Martire, M., Goldstein, M., Grimaldi, R., Bernardi, P., Zini, I., Tatemoto, K. and Mutt, V. (1984b) Evidence for a modulation by neuropeptide Y of the α-2 adrenergic transmission line in central adrenaline synapses. New possibilities for treatment of hypertensive disorders. *Symposium on Neuropeptides and Blood Pressure Control, June 12–14, 1984 in Heidelberg, Germany, Clin. exp. Hypert. Theory Practice*, A6 (10–11): 1951–1956.

Fuxe, K., Agnati, L. F., Andersson, K., Eneroth, P., Härfstrand, A., Goldstein, M. and Zoli, M. (1984c) Studies on neurtensin-catecholamine interactions in the hypothalamus and in the forebrain of the male rat. *Neurochem. Int.*, 6: 737–750.

Fuxe, K., Agnati, L. F., Zoli, M., Härfstrand, A., Grimaldi, R., Bernardi, P., Camurri and Goldstein, M. (1985a) Development of quantitative methods for the evaluation of the entity of coexistence of neuroactive substances in nerve terminal populations in discrete areas of the central nervous system: Evidence for hormonal regulation of cotransmission. In L. F. Agnati and K. Fuxe (Eds.), *Wenner-Gren Symposium on Quantitative Neuroanatomy in Transmitter Research, Stockholm, Sweden, May 3–4, 1984*, Macmillan Press, London, pp. 157–175.

Fuxe, K., Andersson, K., Härfstrand, A., Agnati, L. F., Eneroth, P., Jansson, A. M., Vale, W., Thorner, M. and Goldstein, M. (1985b) Medianosomes as integrative units in the external layer of the median eminence. Studies on GRF/catecholamine and somatostatin catecholamine interactions in the hypothalamus of the male rat. *Neurochem. Int.* (in press).

Goldstein, M., Lew, J. Y., Matsumoto, Y., Hökfelt, T. and Fuxe, K. (1978) Localization and function of PNMT in the central nervous system. In M. A. Lipton, A. DiMascio and K. F. Killiam (Eds.), *Psychopharmacology: A Generation of Progress*, Raven Press, New York, pp. 261–269.

Härfstrand, A., Fuxe, K., Agnati, L. F., Ganten, D., Eneroth, P., Tatemoto, K. and Mutt, V. (1984) Studies on neuropeptide-Y catecholamine interactions in central cardiovascular regulation in the α-chloralose anaesthetized rat. Evidence for a possible new way of activating the α-2 adrenergic transmission line. *Clin. exp. Hypert. Theory Practice*, A6 (10–11): 1947–1950.

Härfstrand, A., Fuxe, K., Agnati, L. F., Grinaldi, R., Ganten,

D. and Karobath, M. (1985) Physiological studies on the neuropeptide Y-adrenaline neuron systems of the medulla oblongata of the male rat. *J. Neurol.*, 232: 192.

Härfstrand, A., Fuxe, K., Agnati, L. F., Wikström, A.-C., Okret, S., Zhao-Ying, Y., Cintra, A., Goldstein, M., Verhofstad, S. and Gustafsson, J.-Å. (1986) Demonstration of glucocorticoid receptor immunoreactivity in monoamine neurons of the rat brain. *Proc. nat. Acad. Sci. USA* (submitted).

Hökfelt, T., Fuxe, K., Goldstein, M. and Johansson, O. (1974) Immunohistochemical evidence for the existence of adrenaline neurons in the rat brain. *Brain Res.*, 66: 235–251.

Hökfelt, T., Goldstein, M., Fuxe, K., Johansson, O., Verhofstad, A., Steinbush, H., Penke, B. and Vargas, J. (1980) Histochemical identification of adrenaline containing cells with special reference to neurons. In K. Fuxe, M. Goldstein, B. Hökfelt and T. Hökfelt (Eds.), *Central Adrenaine Neurons: Basic Aspects and Their Role in Cardiovascular Functions*, Pergamon Press, Oxford and New York, pp. 19–47.

Hökfelt, T., Everitt, B. J., Fuxe, K., Kalia, M. Agnati, L. F., Johansson, O., Theodorsson-Norheim, E. and Goldstein, M. (1984a) Transmitter and peptide systems in areas involved in the control of blood pressure. *Clin. exp. Hyper. Theory Practice*, A6 (1 and 2): 23–41.

Hökfelt, T., Goldstein, M., Foster, G., Johansson, O., Schultzberg, M., Staines, W., Fuxe, K. and Kalia, M. (1984b) Distribution of adrenaline neurons in the rat brain. In G. Racagni, R. Paoletti and P. Kielholz (Eds.), *Clinical Neuropharmacology, Vol. 7, Suppl. 1*, Raven Press, New York, pp. 678–679.

Innis, R. B. and Snyder, S. (1980) Distinct cholecystokinin receptors in brain and pancreas. *Proc. nat. Acad. Sci. USA*, 77: 6917–6921.

Kalia, M., Woodward, D. J., Smith, W. K. and Fuxe, K. (1985) Rat medulla oblongata. IV. Topographical distribution of catecholaminergic neurons with quantitative three-dimensional computer reconstruction. *J. comp. Neurol.*, 233: 350–364.

Paxinos, G. and Watson, C. (1982) *The Rat Brain in Stereotaxic Coordinates*, Academic Press, New York.

Rouot, B. and Snyder, S. H. (1979) ^{3}H-para-aminoclonidine: A novel ligand which binds with high affinity to α-adrenergic receptors. *Life Sci.*, 25: 769–774.

Sternberger, L. A. (1979) *Immunocytochemistry, 2nd edn.*, John Wiley & Sons, New York.

Undén, A. and Bartfai, T. (1984) Regulation of neuropeptide Y (NPY) binding by guanine nucleotides in the rat cerebral cortex. *FEBS Lett.*, 177: 125–128.

Undén, A., Tatemoto, K., Mutt, V. and Bartfai, T. (1984) Neuropeptide Y receptor in the rat brain. *Europ. J. Biochem.*, 145: 525–530.

Zini, I., Merlo Pich, E., Fuxe, K., Lenzi, P. L., Agnati, L. F. Härfstrand, A., Mutt, V., Tatemoto, K. and Moscara, M. (1984) Actions of centrally administered neuropeptide Y on EEG activity in different rat strains and in different phases of their circadian cycle. *Acta physiol. Scand.*, 122: 71–77.

T. Hökfelt, K. Fuxe and B. Pernow (Eds.),
Progress in Brain Research, Vol. 68

CHAPTER 21

Functional consequences of coexistence of classical and peptide neurotransmitters

Tamas Bartfai[1], Kerstin Iverfeldt[1], Ernst Brodin[2] and Sven-Ove Ögren[3]

[1]*Department of Biochemistry, Arrhenius Laboratory, University of Stockholm, S-106 91 Stockholm,* [2]*Department of Pharmacology, Karolinska Institute, S-104 05 Stockholm and* [3]*Astra Läkemedel AB, R and D Laboratories, S-151 85 Södertälje, Sweden*

Introduction

Research of the last 5 years has provided ample examples of coexistence of classical neurotransmitters with peptide neurotransmitters (Hökfelt et al., 1980; Cuello, 1982; Lundberg et al., 1982b; Schultzberg et al., 1982; Lundberg and Hökfelt, 1983). The phenomenon of coexistence is widespread in the central and peripheral nervous system. The purpose of this study was to examine the effect of acute and chronic drug regimens which are known to influence the turnover and tissue level of classical neurotransmitters with respect to their effect on the peptide neurotransmitters which coexist with the affected classical neurotransmitter. It was hypothetized that if these drug regimens change the firing rate or the release per pulse of a neuron then these changes may alter the levels of all neurotransmitters stored and released from the neuron.

The magnitude of change of tissue levels of the classical neurotransmitters and coexisting peptides may be different. Differential action of a drug is made likely by the fact that the mode and site(s) of synthesis of the coexisting classical neurotransmitters and peptides is different (cf. Hökfelt et al., 1980).

It is thus worthwhile to discuss the structural prerequisites of differential drug actions on coexisting classical neurotransmitters and peptides.

Anisotropic distribution of coexisting transmitters

As pointed out by Hökfelt et al. (1980) in their review, the site of synthesis of peptide neurotransmitters is on ribosomes in the soma where the peptides are elaborated in the form of large preprohormones. These are packaged into vesicles alone or together with the classical neurotransmitter, which can be synthetized both in the soma and in the nerve endings. (However, the highest specific activity of synthetizing enzymes is found in the nerve terminals; cf. McGeer et al., 1978.) Vesicle populations containing peptide neurotransmitters or classical neurotransmitters have been found by gradient centrifugation (Lundberg et al., 1981). There are also examples of one and the same vesicle containing peptides and classical neurotransmitters, such as the chromaffin granules which contain opioid peptides in addition to catecholamines and the enzyme dopamine-β-hydroxylase (Viveros et al., 1979).

It is an interesting and important aspect of the function of neurons with classical and peptidergic neurotransmitters that a "pure" peptide containing vesicle once transported from the soma via axonal transport to the terminal and released its content cannot be refilled with the peptide in the terminal since the neurotransmitter(s) elaborated there are the low molecular weight classical neurotransmitters. Thus retrieval of a "peptidergic vesicle" means that it can now be loaded to become a classical neurotransmitter containing vesicle (as was pointed out by R. Kelly, personal communication).

Regulation of release: chemical-frequency coding

Changes in the frequency of stimulation of a neuron containing one signal substance will change the amount of released neurotransmitter at a given synapse *but cannot change the chemical nature of the message*. Changes in the firing frequency of a classical neurotransmitter/peptide neurotransmitter containing neurons however may alter which of the coexisting neurotransmitters is released or in what stoichiometrical proportion they are released: thus the *very chemical nature of the signal may be altered* by changes in the frequency of stimulation. In most peptidergic or peptidergic and classical neurotransmitter containing neurons, the release of the peptide appears to require higher (>2 Hz) frequency of stimulation than that required for release of the classical neurotransmitter. Thus at low frequency stimulation classical neurotransmitter peptide containing neurons may act as classical neurotransmitter releasing neurons (frequency range A in Fig. 1) or as peptide and classical neurotransmitter releasing neurons (frequency range B) or peptidergic neurons (frequency range C). The "purely" peptidergic transmission in frequency range "C" may result from the autoinhibition of the release of the classical neurotransmitter and from the inhibition of the release of the classical neurotransmitter by the coreleased peptide.

It appears that there is a direct translation of the *frequency code into chemical code* at the level of the individual nerve terminals of a neuron with more than one signal substance.

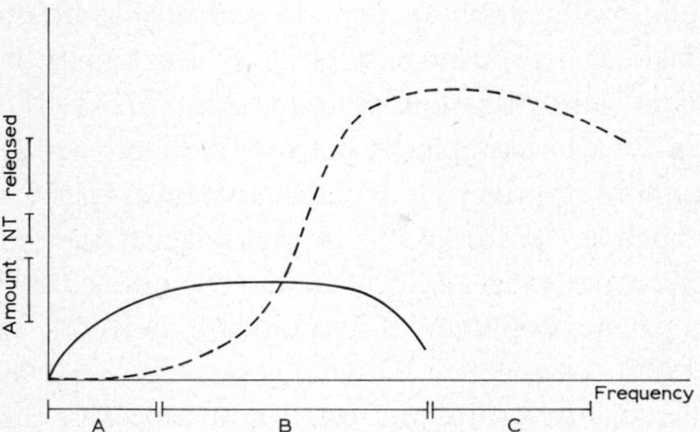

Fig. 1. Dependence of the chemical nature of the signal on frequency of stimulation. Schematic illustration of the release of a classical (———) and a peptide (---------) neurotransmitter from a neuron, at various frequencies of stimulation. In range A (low frequency of stimulation) the neuron releases mainly the classical neurotransmitter, in range B, both neurotransmitters are released and in range C (high frequency of stimulation) the neuron may act as a peptidergic neuron.

Multidimensional neuronal maps

The Ecclesian formulation of Dale's principle (cf. this volume) permitted one to construct neuronal maps assuming that any one neuron acts as a binary unit: when it fires its signal value is one and when it is mute or silent the signal value is zero. The possibility that multiple signals (in any combination) may be released from a neuron which contains more than one neurotransmitter(s) makes these maps redundant. One will have to enlarge the map of any neuron into that many dimensions as it contains meaningful signals or signal combinations for its postsynaptic counterparts. Furthermore, one has to realise that *firing of such neurons may lead to release of different signal substances or different combinations of signal substances at their different synapses* since, e.g. the stimulus may give rise to release conditions which may permit release of both the peptide and the classical neurotransmitter from the axonal nerve terminal while from a dendritic site only the release of the classical neurotransmitter may occur under the same stimulus.

Expansion of the autoreceptor concept

The release per pulse of several neurotransmitters is finely regulated by autoinhibition and facilitation (Stjärne, 1975; Vizi, 1979; Starke, 1981). This has been amply documented in studies on the release of noradrenaline and acetylcholine (ACh) from various preparations and has been found to be applicable to almost every classical neurotransmitter so far studied in both the peripheral and central nervous system.

It is assumed that occupancy of autoreceptors changes the likelihood of release from a terminal or the amount of neurotransmitter released per pulse by changing the resting membrane potential in such a way that the Ca^{2+}-influx upon depolarization by the nerve impulse will be altered. Since the release of peptide and classical neurotransmitters is Ca^{2+}-dependent, it is therefore only to be expected that manipulation of Ca^{2+}-influx into a nerve terminal will influence the release of *all neurotransmitters* (classical and peptidergic) from the nerve terminal. Studies indeed show that the autoreceptors which are best characterized for the classical neurotransmitters will influence the release of not only the classical neurotransmitter but also that of the coexisting peptide. Thus *the autoreceptor concept has to be expanded to involve regulation of release of all transmitters by one of the released transmitters.*

Effects of chronic drug treatment on coexisting classical neurotransmitters and peptide neurotransmitters

Chronic changes in the firing rate of neurons or in the sensitivity of the autoreceptors may affect the tissue levels and turnover of coexisting classical and peptide neurotransmitters differentially because of the differences in the site(s) and mode of their synthesis, storage and release. Rates of biosynthesis of several classical neurotransmitters are regulated by the impulse flow; because the rate-limiting enzymes (e.g. tyrosine hydroxylase or tryptophan hydroxylase) are sensitive to changes in impulse flow at the given nerve ending where most part of monoamine synthesis takes place (Lovenberg et al., 1975; Morgenroth et al., 1975; Salzman and Roth, 1978). The biosynthesis of peptides on ribosomes in the soma does not seem to show the same sensitivity towards changes in impulse patterns in the systems so far studied.

Synergistic effects of coexisting neurotransmitters

The synergistic postsynaptic interactions between receptors for coexisting neurotransmitters have been documented in the case of muscarinic ACh/VIP receptors (Lundberg et al., 1982a; Lundberg and Hökfelt, 1983) SP/5-HT type-1 receptors (Agnati et al., 1983a) NPY/α_2-adrenergic receptors (Agnati et al., 1983b). These synergistic interactions may be of great pharmacological importance since lower doses of drugs acting on classical neurotransmitter receptors can be used to achieve a desired effector response, if synergism with the coexisting peptide is utilized. This may in turn decrease the probability and the time required for development of tolerance. We shall, however, focus on the presynaptic aspects of coexistence in this chapter.

Specific examples: studies on coexistence of ACh and VIP

Most of the above mentioned "theoretical" results are derived from studies on ACh/VIP coexistence in the postganglionic neurons of cat submandibularis gland (Lundberg, 1981; Lundberg and Hökfelt, 1983) and rat submandibularis gland (Hedlund et al., 1983, 1985; Bartfai et al., 1984; Westlind et al., 1984) and in the bipolar cells of rat cerebral cortex (Abens et al., 1984; Eckenstein and Baughman, 1984). The release of ACh from all of these ACh/VIP-containing nerves is feedback regulated via a muscarinic autoreceptor. Atropine treatment leads to enhanced release of ACh because of disinhibition (Polak and Meeuws, 1966; Vizi, 1979; Alberts et al., 1982). It was also found that via muscarinic autoreceptors, ACh inhibited the release of VIP (Lundberg, 1981) as well as VIP acting at VIP receptors inhibited the release of ACh (Lundberg, 1981; Bartfai et al., 1984). Thus blockage or disinhibition of muscarinic autoinhibition of VIP release by atropine, acutely, leads to enhanced release of VIP (Lundberg, 1981). Chronic treatment with atropine, leads to depletion of 60–80% of VIP from the rat submandibularis (Hedlund et al., 1983), probably due to chronic disinhibition of the release of VIP. The increased release of VIP, under conditions of atropine treatment, seems to exceed the amount of VIP transported to the terminal via axonal flow (Fig. 2). Thus treatment with the classical muscarinic antagonist, atropine, causes depletion of VIP, the peptide which coexists with ACh in the terminals. As a consequence, the number of (postsynaptic) VIP receptors is almost doubled in the rat submandibularis (Hedlund et al., 1983) and increased significantly in the rat cerebral cortex (Abens et al., 1984). (Atropine treatment also causes an increase in the number of muscarinic receptors in both tissues.)

Similarly to the release of VIP, the release of ACh from the ACh/VIP terminals is also enhanced in the presence of atropine. The tissue levels of ACh fell only 20% (as compared to the 60–80% loss in VIP) because the accelerated local synthesis of ACh keeps up with the increased release (Karlén et al., 1978).

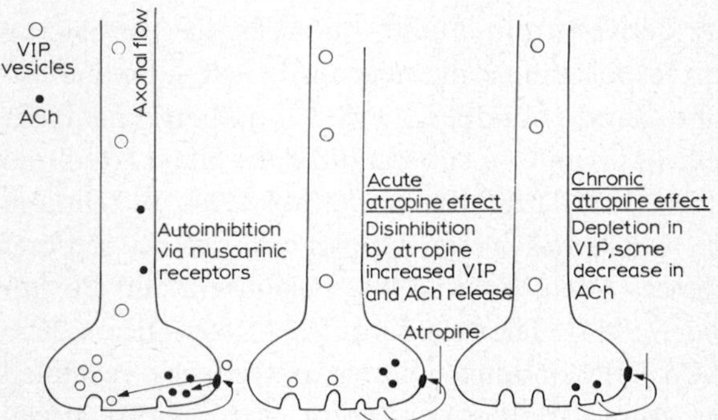

Fig. 2. Schematic model for development of depletion of VIP levels in the submandibularis (and development of supersensitivity of VIP receptors), in a neuron showing coexistence of ACh and VIP, upon treatment with the muscarinic antagonist, atropine. Left panel: control situation, muscarinic autoinhibition of both ACh and VIP-release is effective. Middle panel: acute atropine causes enhanced release. Right panel: axonal flow cannot keep up with the increased release; local ACh synthesis partly balances the increased ACh release during chronic treatment.

Coexistence of serotonin and substance P in the descending neurons in the rat dorsal and ventral spinal cord

Some serotonergic neurons descending from the raphe nucleus contain substance P (SP) (Chan-Palay et al., 1978; Hökfelt et al., 1978) and TRH immunoreactive material in their terminals in the dorsal and ventral spinal cord (Johansson et al., 1981). In this study we have concentrated on 5-HT/SP coexistence and have for the time being neglected measurement of TRH, which could be part of this study on coexistence.

Synthesis, storage and release patterns of 5-HT and SP

5-HT is synthetized both in the soma, in the raphe nucleus and in the terminals in the dorsal and ventral spinal cord.

SP is synthetized on ribosomes in the soma. So far, two mRNA species coding for SP have been isolated from the mammalian brain (Nawa et al., 1983). One of these also codes for another tachykinin: substance K (SK). (Thus our studies could have involved 5-HT/SP/SK and TRH to cover the coexisting neurotransmitters of these descending "serotonergic" neurons known today.)

Gradient centrifugation of isolated synaptic vesicles and synaptosomes shows a distribution of SP-like immunoreactive material and 5-HT which can be interpreted as indicating that at least one population of 5-HT containing vesicles does not contain SP (Fried et al., 1984).

A functional consequence of the existence of separate vesicle population is that chemical manipulations (or physiological stimulus patterns) may be found which cause release of 5-HT without releasing SP (and likely which release SP without releasing 5-HT): low frequency stimulation (below 2–4 Hz) seems to release ^{3}H-5-HT from loaded slices of ventral spinal cord without substantial release of SP.

The known pharmacologic releasing agent *p*-

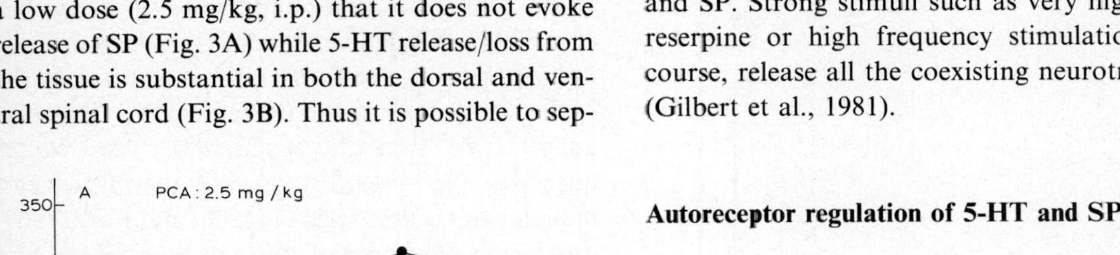

chloroamphetamine (PCA) can also be used in such a low dose (2.5 mg/kg, i.p.) that it does not evoke release of SP (Fig. 3A) while 5-HT release/loss from the tissue is substantial in both the dorsal and ventral spinal cord (Fig. 3B). Thus it is possible to separately manipulate the release of coexisting 5-HT and SP. Strong stimuli such as very high doses of reserpine or high frequency stimulation will, of course, release all the coexisting neurotransmitters (Gilbert et al., 1981).

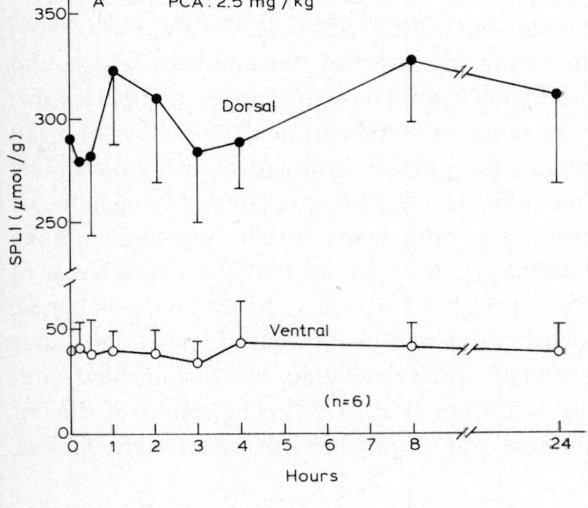

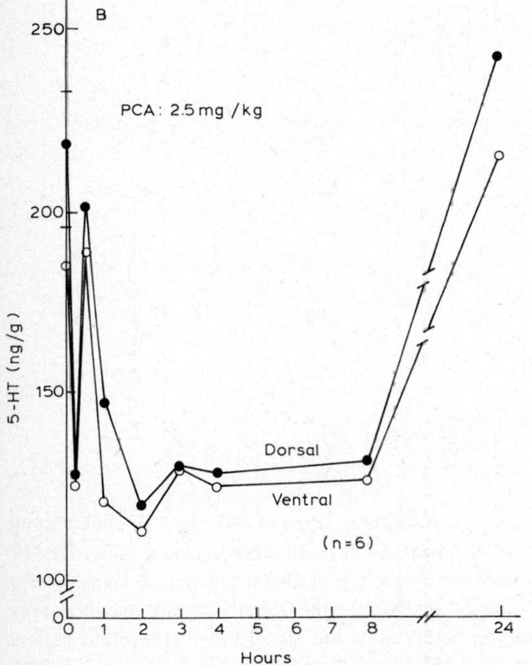

Fig. 3. Time course of changes in SPLI (substance-P like immunoreactivity) levels (A) and in 5-HT levels (B) in dorsal and ventral spinal cord after i.p. administration of PCA (*p*-chloroamphetamine) (2.5 mg/kg).

Autoreceptor regulation of 5-HT and SP release

It is known that in all tissues with serotonergic innervation, 5-HT inhibits 5-HT release via methiotepin sensitive autoreceptors (Cerrito and Raiteri, 1979; Göthert and Weinheimer, 1979; Göthert, 1982).

We have examined whether the serotonin-autoreceptor can also control/influence the release of the coexisting peptide SP. The studies were concentrated on the ventral spinal cord where most of SP occurs in serotonin containing neurones (Chan-Palay et al., 1978; Hökfelt et al., 1978).

Figure 4 shows that serotonin can enhance the K^+-depolarization evoked release of SP from 5-HT/SP nerve terminals in the ventral spinal cord. This effect could be fully blocked by ketanserin, a specific 5-HT type 2 receptor antagonist. The mechanism of 5-HT mediated facilitation is not known in this system, but a well-documented example of 5-HT mediated presynaptic facilitation involving cAMP-dependent protein phosphorylation has been described in *Aplysia* (cf. Kandel and Schwartz, 1982).

In view of the serotonergic autoreceptors regulating both 5-HT and SP release, one may pose the question does SP affect its own release and the release of 5-HT? The question of SP-autoreceptor regulating SP release is not yet solved. With respect to the effect of SP on 5-HT release, there is data from Michell and Fleetwood-Walker (1981) indicating that SP can promote release of 5-HT under conditions of active serotonergic autoinhibition. Thus the concept of autoreceptor has to be expanded to involve regulation of the release of all coexisting neurotransmitters.

With respect to the release of SP/5-HT from these raphe nucleus neurons it should be mentioned that

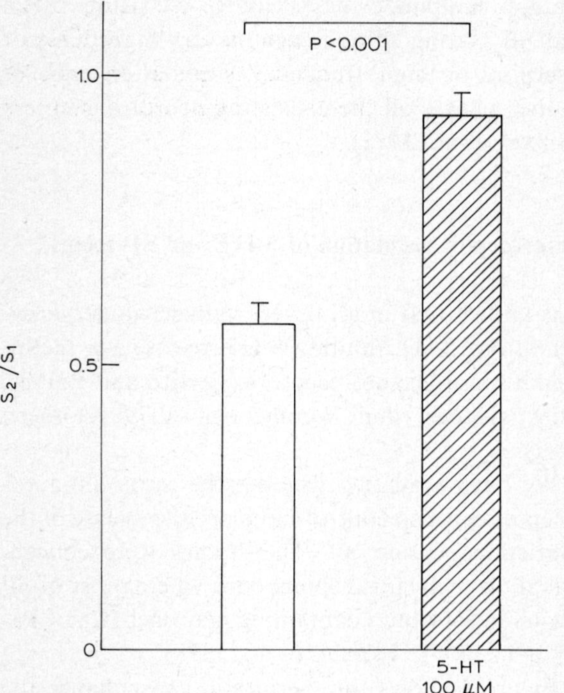

Fig. 4. 5-HT mediated stimulation of K^+-depolarization evoked release of SP in ventral spinal cord. Slices (0.4 mm) of the ventral spinal cord were superfused with Krebs-Ringer's solution (NaCl, 138 mM; KCl, 5 mM; $CaCl_2$, 1 mM; $MgCl_2$, 1 mM; NaH_2PO_4, 1 mM; $NaHCO_3$, 11 mM; glucose, 11 mM) containing ascorbic acid (1 mM), bovine serum albumin (0.2%) and bacitracin (0.3%), pH 7.4 and were stimulated twice with 40 mM K^+ for 3 min, with a 30-min interval between stimulations. The second stimulation in absence or presence of 100 μM 5-HT (5-hydroxy-tryptamine creatinine sulfate). SP-like immunoreactivity was determined using antiserum K 25 (Brodin et al., 1981) (n = 20). (Data from Iverfeldt et al., 1986.)

dendritic release of 5-HT probably plays an important role in the serotonin-autoreceptor mediated control of the firing rate of these neurons (Aghajanian, 1972). (It is not yet known whether SP can be released from dendrites.)

Chronic treatment with serotonin uptake blocking drugs

Several clinically effective antidepressant drugs are potent inhibitors of monoamine uptake into platelets and monoaminergic nerve endings (cf. Hertling et al., 1961; Hamberger and Tuck, 1973; Barchas et al., 1977). Chronic treatment with these drugs is known to lower the firing rate of neurons in the locus coeruleus or in the raphe nucleus (Aghajanian, 1972; de Montigny et al., 1981). As a consequence of the lowered firing rate, the turnover of monoamines is decreased (Corrodi and Fuxe, 1969) due to the sensitivity of tyrosine hydroxylase and tryptophan hydroxylase to changes in impulse flow.

We treated rats subchronically (14 days, 2 × 10 μmol/kg per day, per oral) either with imipramine, a monoamine uptake blocker or with zimelidine or alaproclate, both being specific serotonin uptake blockers. Figure 5 shows that the tissue levels of serotonin fell by 10–20% in the hypothalamus, frontal cortex and in the ventral spinal cord after treatment with zimelidine, as documented previously (Ögren et al., 1984). The results of the imipramine and alaproclate treatment were similar.

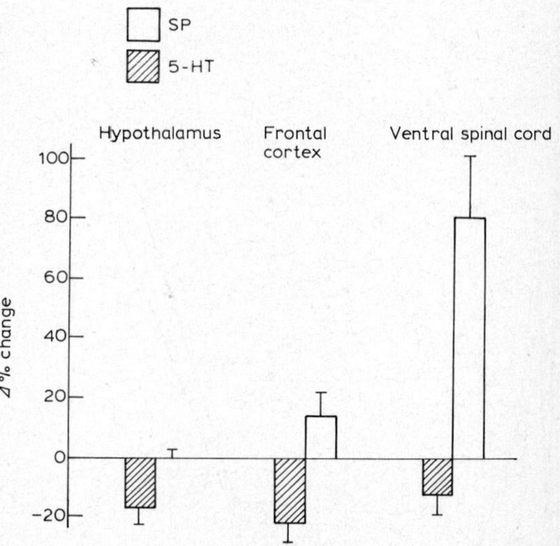

Fig. 5. Changes in the tissue levels of 5-HT and SP upon chronic zimelidine treatment (14 days, 10 μmol/kg, twice daily). The increases in SP levels are significant in the ventral spinal cord $p < 0.01$ and not significant in the frontal cortex or hypothalamus. Decreases in 5-HT levels are significant in the brain regions shown ($p < 0.05$). The data are presented as means ± S.E.M. (n = 8–12). (5-HIAA levels were significantly lower than control in the spinal cord as well as in the hypothalamus and cerebral cortex, indicating lowered firing.) Spinal cord data from Iverfeldt et al., 1986.

The tissue levels of SP were not significantly changed in these brain regions, which are rich in both SP and 5-HT but do not contain these in a coexistence situation. In the dorsal and ventral spinal cord, where 5-HT and SP coexists, the tissue levels of SP were increased highly significantly (Brodin et al., 1984). Thus zimelidine a "serotonergic" drug, designed for selectivity even within the monoaminergic systems, caused highly specific changes in the tissue levels of SP in a region of the nervous system where serotonin coexists with SP.

Several explanations can be offered for this finding (cf. Fig. 6): (a) The build-up of SP levels in the spinal cord may be caused by the decreased firing rate and thereby decreased release of SP from the descending neurons. The biosynthesis of serotonin is adjusted to the chronic change in firing rates whereas SP biosynthesis and axonal transport are uninfluenced, leading to a pile-up of SP in the distal nerve endings in the spinal cord. (b) A change in the sensitivity of the serotonin-autoreceptor mediating enhancement of SP release may be involved. There is data in the literature about development of subsensitivity of serotonin-receptor during chronic antidepressant treatment. Subsensitivity of a stimulatory autoreceptor would lead to a decreased release per pulse and would contribute to the build-up of SP in the nerve endings in the spinal cord, if rates of biosynthesis and axonal transport were unaltered. Finally, the most plausible explanation is a combination of (a) and (b), which takes into account the lowered firing rates of the 5-HT/SP neurons and the lowered release per pulse due to subsensitivity of the serotonergic-autoreceptor (Fig. 6).

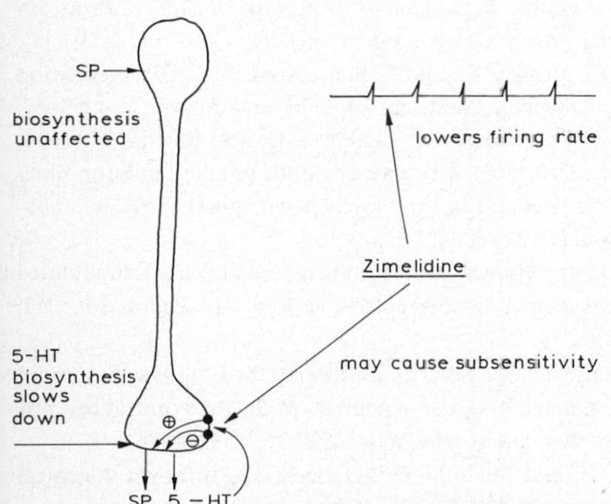

Fig. 6. Possible sites of action of zimelidine bringing about build-up of SP in the ventral spinal cord in the terminals of descending 5-HT/SP neurons.

The build-up of SP increases the amount of SP which can be released upon K^+ stimulation and thus represent a build-up in a releasable pool with functional implications (Iverfeldt et al., 1986).

Experiments are in progress to examine whether changes in the release and size of releasable pool of SP during chronic antidepressant drug treatment are also reflected in changes in the number of SP receptors in the spinal cord. A functional supersensitivity with respect to the postsynaptic serotonin type 1 receptor in the spinal cord, in a tail flick model, has been reported (Ögren et al., 1984).

Coexistence and the action of antidepressant and antipsychotic drugs

Since after chronic treatment with imipramine, zimelidine or alaproclate the changes in tissue levels of the coexisting peptide SP were larger than the changes in the tissue levels of the monoamine, one may hypothetize that part of the therapeutic and side effects of these drugs will have to be explained by their effects on peptides in monoaminergic neurons. The release of the peptide is also altered (here in a differential manner) when the release of the monoamines is altered by chronic drug regimens.

Hökfelt et al. (1980) called attention to the possible involvement of changes in CCK metabolism in the etiology and drug therapy of schizophrenia, based on coexistence of dopamine and CCK in the mesolimbic system. Indeed, chronic treatment with antipsychotic drugs such as chlorpromazine and haloperidol which suppress dopaminergic activity (e.g. lower homovanilic acid and DOPAC levels in CSF), caused a build-up of CCK-8 in the mesolimbic system of rats (Frey, 1983). Thus a differential change is observed in the monoamine versus peptide levels at sites of coexistence similar to that found in the ventral spinal cord. The dopamine/CCK system which is under extensive study also shows "autoreceptor mediated cross-regulation"; CCK release is regulated by dopamine (Meyer and Krauss, 1983) and dopamine release (and change in turnover) is regulated by CCK (Fuxe et al., 1980) similar to the findings discussed with respect to ACh/VIP and 5-HT/SP coexistence.

In the etiology of certain types of depressive and psychotic illness, the primary derangement may thus be of peptidergic rather than of monoaminergic nature and treatments which change firing rates and per pulse release from monoamine/peptide containing neurons may be beneficial partly because it will also alter the peptidergic component of synaptic transmission as well as altering the monoaminergic synaptic transmission (Giller et al., 1985).

Conclusions

Several of the simple concepts arising from the immunohistochemical demonstration of neurons containing more than one signal substance have been formulated and some empirical data from the ACh/VIP, 5-HT/SP and dopamine/CCK coexistence systems have been quoted in support of these concepts. The data are rudimentary, and fragmentary — e.g. we report tissue levels of coexisting peptides rather than measures of turnover etc. — however, they seem to give further impetus for the study of the multidimensional synaptic maps which are the main consequences of the multiplicity of the stored and released signals.

Acknowledgements

The authors wish to acknowledge valuable discussions with Earl Giller, New Haven, R. Kelly, San Francisco, L. L. Peterson, Stockholm, P. Alberts, Umeå, which contributed significantly to the ideas communicated in this paper. T. Bartfai was a fellow at the Neurosciences Institute of the Neurosciences Research Program, New York during the preparation of this chapter.

References

Abens, J., Westlind, A. and Bartfai, T. (1984) Chronic atropine treatment causes increase in VIP receptors in rat cerebral cortex. *Peptides*, 5: 375–377.

Aghajanian, G. K. (1972) Influence of drugs on the firing of serotonin-containing neurons in brain. *Fed. Proc.*, 31: 91–96.

Agnati, L. F., Fuxe, K., Benfenati, F., Zini, I. and Hökfelt, T. (1983a) On the functional role of coexistence of 5-HT and substance P in bulbospinal 5-HT and substance P in bulbospinal 5-HT neurons. Substance P reduces affinity and increases density of ^{3}H-5-HT binding site. *Acta physiol. Scand.*, 117: 299–301.

Agnati, L. F., Fuxe, K., Benfenati, F., Battistini, N., Härfstrand, A., Tatemoto, K., Hökfelt, T. and Mutt, V. (1983b) Neuropeptide Y in vitro selectively increases the number of α_2-adrenergic binding sites in membranes of the medulla oblongata of rat. *Acta physiol. Scand.*, 118: 293–295.

Alberts, P., Bartfai, T. and Stjärne, L. (1982) The effect of atropine on ^{3}H-acetylcholine secretion from guinea pig myenteric plexus evoked electrically or by high potassium. *J. Physiol. (Lond.)*, 322: 93–112.

Barchas, J. D., Berger, P. A., Ciaranello, R. D. and Elliot, G. R. (1977) *Psychopharmacology: From Theory to Practice*, Oxford University Press, New York.

Bartfai, T., Westlind, A., Abens, J., Engström, C. and Alberts, P. (1984) On acetylcholine-vasoactive intestinal polypeptide coexistence and presynaptic interactions. In E. S. Vizi and K. Magyar (Eds.), *Regulation of Transmitter Function*, Proc. 5th Meeting Eur. Soc. Neurochem., pp. 497–500.

Brodin, E., Nilsson, G. and Folkers, K. (1981) Characterization of two substance P antisera. *Acta physiol. Scand.*, 114: 53–57.

Brodin, E., Peterson, L.-L., Ögren, S.-O. and Bartfai, T. (1984) Chronic treatment with the serotonin uptake inhibitor zimelidine elevates substance P levels in rat spinal cord. *Acta physiol Scand.*, 122: 209–211.

Cerrito, F. and Raiteri, M. (1979) Serotonin release is modulated by presynaptic autoreceptors. *Europ. J. Pharmacol.*, 57: 427–430.

Chan-Palay, V., Jonsson, G. and Palay, S. L. (1978) Serotonin and substance P coexist in neurons of the rat's central nervous system. *Proc. nat. Acad. Sci. USA*, 75: 1582–1586.

Corrodi, H. and Fuxe, K. (1969) Decreased turnover in central 5-HT nerve terminals induced by antidepressant drugs of imipramine type. *Europ. J. Pharmacol.*, 7: 56–59.

Cuello, A. C. (1982) *Cotransmission*, MacMillan Press, London.

De Montigny, C., Blier, P., Cailé, G. and Koussi, E. (1981) Pre-

and postsynaptic effects of zimelidine and norzimelidine on the serotoninergic system: Single cell studies in the rat. *Acta psychiatr. Scand.*, 63, Suppl. 290: 79–90.

Eckenstein, F. and Baughman (1984) Two types of cholinergic innervation in cortex, one co-localized with vasoactive intestinal polypeptide. *Nature (Lond.)*, 309: 153–155.

Frey, P. (1983) Cholecystokinin octapeptide levels in rat brain are changed after chronic neuroleptic treatment. *Europ. J. Pharmacol.*, 95: 87–92.

Fried, G., Frank, J. and Brodin, E. (1984) 5-Hydroxytryptamine and substance P coexistence in rat spinal cord: Subcellular distribution and release from synaptosomes. *Abstr. Scand. Physiol. Soc., Lund*, P28.

Fuxe, K., Andersson, K., Locatelli, V., Agnati, L. F., Hōkfelt, T., Skirboll, L. and Mutt, V. (1980) Cholecystokinin peptides produce marked reduction of dopamine turnover in discrete areas in the rat brain following intraventricular injection. *Europ. J. Pharmacol.*, 67: 329–331.

Gilbert, R. F. T., Bennett, G. W., Marsden, C. A. and Emson, P. C. (1981) The effects of 5-hydroxytryptamine-depleting drugs on peptides in the ventral spinal cord. *Europ. J. Pharmacol.*, 76: 203–210.

Giller, E., Bartfai, T. and Peterson, L.-L. (1985) A monoamine-peptide loop hypothesis of depression: models involving neuronal nets and receptor dynamics (in preparation).

Göthert, M. (1982) Modulation of serotonin release in the brain via presynaptic receptors. *Trends Pharmacol. Sci.*, 3: 437–440.

Göthert, M. and Weinheimer, G. (1979) Extracellular 5-hydroxytryptamine inhibits 5-hydroxytryptamine release from rat brain cortex slices. *Naunyn-Schmiedeberg's Arch. Pharmacol.*, 310: 93–96.

Hamberger, B. and Tuck, J. R. (1973) Effect of tricyclic antidepressant on the uptake of noradrenaline and 5-hydroxytryptamine by rat brain slices incubated in buffer or human plasma. *Europ. J. Clin. Pharmacol.*, 5: 1.7.

Hedlund, B., Abens, J. and Bartfai, T. (1983) Vasoactive intestinal polypeptide and muscarinic receptors: supersensitivity induced by long-term atropine treatment. *Science*, 220: 519–521.

Hedlund, B., Abens, J., Westlind, A. and Bartfai, T. (1985) Vasoactive intestinal polypeptide-muscarinic cholinergic interactions. In I. Hanin (Ed.), *Dynamics of Cholinergic Function* (in press).

Hertling, G., Axelrod, J. and Whitby, L. C. (1961) Effect of drugs on the uptake and metabolism of ^{3}H-norepinephrine. *J. Pharmacol. Exp. Ther.*, 134: 146–153.

Hökfelt, T., Ljungdahl, A., Steinbusch, H., Verhofstad, A., Nilsson, G., Brodin, E., Pernow, B. and Goldstein, M. (1978) Immunohistochemical evidence of substance P-like immunoreactivity in some 5-hydroxytryptamine-containing neurons in the rat central nervous system. *Neuroscience*, 3: 517–538.

Hökfelt, T., Johansson, O., Ljungdahl, Å., Lundberg, J. M. and Schultzberg, M. (1980) Peptidergic neurons. *Nature (Lond.)*, 284: 515–521.

Iverfeldt, K., Peterson, L.-L., Brodin, E., Ögren, S.-O. and Bartfai, T. (1986) Serotonin type-2 receptor mediated regulation of substance P release in the ventral spinal cord and the effects of chronic antidepressant treatment. *Naunyn-Schmiedeberg's Arch. Pharmacol.* (in press).

Johansson, O., Hökfelt, T., Pernow, B., Jeffcoate, S. L., White, N., Steinbusch, H. W. M., Verhofstad, A. A. J., Emson, P. C. and Spindal, E. (1981) Immunohistochemical support for three putative transmitters in one neuron: coexistence of 5-hydrotryptamine substance P and thyrotropin releasing hormone-like immunoreactivity in medullary neurons projecting to the spinal cord. *Neuroscience*, 6: 1857–1881.

Kandel, E. R. and Schwartz, J. H. (1982) Molecular biology of learning: modulation of transmitter release. *Science*, 218: 433–443.

Karlén, B., Lundgren, G., Miyata, T., Lundin, J. and Holmstedt, B. (1978) Effect of atropine on acetylcholine metabolism in the mouse brain. In D. J. Jenden (Ed.), *Cholinergic Mechanisms and Psychopharmacology*, Plenum Press, New York, pp. 643–655.

Lovenberg, W., Bruckwick, E. A. and Hanbauer, O. (1975) ATP, cyclic AMP and magnesium increase the affinity of rat striatal tyrosine hydroxylase for its cofactor. *Proc. nat. Acad. Sci. USA*, 72: 2955–2958.

Lundberg, J. M. (1981) Evidence for coexistence of vasoactive intestinal polypeptide (VIP) and acetylcholine in neurons of cat exocrine glands. *Acta physiol. Scand.*, 112, Suppl. 496: 1–57.

Lundberg, J. M. and Hökfelt, T. (1983) Coexistence of peptides and classical neurotransmitters. *Trends Neurosci.*, 6: 325–333.

Lundberg, J. M., Fried, G., Fahrenkrug, J., Holmstedt, B., Hökfelt, T., Lagercrantz, H., Lundgren, G. and Änggård, A. (1981) Subcellular fractionation of cat submandibular gland: comparative studies on the distribution of acetylcholine and vasoactive intestinal polypeptide (VIP). *Neuroscience*, 6: 1001–1010.

Lundberg, J. M., Hedlund, B. and Bartfai, T. (1982a) Vasoactive intestinal polypeptide enhances muscarinic ligand binding in cat submandibular salivary gland. *Nature (Lond.)*, 295: 147–149.

Lundberg, J. M., Hedlund, B., Änggård, A., Fahrenkrug, J., Hökfelt, T., Tatemoto, K. and Bartfai, T. (1982b) Costorage of peptides and classical transmitters in neurons. In S. R. Bloom, J. M. Polak and E. Lindenlaub (Eds.), *Systemic Role of Regulatory Peptides*, F. K. Schattauer-Verlag, Stuttgart and New York, pp. 93–119.

McGeer, P. L., Eccles, Sir J. C. and McGeer, E. G. (1978) *Molecular Neurobiology of the Mammalian Brain*, Plenum Press, New York, 644 pp.

Meyer, D. K. and Krauss, J. (1983) Dopamine modulates cholecystokinin release in neostriatum. *Nature (Lond.)*, 301: 338–340.

Mitchell, R. and Fleetwood-Walker, S. (1981) Substance P, but not TRH, modulates the 5-HT autoreceptor in ventral lumbar spinal cord. *Europ. J. Pharmacol.*, 76: 119–120.

Morgenroth, III, V. A., Hegstrand, L. R., Roth, R. H. and Greengard, O (1975) Evidence for involvement of protein kinase in the activation by adenosine 3′5′-monophosphate of brain tyrosine 3-monooxygenase. *J. Biol. Chem.*, 250: 1946–1948.

Nawa, H., Hirose, T., Takashima, H., Inayama, S. and Nakanishi, S. (1983) Nucleotide sequences of cloned cDNAs for two types of bovine brain substance P precursor. *Nature (Lond.)*, 306: 32–36.

Ögren, S. O., Ross, S. B., Hall, H., Holm, C. and Renyi, A. L. (1984) The pharmacology of zimelidine: A 5-HT selective reuptake inhibitor. *Acta psychiat. Scand.*, Suppl. 290, 63: 127–151.

Polak, R. L. and Meeuws, M. M. (1966) The influence of atropine on the release and uptake of acetylcholine by the isolated cerebral cortex of the rat. *Biochem. Pharmacol.*, 15: 989–992.

Salzman, P. M. and Roth, R. H. (1978) Noradrenergic neurons: Poststimulation increase in catecholamine biosynthesis. In P. Deniker, C. Radouco-Thomas and A. Villeneuve (Eds.), *Neuropsychopharmacology, Vol. 2,* Pergamon Press, New York, pp. 1439–1455.

Schultzberg, M., Hökfelt, T. and Lundberg, J. M. (1982) Coexistence of classical transmitters and peptides in the central and peripheral nervous systems. *Brit. Med. Bull.*, 38: 309–313.

Starke, K. (1981) Presynaptic receptors. *Ann. Rev. Pharmacol. Toxicol.*, 21: 7–30.

Stjärne, L. (1975) Basic mechanisms and local feedback control of secretion of adrenergic and cholinergic neurotransmitters. In L. L. Iversen, S. D. Iversen and S. H. Snyder (Eds.), *Handbook of Psychopharmacology, Vol. 6,* Plenum Press, New York, pp. 179–233.

Viveros, O. H., Diliberto, E. L., Hazum, E. and Chang, K.-J. (1979) Opiate-like materials in the adrenal medulla: evidence for storage and secretion with catecholamines. *Mol. Pharmacol.*, 16: 1101–1108.

Vizi, E. S. (1979) Presynaptic modulation of neurochemical transmission. *Prog. Neurobiol.*, 12: 181–290.

Westlind, A., Abens, J. and Bartfai, T. (1984) Functional aspects of the coexistence of classical neurotransmitters and peptide neurotransmitters. In J. E. Dumont and J. Nunex (Eds.), *Hormones and Cell Regulation, Vol. 8,* Elsevier Science Publishers, Amsterdam, pp. 195–211.

T. Hökfelt, K. Fuxe and B. Pernow (Eds.),
Progress in Brain Research, Vol. 68

CHAPTER 22

Characterization of central neuropeptide Y receptor binding sites and possible interactions with α_2-adrenoceptors

Menek Goldstein[1], Norifumi Kusano[1], Charles Adler[1] and Emanuel Meller[2]

Department of Psychiatry, New York University Medical Center, [1]Neurochemistry Research Laboratories and [2]Millhauser Laboratories New York, NY 10016, U.S.A

Introduction

Immunohistochemical studies show that some neurons contain both a classical transmitter, such as a catecholamine, and a peptide (Hökfelt et al., 1984). Studies with antisera raised against neuropeptide Y (NPY) and tyrosine hydroxylase (TH) demonstrate that peripheral and central catecholamine neurons contain an NPY-like peptide (Everitt et al., 1984). Subcortical regions, in particular the nucleus accumbens, amygdala and hypothalamus, were found to be relatively rich in NPY. A population of noradrenergic cell bodies within the locus ceruleus, as well as a noradrenergic population of the A1/C1 cell group in the ventrolateral medulla oblongata, contain NPY. The majority of the adrenergic cell bodies of the C2 cell group also contain NPY (Everitt et al., 1984). Furthermore, the findings that NPY induces a dose-dependent vasoconstriction (Lundenberg and Tatemoto, 1982) and that it is involved in the central adrenergic control of blood pressure (Fuxe et al., 1983), suggest a possible functional interaction between norepinephrine (NE) and/or epinephrine (E) and NPY.

* *Address for correspondence:* Menek Goldstein, New York University Medical Center, Neurochemistry Research Laboratories, Rm. H-544, New York, NY 10016, U.S.A.

The widespread distribution of NPY in the CNS indicates that it may be involved in various regulatory functions. We have therefore investigated the specific receptor binding sites for NPY which might be involved in mediation of these functions and studied the regulation of these binding sites by α_2-adrenoceptors. Since neuropeptides carry out a number of cellular actions by mobilizing intracellular Ca^{2+} (Gardner, 1979), we studied the effects of Ca^{2+} and of various agents that work through Ca^{2+} on NPY receptor binding sites.

Binding studies with [^{3}H]NPY and [^{125}I]NPY

The availability of two radioligands with high specific activity, namely [^{3}H]NPY and [^{125}I]NPY has made it possible to develop a procedure for measuring the specific binding of this peptide to cerebral membrane sites. NPY was iodinated using the Bolton Hunter reagent (New England Nuclear, 2000 Ci/mmol) and the iodinated peptide was isolated by HPLC. We have also used the commercially available [^{125}I]NPY (sp. act. 2000 Ci/mmol; diluted 16 times with nonradioactive NPY) and [^{3}H]NPY (sp. act. 70 Ci/mmol), both obtained from Amersham or New England Nuclear. The procedure for measuring the binding of [^{3}H]NPY and of [^{125}I]NPY to rat cerebral cortical membranes is summarized in

TABLE I

Schematic representation of the procedure for measuring the binding of [^{125}I]NPY or [^{3}H]NPY to cerebral cortical membrane sites

(1) Rat cerebral cortex: homogenization in 40 vol of Tris-HCl (50 mM, pH 7.6); centrifugation at 48,000 × *g* for 10 min
(2) Suspension of the 48,000 × *g* sediment in 80 vol of Tris-HCl (50 mM, pH 7.6) containing 5 mM $MgCl_2$, 5 mM $CaCl_2$, 0.1 mM bacitracin, 0.065 TIU/ml aprotinin, 10 μg/ml leupeptin and 5 mM DL-dithiothreitol (DTT)
(3) Incubation mixture: 400 μl of membrane suspension, 50 μl of various concentrations of radioactive NPY, or 1 μM nonradioactive NPY (for nonspecific binding), and 50 μl of 0.1% BSA. The incubation was carried out at room temperature for 90 min
(4) Termination of the incubation: the incubation was terminated by adding 2 ml of 50 mM Tris-HCl (pH 7.6) containing 2.5 mM $MgCl_2$, 2.5 mM $CaCl_2$ and 0.02% BSA, and the mixture was centrifuged at 10,000 × *g* for 15 min
(5) Determination of radioactivity: [^{125}I]NPY radioactivity was determined in the pellet using a Beckman 400 gamma counter. [^{3}H]NPY was determined by sonicating the pellet in 1 ml solution containing 10% SDS and by measuring the radioactivity in a beta-scintillation counter.

Table I. Both radioligands are displaced from the cerebral membranes with low concentrations of NPY. However, NPY fragments 14–36 and 19–36 did not inhibit the binding of [^{125}I]NPY (Kusano et al., 1985), suggesting that the receptor recognition site resides in the N-terminal region of the molecule. Specific binding was determined as the difference between total and nonspecific binding (in the presence of 10^{-6} M NPY) and the specific binding was approximately 70% of the total binding. Scatchard plots of [^{125}I]NPY binding to cerebral cortical membranes revealed an apparently homogeneous population with a dissociation constant (K_d) of 0.39 ± 0.08 nM and a maximum number of binding sites (B_{max}) of 405 ± 47 fmol/mg of protein, while Scatchard plots of [^{3}H]NPY revealed a slightly higher K_d (0.53 ± 0.08 nM) and a slightly lower B_{max} (382 ± 35 fmol/mg protein).

Effect of Ca^{2+} on the specific binding of radioactive NPY

The specific binding of radioactive NPY is influenced by the concentration of divalent cations in the incubation mixture. The specific binding of [^{3}H]NPY was approximately 85% inhibited in absence of Ca^{2+} in the medium. Scatchard plots of [^{3}H]NPY binding to cerebral cortical membranes in presence and absence of Ca^{2+} show that the K_d decreases and the B_{max} increases in presence of Ca^{2+}. The maximum specific binding of [^{3}H]NPY or of [^{125}I]NPY to cerebral membranes was obtained in presence of 5 mM Ca^{2+}, and therefore if not otherwise stated, all the experiments were carried out at this concentration of the divalent cation.

Effect of Ca^{2+} antagonists on [^{3}H]NPY binding to cerebral cortical membranes

The results presented in Table II show that various agents which interfere with the cellular activation mediated by Ca^{2+} inhibit the binding of NPY to cerebral cortical membranes at high concentrations. Thus, the Ca^{2+} channel antagonist felodipine, which also interacts with calmodulin (Bostrom et

TABLE II

The effects of various Ca^{2+} antagonists on the specific binding of NPY to rat cerebral cortical membranes

Ca^{2+} antagonist (10^{-4} M)	Specific NPY binding (%)
Control	100
Ca^{2+}-free medium	15
Felodipine	60
Trifluoperazine	75
W-7	70
W-5	110

The experimental conditions are described in the text. The results are the means from three experiments ± S.E.M. of 2–5%.

al., 1981), significantly inhibits the specific binding of NPY. Several drugs that are known to inhibit the activity of Ca^{2+}/calmodulin and/or Ca^{2+} and phospholipid-dependent kinase (kinase C) also inhibit the specific binding of NPY. Trifluoperazine (TFP), as well as the known Ca^{2+}/calmodulin antagonist *N*-(6-aminohexy)5-(chloronaphthalene)-1-sulfonamide (W-7), inhibit the specific binding of NPY. The compound with a closely related structure to W-7, namely *N*-(6-aminohexyl)-1-(naphthalene) sulfonamide (W-5) does not interfere with the action of calmodulin and does not inhibit the specific binding of NPY.

Effect of chronic treatment with clonidine on [^{125}I]NPY binding to rat cerebral cortical membranes

Treatment of rats with the α_2-adrenoceptor agonist clonidine (100 μg/kg, i.p.) twice daily for 11 days resulted in an increased specific binding of [^{125}I]NPY to cerebral cortical membranes. Scatchard plots of [^{125}I]NPY binding to cerebral cortical membranes revealed that following chronic treatment with clonidine, the B_{max} increased from 410 fmol/mg protein to 529 fmol/mg protein, while the K_d did not change significantly.

TABLE III

Effect of chronic inhibition of PNMT by LY 134046 on [^{125}I]NPY binding to membrane isolated from the rat hypothalamus

Conc. of [^{125}I]NPY	Specific binding (f/mg protein)	
	Control	Treated
0.07 nM	13.7	17.4
0.78 nM	124.7	160.0

Treatment of the animals is described in the text. The results were obtained from a single experiment at each concentration of [^{125}I]NPY in triplicate.

Effects of chronic treatment with the PNMT inhibitor LY 134046 on [^{125}I]NPY binding to rat hypothalamic membranes

To determine the effects of central E depletion on specific NPY binding, we treated animals with the PNMT inhibitor LY 134046. The animals were treated subcutaneously (18 mg/kg per day) by a minipump for 7 days. The results presented in Table III show that chronic treatment with the PNMT inhibitor resulted in an increased specific binding of [^{125}I]NPY to rat hypothalamic membrane sites.

Irreversible inactivation and recovery of α_2-adrenoceptors

Recently we have shown that *N*-ethoxycarbonyl-2-ethoxy-1,2-dihydroquinoline (EEDQ) irreversibly inactivates α_2-adrenoceptors (Mellet et al., 1985) and that the NPY binding is not affected by this reagent. Thus it might be possible to study the relationships between α_2-adrenoceptors and NPY receptors by measuring the effects of the gradual inactivation of the latter receptor on the binding characteristics of NPY. The kinetics of repopulation of α_2-adrenoceptor binding sites following inactivation by EEDQ show a nonexponential pattern with a half life ($t_{\frac{1}{2}}$) of 4.1 days. The functional recovery for restoration of α_2-adrenoceptor-mediated inhibition of [^{3}H]NE release (mediated by autoreceptors) and of [^{3}H]5-HT release (mediated by heteroreceptors) follows a nonexponential pattern with a $t_{\frac{1}{2}}$ of 2.4 days and 4.6 days, respectively (Adler et al., 1985). These results indicate that the recovery of the binding sites parallels the functional recovery of the heteroreceptor. The difference between the functional recoveries of α_2-adrenoceptor agonist-mediated inhibition of [^{3}H]NE release and that of [^{3}H]5-HT release may reflect the presence of a larger population of receptor reserve for α_2-autoreceptors than for α_2-heteroreceptors.

Discussion

The potential role of NPY in various brain functions prompted us to investigate the characteristics of NPY receptor binding sites. We have developed a procedure for measuring the specific binding of NPY to cerebral membranes (Kusano et al., 1985) which is similar to the procedure developed independently by Unden et al. (1984). The results of our study show that the specific NPY binding is dependent on extracellular Ca^{2+} and that various agents which interfere with the action of Ca^{2+} inhibit the binding of NPY.

Under our experimental conditions, high concentrations of Ca^{2+} were required for maximum specific binding of NPY and the inhibition of the binding was only achieved with high concentrations of Ca^{2+} antagonists. The requirements for these high concentrations might be due to the presence of Ca^{2+} binding proteins in the crude membrane preparations and these proteins could compete with the NPY receptor binding protein for the extracellular Ca^{2+}. It is noteworthy that the Ca^{2+}-influx blocker felodipine inhibits the specific binding of NPY at high concentrations, and that verapamil in vitro reverses at high doses the vasoconstrictor response of NPY (Edvinsson et al., 1983). Since several drugs that are known to inhibit the activity of Ca^{2+}/calmodulin and/or Ca^{2+} and phospholipid-dependent kinase also inhibit the specific binding of NPY, one is tempted to suggest that the NPY receptor might be linked to a Ca^{2+}-dependent protein kinase. Phosphorylation of receptors is, in many instances, important in controlling cell responsiveness following ligand-receptor interactions. Evidence has been obtained that several receptors are susceptible to phosphorylation by kinases and our data suggest that the NPY receptor might also be affected by a Ca^{2+}-dependent kinase. It should be noted that the activity of kinase C is linked with the phosphatidyl inositol turnover and mobilization of Ca^{2+}, and therefore it would be of interest to determine whether the activation of the NPY receptor promotes the hydrolysis of phospholipids.

Chronic treatment of rats with the α_2-adrenoceptor agonist clonidine resulted in a small increase in the number of maximum binding sites (B_{max}) for NPY in cerebral cortical membranes. In view of the findings that the co-localization of NPY with NE in the CNS is restricted only to a small fraction of the neuronal population containing either the peptide or NE alone, it is not surprising that α_2-adrenoceptor agonists only marginally affect the NPY binding in the cerebral cortex. On the other hand, the majority of E-containing neurons seem to be colocalized with NPY, and lowering of central E levels by chronic treatment with a specific PNMT inhibitor significantly affects the specific binding of NPY in the hypothalamic membranes. Preliminary studies with EEDQ indicate that it is possible to study the relationships between functional α_2-adrenoceptors and NPY receptors. These studies may reveal whether interactions between these two receptor systems occur and whether these mechanisms play a role in the modulation of their functional activities.

Summary

[^{125}I]NPY or [^{3}H]NPY binds with high affinity to a single site in homogenates of rat cerebral cortex and hypothalamus. The specific binding of NPY requires extracellular Ca^{2+}, and various Ca^{2+} antagonists inhibit the specific binding. It is suggested that the NPY receptor might be linked to a Ca^{2+}-dependent protein kinase and phosphorylation may play a role in the regulation of the receptor activity state. Chronic treatment with the α_2-adrenoceptor agonist clonidine slightly increases the maximal binding sites of NPY to cerebral cortical membranes. Depletion of central epinephrine by chronic treatment with a PNMT inhibitor increases the maximal binding sites of NPY to the hypothalamic membrane sites. The relationships between α_2-adrenoceptors and NPY is being investigated by determining the effects of irreversible inactivation of the latter on the binding characteristics of the former receptor.

Acknowledgements

These studies were supported by NIMH Grant MH-02717 and NIH Grant NINCDS-06801. We wish to thank Ms. Judith Scheer for her excellent secretarial assistance.

References

Adler, C. A., Meller, E. and Goldstein, M. (1985) Recovery of α_2-adrenergic receptor binding and function after irreversible inactivation by *N*-ethoxycarbonyl-2-ethoxy-1,2-dihydroquinoline (EEDQ). *Europ. J. Pharmacol.* (in press).

Bostrom, S.-L., Ljung, B., Mardh, S., Forsen, S. and Thulin, E. (1981) Interaction of the antihypertensive drug felodipine with calmodulin. *Nature (Lond.)*, 292: 777–778.

Edvinsson, L., McCullock, J., Tatemoto, K. and Uddman, R. (1983) Neuropeptide Y: A unique system of perivascular nerves mediating contraction of cerebral vessels. *J. cereb. Blood Flow Metab.*, 3: 5182–5183.

Everitt, B. J., Hökfelt, T., Terenius, L., Tatemoto, K., Mutt, V. and Goldstein, M. (1984) Differential co-existence of neuropeptide Y (NPY)-like immunoreactivity with catecholamines in the central nervous system of the rat. *Neuroscience*, 11: 443–462.

Fuxe, K. Agnati, L., Harfstand, A., Zini, I., Tatemoto, K., Pich, E. M., Hökfelt, T., Mutt, V. and Terenius, L. (1983) Central administration of neuropeptide Y induces hypotension, bradycardia and EEG synchronisation in the rat. *Acta physiol. Scand.*, 117: 315–318.

Gardner, J. P. (1979) Regulation of pancreatic exocrine function in vitro: Initial step in the action of secretagogues. *Ann. Rev. Physiol.*, 41: 55–66.

Hökfelt, T., Johansson, O. and Goldstein, M. (1984) Chemical anatomy of the brain. *Science*, 225: 1326–1334.

Kusano, N., Schlesinger, D. and Goldstein, M. (1985) The binding of ^{125}I-NPY to rat cerebral cortical receptor membrane sites. *Fed. Proc.*, 44: Abst. 4853.

Lundberg, J. M. and Tatemoto, K. (1982) Pancreatic polypeptide family (APP, BPP, NPY and PYY) in relation to sympathetic vasoconstriction resistant to alpha adrenoceptor blockade. *Acta physiol. Scand.*, 116: 393–402.

Meller, E., Bohmaker, K., Goldstein, M. and Friedhoff, A. J. (1985) Inactivation of D_1 and D_2 dopamine receptors by *N*-ethoxycarbonyl-2-ethoxy-1,2-dihydroquinoline in vivo: Selective protection by neuroleptics. *J. Pharmacol. exp. Ther.*, 233: 656–662.

Unden, A., Tatemoto, K., Mutt, V. and Bartfai, T. (1984) Neuropeptide Y receptor in the rat brain. *Europ. J. Biochem.*, 145: 525–530.

T. Hökfelt, K. Fuxe and B. Pernow (Eds.),
Progress in Brain Research, Vol. 68
© 1986 Elsevier Science Publishers B.V. (Biomedical Division)

CHAPTER 23

Neuropeptide Y receptor interaction with beta-adrenoceptor coupling to adenylate cyclase

Marjut Olasmaa and Lars Terenius

Department of Pharmacology, University of Uppsala, Box 591, 751 24 Uppsala, Sweden

Introduction

The complexity of the central nervous system (CNS) is not only formidable at an anatomical level, there is also increasing evidence that a very large number of substances are involved in synaptic communication (Bloom, 1984). A newly discovered principle, co-existence in one neuron between so-called classic transmitter and neuropeptide(s) (Hökfelt et al., 1984, and central theme of this volume) adds to the possibilities for signal expression. Substances acting as modulators may reach extrasynaptic targets, subtly modulating the transmission process. This plethora of substances involved in communication is matched by a large number of receptors; not uncommonly one signal substance may interact with several receptor types.

However, some of this diversity breaks down in the receptor-effector coupling. One cell may have several receptors which work through a common effector system. The receptors coupled to adenylate cyclase are the classic example. These receptors are known to have three components: (1) a molecule with a recognition site for a signal substance, the receptor component; (2) the GTP-binding protein (N-protein), the transducer; and (3) the catalytic unit (C) which is the enzyme adenylate cyclase, the effector. This system is sensitive to both positive and negative signals via functionally different transducers; an N_s-protein mediates the stimulatory signaling and an N_i-protein mediates the inhibitory coupling to the C-unit. Thus, when an agonist interacts with a receptor component which couples to the N_s-protein, the C-unit becomes activated to form cAMP, if the receptor component couples to the N_i-protein, the C-unit is deactivated (Rodbell, 1980).

A good example is a mouse anterior pituitary cell line which secretes ACTH. This cell is stimulated by several ligands which activate adenylate cyclase, corticotrophin-releasing factor, noradrenaline (NA), vasoactive intestinal polypeptide (VIP) and is inhibited by somatostatin through deactivation of adenylate cyclase (Axelrod and Reisine, 1984). It is likely that the different receptor components couple with the same pool of N_s- and N_i-proteins, respectively. Schramm and co-workers (Schramm, 1979) were in fact able to show that receptor components of foreign cell membrane could be introduced into a cell line by membrane fusion and become functionally competent by coupling to the adenylate cyclase system of the recipient cell. Receptor components in this system are interchangeable and in dynamic exchange with the N-proteins; interactions between receptor components could be understood as obeying mass-action laws.

Receptor-receptor interactions

Recent experimental work has, however, indicated that receptor-receptor interactions may be more complex. Such observations have been done both in receptor systems which couple to adenylate cyclase and in other systems. Receptors are highly flexible molecules and sensitive to ionic and lipid environment (Kirilovsky et al., 1985), but probably also to the presence of other proteins and particularly to other receptors. Several receptors seem to be oligomers; it has even been suggested that different receptor types (sharing the same signal substance) may arise through recombinations of dissimilar receptor subunits (heteromers). Interactions *between* receptors have been indicated by binding analysis. Like other receptors which activate adenylate cyclase, the beta-adrenoceptor has lower affinity for agonist in the presence of GTP. Interestingly, this so-called GTP-shift in agonist binding affinity is reversed in the presence of muscarinic agonists. The muscarinic agonists also inhibited isoprenaline-induced activation of adenylate cyclase. Apparently, the muscarinic agonists affected the coupling efficacy of the adrenoceptors (Watanabe et al., 1978). Lundberg et al. (1982) reported that VIP decreased the binding affinity of a muscarinic antagonist in salivary gland membranes by several orders of magnitude. This is of particular interest since VIP and acetylcholine (ACh) coexist in the parasympathetic nerves innervating this organ. Fuxe and collaborators (1983) have systematically studied the interaction between signal substances co-existing in CNS neurons. They observed more modest changes in affinity and/or maximum binding capacity of various radioactive ligands, when ligands of other receptors were present simultaneously. Indirect functional correlates between receptor-receptor interactions and pharmacologic interactions were also observed. In a rat strain with hypertension, neuropeptide Y (NPY) failed to show interaction with α_2-receptor agonist binding, suggesting faulty receptor regulation in this rat strain (Agnati et al., 1983a).

In other series of experiments, Magistretti and Schorderet (1984) observed a potentiation of VIP stimulated adenylate cyclase activity by NA in mouse frontal cortex slices. VIP is present in bipolar interneurons, whereas the NA fibers originate extrinsically, mainly in the locus coeruleus. Local activity in VIP cells may then amplify the actions of global NA release. Mudge and co-workers have observed interactions with the AC-system in cellular systems. In astrocytes, synergistic interactions were observed between NA and the neuropeptide somatostatin which potentiates the NA effect whereas, enkephalin inhibited the NA response. These and similar observations were interpreted in terms of either changes in NA-receptor affinity or effects on receptor-effector coupling efficacy introduced by the respective peptide (Rougon et al., 1983).

Membrane fusion transfer of receptors

The mechanisms behind the apparent receptor-receptor interactions discussed above remain unclear.

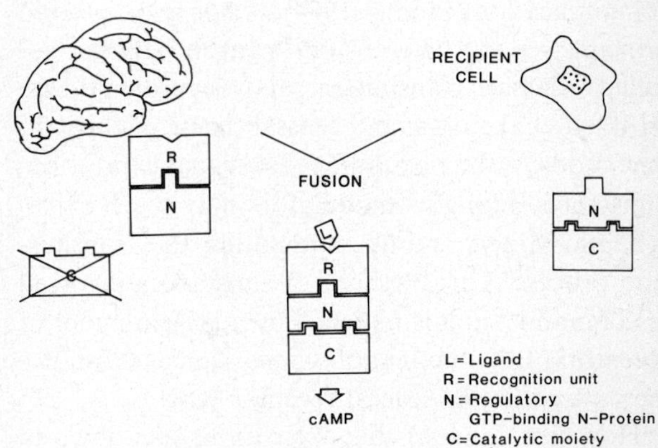

Fig. 1. Fusion transfer of receptors. The figure illustrates the principle. Experimentally, tissue specimens from CNS are homogenized in 0.32 M sucrose including 20 mM Tris-HCl pH 7.4 and 2 mM EGTA. The mitochondrial pellet (P_2) with synaptosomes is subjected to osmotic shock, whereafter centrifugation is used to separate the mitochondria and brain membranes. Prior to the fusion the brain membranes are treated with 5 mM *N*-ethylmaleimide (NEM) and then with phospholipids. A mouse tumor cell line, Friend erythroleukemia (F_c), is used as recipient. F_c cells are sedimented on top of a NEM-treated brain membrane pellet, and membranes and F_c cells are fused together in the presence of 52% polyethylene glycol (Schramm, 1979). Then, the adenylate cyclase activity is determined by incubation at 37° for 10 min and cAMP is measured according to the method of Salomon et al. (1974).

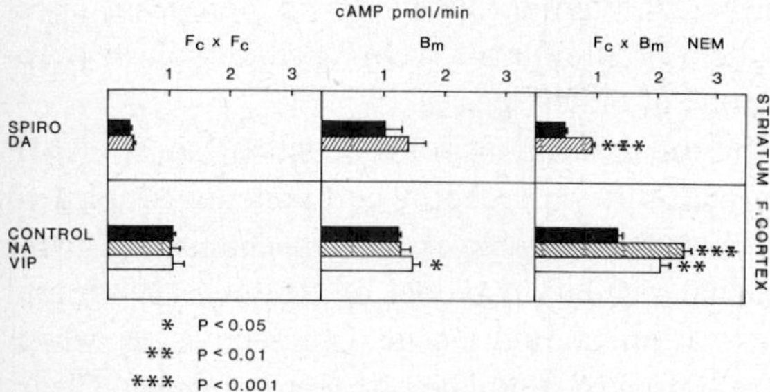

Fig. 2. The upper panel shows the effect of dopamine (DA) on the adenylate cyclase activity measured both directly on the brain membranes (B_m), prepared from rat striatum, and after fusion with Friend erythroleukemia cells ($F_c \times B_m$ NEM). In the lower panel, the data demonstrates the stimulation of adenylate cyclase by noradrenaline (NA) and vasoactive intestinal polypeptide (VIP) in rat frontal cortex membranes (B_m) and the potentiation of the signals after fusion ($F_c \times B_m$ NEM). The adenylate cyclase activity is given as pmoles cAMP generated per min; the values are means ± S.E.M. of duplicates from three independent experiments.

Studies on intact brain tissue are also complicated by the anatomical organization. We have seen certain advantages in using the membrane fusion procedure of Schramm and collaborators (Schramm, 1979). According to this technique the brain membranes are first treated with *N*-ethylmaleimide, to irreversibly inactivate their adenylate cyclase system. After this treatment the brain membranes, bearing the receptor components, are fused to a recipient cell line that possesses a functional effector system, but lacks the receptor components for neurotransmitters of study. This method offers the advantage that the transferred receptor components will have equal chances to become coupled to a well-defined homogeneous effector system. The principle of the method is outlined in Fig. 1.

The optimum experimental conditions for fusion transfer of receptors, were worked out for the DA_1-receptor of rat striatum (Olasmaa and Terenius, 1985). The effect of exogenous protein was observed by the response of the PGE_1 receptor of the recipient cell; it was found that about 200 μg of membrane protein could be fused into about 10^7 cells with retention of at least 50% of the indigenous PGE_1 receptor function. This amount of membrane protein was also quite sufficient for observing a signal from the DA_1 receptor after fusion (Fig. 2). Even 100 μg membrane protein gave a clear signal after DA stimulation.

This method allowed studies of DA_1 receptor from rat, rhesus monkey and human striatum (Olasmaa and Terenius, 1985). The magnitude of the signal in relation to membrane protein was comparable, suggesting that coupling efficiency is similar across species. A definite statement to this effect would require comparison of receptor numbers in the different preparations, which has not been done.

Receptor-receptor interactions studied by membrane fusion

To study potential receptor-receptor interactions in the adenylate cyclase system, the frontal cerebral cortex was chosen. This area has dense representation of postsynaptic beta-adrenoceptors (Mobley and Greengard, 1985) and of VIP receptors (Magistretti and Schorderet, 1984). Both NA and VIP receptor components couple via the stimulatory N_s-protein to cyclase. As indicated above, VIP amplifies activation of adenylate cyclase via beta-adrenoceptors in slice preparations of cerebral cortex. Another peptide which occurs in large quantities in the CNS and in the peripheral nervous system is NPY. It is known to co-exist with NA in both. In the cerebral cortex, NPY is a major neuropeptide, although it is apparently not present in the NA neurons (Everitt et al., 1984). Receptors for NPY have recently been identified in rat cerebral cortex membranes with the use of radioactive ligand binding techniques. The receptor binding capacity (which is very high) was reduced in the presence of GTP without any changes in the equilibrium binding constant of the receptor-ligand complex (Undén and Bartfai, 1984). This is unusual, since as discussed earlier, GTP-shifts to lower receptor-binding of agonist usually involve conversion of high affinity to low affinity sites and are indicative of receptor

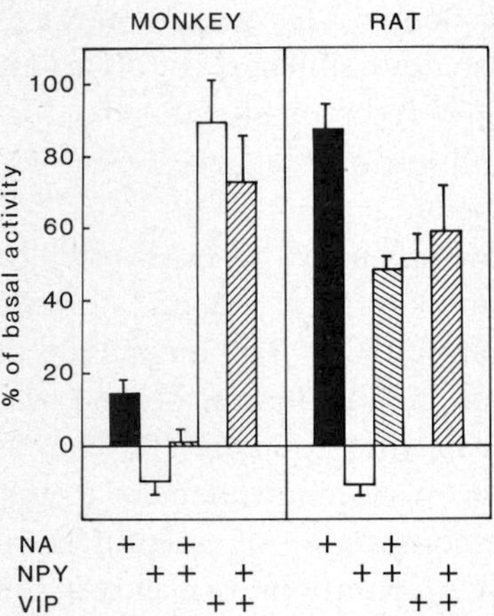

Fig. 3. The effects of noradrenaline (NA), vasoactive intestinal polypeptide (VIP), neuropeptide Y (NPY) and certain combinations on adenylate cyclase activity of rhesus monkey and rat brain membranes fused with Friend erythroleukemia cells. The data are presented as % of basal activity, and all values are means ± S.E.M. of duplicates from three independent experi-

coupling to adenylate cyclase (Watanabe et al., 1978).

The conditions developed for transfer of functionally competent DA_1-receptor were successfully applied to the study of NA and VIP receptors in rat frontal cortex. Whereas NA had no effect and VIP had a barely significant effect when added directly to brain membranes, the same membranes with inactivated C-unit gave highly significant substantial stimulation of cAMP formation after fusion (Fig. 2). Thus, both the beta-adrenoceptor and the VIP receptor components are transferable by membrane fusion and are able to form a functional unity with their new effector system.

In another series of experiments, frontal cortex membrane preparations from either rhesus monkey or rat, were transferred by fusion to the F_c cells. The effects of NA, NPY, VIP and certain combinations were tested (Fig. 3). NA gave a much larger response in rat than in the monkey preparation, and the opposite was observed with VIP. NPY alone gave a slight but significant inhibition of "basal" cAMP production. NPY obliterated the NA response in the monkey preparation and strongly attenuated the NA response in the rat preparation. On the other hand, NPY had no significant effect on the VIP stimulated cAMP production in preparations of either species.

The usual mechanism for deactivation of cAMP production is via receptor components coupled to inhibitory N_i (see above). This mechanism assumes the dual regulation model of Rodbell (1980) and deactivation should occur irrespective of which agent is used to stimulate cAMP production. Clearly this is not observed here; NPY inhibits NA *but not* VIP activation of cAMP production. It would be interesting to know whether NPY interacts with other activating receptors. Pilot experiments indicate that it does not interfere with the function of PGE_1 receptors of the F_c cells.

At present, one can only speculate how NPY affects the beta-adrenoceptor response. The sensitivity of the interaction between NPY and its receptor to GTP (Undén and Bartfai, 1984) points to the transducing step. If NPY uniquely interacts with NA receptors including the α_2-receptor (Agnati et al., 1983b) it does not seem unreasonable to associate to the co-existence of NA and NPY in sympathetic nerves and in central neurons, or to topological apposition of NA and NPY receptors in the cerebral cortex.

Acknowledgements

This work was supported by the Swedish Medical Research Council (04X-3766).

References

Agnati, L. F., Fuxe, K., Benfenati, F., Battistini, N. Härfstrand, A., Hökfelt, T., Cavicchioli, L., Tatemoto, K. and Mutt, V. (1983a) Failure of neuropeptide Y in vitro to increase the number of alpha$_2$-adrenergic binding sites in membranes of medulla oblongata of the spontaneous hypertensive rat. *Acta physiol. Scand.*, 119: 309–312.

Agnati, L. F., Fuxe, K., Benfenati, F., Battistini, N., Härfstrand, A., Tatemoto, K., Hökfelt, T. and Mutt, V. (1983b) Neuropeptide Y in vitro selectively increases the number of alpha$_2$-adrenergic binding sites in membranes of the medulla oblongata of the rat. *Acta physiol. Scand.*, 118: 293–295.

Axelrod, J. and Reisine, T. D. (1984) Stress hormones: Their interaction and regulation. *Science,* 224: 452–459.

Bloom, F. E. (1984) The functional significance of neurotransmitter diversity. *Amer. J. Physiol.,* 246: C184–C194.

Everitt, B. J., Hökfelt, T., Terenius, L., Tatemoto, K., Mutt, V. and Goldstein, M. (1984) Differential co-existence of neuropeptide Y (NPY)-like immunoreactivity with catecholamines in the central nervous system of the rat. *Neuroscience,* 11: 443–462.

Fuxe, K. Agnati, L. F., Benfenati, F., Celani, M. F., Zini, I., Zoli, M. and Mutt, V. (1983) Evidence for the existence of receptor-receptor interaction in the central nervous system. Studies of the regulation of monoamine receptors by neuropeptides. *J. Neural. Trans.* 18, Suppl., 165–179.

Hökfelt, T., Johansson, O. and Goldstein, M. (1984) Chemical anatomy of the brain. *Science,* 225: 1326–1334.

Kirilovsky, J., Steiner-Mordoch, S., Selinger, Z. and Schramm, M. (1985) Lipid requirements for reconstitution of the delipidated beta-adrenergic receptor and the regulatory protein. *FEBS Lett.,* 183: 75–80.

Lundberg, J. M., Hedlund, B. and Bartfai, T. (1982) Vasoactive intestinal polypeptide enhances muscarinic ligand binding in cat submandibular salivary gland. *Nature (Lond.),* 295: 147–149.

Magistretti, P. J. and Schorderet, M. (1984) VIP and noradrenaline act synergistically to increase cyclic AMP in cerebral cortex. *Nature (Lond.),* 308: 280–282.

Mobley, P. and Greengard, P. (1985) Evidence for widespread effects of noradrenaline on axon terminals in the rat frontal cortex. *Proc. nat. Acad. Sci. (Wash.),* 82: 945–947.

Olasmaa, M. and Terenius, L. (1985) Fusion transfer of dopamine DA_1 receptors to Friend erythroleukemia cells. *Neurosci. Lett.,* 53: 209–214.

Rodbell, M. (1980) The role of hormone receptors and GTP-regulatory proteins in membrane transduction. *Nature (Lond.),* 284: 17–22.

Rougon, G., Noble, M. and Mudge, A. W. (1983) Neuropeptides modulate the beta-adrenergic response of purified astrocytes in vitro. *Nature (Lond.),* 305: 715–717.

Salomon, Y., Londos, C. and Rodbell, M. (1974) A highly sensitive adenylate cyclase assay. *Analyt. Biochem.,* 58: 541–548.

Schramm, M. (1979) Transfer of glucagon receptor from liver membranes to a foreign adenylate cyclase by a membrane fusion procedure. *Proc. nat. Acad. Sci. (Wash.),* 76: 1174–1178.

Undén, A. and Bartfai, T. (1984) Regulation of neuropeptide Y (NPY) binding by guanine nucleotides in the rat cerebral cortex. *FEBS Lett.,* 177: 125–128.

Watanabe, A. M., McConnaughey, M. M., Strawbridge, R. A., Fleming, J. W., Jones, L. R. and Besch, H. R. (1978) Muscarinic cholinergic receptor modulation of beta-adrenergic receptor affinity for catecholamines. *J. biol. Chem.,* 253: 4833–4836.

T. Hökfelt, K. Fuxe and B. Pernow (Eds.),
Progress in Brain Research, Vol. 68

CHAPTER 24

Cotransmission at GABAergic synapses

E. Costa, H. Alho, M. R. Santi, P. Ferrero and A. Guidotti

Laboratory of Preclinical Pharmacology, National Institute of Mental Health, Saint Elizabeths Hospital, Washington, D.C. 20032, U.S.A.

Introduction

Coexistence in the same axon of more than one putative neuromodulator has been taken as evidence for the participation of multiple signals in synaptic communication. However, the strategy to gather evidence for coexistence in order to create experimental support for cotransmission does not seem to be the only avenue to be pursued. Actually, we believe that sometimes this strategy may focus on a type of cotransmission that in the final evaluation may not even be substantiated. In fact, if cotransmission indicates the participation of two or more signals in the transduction of synaptic communication, then it is not compulsory that these signals originate from the same axon. In fact, they could be located in different axons and participate in the modulation of synaptic events by bringing information resulting from an elaboration that has occurred in two different neuronal fields. This model implies that coexistence of two putative neuromodulators may indicate participation of each modulator in one of the two adjacent synapses. Thus, coexistence of cholecystokinin (CCK) with dopamine or that of vasoactive intestinal polypeptide (VIP) with acetylcholine may not necessarily mean that CCK participates in dopaminergic transmission or that VIP participates in cholinergic transmission. As illustrated in the drawing of Fig. 1 for the cotransmission at GABAergic synapses, the convergence of different chemical signals at postsynaptic receptor sites may occur with different modalities. Hence, since in cotransmission the action is at postsynaptic receptors, it seems to us that these receptors could be the departure point to gather information on cotransmission.

We have incorporated this line of thinking into the conceptual frame of reference that postsynaptic receptors are supramolecular structures including at least three operational subunits: the signal recognition site, the coupling system and the transducer. The signal recognition site may include a primary site for the action of the signal that has the capability to activate the transducer and a secondary site(s) for the action of the signal(s) that cannot activate the transducer but can change by an allosteric receptor-receptor interaction the characteristics of the recognition site for the primary transmitter. Through this mechanism the secondary signal would modulate the efficiency of the transduction elicited by the primary transmitter. This secondary signal could regulate the response to the primary signal by acting on the coupling mechanism or at the level of the enzyme or ionophore functioning as the effector in signalling transduction.

The question then arises, does this model reflect anything known in synaptic communication? The answer to this question is yes. In fact, the modulation of GABAergic transmission exemplifies the brain events from which the inferences operative in this model were made.

MODELS OF COTRANSMISSION AT GABAERGIC SYNAPSE

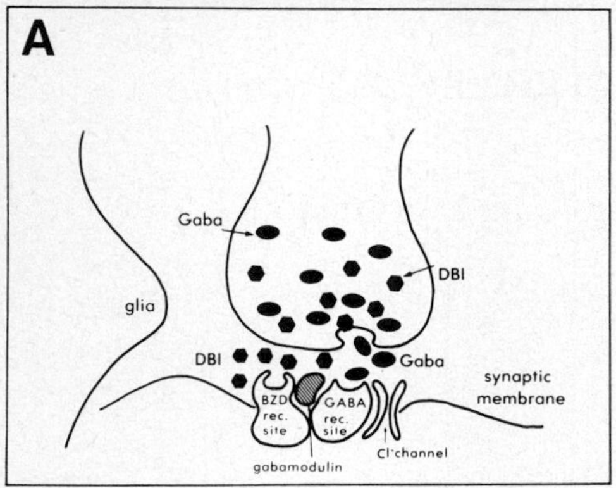

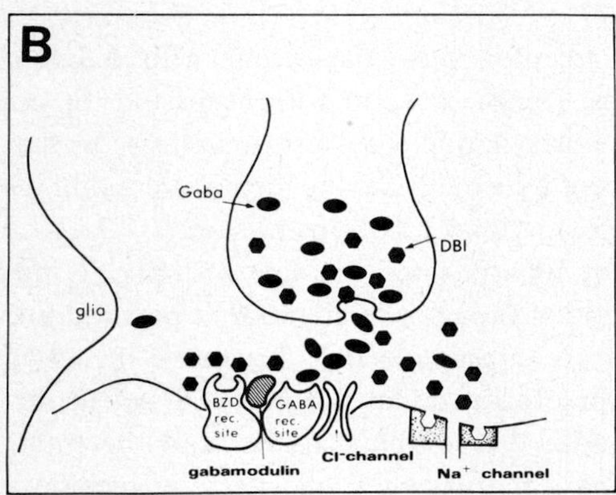

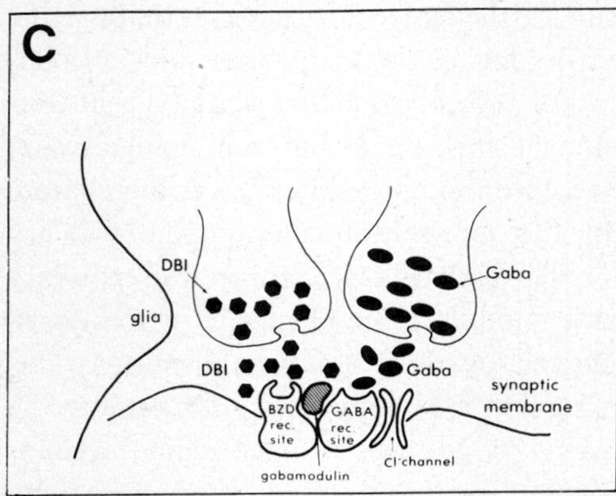

Fig. 1. (A) Primary transmitter (GABA) and cotransmitter (DBI) coexist in the same neuron and after release may interact with the same postsynaptic receptor (the GABA/benzodiazepine/Cl^-ionophore complex). (B) Primary transmitter and cotransmitter coexist, but after release they interact with more than one type of postsynaptic receptor complex. (C) Primary transmitter and cotransmitter are located in different neurons, but after release they converge on the same postsynaptic receptor complex.

GABAergic receptors as a focus for transmitter and cotransmitter interaction

Mao et al. (1975) reported that changes in cerebellar cyclic GMP content observed in rats receiving either GABA mimetics, or inhibitors of GABA synthesis or benzodiazepines or a combination of these drugs are in keeping with the concept that benzodiazepines facilitate GABAergic transmission by acting at postsynaptic GABA receptors. This evidence cast some light on an earlier report by Schmidt et al. (1967) that diazepam selectively enhances the presynaptic inhibition of spinal motor neurons in the cat. When Schmidt et al. (1967) reported this finding it was not known that GABA was an inhibitor of motor neurons acting presynaptically. Today because of a better understanding of the mode of action of GABA in spinal cord, the enhancement of presynaptic inhibition by benzodiazepines can be interpreted as an involvement of GABA in the action of benzodiazepines. A similar GABA/benzodiazepine interaction was found to be operative in the facilitation of the presynaptic inhibition by benzodiazepines in many brain areas (Haefely et al., 1975), thereby leading to the generalization that the pharmacological actions of benzodiazepines (anxiolytic, muscle relaxant and anticonvulsant) can be explained by their facilitatory action on GABA receptor function (Costa et al., 1975). This possibility acquired more consistency when Squires and Braestrup (1977) and Mohler and Okada (1977) showed that benzodiazepines bind with high affinity to sites present in brain synaptic membranes. Using flunitrazepam as a photoaffinity label for this recognition site, Mohler et al. (1981) showed that the benzodiazepine recognition site is located in contiguity with GABAergic axon terminals. More recently, Smart et al. (1983) could show that by injecting xenopus oocytes with a preparation of chick brain mRNA they could obtain the expression in the oocyte surface of a GABA mediated conductance increase and depolarization believed to be maintained by Cl^-. These GABA responses were reversibly antagonized by bicuculline and were clearly enhanced by a benzodiazepine in accordance with previous data on native GABA receptors. Finally, when the GABA recognition site was purified to physical homogeneity from the brain of various species (Siegel et al., 1983; Barnard et al., 1984; Schoch et al., 1985), it preserved the binding site for GABA agonists and antagonists, benzodiazepine agonists and antagonists, beta-carbolines, pentobarbital and bicyclophosphate Cl^- channel modulators. Moreover, these sites presented the characteristic interactions among each other.

This evidence taken together support the contention that GABA recognition sites (primary transmitters) are modulated by accessory sites linked to the GABA recognition site, allosterically (Costa and Guidotti, 1979; Olsen, 1982).

GABA/benzodiazepine interactions as a model for primary transmitter cotransmitter interactions

It is known that crude synaptic membranes contain two populations of GABA recognition sites with 22 nM and 160 nM K_D, respectively (Enna and Snyder, 1977). We proposed that these two sites expressed two conformational states of the GABA recognition site and that the expression of these states was regulated by an endogenous peptide (molecular weight around 1×10^4 daltons) which was thermostable (Costa et al., 1978; Guidotti et al., 1978; Costa and Guidotti, 1979). This peptide appears to function as a down regulator of the high affinity characteristics of the GABA recognition sites. In the presence of this peptide the benzodiazepines lose their capability to increase the efficiency of the interaction of GABA with its own receptor. In binding studies it could be shown that benzodiazepines increase the B_{max} of high affinity GABA recognition sites and that the peptide could displace benzodiazepines from their specific recognition sites (Guidotti et al., 1978, 1983). For this reason the peptide was termed DBI (diazepam binding inhibitor) (Guidotti et al., 1983). At that time, we also proposed that drugs could be found that mimic the action of the endogenous peptide and thereby exert a new type of CNS stimulation (Costa et al., 1978). The prediction that the recognition site for benzodiazepines could accept ligands with a pharmacological action opposite to that expressed by benzodiazepines was verified later by Braestrup et al. (1982) when they reported that beta-carboline-3-carboxylate esters possess a high affinity for benzodiazepine recognition sites and could be down regulated by GABA. When metabolically stable derivatives of beta-carboline-3-carboxylate esters were injected in rodents they caused convulsions (Braestrup et al., 1982) or elicited proconflict responses in the operant behavioral paradigm proposed by Vogel et al. (1971) as modified by Corda et al. (1983) to assay anxiogenic compounds. In fact, some of these beta-carboline derivatives injected into humans elicit anxiety (Dorow et al., 1983). In the light of these results and based on our original working hypothesis (Costa et al., 1978) we inferred that DBI could participate in GABAergic transmission as an additional chemical signal with modulatory capability (Costa et al., 1983). This inference was considered by others an unlikely probability because it contraverted the then popular belief that synaptic transmission was transacted by a single chemical signal (Polc et al., 1982). Meanwhile the structural complexity of the benzodiazepine recognition site that was implicit in our proposal became more evident. Thomas and Tallman (1981) repeating the photoaffinity labeling of GABA/benzodiazepine recognition sites with flunitrazepam reported that this procedure, as expected, decreased the B_{max} of benzodiazepine binding. However, when the binding of β-[^{3}H]carboline was tested after flunitrazepam photoaffinity labeling, the B_{max} of this ligand binding remained unaffected. This was surprising because in normal synaptic membranes beta-carboline derivatives displace flunitrazepam completely from their specific binding sites. A current interpretation of these findings is that the recognition sites for benzodiazepines and beta-carbolines include two domains. One which is shared by the two compounds and is devoid of functional significance and the other which expresses the intrinsic activity of a ligand and is specific for each compound. The latter is a specific receptor domain which is responsible for the modulation of GABA receptors and expresses the pharmacological profile of the compounds.

The search for an endocoid for benzodiazepine-beta-carboline recognition site

While this research was unfolding, a number of laboratories following different research strategies, searched for specific putative endocoids for the benzodiazepine recognition sites. Mohler et al. (1979) reported that in brain extracts purified by gel chromatography, three peaks which displaced [^{3}H]diazepam from specific binding sites could be detected. Each peak appeared to be rich in one of the three compounds, inosine, hypoxanthine and nicotinamide, respectively. A study of these three compounds suggested that nicotinamide was the best candidate for the benzodiazepine recognition site endocoid. However, a more careful investigation of nicotinamide brain distribution and binding characteristics suggested that this compound could not be considered further as a benzodiazepine recognition site endocoid. This trend of looking for an endogenous neuromodulator acting on benzodiazepine recognition sites was pursued also by Skolnick et al. (1978), Asano and Spector (1978) and Davis and Cohen (1980). Their efforts failed to lead to any major breakthrough. In contrast, DBI remained an attractive possibility as the benzodiazepine endocoid and its study was continued in our laboratory.

DBI as the endocoid for benzodiazepine recognition site

Chemistry

DBI was isolated and purified to physical homogeneity from human and rat brain. In both instances, the peptide appeared to include 104 amino acid residues with the terminal amino acid group blocked. This blockade has created some difficulties in obtaining the amino acid sequence by standard techniques. Hence, we have established the partial sequence of rat DBI by fragmenting the peptide with trypsin digestion and since the peptide contained 2 methionines also, by CNBr cleavage at the peptidic bonds containing methionine. This has allowed us to establish the sequence of 58 amino acid residues by conventional methods (Guidotti et al., 1983). In collaboration with Dr. Seeburg of Genentech (San Francisco, CA) we are now establishing the amino acid sequence of rat and human DBI by obtaining the DBI cDNA sequence. So far, using the molecular biological approach, the sequence obtained with a conventional method is essentially confirmed. We have obtained substantial evidence to believe that the epicenter of the biological activity resides in the following sequence:

Lys-Gln-Ala-Thr-Val-Gly-Asp-Val-Asn-Thr-Asp-Arg-Pro-Gly-Leu-Leu-Asp-Leu-Lys-Gly-Lys-Ala-Lys-Trp. A B C

This sequence is located in the residues (51–74) of DBI. We have confirmed its biological importance by synthesizing and studying the following octadecaneuropeptide (ODN): Gln-Ala-Thr-Val-Gly-Asp-Val-Asn-Thr-Asp-Arg-Pro-Gly-Leu-Leu-Asp-Leu-Lys (Ferrero et al., 1984). This compound was found to be biologically active and its biological profile will be discussed later on in this chapter.

We raised antibodies against human and rat DBI and against ODN. The rat DBI binds with high affinity to its antibody and this antibody reacts also with human DBI but this cross-reactivity is rather poor. The antibody against human DBI reacts better with its antigen than with rat DBI. This suggests that the sequences of rat and human DBI are not homologous. This inference is supported by a number of differences found in the peptide fingerprint of the tryptic digest of human and rat DBI. The antibody against ODN cross-reacts poorly with human and rat DBI but the antibodies against the two types of DBI do not cross-react with ODN.

Using the antibody against ODN, we studied whether ODN is present in rat brain extracts. As shown in Fig. 2, a Bio-Gel P-6 chromatogram shows the presence of two peaks of immunoreactivity. One of them can be ascribed to DBI and the other to ODN. The latter peak was rechromatographed on reverse phase HPLC yielding at least three peaks of immunoreactivity. Of this, one can be ascribed to ODN, the molecular nature of the other two peaks was not identified yet. This evidence indicates that DBI is processed in the brain to produce ODN-like material.

Tissue distribution

By using rat DBI as a reference standard and RIA it was established that DBI-like material can be assayed in brain. This material present in various brain structures can be identified with authentic DBI on the basis of Western blot and HPLC studies. The content of DBI-like immunoreactive material of some regions of rat brain is reported in Table I. The highest content was found in arcuate nucleus of the hypothalamus followed by the ventral medial, supraoptic and other hypothalamic nuclei, the periaqueductal gray and the cerebellar cortex. Much lower concentrations were found in caudatus-putamen, the lowest concentrations were detected in anterior pituitary. The difference in DBI content between the lowest and the highest brain region was about 7-fold. DBI-like immunoreactivity is present also in spinal fluid of man and rat. In man, this material has been shown to have an HPLC profile similar to authentic DBI. The content of spinal fluid DBI seems to be higher in male than in female, increases with age and on alcohol withdrawal, DBI does not appear to have a gradient distribution. The presence of DBI in spinal fluid indicates that the peptide could be secreted extracellularly.

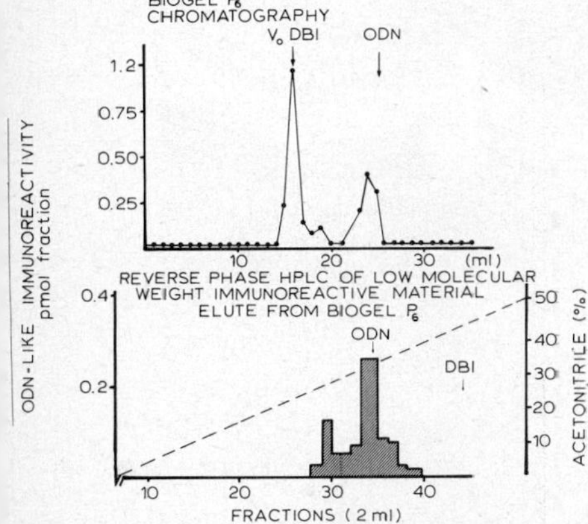

Fig. 2. Immunological identification of ODN in rat brain extracts. Rat brain was homogenized in 1 N acetic acid. In the upper panel, the 48,000 × *g* supernatant was applied to a Bio-Gel P6 column (1 × 70 mm) equilibrated with 1 N acetic acid. In the lower panel the low molecular weight immunoreactive material emerging from the Bio-Gel P6 column was applied to a μ Bondapack C18 reversed phase HPLC column equilibrated with 0.1% TFA in H_2O. The sample was eluted with a gradient (0–60% in 60 min) of 0.1% TFA in acetonitrile. After lyophilization the fractions were immunoreacted with ODN antiserum (1:2000 dilution) and ODN-like material was detected with ELISA method.

TABLE I

Brain distribution of DBI-like immunoreactivity in rat brain

Brain region	DBI-like immunoreactivity (pmol/mg protein)
Hypothalamus	
Arcuate nucleus	350 ± 24
Ventral medial nucleus	190 ± 14
Supraoptic nucleus	170 ± 14
Medial preoptic area	145 ± 18
Posterior nucleus	120 ± 16
Central periaqueductal gray	185 ± 15
Cerebellar cortex	170 ± 12
Septohippocampal nucleus	120 ± 12
Lateral septal nucleus	95 ± 9
Substantia nigra	105 ± 10
Caudate-putamen	57 ± 7.2
Nucleus accumbens	60 ± 8.0
Frontal cortex	45 ± 3.6
Anterior pituitary	12 ± 1.0

Neuronal location

A study of the histochemical location of the DBI-like immunoreactivity was carried out with antisera directed against rat DBI and synthetic ODN. Using ODN antisera (1:2000) and DBI antisera (1:40,000)

coupled with peroxidase reaction, immunostaining was detected in fibers and cell bodies of many brain regions (Fig. 3). The immunoreactivity was evident in several hypothalamic nuclei, some thalamic nuclei, cortex, hippocampus and in cerebellum. The cell body location of the immunostaining was intensified with intraventricular injections of colchicine. In the hippocampus the immunoreactive neurons were mainly located sparsely in all the CA areas and in dentate gyrus (Fig. 4). Figure 5 shows details of the hippocampal location of immunoreactive material visualized with antibodies directed against rat DBI and synthetic ODN. The distribution of the immunoreactive neurons were identical with both antisera and was mainly found in pyramidal cells (Fig. 5) but also in smaller cells in the subgranular zone of dentate gyrus. In cortex, both DBI and ODN immunoreactive neurons were located mainly in layer VI (Fig. 6a). The majority of the cells were small pyramidal cells but also smaller cells, probably stellate cells, were stained (Fig. 6b).

It is possible to note that using ODN antiserum immunoreactivity was located predominantly with neurons; glial cells contain little or no immunostaining (i.e. Fig. 4). By using low dilution of DBI antisera (1:10,000) also glial staining was present (Fig. 7a); however, higher dilutions of this antisera (1:40,000) produced only neuronal staining (Fig.

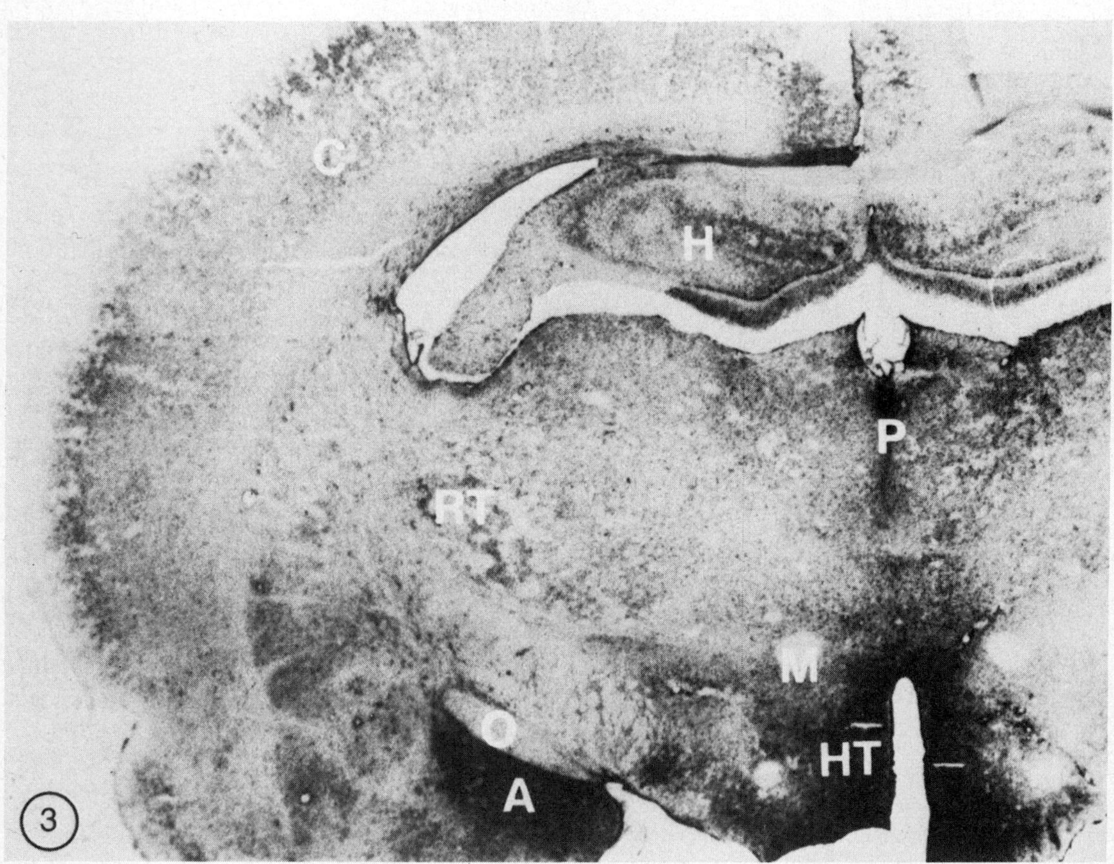

Fig. 3. DBI immunostaining in a coronal section of normal rat brain. Note the high immunoreactivity in the hypothalamus (HT), medial amygdaloid nucleus (A) and in paraventricular thalamic nucleus (P), and the moderate immunoreactivity in cortex (C), hippocampus (H), and in reticular thalamic nucleus (RT). A low or virtual absence of immunoreactivity, i.e. in optic tract (O) and in mamillothalamic tract (M).

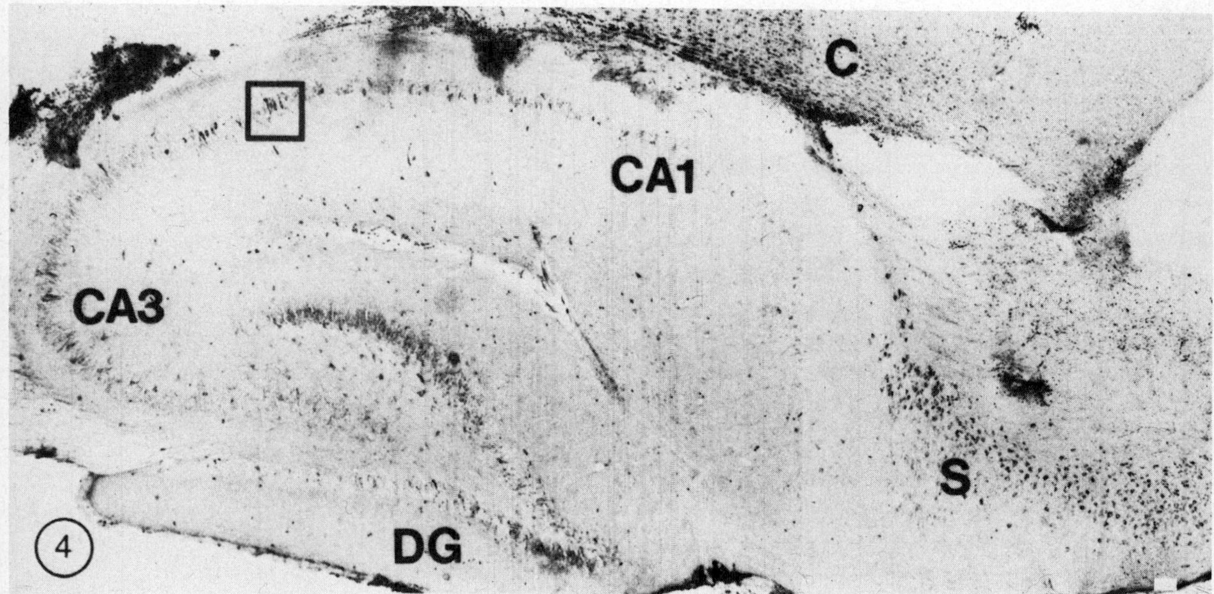

Fig. 4. ODN immunostaining in dorsal hippocampus of colchicine treated rat (colchicine, 70 μg i.c.v.). ODN positive cells are located sparsely in all CA areas and in dentate gyrus. Note also the immunoreactive cells in cortex (C) and in subiculum (S). Square represents the area shown in Fig. 5a. Bar = 100 μm.

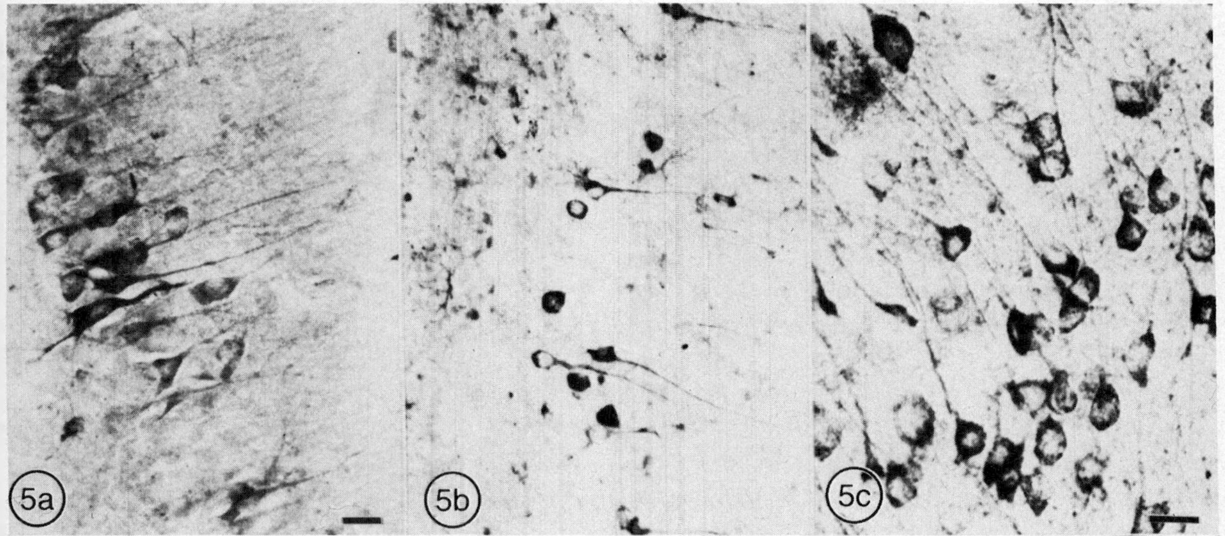

Fig. 5. ODN and DBI immunostaining in selected areas of dorsal hippocampus. (A) ODN immunoreactive cells in CA2 area of dorsal hippocampus showing ODN positive pyramidal cells. (B) DBI positive pyramidal cells in CA1 area of the hippocampus. (C) DBI immunoreactive cells, in subiculum; animals were colchicine treated. Bar = 20 μm.

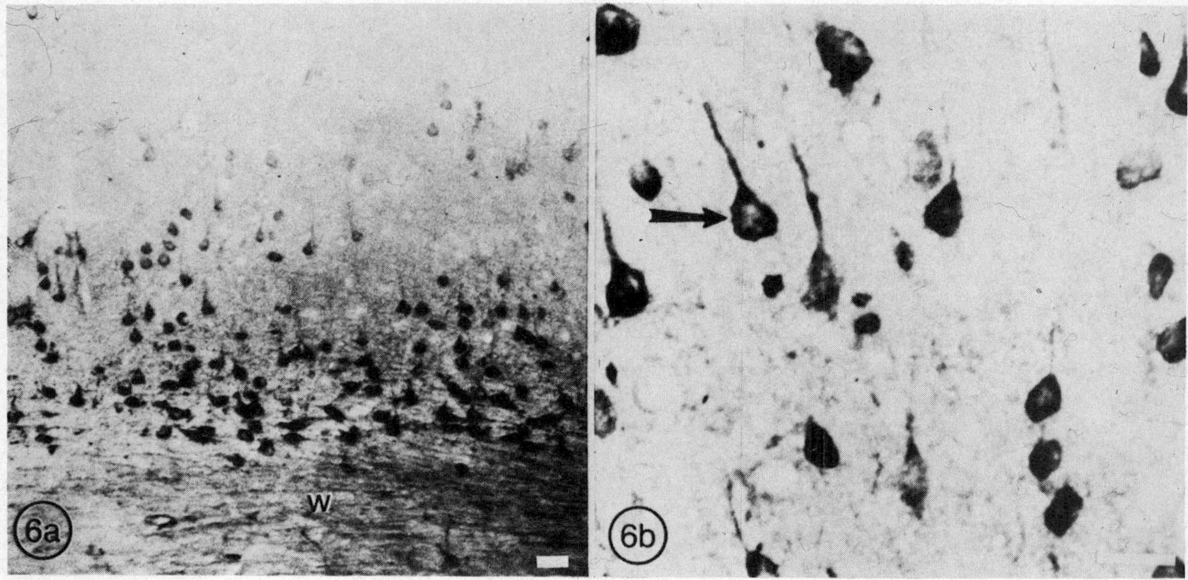

Fig. 6. ODN and DBI immunostaining in parietal cortex. (a) ODN immunoreactivity in parietal cortex showing that the positive cells are mainly located in VI layer of cortex (w = white matter). (b) DBI immunoreactive cells in VI layer of frontal cortex demonstrating that the cells are mainly pyramidal cells. Animals were colchicine treated. Bar = 20 μm.

7b). The immunostaining of neuronal fibers tends to disappear with colchicine treatment while the immunoreactive material becomes very dense in the neuronal cell bodies (Fig. 7b–d). In contrast, the staining of glial cells is not affected by the injections of colchicine.

In hippocampus and cortex the DBI and ODN positive cells were mainly pyramidal cells. Since

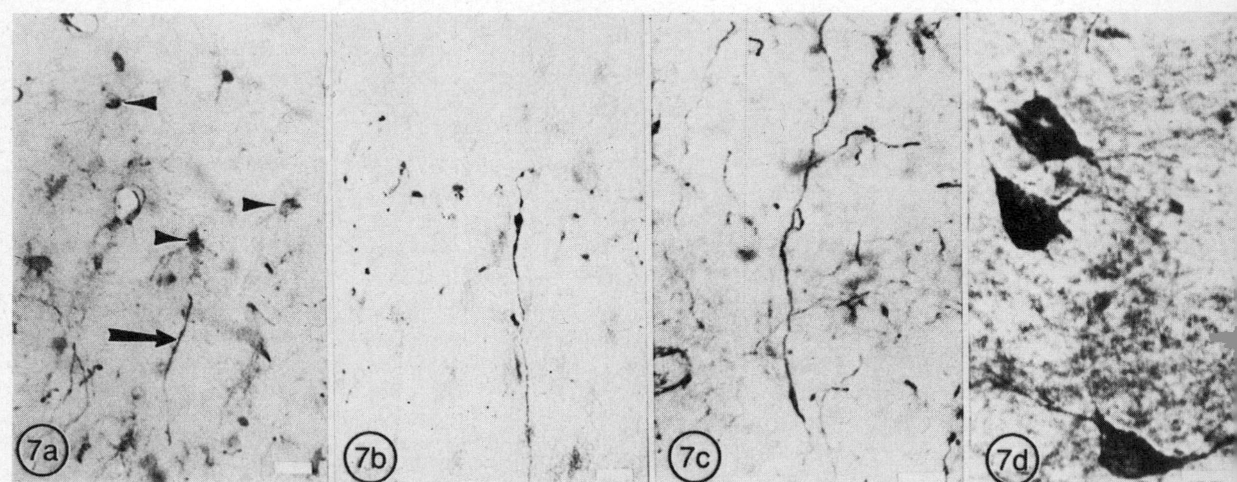

Fig. 7. DBI and ODN immunostaining in amygdaloid nucleus. (a) DBI immunoreactivity in cortical amygdaloid nucleus of normal rat brain when the antisera is diluted 1:10,000. Note the nerve fibers (arrow) but also staining in the astrocytes (arrowheads). Bar = 10 μm. (b) DBI immunoreactivity in the same area when the antisera is diluted 1:40,000, only the nerve fibers can be seen and the glial staining is absent. (c) ODN immunostaining (1:2000) in the same area showing only nerve fibers. (d) DBI immunostaining (1:30,000) in the same area in colchicine-treated animal demonstrating the cell bodies. Bar = 20 μm.

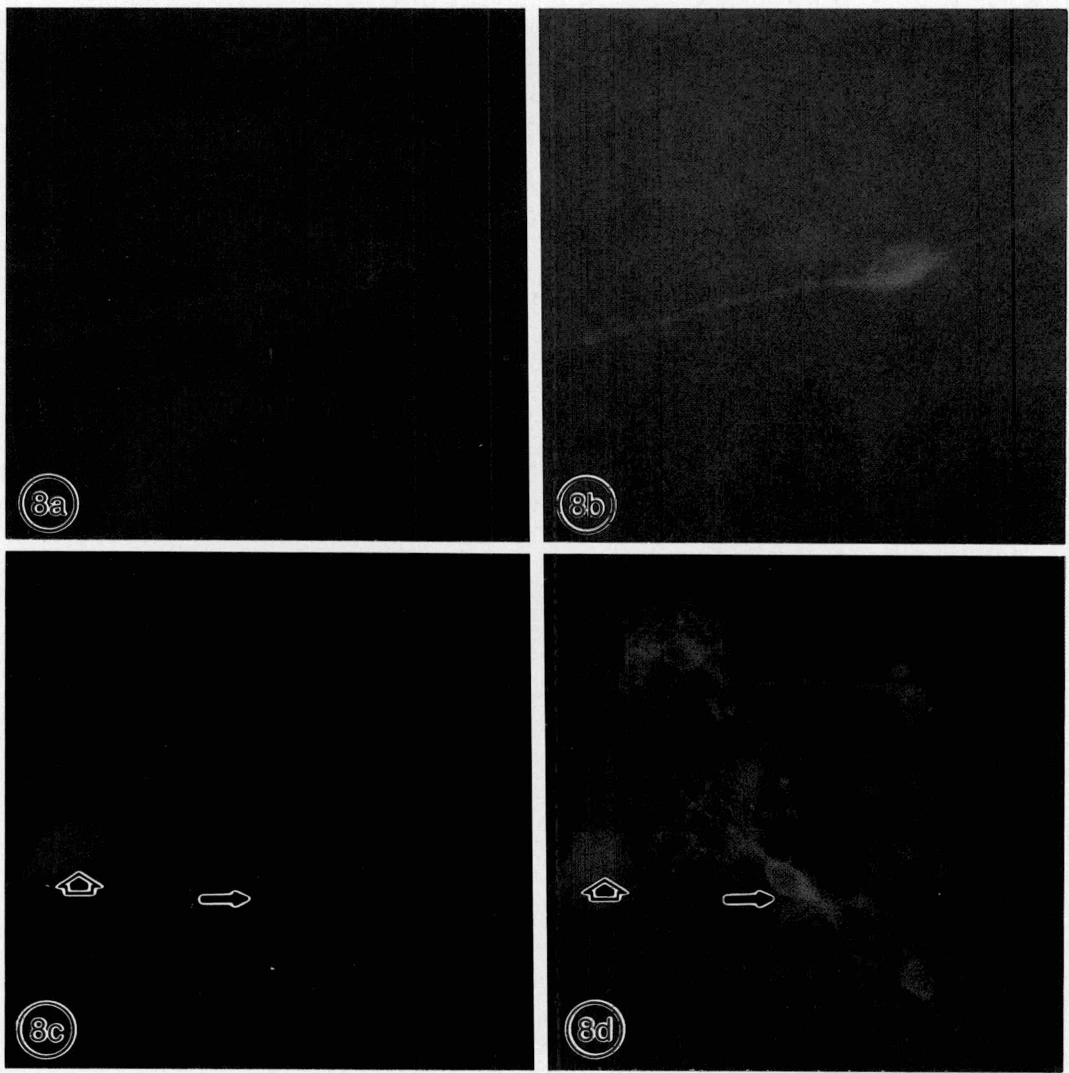

Fig. 8. Fluorescence micrographs from primary cultures of hippocampal cells. (a) DBI immunostaining and (b) the same cell double labeled with GAD antiserum showing the labeling in the same cell. (c) DBI positive cell (large arrow) which is not labeled with the GAD antiserum (d), GAD immunoreactive cell (long arrow) in (d) is not labeled with DBI antiserum in (c).

these cells are not GABAergic it is evident that DBI is not exclusively present in GABAergic neurons. That not all of the GABAergic cells contain DBI is also shown by the absence of DBI-like immunoreactivity in Purkinje cells of cerebellum which are known to be GABAergic. The data raised the question as to whether DBI and GABA coexist in the same neurons. To answer this question, we have used primary cultures of hippocampal cells. In some cells, DBI and glutamic acid decarboxylase (GAD) coexist (Fig. 8a,b) but in many cells no such coexistence is detectable (Fig. 8c,d). These results corroborate the impression emerged from the study of cerebellum, substantia nigra and striatum that the brain distribution of GABA and DBI is not strictly homologous. The relatively low density of DBI containing neurons in striatum and substantia nigra which are areas rich in GABA containing neurons suggests that not all the GABAergic cells contain DBI, or that the gene(s) that code for DBI is (are) expressed differently in different GABAergic neurons.

Action of DBI in conflict situations

The test proposed by Vogel to estimate anxiolytic action of drugs in rats is based on the concept that anxiolytic agents abolish the behavioral inhibition caused by punishment (Vogel et al., 1971). Hence, thirsty rats placed in a cage with water are compelled to drink. When the water spout is connected with a device that delivers a shock when the rat drinks the behavior of the rat can be inhibited as a function of the shock intensity. Anxiolytic drugs such as benzodiazepines can lessen the behavioral inhibition elicited by electric shock whereas anxiogenic drugs such as the esters of beta-carboline-3-carboxylate can increase the behavioral inhibition elicited by weak stimuli (Corda et al., 1983). There is another class of drugs that are partial agonists of the benzodiazepine-beta-carboline recognition site. When these drugs occupy the site very little happens because of their low intrinsic activity. However because of their high affinity for the recognition site they can prevent the action of either anxiolytic or anxiogenic drugs. One such partial agonist is an imidazobenzodiazepine derivative known as Ro 15-1788 (Hunkeler et al., 1981). This drug and its congeners are very useful because they can detect the participation of benzodiazepine-beta-carboline recognition sites in the behavioral and other physiological modifications elicited by various compounds. Ro 15-1788 fails to modify the Vogel test in a wide dose range, but it acts facilitating the behavioral effect of punishment when tested during a perturbation of GABAergic transmission (Costa et al., 1984). Such a deficiency can be elicited by inhibiting the synthesis of GABA with isoniazid. Thus, it is necessary to change the balance of the GABAergic tone in order to reveal the weak partial agonist action of Ro 15-1788. DBI injected intraventricularly in the thirsty rat operating in the Vogel test facilitates the behavioral inhibition by punishment and antagonizes the anticonflict action of diazepam (Guidotti et al., 1983). Thus, as shown in Fig. 9, DBI facilitates the behavioral inhibition elicited by punishment in a dose-related manner. The action of DBI can be differentiated from the anticonflict action of benzodiazepines and was termed proconflict effect. Since this proconflict effect can be inhibited by Ro 15-1788 (Guidotti et al., 1983) the participation of the benzodiazepine-beta-carboline recognition site can be suggested. Further studies have suggested that ODN is the epicenter in the DBI sequence responsible for the biological activity of DBI. ODN not only can be generated in vitro as the only biologically active fragment formed by the tryptic digestion of DBI (Ferrero et al., 1984) but ODN-like material is present in the brain of rat (Fig. 2). Presumably DBI functions as the precursor of an ODN-like compound which is the biologically active ligand modulating GABAergic transmission. ODN similarly to DBI elicits a dose-related proconflict action (Fig. 9). Its intrinsic activity is greater than that of DBI. Since this

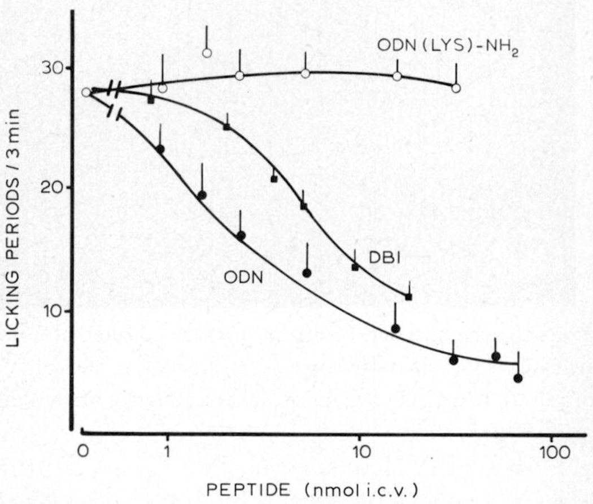

Fig. 9. Proconflict properties of DBI, octadecaneuropeptide (ODN) and octadecaneuropeptide-amide (ODN-Lys-NH_2) in shock-induced suppression of water drinking in thirsty rats. The conditions of the experiments were as follows: (a) current intensity 0.25 mA; (b) rat, 175 g were deprived of water 72 h prior to test; (c) the peptides were injected intraventricularly (i.c.v.) 3 min before the test; (c) one licking period is equal to 3 sec of continuous licking. The conditions of the test are the ones described by Corda et al. (1983). Each value is the mean of 5–6 animals ± S.E.M.

action is inhibited by Ro 15-1788 the participation of benzodiazepine recognition sites can be considered.

DBI-GABA interaction at the Cl^- channel

When neuronal GABA is released, it induces a receptor mediated transient increase of the postsynaptic membrane conductance to Cl^- ions. This function of GABA occurs in burst of duration proportional to the GABA concentrations. Various ligands of benzodiazepine recognition sites prolong (benzodiazepines) or shorten (beta-carboline-3-carboxylate esters) the bursts of Cl^- channel opening elicited by GABA. When DBI is tested in primary cultures of spinal cord cells from mouse embryo patched clamped for the recording of Cl^- currents, this peptide inhibits the Cl^- currents generated by GABA (Bormann et al., 1985). The peptide is devoid of action in absence of GABA. The inhibition of the Cl^- currents generated by GABA is due to an action on benzodiazepine recognition sites because it is inhibited by Ro 15-1788 which per se is inactive (Bormann et al., 1985). These electrophysiological results indicate that DBI down regulates the efficiency whereby the activation of GABA receptors triggers the burst opening of Cl^- channel. However, the molecular mechanism underlying the reduction of GABA-induced Cl^- currents elicited by DBI is not understood and needs further investigation with single channel recording methods.

Displacement by DBI and ODN of specific ligands of benzodiazepine recognition sites

DBI was shown to displace [^{3}H]benzodiazepines from their binding sites located in crude synaptic membranes (Guidotti et al., 1983). In this model, DBI displaces both [^{3}H]benzodiazepines or β-[^{3}H]carboline-3-carboxylate esters. However, its efficiency in displacing beta-carboline is greater than that for [^{3}H]benzodiazepines. ODN was studied in the same preparation but it was weaker than DBI and the results were erratic. Because these major difficulties in studying ODN binding using crude synaptic membranes could be accounted for

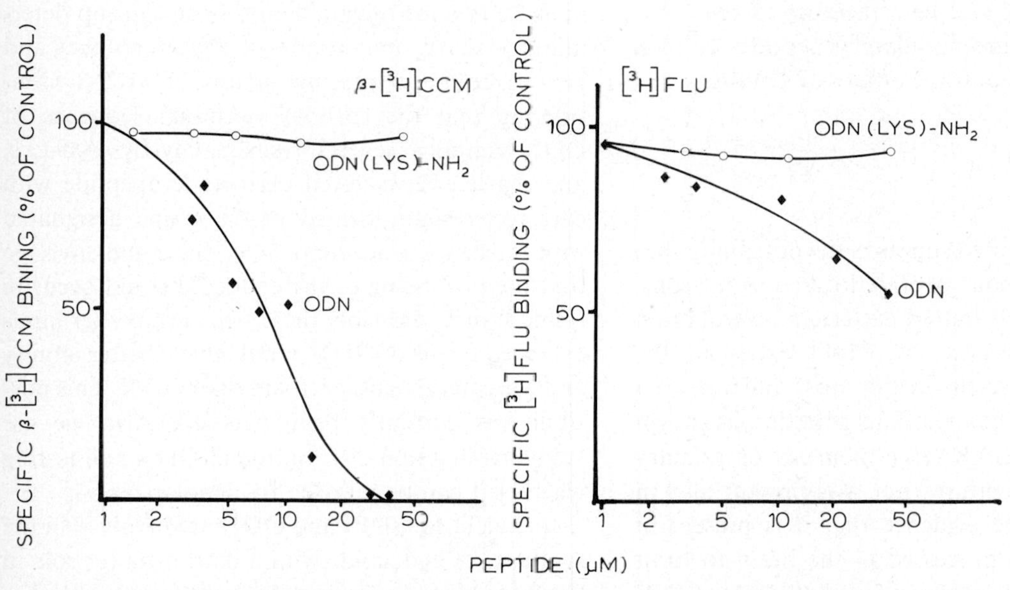

Fig. 10. Inhibition of β-[^{3}H]CCM and [^{3}H]flunitrazepam binding to primary culture of cerebellar granule cells by the octadecaneuropeptide (ODN) or ODN(Lys)-NH_2. Binding was carried out at 18° in intact cells grown in monolayer and maintained in Locke's solution (pH 7.4). The concentration of β-[^{3}H]CCM and [^{3}H]FLU was 3 nM. Experimental conditions as described by Gallo et al. (1985).

in part by the high peptidase activity of this preparation, we have attempted to find a preparation with lower levels of peptidase activity which would allow the study of [^{3}H]benzodiazepine displacement by peptides in standardized conditions. Such a preparation was the primary culture of cerebellar granule cells which have on their surface a significant number of GABA recognition sites (Vaccarino, personal communication). These intact cells maintained in a physiological milieu bind with high affinity and in a saturable fashion different benzodiazepine receptor ligands at 4 or 18°. As shown in Fig. 10, ODN completely displaces β-[^{3}H]carboline bound to granule cells with an EC_{50} of 5–10 μM. The alpha-amide of the terminal lysine of ODN is devoid of displacing action. When ODN is tested for its ability to displace [^{3}H]flunitrazepam the EC_{50} is about 10-fold greater than that which displaces β-[^{3}H]carboline-3-carboxylate esters (Fig. 10). The alpha-amide of the terminal lysine of ODN is inactive in displacing benzodiazepines. These data suggest that ODN could be a ligand of benzodiazepine/beta-carboline recognition site, and since it is present in brain it could be formed from DBI. Thus, ODN might well be a member of new class of endogenous neuromodulatory peptides formed by DBI acting as contransmitters of GABA.

Conclusions

The evidence presented supports the possibility that DBI is an endogenous peptide located in neurons. It has a specific distribution pattern in several brain structures; a difference of 7-fold exists in the amount of DBI present in the most and the least abundant brain structures. This peptide was shown to be located in GABAergic neurons of primary hippocampal cell cultures but it is present also in other neurons. The evidence that it is present in spinal fluid and is processed in the brain to form ODN-like material speaks in favor of a role of DBI in neuronal secretion. However, we have not yet obtained evidence that DBI or ODN is released by depolarization from neuronal stores and plays a physiological role in the modulation of neuronal transmission. We have shown that DBI and ODN can displace beta carbolines with an EC_{50} smaller than that for the benzodiazepines. DBI can reduce the action of GABA on Cl^- fluxes; moreover, DBI and ODN can elicit a proconflict action in rats. This action is dose-dependent and can be antagonized by partial agonists of the imidobenzodiazepine series such as Ro 15-1788, a specific partial agonist of benzodiazepine-beta-carboline recognition site. DBI and ODN are present in human brain, their cDNA is now being studied in rat and human brain. Though DBI and ODN bind to the benzodiazepine-beta-carboline recognition site their affinity is rather low and appears to be in the μM range. The low affinity of DBI is not surprising because it could function as the precursor of the benzodiazepine recognition site endocoid rather than being the endocoid itself. Actually, all the data available speak in support of this possibility. The low affinity binding of ODN is surprising. The evidence available indicates that the alpha carboxy terminus of the ODN must be free for the amidation of this group determines a sharp obliteration of the proconflict and beta-carboline displacing action of ODN. Considering that the carboxyl terminal sequence of ODN contains several lysines: Gly-Lys-Ala-Lys, and that we have tested the octadecapeptide with carboxyterminus located in the lysine designated with A (see sequence on p. 346), one could envisage that the processing of the endocoid could occur in lysine B or C. Possibly these two carboxy terminus extended forms of ODN could have a better affinity and a greater intrinsic activity than ODN. This possibility is currently being studied. Also we are studying the brain distribution of ODN and testing whether it can be released by depolarization.

In conclusion, DBI and ODN are involved in the synthesis of endocoids with a cotransmitter role in GABAergic transmission. However, their role has not been defined thoroughly.

References

Asano, T. and Spector, S. (1978) Identification of inosine and hypoxanthine as endogenous ligands for the brain benzodiazepine binding sites. *Proc. nat. Acad. Sci. USA*, 76: 977–981.

Barnard, E. A., Stephenson, F. A., Sigel, E., Mamalaki, G. and Bilbe, G. (1984) The purified GABA/benzodiazepine complex: retention of multiple functions. *Neuropharmacology*, 23: 813–814.

Bormann, J., Ferrero, P., Guidotti, A. and Costa, E. (1985) Neuropeptide modulation of GABA receptor Cl^- channels. *Regul. Peptides*, Suppl. 4, 33–38.

Braestrup, C., Schmiechen, R., Neef, G., Nielsen, M. and Petersen, E. N. (1982) Interaction of convulsive ligands with benzodiazepine receptors. *Science*, 216: 1241–1243.

Corda, M. G., Blacker, W. D., Mendelson, W. B., Guidotti, A. and Costa, E. (1983) Beta carbolines enhance shock induced suppression of drinking in rats. *Proc. nat. Acad. Sci. USA*, 80: 2072–2076.

Costa, E. and Guidotti, A. (1979) Molecular mechanisms in the receptor action of benzodiazepines. *Ann. Rev. Pharmacol. Toxicol.*, 19: 531–545.

Costa, E., Guidotti, A., Mao, C. C. and Suria, A. (1975) New concepts on the mechanism of action of benzodiazepines. *Life Sci.*, 17: 167–186.

Costa, E., Guidotti, A. and Toffano, G. (1978) Molecular mechanisms mediating the action of diazepam on GABA receptors. *Brit. J. Psychiat.*, 133: 239–248.

Costa, E., Corda, M. G. and Guidotti, A. (1983) On a brain polypeptide functioning as a putative effector for the recognition sites of benzodiazepines and beta-carboline derivatives. *Neuropharmacology*, 22: 1481–1492.

Costa, E., Ferrari, M., Ferrero, P. and Guidotti, A. (1984) Multiple signals in GABAergic transmission: pharmacological consequences. *Neuropharmacology*, 23: 989–991.

Davis, L. G. and Cohen, R. K. (1980) Identification of an endogenous peptide-ligand for the benzodiazepine receptor. *Biochem. Biophys. Res. Commun.*, 92: 141–148.

Dorow, R., Horowski, R., Paschelke, G., Amin, M. and Braestrup, C. (1983) Severe anxiety induced by FG 7142, a beta carboline ligand for benzodiazepine receptors. *Lancet*, II: 98–99.

Enna, S. J. and Snyder, S. J. (1977) Influence of ions, enzymes and detergents on gamma-aminobutyric acid receptor binding in synaptic membranes of rat brain. *Mol. Pharmacol.*, 13: 442–453.

Ferrero, P., Guidotti, A., Conti-Tronconi, B. and Costa, E. (1984) A brain octadecaneuropeptide generated by tryptic digestion of DBI (diazepam binding inhibitor) functions as a proconflict ligand of benzodiazepine recognition sites. *Neuropharmacology*, 23: 1339–1362.

Gallo, V., Wise, B. C., Vaccarino, F. and Guidotti, A. (1985) GABA and benzodiazepine-induced modulation of ^{35}S-t-bicyclophosphorotionate binding to cerebellar granule cells. *J. Neurosci.*, 5: 2432–2438.

Guidotti, A., Toffano, G. and Costa, E. (1978) An endogenous protein modulates the affinity of GABA and benzodiazepine receptors in rat brain. *Nature (Lond.)*, 257: 553–555.

Guidotti, A., Forchetti, C. M., Corda, M. G., Konkel, D., Bennett, C. D. and Costa, E. (1983) Isolation, characterization and purification to homogeneity of an endogenous polypeptide with agonistic action on benzodiazepine receptors. *Proc. nat. Acad. Sci. USA*, 80: 3531–3535.

Haefely, W., Kulcsar, A., Mohler, H., Pieri, L., Polc, P. and Schaffner, R. (1975) Possible involvement of GABA in the central actions of benzodiazepines. In E. Costa and P. Greengard (Eds.), *Mechanisms of Action of Benzodiazepines*, Raven Press, New York, pp. 131–151.

Hunkeler, W., Mohler, H., Pieri, L., Polc, P., Bonetti, E. P., Cumin, R., Schaffner, R. and Haefely, W. (1981) Selective antagonists of benzodiazepines. *Nature (Lond.)*, 290: 514–516.

Mao, C. C., Guidotti, A. and Costa, E. (1975) Evidence for an involvement of GABA in the mediation of cerebellar cGMP decrease and the anticonvulsant action of diazepam. *Naunyn--Schiedeberg's Arch. Pharmacol.*, 289: 369–378.

Mohler, H. and Okada, T. (1977) Benzodiazepine receptors: demonstration in central nervous system. *Science*, 198: 849–851.

Mohler, H., Polc, P., Cumin, R., Pieri, L. and Ketter, R. (1979) Nicotinamide is a brain constituent with benzodiazepine-like action. *Nautre (Lond.)*, 278: 563–565.

Mohler, H., Richards, J. G. and Wu, J.-Y. (1981) Autoradiographic localization of benzodiazepine receptors in immunocytochemically identified gamma aminobutyrergic synapses. *Proc. nat. Acad. Sci. USA*, 78: 1935–1938.

Olsen, R. W. (1982) Drug interactions at the GABA receptor-ionophore complex. *Ann. Rev. Pharmacol. Toxicol.*, 22: 245–277.

Polc, P., Bonetti, E. P., Schaffner, R. and Haefely, W. (1982) A three state model of the benzodiazepine receptor explains the interaction between the benzodiazepine antagonist RO 15 1788, benzodiazepine tranquilizers, beta-carbolines and phenobarbitone. *Naunyn-Schmiedeberg's Arch. Pharmacol.*, 321: 260–264.

Schoch, P., Richards, J. G., Haring, P., Takacs, B., Stahli, C., Staehelin, T., Haefely, W. and Mohler, H. (1985) Colocalization of $GABA_A$ receptors and benzodiazepine receptors in the brain shown by monoclonal antibodies. *Nature (Lond.)*, 314: 168–171.

Schmidt, R. F., Vogel, M. E. and Zimmermann, M. (1967) Die Wirkung von Diazepam auf die prasynaptische Hemmung und andere Rückenmarksreflexe. *Naunyn-Schmiedeberg's Arch. Pharmacol.*, 258: 69–82.

Skolnick, P., Marangos, P. and Goodwin, F. K. (1978) Identification of inosine and hypoxanthine as endogenous inhibitors of ^{3}H-diazepam binding in the central nervous system. *Life Sci.*, 23: 1473–1480.

Siegel, E., Stepheson, F. A., Mamalaki, C. and Barnard, E. A. (1983) A GABA/benzodiazepine receptor complex of bovine cerebral cortex. *J. Biol. Chem.*, 258: 6965–6971.

Smart, T. G., Constanti, A., Bilbe, G., Brown, D. A. and Barnard, E. A. (1983) Synthesis of functional chick brain GABA/benzodiazepine-barbiturate/receptor complexes in mRNA injected xenopus oocytes. *Neurosci. Lett.*, 70: 55–59.

Squires, R. F. and Braestrup, C. (1977) Benzodiazepine receptors in rat brain. *Nature (Lond.)*, 266: 732–734.

Thomas, J. W. and Tallman, J. F. (1981) Characterization of photoaffinity labeling of benzodiazepine binding sites. *J. Biol. Chem.*, 256: 9838–9842.

Vogel, J. R., Beer, B. and Clody, D. E. (1 971) A simple and reliable conflict procedure for testing antianxiety agents. *Psychopharmacologia*, 21: 1–7.

T. Hökfelt, K. Fuxe and B. Pernow (Eds.),
Progress in Brain Research, Vol. 68

CHAPTER 25

Functional studies of cholecystokinin-dopamine co-existence: electrophysiology and behavior

L. R. Skirboll, J. N. Crawley and D. W. Hommer

Electrophysiology and Behavioral Neuropharmacology Units, Clinical Neuroscience Branch, NIMH, Bethesda, MD, U.S.A.

Introduction

Immunohistochemical maps have shown cholecystokinin (CCK) to be present in diverse areas of rat brain including cortex, hippocampus, hypothalamus, amygdala and midbrain (Innis et al., 1979; Loren et al., 1979; Vanderhaegen et al., 1980). Interest in the functional significance of CCK has arisen from evidence that CCK has transmitter-like properties. It is released from synaptic vesicles after electrical stimulation in a calcium-dependent manner (Meyer and Krauss, 1983; Pinget et al., 1979). Specific binding sites in brain have been characterized, including descriptions of regional distribution (Hays et al., 1980; Saito et al., 1980; Zarbin et al., 1983; Gaudreau et al., 1983a,b).

Immunohistochemical evidence for the co-existence of CCK and dopamine (DA) has been described in detail (Hökfelt et al., 1980a,b). This co-existence has been based on several lines of evidence: (1) data from experiments using either adjacent sections or the elution-restaining method showed cell bodies in the ventral mesencephalon which were both CCK and tyrosine hydroxylase (TH) immunoreactive; (2) CCK and TH immunoreactive nerve terminals showed close overlap in the accumbens, olfactory tubercle, and central nucleus of the amygdala; (3) injections of intracerebral colchicine or 6-OHDA induced an accumulation of both CCK and TH immunoreactivity in axons caudal to the injection; (4) intracerebral 6-OHDA produced a marked reduction in CCK and TH immunoreactive cell bodies and nerve terminals in the mesencephalon and limbic forebrain; and (5) retrograde tracing combined with immunohistochemistry verified CCK-DA projections from the mesencephalon to the limbic forebrain (Hökfelt et al., 1980a,b). These data suggest that, at least in the rat, the CCK-DA co-existence is confined primarily to the mesolimbic system (see Hökfelt et al., this volume). In this regard, Williams et al. (1981) and Meyer et al. (1982) have shown that cutting the median forebrain bundle has no effect on CCK levels in the caudate, thus, confirming that the CCK-DA neurons, at least in the rat, appear to be primarily limited to the mesolimbic areas.

This finding raised many questions about the functional role of the co-existence of CCK and DA. In an effort to explore some of these questions, we used several techniques. First, in a series of electrophysiological experiments, we examined whether i.v. or locally applied CCK altered DA cell activity in the substantia nigra (SN) and ventral tegmentum (VT). In an effort to examine in more detail the central versus peripheral components of these responses, we lesioned the major sensory pathway into the brain and examined the effects of CCK under these conditions. Finally, we examined the effect of CCK and its fragments on the ability of DA to act as an inhibitory transmitter (Skirboll et al., 1981; Hommer and Skirboll, 1983; Hommer et al., 1985, 1986).

In a second series of experiments, behavioral approaches were used to investigate the functional significance of CCK-DA co-existence at the post-synaptic site. Since terminals of the VT neurons containing both CCK and DA have been localized in the medial posterior region of the accumbens (Hökfelt et al., 1980a,b; Fallon et al., 1983) this region was chosen as the site of analysis. In particular, the behavioral effects of DA and dopaminergic agents administered into the accumbens have been previously characterized in rats; DA and amphetamine elicit hyperlocomotion (Creese and Iversen, 1974) while DA and apomorphine (APO) elicit stereotyped sniffing (Costall et al., 1977; Joyce, 1983; Van Ree et al., 1983). We began by testing three hypotheses: (1) CCK administered into the accumbens could mimic the behavioral actions of DA; (2) CCK administered into the accumbens in combination with DA could potentiate the behavioral actions of DA; (3) CCK administered into the accumbens could inhibit the behavioral actions of DA (Crawley et al., 1984). Finally, we will report the effects of CCK antagonists on the electrophysiological and behavioral effects of this peptide.

Electrophysiological studies

Methods

Recordings were performed on male Sprague-Dawley rats weighing 250–350 g and have been described in detail elsewhere (Skirboll et al., 1981; Hommer et al., 1985). Briefly a 3 mm burr hole was drilled at co-ordinates overlying the SN zona compacta (SNZC) and VT in rats anesthetized with chloral hydrate (400 mg/kg i.p.). Recordings were obtained from DA containing neurons based on waveform, firing rate and pattern (Bunney et al., 1973). Intravenously administered drugs and supplemental chloral hydrate were given through the lateral tail vein.

In one series of experiments, the effects of i.v. administered CCK-like peptides (CCK-7, CCK-8 sulphated (CCK-S) and unsulphated (CCK-US), CCK-4, CCK-3) on single units were assessed by recordings made with single barrel micropipettes (4–7 Mohms resistance at 60 Hz). The DA agonist, APO HCl, was administered i.v. in doses calculated according to the weight of its salt (1–32 μg/kg). In another series of experiments, five barrel glass microelectrodes were used; recordings were obtained from the central barrel while iontophoretically administering CCK-8 (S and US), glutamate, or substance P. In both series of experiments, electrode potentials were passed through a high input impedance amplifier and monitored on an oscilloscope and audio monitor. The firing rate of single neurons was measured by means of a rate-averaging computer visually displayed on a chart recorder as a continuous histogram of discharge rate. At the end of each experiment, the site of the electrode tip was marked. In some cases, animals were treated with colchicine and processed for immunohistochemistry (for details see Hökfelt et al., 1980a,b).

In lesion experiments, acute vagotomies and acute Cl transections were performed during the recording procedure under chloral hydrate anesthesia. In order to lesion afferents and efferents of the nucleus tractus solitarius (NTS), bilateral subdiaphragmatic vagotomies as well as unilateral and bilateral lesions of the medulla were performed under halothane anesthesia 8–10 days prior to recording.

Effects of CCK

In the first series of experiments (Skirboll et al., 1981), the effects of intravenously administered CCK in doses of 1–16 μg/kg injected into the tail vein of the rat were analysed while recording from either SNZC or VT/DA neurons. In SNZC, 63% of the cells showed an increase in firing rate in response to CCK-S (Fig. 1) while 37% had no response. In VT, 29% of the cells showed an increase, 48% a decrease and 23% no response. The unsulphated form of the peptide was used as a control. It has been shown that 90% of the CCK in the brain is in the sulphated form (Dockray, 1980) and in peripheral bioassay the unsulphated form has been

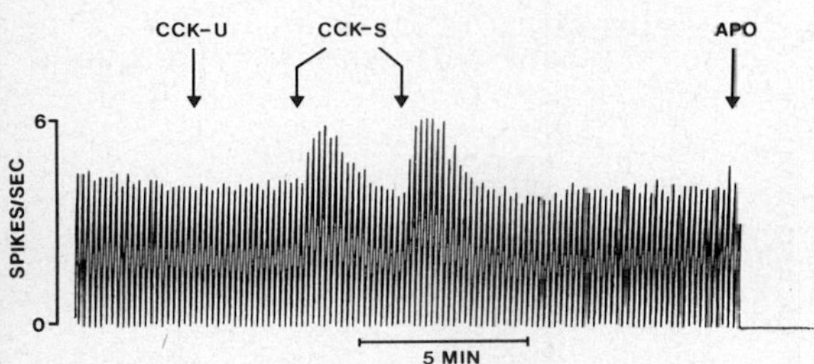

Fig. 1. Representative response of a DA neuron in the ventral tegmental area to i.v. administered CCK. Sulphated CCK-8 (10 μg/kg) administered at the arrows resulted in a transient increase in the firing rate of this DA neuron. Apomorphine, a direct acting DA agonist, inhibited cell firing (dose = 0.1 mg/kg i.v.) in its normal manner (Bunney et al., 1973).

shown to be up to 300 times less potent (Thomson, 1973). As would be expected, CCK-US had no effect on the firing rate of midbrain DA neurons.

There is a continuing debate in peptide research as to the ability of peripherally administered peptides to cross the blood-brain barrier. With regard to our i.v. data, several questions must be asked: (1) does the ability of CCK to excite these neurons reflect a central or peripheral site of action? and (2) even if CCK is acting centrally, is it acting directly on DA neurons or on some site distal to the cells themselves, i.e. on neurons which subsequently impinge on these cells?

The first question is of particular interest in light of data revealing that CCK-induced satiety and exploratory behavior which were initially thought to be mediated centrally was instead shown in several labs to be blocked by vagotomy (Anika et al., 1977; Crawley et al., 1981; Smith et al., 1981; Morley et al., 1982). In this regard, CCK immunoreactive fibers have been found in the NTS and CCK containing axons and CCK receptors have been demonstrated along the vagus (Rehfeld et al., 1983; Uvnas-Wallenstein et al., 1977; Zarbin et al., 1981). In addition, Palkovits and collaborators (1982) have shown significant amounts of CCK in the NTS and that the peptide is extrinsic and vagal in origin. Thus, we sought to examine whether the excitatory effects of CCK on DA cells were peripheral or central in origin. The effects of peripherally administered CCK were examined in animals who were subjected to various lesions of the primary and secondary neurons of the vagal pathway in order to alter visceral afferents which relay information to the brain (Hommer et al., 1985).

There were several treatment groups: (1) acute: and (2) chronic vagotomy; (3) acute cervical Cl transections. In addition, since the central terminal sensory relay nuclei of the vagus is the NTS, unilateral; and (4) bilateral lesions of the medulla. We found that neither acute nor chronic vagotomy had any effect on the excitatory response of nigral DA neurons to systemically administered CCK. High cervical spinal cord transections (Cl) were similarly without result. In contrast, lesions of either vagal fibers in the medulla or of efferent pathways from the NTS, the primary sensory nucleus of the vagus, produced significant attenuations of the excitatory effects of CCK (Fig. 2). Thus, unilateral intramedullary lesions of both afferents and efferents of the NTS were effective in reducing the effects of CCK. On the lesioned side, CCK increased cell activity by 34% while on the unlesioned side, cells increased their rate by 76%. Bilateral intramedullar lesions of efferents from the NTS also produced a significant reduction in the ability of CCK to affect nigral DA neurons. CCK induced a 34% increase on the lesioned side while increasing the firing rate by 66% in sham lesioned animals.

In sum, lesions of the NTS afferents and efferents as well as efferents alone significantly reduced CCK-induced excitation while vagotomy had no effect on this phenomenon. These data suggest that CCK's excitatory action is not dependent on primary vagal neurons but rather has its site at the efferent fibers of the NTS. With regard to the question of whether the action of systemically administered CCK is central or peripheral in origin, it is important to note that NTS lesions were capable of attenuating but not abolishing the ability of CCK to excite DA cells. This finding suggests that there may well be two components to the effect of peripherally administered CCK; one mediated peripherally through fibers from the NTS and a second, central action on the nigral cells.

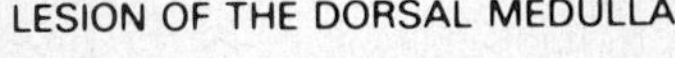

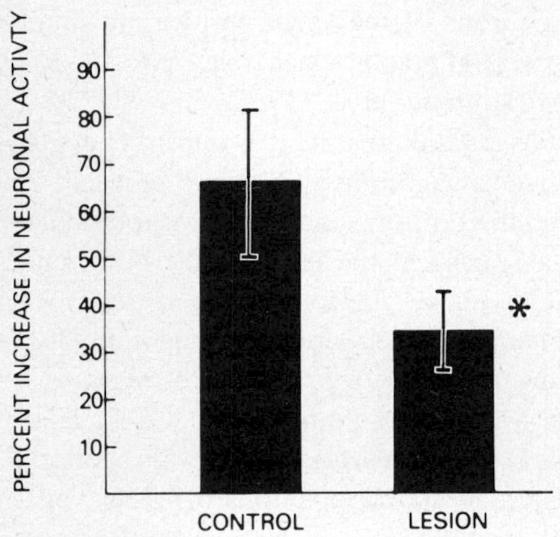

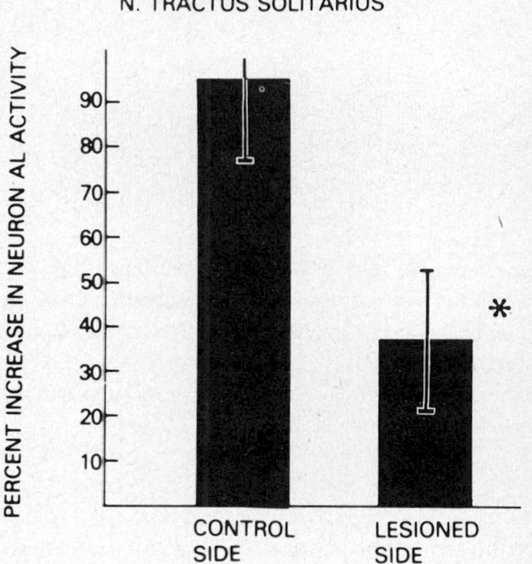

Fig. 2. Histograms comparing change in firing rate of DA neuron in lesioned and unlesioned animals following i.v. administration of CCK-8-S (20 μg/kg). (A) Unilateral lesion of the vagal afferent of the nucleus tractus solitarius (NTS) in the medulla produced a significant attenuation of the effect of CCK on nigral DA neurons (* $t = 2.81$, $p < 0.05$, t-test for independent groups; $n = 9$). Bars indicate standard error of the mean. (B) Lesions through the dorsal medulla of the efferents from the NTS produced a significant decrease in the response of DA neurons to peripherally administered CCK (* $t = 2.22$, $p < 0.05$, t-test for independent groups; $n = 6$). Bars indicate standard error of the mean.

We next asked whether this presumed central component of CCK excitation reflected an action directly on the DA cells or on some central site distal to the substantia nigra? In order to examine this, we turned to iontophoretic techniques (Skirboll et al., 1981). In response to up to 40 nA CCK-S, 76% of SNZC cells were excited while 24% showed no response. In VT, 100% of the cells were excited by CCK-S. CCK-US had no effect in either area. The excitatory effect of CCK-S was delayed 20–30 sec to onset. The biological significance of this delay is, however, unclear. Similar work with substance P has shown that its slow onset reflects the slow ejection of the peptide from the micropipette rather than a function of true delayed pharmacological response (Guyenet et al., 1979).

In order to examine the specificity of this response, the responses to iontophoretically administered CCK were compared to that of substance P and glutamate (GLU). Although substance P had no effect on nigral DA cells, the effects of GLU were distinct from those of CCK. In both SNZC and VT, all cells were effectively turned on by the iontophoretic administration of GLU; thus in SNZC, both CCK-responsive and CCK-unresponsive cells were excited by GLU. GLU excitation was observed promptly after the start of drug application as compared to the slow CCK onset. GLU excitation also halted abruptly after current cessation while the CCK response was slow to offset. One of the most distinctive features of CCK administration was its ability to cause a bursting pattern of activity; GLU effectively increased the rate of cell activity without affecting pattern. Finally, both CCK and GLU were potent excitatory agents; they were effective in eliciting activity from quiescent cells. CCK, in microgram doses, was shown to produce depolarization inactivation which could be reversed by the application of the inhibitory transmitter, GABA. Similar excitatory effects of CCK have been reported by others. Studies by Dodd and Kelly (1981) in hippocampal slices and spinal cells in culture by Rogawski (1982) have shown that CCK induces a decrease in membrane resistance, a short latency depolarization and an increase in excitability. Similarly, CCK showed excitatory effects in the nucleus accumbens (De France et al., 1984; White and Wang, 1984) and the cat trigeminal nucleus (Salt and Hill, 1982).

Finally, topographical analysis of the site of CCK action within the midbrain was made by combining immunohistochemistry with electrophysiology. When CCK-responsive and unresponsive cells were matched to sites within the SNZC/VT recording area, cells which were responsive were found to be limited to co-existent areas while unresponsive cells were found in the medial areas of SNZC in which limited co-existence has been reported (see Hökfelt et al., this volume). In addition, activity in the zona reticulata of the SN, an area which does not contain CCK, was unaltered following CCK injection.

These findings suggest that CCK is a potent excitatory agent on a majority of cells in the VT and a discrete population of cells in SNZC. The inability of CCK-US to mimic the effects of CCK-8 combined with data that substance P is ineffective suggest that these effects are specific. The uniqueness of its action is also demonstrated by its dissimilarity with the endogenous excitatory agent, GLU. The mechanism of action is, at present, unknown. This increase in firing rate could be mediated through one or any combination of events. For example, a direct depolarizing action may account for the excitatory effect. This possibility is consistent with the findings of Dodd and Kelly (1981) and Rogawski (1982). CCK may be acting presynaptically to increase the release or potentiate the postsynaptic actions of an excitatory transmitter such as GLU, although our data that CCK and GLU are dissimilar would dispute this possibility. Finally, CCK may act to block the release or the effects of an inhibitory transmitter such as GABA. In this regard, however, studies by Sheehan and Belleroche (1983) have shown that CCK facilitates rather than inhibits the release of GABA in the rat cortex.

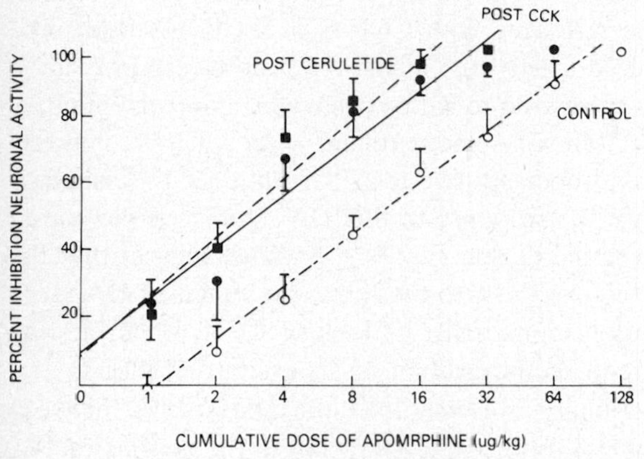

Fig. 3. Dose-response curve for apomorphine-induced inhibition of DA neuronal activity under control versus CCK or ceruletide pretreatment conditions. Pretreatment with either peptide significantly shifted the APO curve to the left ($p < 0.001$, test for common intercept). The effects of CCK and ceruletide were not significantly different from each other. The bars indicate standard error of the mean. Graphs were plotted using linear regression.

Interaction between CCK and DA

Since CCK and DA co-exist, we next explored the functional interaction between these putative transmitters. The ability of peripherally administered CCK to modulate the response of neurons in both SNZC and VT to a classical DA agonist, APO was examined. Pretreatment with doses of CCK as low as 4 μg/kg i.v. produced a significant left shift in the APO dose-response curve suggesting the development of DA supersensitivity (Fig. 3). Iontophoretic studies addressed the question of whether this effect was central or peripheral; CCK again potentiated the inhibitory actions of DA. These findings were unexpected. It was reasoned that as an excitatory agent, CCK would be expected to block the effects of an inhibitory transmitter such as DA. Thus, CCK appears to have two distinct actions on cell bodies: intrinsic excitation and facilitation of the effects of DA.

Our next question asked whether the differential effects of CCK were a reflection of CCK modulation at two independent sites, e.g. different receptors. The localization of CCK in the brain has been

TABLE I

Comparison of the electrophysiological and biochemical effects of CCK-like peptides

	Electrophysiology		Biochemistry*	
	Potentiation of apomorphine	Excitation	Affinity for central site	Affinity for peripheral site
CCK-S	+++	+++	+++	+++
CCK-US	+++	–	+++	–
CCK-4	++	–	++	–
CCK-3	–	–	–	–

* From Hays et al., 1980; Saito et al., 1981; Gaudreau et al., 1983a,b; Van Dijk et al., 1984; Wennogle et al., 1984; Steigerwalt and Williams, 1984; Knight et al., 1984.

shown by several laboratories to be paralleled to a large extent by the distribution of specific binding sites (Hays et al., 1980; Saito et al., 1980; Zarbin et al., 1983). Studies on the autoradiographic distribution of CCK binding sites using tritiated pentagastrin (which represents a more selective ligand than CCK-33 for brain receptors) reveal a high density of CCK receptors in the midbrain areas (Gaudreau, 1983a,b) which are rich in CCK-like immunoreactivity (Hökfelt et al., 1980a,b). It has in fact, been suggested that there are multiple CCK receptors (Innis and Snyder, 1980; Moran et al., 1985). More recently, the detailed structural requirements for octapeptide binding to central CCK receptors has been studied by several groups (Gaudreau et al., 1983a,b; Knight et al., 1984). Gaudreau studied the ability of various CCK peptides to inhibit specific [^{125}I]CCK1-33, [^{125}I]CCK-8 or [^{3}H]CCK-5 binding to rat striatal tissues. She reported that CCK-8-S was approximately equipotent to CCK-8-US which was slightly more potent than CCK-7-S, US followed by CCK-4. Finally, ligands smaller than CCK-4 failed to displace binding. These findings are similar to those of Knight et al. (1984) who found that CCK-8 bound more potently to brain sites than CCK-4 or CCK-3 and that sulfation was not necessary for maximal interaction with the CNS receptor.

Thus, in an effort to address the question of whether the excitatory and facilitatory actions of CCK were mediated at two receptor sites, we tested several CCK analogues to examine their ability to induce either excitation or DA facilitation or both. As with earlier studies, CCK-S excited neurons in the A10 area of the brain. CCK-US, CCK-4 and CCK-3, however, failed to alter the activity of these neurons. In contrast, pretreatment of DA cells in the A10 area with CCK-S or CCK-US both produced a left shift in the APO dose-response curve as compared to saline pretreated controls. Similarly, following pretreatment with CCK-4, neurons were supersensitive to APO; while CCK-3 failed to shift the response to this DA agonist as compared to saline (Table I). These findings suggest that the ability of CCK to modulate the effects of DA more closely mimics the actions of CCK at its binding site in the brain than do its excitatory effects.

Finally, we examined the relationship between the ability of CCK to facilitate the actions of DA and the site of action within the SN. Similar to our finding with regard to the excitatory effects of CCK, the facilitatory actions of this peptide were limited to areas of the SN in which CCK and DA are coexistent, i.e. VT and the medial aspects of SNZC.

Behavioral studies

Methods

Having established electrophysiological evidence for an interaction between CCK and DA we turned to some behavioral paradigms to examine this interaction in awake, unrestrained animals. Male Sprague-Dawley rats, 200–250 g, were stereotaxically implanted under sodium pentobarbital anesthesia with bilateral 24 gauge hypodermic stainless steel guide cannulae into the nucleus accumbens or caudate nucleus one week before behavioral testing. Guide cannulae were placed 1 mm dorsal to the intended site of injection, and closed with 31 gauge stylets. Drugs were microinjected through a 31 gauge injection tube, after removal of the stylet at a site 1 mm ventral to the ventral tip of the guide cannula, in a volume of 0.2 μl (accumbens) or 0.5 μl (caudate) over a one minute infusion period, using a Sage microinfusion pump. This procedure is designed to minimize tissue damage within the site of injection and to minimize spread of drug away from the intended injection site. After each experiment, fast green dye was identically injected and brains were removed, frozen, sectioned and stained with cresyl violet for histological analysis of the injection site. Rats with injection sites outside the medial posterior accumbens or head of the caudate were eliminated post facto from the statistical analysis of the behavioral data. Locomotor activity was scored over a 15-min session beginning immediately after microinjection in an automated photocell-equipped Digiscan locomotor activity monitor. Stereotyped sniffing and grooming activity was scored by an observer uninformed of treatment condition using the standard 0–5 rating scale developed by Creese and Iversen (1974). We chose to look at two different areas of the brain, accumbens and caudate. These represent: (1) an area in which CCK and DA co-exist and; (2) an area in which CCK is present but not co-existent with DA (Hökfelt et al., 1980a,b; Williams et al., 1981; Meyer et al., 1982). Behavioral actions of DA in the mesolimbic and nigrostriatal pathways have been well described (Creese and Iversen, 1974; Costall et al., 1977; Joyce, 1983; Van Ree, 1983).

Effects of CCK and interaction with DA-mediated behaviors

In the first series of experiments, CCK-8-S was microinjected into the accumbens at doses of 20 pg–200 ng either alone, in combination with DA (20 μg) or 15 min after subcutaneous APO (0.2 mg/kg, s.c.). CCK administered alone into the accumbens

TABLE II

Systemic administration of CCK antagonists blocks the behavioral actions of centrally administered CCK

Treatment (intraperitoneal)	Intra-accumbens	Locomotion (ambulation/15 min)
Saline	Saline	832 ± 83
Proglumide (5 mg/kg i.p.)	Saline	461 ± 95
Benzotript (10 mg/kg i.p.)	Saline	477 ± 118
Saline	Dopamine (20 μg)	1854 ± 249
Proglumide (5 mg/kg i.p.)	Dopamine (20 μg)	2044 ± 535
Benzotript (10 mg/kg i.p.)	Dopamine (20 μg)	1460 ± 383
Saline	Dopamine (20 μg) + CCK (1 ng)	2719 ± 205
Proglumide (5 mg/kg i.p.)	Dopamine (20 μg) + CCK (1 ng)	1847 ± 220 * $p < 0.05$
Benzotript (10 mg/kg i.p.)	Dopamine (20 μg) + CCK (1 ng)	1833 ± 417 * $p < 0.05$

had no effect on either locomotion or stereotypy over the wide dose range tested. However, CCK (200 pg–200 ng) administered in combination with DA significantly increased the hyperlocomotion response to DA (Table II). Similarly, CCK (20 pg–200 ng) administered in combination with APO significantly increased the stereotypy response to APO (Crawley et al., 1984a, 1985b).

It is of interest to note that the dose-response curves for CCK potentiation of DA-induced hyperlocomotion and APO-induced stereotypy appeared to be biphasic; high doses of CCK were ineffective in producing potentiation. In light of this, the possibility that even higher doses of CCK, in the μg range, might inhibit the behavioral actions of DA and APO should be raised. Due to CCK solubility limits in the small injection volume used in these studies, we could not test this hypothesis. In support of this notion, however, μg doses of CCK have been reported elsewhere to have no effect or to inhibit the behavioral effects of DA, APO, and amphetamine (Kovacs et al., 1981; Ellinwood et al., 1983; Schneider et al., 1983; Widerlov et al., 1983; Hamilton et al., 1984). In addition, we have reported that mg doses of CCK produce depolarization block (Skirboll et al., 1981; White and Wang, 1984). The pg-ng dose range, at which potentiation of DA-mediated behaviors was seen in the present studies, may therefore represent a more physiological action of CCK. Thus, these data suggest that CCK acts as modulator of DA, i.e. CCK alone had no behavioral effects while it effectively potentiated the behavioral effects of DA and APO.

The second series of experiments was designed to test the hypothesis that CCK potentiation of DA-mediated behaviors occurs specifically at anatomical sites at which co-existing CCK-DA terminals are localized. Using the surgical procedure described above, CCK-8-S was injected either into the caudate nucleus or in regions within or 1 mm away from the medial posterior accumbens where CCK and DA are found in separate nerve terminals (Hökfelt et al., 1981; Fallon et al., 1983). CCK-8-S was microinjected into the caudate at doses of 40 pg–400 ng, either alone or in combination with DA (20 μg), or 15 min after the s.c. injection of APO (0.2 mg/kg). CCK into the caudate had no effect when administered alone and had no effect on either locomotion or stereotypy when administered in combination with DA or after APO (Crawley et al., 1984a, 1985b). Analysis of the effects of regional injection of CCK into the accumbens revealed a correlation between the injection sites at which CCK effectively potentiated DA-induced hyperlocomotion and sites at which CCK and DA reportedly co-exist (Fig. 4) (Crawley et al., 1985a). In this regard, Studler et al. (1985) have shown that CCK potentiates DA stimulation of adenylate cyclase in posterior accumbens and inhibits DA-induced adenylate cyclase stimulation in anterior accumbens. Thus, evidence that CCK is ineffective in the caudate and regions of the accumbens absent where CCK-DA terminals are suggests that CCK acts as a modulator of DA specifically at sites of co-existence.

Antagonists

Pharmacological studies of the functions of CCK have been hindered by the lack of potent and specific CCK antagonists. Three compounds have been identified which block the ability of CCK to stimulate pancreatic amylase secretion: proglumide (PRO), benzotript (BZT) and dbGMP (Davison and Najafi-Garashah, 1981; Hahne et al., 1981; Jensen et al., 1983). There has been a question, however, as to whether peripherally active antagonists

Fig. 4. Comparison of the anatomical sites at which CCK potentiates DA-induced hyperlocomotion and sites which immunohistochemical studies have shown contain both CCK and DA (Hökfelt et al., 1981). Co-existent sites are designated as hatched lines on the right sides of three frontal cross-sections of brain. Injection sites for DA (20 μg) + CCK (1 ng) are illustrated as circles on the left. ●, Sites of strong potentiation; ○, sites of weak potentiation; ○, eliciting no potentiation. Strong potentiation was observed primarily in regions of CCK-DA co-existence.

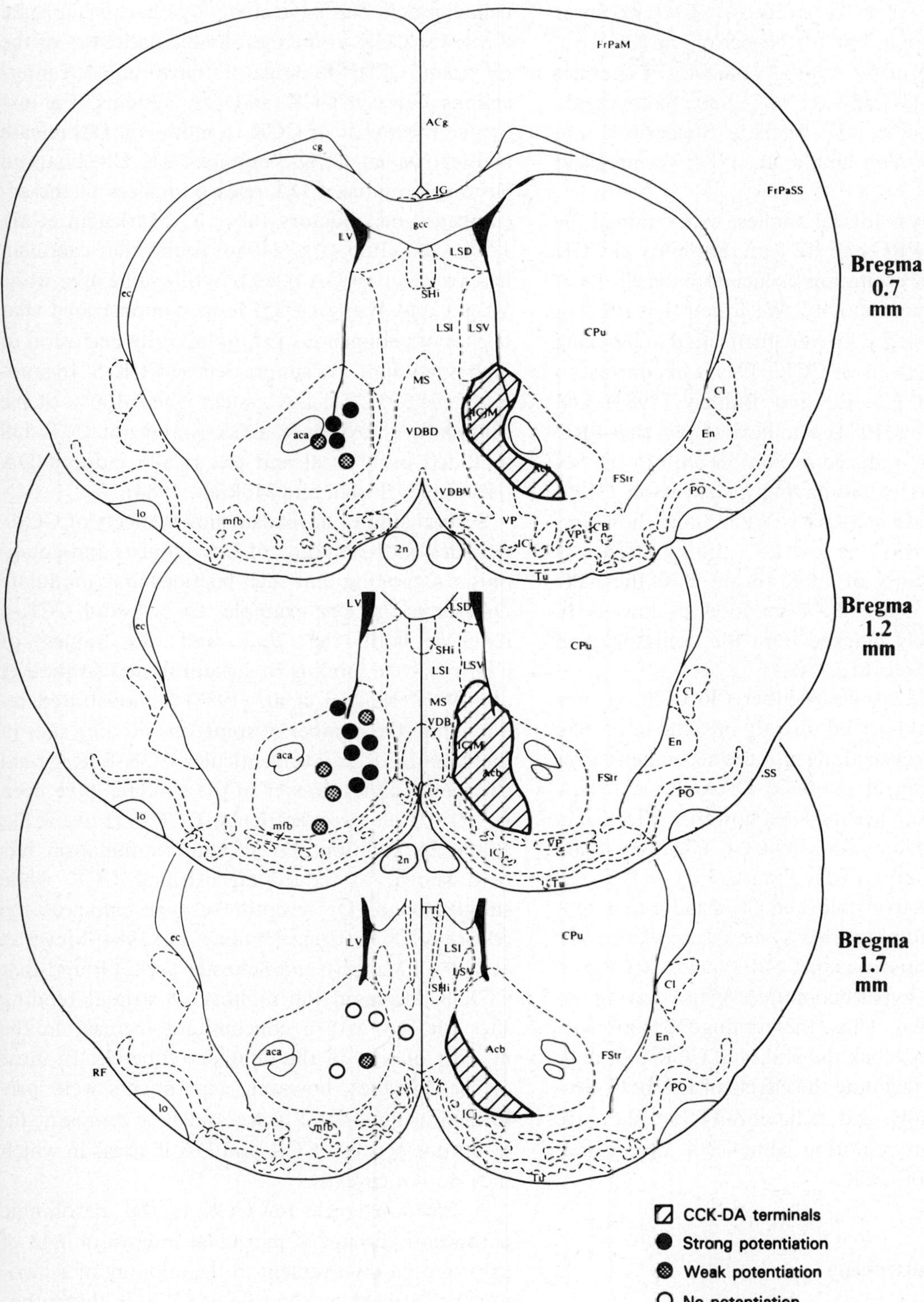
FrPaM
ACg
cg
IG
FrPaSS
gcc
LV
LSD
SHi
ec
LSI
LSV
CPu
MS
ICjM
Cl
aca
VDBD
En
Acb
FStr
VDBV
PO
lo
mfb
VP
2n
ICj
VP
CB
Tu
Bregma
0.7
mm
LV
LSD
ec
SHi
CPu
LSI
LSV
MS
VDB
Cl
ICjM
En
aca
Acb
FStr
SS
PO
lo
mfb
VP
2n
ICj
Tu
Bregma
1.2
mm
TT
LV
LSI
ec
LSV
CPu
SHi
Cl
Acb
En
aca
FStr
RF
PO
lo
mfb
ICj
Tu
Bregma
1.7
mm
CCK-DA terminals
Strong potentiation
Weak potentiation
No potentiation

are also active centrally; the central CCK receptor may not be equivalent to the peripheral CCK receptor in terms of the relative potencies of agonists and antagonists (Hays et al., 1980; Saito et al., 1981; Gaudreau et al., 1983a,b; Steigerwalt and Williams, 1984; Van Dijk et al., 1984; Wennogle et al., 1984).

In electrophysiological studies, we examined the effects of both PRO and BZT on the ability of CCK to either induce excitation or facilitate the effects of DA on single unit activity. We found that PRO in doses of up to 80 mg/kg were ineffectual in blocking the excitatory effects of CCK. This is in contrast to the reports of Chiodo and Bunney (1983) and White and Wang (1984) who have shown that PRO can block CCK-induced excitation both in the SN and accumbens, while having no effect on GLU-induced increases in activity. We did find, however, that doses of PRO as low as 2 mg/kg effectively blocked the ability of CCK to left shift the APO dose-response curve. BZT in doses as low as 16 mg/kg effectively blocked both the excitatory and facilitatory actions of CCK.

In behavioral studies, neither PRO (20 μg) nor BZT (10 μg/kg) injected directly into the brain had an effect when given alone into the accumbens; similarly, neither agent modified DA-induced hyperlocomotion. Both agents were, however, effective in blocking DA potentiation by CCK (Crawley et al., 1984b). In addition, PRO (5 mg/kg i.p.) or BZT (10 mg/kg i.p.) effectively blocked CCK-induced potentiation when administered systemically (Table II). In addition, antiserum to CCK blocked CCK-potentiated DA hyperlocomotion while having no effects of its own. Thus, these antagonists are specific in that they block the ability of CCK to induce excitation and facilitate the effects of DA both electrophysiologically and behaviorally but they are not very potent requiring some 1000 times more than the dose of CCK.

Summary and discussion

Immunohistochemical, electrophysiological and behavioral studies have come together to implicate a role for CCK in the mesolimbic pathways of the rat brain. Other investigators have reported interactions between CCK and DA systems. For example, the ability of CCK to modulate DA release is controversial. CCK-S but not CCK-US enhanced electrically induced DA release in slices of the accumbens and olfactory tubercle (Markstein et al., 1985). Hamilton et al. (1984) found that caerulein had no effect on DA release in this same area while Voight and Wang (1985) have demonstrated that release of endogenous DA induced by perfusion of high potassium was suppressed by CCK-S. In studies of the cat CCK-DA system where 100% of the cells show co-existence, CCK-S and not CCK-US inhibited both basal and electrically induced DA release (Markstein and Hökfelt, 1984).

Several studies have also shown effects of CCK-peptides on the binding of DA agonists and antagonists suggesting that such peptides may modulate DA receptors. For example, CCK-8 and CCK-4 reduced both the $B_{\max}$ and K_d values of [^{3}H]spiperone binding in striatal tissues (Agnati et al., 1983). Mashal et al. (1983) demonstrated reduction in the number of spiperone binding sites in the striatum after intraventicular CCK-8. Regional changes in DA turnover in the caudate have been reported after intraventricular CCK-S (Fuxe et al., 1981). In addition, D_1 receptor stimulation has been shown to reduce nigrostriatal CCK while stimulation of D_2 receptor subtype enhances the release of CCK (Conzelmann et al., 1984; Meyer et al., 1984). Murphy and Schuster (1982) found that CCK-8 decreased the number of striatal binding sites for DA with a concomitant increase in the number of sites in the olfactory tubercle. In most of these studies, however, experiments were performed using striatal tissue and thus represent interactions between CCK and DA in areas in which they do not co-exist.

A functional role for CCK in the mesolimbic pathway is perhaps of particular interest in light of its proposed involvement in the etiology of schizophrenia. Studies on the role of CCK in the pathophysiology of the human brain are contradictory.

In studies of CCK's ability to treat or modify schizophrenic symptoms, Moroji et al. (1982) and Nair et al. (1982) initially reported that peripherally administered CCK and CCK analogs may have caused a beneficial effect in patients with schizophrenia. According to the DA hypothesis of schizophrenia, at least some of the symptoms of this disease are related to an overactivity of the mesolimbic DA system. The results of these clinical investigators might be explained by actions similar to those reported by Markstein and Hökfelt (1984), i.e. a decrease in DA release. However, our electrophysiological and behavioral data suggest, to the contrary, that CCK serves to potentiate the effects of DA. In this regard, Hommer et al. (1984) reported no changes in either positive or negative symptoms of schizophrenia following two paradigms of either i.v. or i.m. CCK or caeruletide; there was no tendency for the patients' conditions to either improve or worsen as a result of treatment. One possible explanation for CCK's failure to influence psychosis is that these peptides do not cross the blood-brain barrier. In animals, peripherally administered CCK cannot be detected in the CSF (Passaro et al., 1982). Given our electrophysiologic findings that some, but not all, of the effects of CCK may be mediated through the NTS, it is possible that CCK may cross the blood-brain barrier in amounts that are too small to be detected. It is also possible that the effects of peptides are not long lasting enough to induce behavioral changes in humans.

Our electrophysiologic and behavioral data support the idea that there is a functional role for CCK in brain. More specifically, CCK appears to act as modulator of the actions of DA primarily in areas of co-existence. The clinical significance of this interaction may rest with the DA hypothesis of schizophrenia. Thus, our finding that CCK-like peptides potentiate the effects of DA suggests that a likely candidate for the treatment of schizophrenia might well be an agent which acts as a potent and specific CCK antagonist.

Acknowledgements

The authors would like to thank Robert Long and Jill Stivers for their expert technical assistance. Special thanks should also be extended to Gene Stoner for his valuable assistance in the preparation of this data.

References

Agnati, L. F., Fuxe, K., Benfenati, F., Celani, M. F., Battistini, N., Mutt, V., Cavicchioli, L., Galli, G. and Hökfelt, T. (1983) Differential modulation of CCK-8 and CCK-4 of ^{3}H-spiperone binding sites linked to dopamine and 5-hydroxytryptamine receptors in the brain of the rat. *Neurosci. Lett.*, 35: 179–183.

Anika, S. M., Houpt, T. R. and Houpt, K. A. (1977) Satiety elicited by cholecystokinin in intact and vagotomized rats. *Physiol. Behav.*, 19: 761–766.

Bunney, B. S., Walters, J. R., Roth, R. H. and Aghajanian, G. K. (1973) Dopaminergic neurons: effects of antipsychotic drugs and amphetamine on single cell activity. *J. Pharmacol. exp. Ther.*, 185: 560–571.

Chiodo, L. A. and Bunney, B. S. (1983) Proglumide: Selective antagonism of excitatory effects of cholecystokinin in central nervous system. *Science*, 219: 1449–1451.

Costall, B., Naylor, R. J., Cannon, J. G. and Lee, T. (1977) Differentiation of the dopamine mechanisms mediating stereotyped behaviors and hyperactivity in the nucleus accumbens and caudate-putamen. *J. Pharm. Pharmacol.*, 29: 337–342.

Crawley, J. N. (1985) Cholecystokinin potentiation of dopamine mediated behaviors in the nucleus accumbens. In *Neuronal Cholecystokinin, NY Acad.* Vanderhaeghen, J. J. and Crawley, J. N. (Eds.), 448, pp. 283–292.

Crawley, J. N., Hays, S. E. and Paul, S. M. (1981) Vagotomy abolishes the inhibitory effects of cholecystokinin on rat exploratory behaviors. *Europ. J. Pharmacol.*, 73: 379–380.

Crawley, J. N., Hommer, D. W. and Skirboll, L. R. (1984a) Behavioral and neurophysiological evidence for a facilitatory interaction between coexisting transmitters: cholecystokinin and dopamine. *Neurochem. Int.*, 6: 755–760.

Crawley, J. N., St. Pierre, S. and Gaudreau, P. (1984b) Analysis of the behavioral activity of C$^-$ and N-terminal fragments of cholecystokinin octapeptide. *J. Pharmacol. exp. Ther.*, 230: 438–444.

Crawley, J. N., Hommer, D. W. and Skirboll, L. R. (1985a) Topographical analyses of nucleus accumbens sites at which cholecystokinin potentiates dopamine-induced hyperlocomotion in the rat. *Brain Res.*, 335: 337–341.

Crawley, J. N., Stivers, J. A., Blumstein, L. K. and Paul, S. M. (1985b) Cholecystokinin potentiates dopamine-mediated behaviors: evidence for modulation specific to a site of co-existence. *J. Neurosci.*, 5, 8: 1972–1983.

Creese, I. and Iversen, S. D. (1974) The role of forebrain dopamine systems in amphetamine induced stereotyped behavior in the rat. *Psychopharmacologia*, 39: 345–357.

Davison, J. S. and Najafi-Farashah, A. (1981) Dibutyryl cyclic GMP, a competive inhibitor of cholecystokinin/pancreozymin and related peptides in the gall bladder and ileum. *Canadian J. Physiol. Pharmacol.*, 59: 1100–1104.

DeFrance, J., Sikes, R. W. and Chronister, R. B. (1984) Effects of CCK-8 in the nucleus accumbens. *Peptides*, 5: 1–6.

Dockray, G. J. (1980) Cholecystokinin in rat cerebral cortex: identification, purification and characterization by immunochemical methods. *Brain Res.*, 188: 155–165.

Dodd, J. and Kelly, J. S. (1981) The actions of cholecystokinin and related peptides on pyramidal neurones of the mammalian hippocampus. *Brain Res.*, 205: 337–350.

Ellinwood, E. H., Rockwell, K. and Wagoner, N. (1983) Apomorphine behavioral effect is facilitated by dibutyryl/cAMP and inhibited by caerulein. *Psychopharmacol. Bull.*, 29: 352–354.

Fallon, J. H., Hicks, R. and Loughlin, S. E. (1983) The origin of cholecystokinin terminals in the basal forebrain of the rat: evidence from immunofluorescence and retrograde tracing. *Neurosci. Lett.*, 37: 29–35.

Fuxe, K., Agnati, L., Benefenati, F., Cimmino, M., Algeri, S., Hökfelt, T. and Mutt, V. (1981) Modulation by cholecystokinin of ^{3}H-spiropendol binding in rat striatum: evidence for increased affinity and reduction in number of binding sites. *Acta physiol. Scand.*, 113: 567–569.

Gaudreau, P., Morell, J. L., St. Pierre, S., Quirion, R. and Pert, C. B. (1983a) Cholecystokinin octapeptide fragments: synthesis and structure-activity relationship. In: V. Hruby and D. Rich (Eds.), *Proceedings of the Eighth American Peptide Symposium*, Pierce Chemical Company, Rockford, Illinois, pp. 441–444.

Gaudreau, P., Quirion, R., St. Pierre, S. and Pert, C. B. (1983b) Tritium-sensitive film autoradiography of [^{3}H]cholecystokinin-5/Pentagastrin receptors in rat brain. *Europ. J. Pharmacol.*, 87: 173–174.

Gonzelmann, Ute, Holland, A. and Meyer, D. K. (1984) Effects of selective dopamine D_2-receptor agonists on the release of cholecystokinin like-immunoreactivity from rat neostratum. *Europ. J. Pharmacol.*, 101: 119–125.

Guyenet, P., Mroz, E. A., Aghajanian, G. and Leeman, S. E. (1979) Delayed iontophoretic ejection of substance P from glass micropipettes: correlation with time-course of excitation in vivo. *Neuropharmacology*, 18: 553–558.

Hahne, W. F., Jensen, R. T., Lemp, G. F. and Gardener, J. D. (1981) Proglumide and benzotript: members of a different class of cholecystokinin receptor antagonists. *Proc. nat. Acad. Sci. USA*, 78: 6304–6308.

Hamilton, M., Sheehan, M. J., DeBelleroche, J. and Herberg, L. J. (1984) The cholecystokinin analogue, caerulein, does not modulate dopamine release or dopamine-induced locomotor activity in the nucleus accumbens of rat. *Neurosci. Lett.*, 44: 77–82.

Hays, S. E., Goodwin, F. K. and Paul, S. M. (1981) Cholecystokinin receptors are decreased in basal ganglia and cerebral cortex of Huntington's disease. *Brain Res.*, 225: 452–456.

Hökfelt, T., Rehfeld, J. F., Skirboll, L., Ivemark, B., Goldstein, M. and Markey, K. (1980a) Evidence for coexistence of dopamine and CCK in meso-limbic neurones. *Nature (Lond.)*, 285: 476–478.

Hökfelt, T., Skirboll, L., Rehfeld, J. F., Goldstein, M., Markey, K. and Dann, O. (1980b) A subpopulation of mesencephalic dopamine neurons projecting to limbic areas contain a cholecystokinin-like peptide: evidence from immunohistochemistry combined with retrograde tracing. *Neuroscience*, 5: 2093–2124.

Hommer, D. W. and Skirboll, L. R. (1983) Cholecystokinin-like peptides potentiate apomorphine-induced inhibition of dopamine neurons. *Europ. J. Pharmacol.*, 91: 151–152.

Hommer, D. W., Pickar, D., Roy, A., Ninan, P., Boronow, J. and Paul, S. M. (1984) The effects of ceruletide in schizophrenia. *Arch. Gen. Psychiatr.*, 41: 617–619.

Hommer, D. W., Palkovits, M., Crawley, J. N., Paul, S. M. and Skirboll, L. R. (1985) Cholecystokinin-induced excitation in substantia nigra: evidence for peripheral and central components. *J. Neurosci.*, 5: 1387–1392.

Hommer, D. W., Stoner, G., Crawley, J. N., Paul, S. M. and Skirboll, L. R. (1986) CCK-DA coexistence: electrophysiological evidence for selective sites of action. *J. Neurosci.* (in press).

Innis, R. B. and Snyder, S. H. (1980) Cholecystokinin receptor binding in brain and pancreas: Regulation of pancreatic binding by cyclic and acyclic guanine nucleotides. *Europ. J. Pharmacol.*, 65: 123–124.

Jensen, R. T., Jones, S. W. and Gardner, J. D. (1983) COOH-terminal fragments of cholecystokinin, a new class of cholecystokinin receptor antagonists. *Biochem. Biophys. Acta*, 757: 250–258.

Joyce, J. N. (1983) Multiple dopamine receptors and behavior. *Neurosci. Biobehav. Rev.*, 7: 227–256.

Jurna, I. and Zetler, G. (1981) Antinociceptive effect of centrally administered caerulein and cholecystokinin octapeptide (CCK-8). *Europ. J. Pharmacol.*, 73: 323–331.

Knight, M., Tamminga, C. A., Steardo, L., Beck, M. E., Barone, P. and Chase, T. N. (1984) Cholecystokinin-octapeptide fragments: binding to brain cholecystokinin receptors. *Europ. J. Pharmacol.*, 105: 49–55.

Kovacs, G. L., Szabo, G., Penke, B. and Telegdy, G. (1981)

Effects of cholecystokinin octapeptide on striatal dopamine metabolism and on apomorphine-induced stereotyped cage-climbing in mice. *Europ. J. Pharmacol.*, 69: 313–319.

Loren, I., Alumets, J., Hakanson, R. H. and Sundler, F. (1979) Distribution of gastrin and cholecystokinin-like peptides in rat brain. *Histochemistry*, 59: 249.

Markstein, R. and Hökfelt, T. (1984) Effect of cholecystokinin-octapeptide on dopamine release from slices of cat caudate nucleus. *J. Neurosci.*, 4: 570–575.

Markstein, R., Skirboll, L. and Hökfelt, T. (1984) Cholecystokinin-like peptides increase dopamine release from brain slices. *Europ. J. Pharmacol.* (submitted).

Meyer, D. K. and Krause, J. (1983) Dopamine modulates cholecystokinin release in neostriatum. *Nature (Lond.)*, 301: 338–340.

Meyer, D. K., Beinfeld, M. C., Oertel, W. H. and Brownstein, M. J. (1982) Origin of the cholecystokinin-containing fibers in the rat caudatoputamen. *Science*, 215: 187.

Meyer, D. K., Holland, A. and Conzelmann, O. (1984) Dopamine D_1-receptor stimulation reduces neostratal cholecystokinin release. *Europ. J. Pharmacol.*, 104: 387–388.

Moran, T. H., Robinson, P. H. and McHugh, P. R. (1985) Differentiation of two CCK receptor types within the brain. Abstract presented at *Neural and Endocrine Peptides and Receptors Conference*, Washington, D.C.

Morley, J. E., Levine, A., Kneip, J. and Grace, M. (1982) The effect of vagotomy on the satiety effects of neuropeptides and naloxone. *Life Sci.*, 30: 1943–1947.

Moroji, T., Watanabe, N., Aoki, N. and Itoh, S. (1982) Antipsychotic effects of ceruletide (caerulein) on chronic schizophrenia. *Arch. gen. Psychiat.*, 39: 485–486.

Murphy, R. B. and Schuster, D. I. (1983) Modulation of [^{3}H]dopamine binding by cholecystokinin octapeptide (CCK-8). *Peptides*, 3: 539–543.

Nair, N. P. V., Bloom, D. M. and Nestoros, J. N. (1982) Cholecystokinin appears to have antipsychotic properties. *Prog. Neuro-Psychopharmacol. biol. Psychiat.*, 6: 509–512.

Palkovits, M., Kiss, J. Z., Beinfeld, M. C. and Williams, T. H. (1982) Cholecystokinin in the nucleus of the solitary tract of the rat: Evidence for its vagal origin. *Brain Res.*, 252: 386–390.

Passaro, E., Bebas, H., Oldendorf, W. and Yamado, T. (1981) Rapid appearance of intraventricularly administered neuropeptides in the peripheral circulation. *Brain Res. Eur. J. Pharmacol.*, 73: 379–380.

Paxinos, G. and Watson, C. (1982) *The Rat Brain*, Academic Press, N.Y.

Pinget, M., Straus, E. and Yalow, R. S. (1979) Release of cholecystokinin peptide from a synaptosome-enriched fraction of rat cerebral cortex. *Life Sci.*, 25: 339–342.

Rehfeld, J. F. and Lundberg, J. M. (1983) Cholecystokinin in feline vagal and sciatic nerves: Concentration, molecular form and transport velocity. *Brain Res.*, 275: 341–347.

Rogawski, M. A. (1982) Cholecystokinin octapeptide: Effects on excitability of cultured spinal neurons. *Peptides*, 3: 545–551.

Saito, A., Sankaran, H., Goldfine, I. D. and Williams, J. A. (1980) Cholecystokinin receptors in brain: characterization and distribution. *Science*, 208: 1155–1156.

Salt, T. E. and Hill, R. G. (1982) The effects of C-terminal fragments of cholecystokinin on the firing of single neurons in the caudal trigeminal nucleus of the rat. *Neuropeptides*, 2: 301–306.

Schneider, L. H., Alpert, J. E. and Iversen, S. D. (1983) CCK-8 modulation of mesolimbic dopamine: antagonism of amphetamine-stimulated behaviors. *Peptides*, 4: 749–753.

Shechan, M. and deBelleroche, J. (1983) Facilitation of GABA release by cholecystokinin and caerulein in rat cerebral cortex. *Neuropeptides*, 3: 429–434.

Skirboll, L. R., Grace, A. A., Hommer, D. W., Rehfeld, J., Goldstein, M., Hökfelt, T. and Bunney, B. S. (1981) Peptide-monoamine coexistence: studies of actions of cholecystokinin-like peptide on the electrical activity of midbrain dopamine neurons. *Neuroscience*, 6: 2111–2124.

Smith, G. P., Jerome, C., Cushin, B., Eterno, R. and Simansky, K. (1981) Abdominal vagotomy blocks the satiety effect of CCK in the rat. *Science*, 213: 1036–1037.

Steigerwalt, R. W. and Williams, J. A. (1984) Binding specificity of the mouse cerebral cortex receptor for small cholecystokinin peptides. *Regul. Peptides*, 8: 51–59.

Thomson, J. C. (1973) In P. Holton (Ed.), *Pharmacology of Gastrointestinal Motility and Secretion, Int. Encyclop. Pharmacol. Ther. Sec.*, 39A 261–286.

Uvnas-Wallensten, K., Rehfeld, J. F., Larsson, L. and Uvnas, B. (1977) Heptodecapeptide gastrin in the vagal nerve. *Proc. nat. Acad. Sci. USA*, 74: 5707–5710.

Vanderhaeghen, J. J., Lotstra, F., DeMay, J. and Gillis, C. (1980) Immunohistochemical localization of cholecystokinin- and gastrin-like peptides in the brain and hypophysis of the rat. *Proc. nat. Acad. Sci. USA*, 77: 1190.

Van Dijk, A., Richards, J. G., Trzeciak, A., Gillessen, D. and Möhler, H. (1984) Cholecystokinin receptors: biochemical demonstration and autoradiographical localization in rat brain and pancreas using [^{3}H]cholecystokinin 8 as radioligand. *J. Neurosci.*, 4: 1021–1033.

Van Ree, J. M., Gaffori, O. and DeWied, D. (1983) In rats, the behavioral profile of CCK-8 related peptides resembles that of antipsychotic agents. *Europ. J. Pharmacol.*, 93: 63–78.

Voight, M. M. and Wang, R. Y. (1985) In vivo release of dopamine in nucleus accumbens of the rat: modulation by cholecystokinin. *Brain Res.* (in press).

Wennogle, L., Steel, D. J. and Petrack, B. (1985) Characterization of central cholecystokinin receptors using a radioactivated octapeptide probe. *Life Sci.*, 36: 1485–1492.

White, F. J. and Wang, R. Y. (1984) Interactions of cholecystokinin octapeptide and dopamine on nucleus accumbens neurons. *Brain Res.*, 300: 161–166.

Widerlov, E., Kalivas, P. W., Lewis, M. H., Prange, A. J. and Breese, G. R. (1983) Influence of cholecystokinin on central monoaminergic pathways. *Regul. Peptides,* 6: 99–109.

Williams, R. G., Gayton, R. J., Zhu, W.-Y. and Dockray, G. J. (1981) Changes in brain cholecystokinin octapeptide following lesions of the medial forebrain bundle. *Brain Res.,* 213: 227.

Zarbin, M. A., Innis, R. B., Wamsley, J. K., Snyder, S. H. and Kuhar, M. J. (1983) Autoradiographic localization of cholecystokinin receptors in rodent brain. *J. Neurosci.,* 3: 877–906.

SECTION VII

Synthesis

T. Hökfelt, K. Fuxe and B. Pernow (Eds.),
Progress in Brain Research, Vol. 68

CHAPTER 26

Coexistence of neuronal messengers and molecular selection

Jean-Pierre Changeux

Institut Pasteur, Paris, France

'Tout le cerveau n'est autre chose qu'un tissu composé d'une certaine façon particulière ...'
René Descartes — l'Homme 1677 2ème édition p. 56.

Introduction

The exceptional interest and success of the Symposium splendidly organized by Tomas Hökfelt, Kjell Fuxe and Bengt Pernow, with the help of the Marcus Wallenberg Foundation represented by David Ingvar, resides in the content of its title "Coexistence of neuronal messengers: a new principle in chemical transmission". This title is built out of two distinct propositions. The first, "coexistence of neuronal messengers", makes explicit an anatomical fact: the simultaneous presence at the level of a given nerve cell of *several* compounds referred to here as "messengers" because of their potential role in information transfer. The second, "a new principle of chemical transmission", is a theoretical proposal about the functional significance of the coexisting messengers: this anatomical disposition offers new possibilities of signalling within the nervous system and between the nervous system and the peripheral organs.

In this Synthesis, I shall attempt to summarise the wealth of new findings reported at the Meeting which, in a consistent manner, bring substantial support to the proposed hypothesis. Also, I shall try to discuss further some of the theoretical consequences and problems that these observations raise.*

"Dale principle" reconsidered

Importance of model building

In chemistry and physics, theory has acquired full rights as a fundamental research issue. Yet, this is not always the case in biological sciences, where theory is sometimes considered as useless or even misleading compared to the concrete attempts to observe and to experiment. In reality, even the simplest description of a biological object requires a minimum of theoretical treatment. "Nature answers only in the language in which the questions are asked" wrote W. Shea. In practice, biologists, as any other category of scientists, elaborate *models* which create the language necessary to raise pertinent questions and which constitute "representa-

* Reference to a chapter of the book and bibliography therein is indicated by the first author name between brackets.

tions" in a coherent but simplified form of the investigated object or phenomenon.

Jöns-Jacob Berzelius, in the second chapter of his "Theory of chemical proportions" (1835, 2nd French edition), stressed the importance of theory but also drew attention to its limitations. He wrote (p. 12) "Theory is only a way to represent the inside of phenomena. It is acceptable and sufficient as long as it may explain known facts. It may however be wrong, although within a given period of science development, it might be as *useful* as a right theory. The experiments increase in number, one discovers facts which are no longer consistent with the theory, and one then has to look for another explanation equally applicable to these new facts" (author's translation from the French edition).

Dale "physiological model" of the neuron

"Dale's principle", as it emerged from the work of Sir Henry Dale and his associates and as stated by Sir John Eccles (1957) [Eccles], should be discussed in the spirit of Berzelius' remarks. In particular, one should keep in mind the historical context in which it was first enunciated and thus view it as some kind of "model" expressing, in a condensed form, and as a "provisional hypothesis" (Eccles, 1962), the state of knowledge available about the physiology and pharmacology of the neuron from the 30's to the late 60's.

At the end of the 19th century, S. Ramon y Cajal opposes to the "reticular theory", the "neuron theory", in which he stresses the *anatomical unity* of the nerve cell. For him, neurons are "individual *units,* completely independent, simply in contact with each other". In retrospect, the Dale model appears as the physiological or "metabolic" counterpart of the Cajal anatomical model. In several well-defined instances, such as the spinal cord motor neurons, the same neurotransmitter was found to be liberated at the center *and* at the periphery [Eccles] leading to the statement that "any one class of nerve cells operates at all its synapses by the same chemical transmission mechanism", a notion that "stems from the metabolic *unity* of a single cell which extends to all its branches" (Eccles, 1957). Clearly, for Dale the metabolic unity of the neuron coincides with its anatomical unity for he writes [quoted by Eccles] that "like a cytoplasmic process of any other cell, the axon and its endings must be dependent of the nucleus of the cell body for the maintenance of their integrity and special constituents". The *biochemical unity* of the neuron results from its cellular organisation.

For a while, this formulation led to divergent interpretations (see Potter et al., 1981). The statement that "the same chemical transmission mechanism operates at all nerve endings" was sometimes taken as meaning that *"only one* transmitter" is synthesized and liberated by any given nerve cell. The small number of transmitters known at the time left this possibility open despite the fact that Sir Henry Dale himself might have considered the eventuality of multiple transmitters (see Potter et al., 1981).

In any case, as emphasized by both Sir John Eccles [this volume] and Potter et al. (1981) [this volume], one should no longer perpetuate this confusion but should clearly distinguish:

(1) the single transmitter status of the neuron, and
(2) the metabolic unity, of the nerve cell.

These two notions have to be discussed separately and their validity challenged on the basis of the relevant data. Anticipating the conclusions of this Synthesis, one may say that the first one no longer holds and that the second may suffer limitations.

Selection versus instruction in the nervous system

Living organisms possess two characteristic albeit, at a glance, contradictory properties. They possess the capacity to perpetuate their internal order but preserve the ability to modify this order in response to changes of their environment. The first is linked to the self-replication of DNA, the second, either to alterations in the sequence of the DNA (*genetic* process) or to a regulation of the expression of its constituent genes (*epigenetic* process).

Three main theses have served as theoretical

framework in the debate about the second group of processes:

(1) According to the Rationalist or "inneist" thesis, the organisation of living organisms, in particular their brain, is entirely submitted to a strict genetic determinism, their intrinsic structure is rich and the interaction with the outside world does *not* bring any new order.

(2) On the other hand, the Empiricist view is that, at birth, the brain is a *tabula rasa* and that all its internal order results from experience.

(3) In between, stands the Selectionist or Darwinist thesis according to which the increase of internal order is *indirect*. The organism spontaneously generates a multiplicity of internal variations and the interaction with the environment merely selects or "selectively stabilizes" some of these endogenous variations.

A selective machine thus contains two basic devices:

(1) a generator of internal diversity, utilizing a combinatorial process, and

(2) a mechanism for selection of privileged combinations (and/or elimination or rejection of the others) associated with the exchange of signals with the environment (for discussion see Changeux et al., 1984b).

Selectionist models have encountered success in several major domains of biological research such as the Evolution of species or the biosynthesis of antibodies (see Jerne, 1985). In the Neurosciences, the Empiricist mode of thinking has been traditional in the field of Learning theory since Thorndike and Pavlov (Hebb, 1949; Stent, 1973; Rescorla and Wagner, 1972; Hopfield, 1982; see Marler and Terrace, 1984, for discussion). On the other hand, Selectionist theories have recently been revived, in particular with the extension of the antibody synthesis model to the problem of learning (Jerne, 1967) and with the proposal and mathematical formalization of a cellular mechanism for the active "epigenesis" of synaptic connections during development (Changeux, 1972; Changeux et al., 1973; Changeux and Danchin, 1974, 1976, review Changeux et al., 1984b; Marler and Terrace, 1984). According to this last model, selection would operate among multiple and labile connections that occur spontaneously at critical stages (or sensitive periods) of development via the selective stabilization by spontaneous and/or evoked activity of matching patterns of connections accompanied by the correlative elimination of the others. Among other consequences, the model accounts (at least as one among many plausible mechanisms) for two paradoxes raised by the comparison of the "complexity" of the nervous system with that of the genome (Changeux, 1983a,b):

(1) the number of genes available for coding is small (gene parsimony), and

(2) this number does not increase linearly with the complexity of the anatomy in the course of phylogenesis, particularly in mammals.

As mentioned, "the model presents evident analogies with the classical neodarwinist theories of evolution. In both cases, selection operates in a system in growth and the fluctuations are introduced either by the modalities of growth and motion of nerve endings, or by mutations in the DNA" (Changeux and Danchin, 1974).

Selectionist theories have been subsequently extended to higher brain functions in the form of a "group-selection and phasic re-entrant mechanism" (Edelman, 1978; Finkel and Edelman, 1985) and of a mechanism of high level learning by selection of mental "pre-representations" by "resonance" (Changeux, 1983a,b; Changeux et al., 1984b; Heidmann et al., 1984; see also Marler and Terrace, 1984; Freeman, 1983; Toulouse et al., 1986). They have also been applied to the formation of neural maps (Schmidt, 1985; Fraser, 1985; see also Edelman and Finkel, 1984).

A question we shall ask in this Synthesis is to what extent such selectionist models may be useful in discussing the problems raised by the chemical diversity and variability of the nerve cell as they emerge from the analysis of coexisting messengers.

Anatomical evidence for coexistence of neuronal messengers

Exocrine or endocrine glands classically synthesize and release batteries of peptide hormones and/or enzymes [see Pearse] sometimes even from different points of their cell surface. Despite its well-established secretory properties, the nerve cell has been, and is still sometimes, viewed as producing and liberating a unique neurotransmitter. The demonstration that this single transmitter status of the neuron no longer holds [Hökfelt et al.; Potter et al.] relies on several recent technical and methodological developments.

In Dale's time, only a few neuronal messengers were known. Since then, in particular by including peptides among them (see Hökfelt et al., 1980), the number of *potential* neurotransmitters has increased to about 50 [Iversen]. Initiated by the histofluorescence studies of Hillarp, Falk and their associates (Carlsson et al., 1962; Dahlström and Fuxe, 1964, 1965; Fuxe, 1965), methods for the cellular localisation of known chemical substances became almost universal with the development of immunocytochemistry [Hökfelt et al.] which has even been made quantitative [Fuxe et al.] and extended to the electron microscopy level [Brownstein and Mezey]. Moreover, the simultaneous detection on the same neuron of several putative neurotransmitters has been made possible in particular, by the double or multiple labelling of the same section with probes easy to distinguish from one another [Hökfelt et al.].

Another particularly elegant method for exploring coexistence of neurotransmitters has consisted of the microculture of single (sympathetic) neurons, where the presence of given neurotransmitters as a function of the time of culture (up to 1–3 months) is monitored by the electro-physiological response of underlying cardiac muscle cells [Potter et al.].

Finally, in situ hybridization techniques with specific DNA probes [Brownstein and Mezey] give access to the localisation of a given mRNA species at the single neuron level, and its joint utilisation with immunocytochemistry at the same level (see Brahic et al., 1984) leads to the interesting possibility of comparing in the same cell, the level of a given neurotransmitter or hormone and that of the mRNA which codes for it or for its biosynthetic enzymes.

A large number of neuronal systems have been investigated by these methods and the general conclusion which emerges from this Symposium is the widespread coexistence of neuronal messengers [Hökfelt et al; Lundberg and Hökfelt; Potter et al.; Stjärne and Lundberg; Brownstein and Mezey; Swanson et al.; M. Costa et al. and others] in a variety of combinations [see Hökfelt et al. for review]. For instance, a classical transmitter may coexist together with one or more peptides. Up to seven neuropeptides may be produced by the same neurosecretory neuron in the rat hypothalamic paraventricular nucleus [Swanson et al.]. ATP [Burnstock; Lundberg and Hökfelt; Stjärne and Lundberg] coexists as a putative transmitter with noradrenaline and neuropeptide Y in sympathetic neurons, and several classical transmitters like 5-HT (dopamine) and GABA can be found in the same neurons. Even a leukotriene (LTC4-like compound) (see Samuelsson, 1983) might be produced by LHRH neurons from the anterior pituitary gland [Hökfelt et al.]. In cultured sympathetic neurons, the number of effective transmitters potentially released by the same cell may reach a dozen [Potter et al.]. Finally, coexistence of neuronal messengers has also been reported in several species of Invertebrates [Castellucci et al.]. The single transmitter status of the neuron thus looks exceptional, and one may even wonder if it exists at all in the nervous system. Coexistence, on the contrary, appears to be the rule.

Moreover, an important feature which arises from the analysis of coexistence at the tissue level is that subpopulations of neurons may display different combinations of chemical messengers. This happens, among the many other examples presented by Hökfelt et al. [this volume], in the medullary raphe nuclei where the proportions of 5-HT neurons containing substance P and TRH-like immunoreactivities vary depending on the subregion studied, in the paraventricular nucleus [Swanson et al.] where distinct subpopulations of CRF neurons stain for oxytocin and for vasopressin (or neurotensin or enkephalin or CCK), in the guinea pig gut [M. Costa et al.] where diverse combinations of as many as eight putative messengers (of which up to five may coexist) have been assigned to distinct groups of neurons with different distributions.

Even though the exact significance of this diversity is debated, correlation has often been noted between the content of chemical messengers of a given neuron and the target areas of its *projections.* For example, the noradrenergic neurons in the locus coeruleus that contain neuropeptide Y preferentially project to the hypothalamus [Hökfelt et al.] and a similar regularity exists within the guinea pig gut [M. Costa et al.] and in the paraventricular neurons of the hypothalamus [Swanson et al.]. The possibility has even been mentioned — though conclusive evidence is still lacking — that in this last case *afferent* fibres with different chemical specificity may end on cell types with different chemical messenger patterns [Swanson et al.]. In other words, a definite relationship exists between the precise connectivity of a given neuron and its content of chemical messengers. Thus, the definition of the *"singularity"* (Changeux, 1983) of a given individual neuron within a category should include, in addition to its precise connectivity, the repertoire of the putative neuronal messengers it synthesizes.

Coexistence as a selected state of neuronal differentiation

"Determination" and "differentiation" of the nerve cell

As underlined by Sir Henry Dale [Eccles], the nerve cell exhibits the rather unique property of being able to establish a large number of defined synaptic contacts with a variety of target cells, but nevertheless possesses a unique nucleus and this nucleus contains the genes coding for all these synapses. The problem of coexistence of chemical messengers thus becomes a problem of nuclear gene expression and regulation.

A given nerve cell synthesizes proteins which are common to many other cell types and thus referred to as "house keeping". In addition, it synthesizes proteins which characterize a given neuronal type and are referred to as "specific". Coexistence of neuronal messengers thus simply means that a given nerve cell synthesizes among its specific proteins, several potential messengers (and their biosynthetic enzymes) and thus that the particular set of specific genes which code for them is actively expressed into proteins.

The *phenotype* of the mature nerve cell "labelled" by the coexisting messengers represents the terminal state of a cascade of cellular processes beginning with the cleavage of the fertilized egg and including multiple divisions according to well-defined lineages [see for *Caenorhabditis elegans,* Sulston (1983); for the mouse, Johnson et al. (1984)]. Some of these embryonic divisions are *asymmetrical* and lead to an irreversible, in general epigenetic, commitment referred to as *determination* (see Brown, 1984) of one cell into a lineage different from that of the daughter cell. This occurs, for instance, when the neuro-epithelial cells segregate into neuronal vs. glial cells or, at a more terminal stage, when the Purkinje cell and granular cell precursors form in the developing cerebellum. The asymmetrical divisions may be followed by *symmetrical* ones which preserve the determined state of the cell. After the divisions have ceased and the neuroblasts have reached their final location by eventual migrations, then they express the proteins characteristic of their *differentiated* state (see Brown, 1984).

The mechanisms engaged in embryonic determination and differentiation are actively investigated by molecular biologists and it is out of the scope of this Synthesis even to review them briefly (see Breathnach and Chambon, 1981; Brown, 1984; Yaniv, 1984). Among the multiple successive molecular events identified, one may mention: (1) the local conformational transition of the chromatin which switches a specific gene from a "buried, closed" state to an "open" or "ready to be transcribed" configuration (and conversely); (2) the actual transcription of the open gene into RNA and the processing (capping, poly A addition, splicing), export and stabilization/destabilization of the mature messenger RNA (mRNA); (3) the translation of the mature mRNA into protein and, in some cases, post-translational modification of the synthesized protein.

Determination is in general viewed as involving mechanisms of the first type, differentiation of the second. Opening and closing of structural genes have been monitored in several somatic systems such as the red blood cells in chick embryo (Groudine and Weintraub, 1981; Weintraub et al., 1981), chick oviduct or frog liver (see Burch and Weintraub, 1983; Brown, 1984; Yaniv and Cereghini, 1985). In these systems, "opening" of a gene is characterized by an hypersensitivity to DNAse I, an unmethylated state and an enhanced capacity to bind nuclear proteins; "closing" by the reverse reactions. Acquisition of the final state of differentiation *sensu stricto* would then correspond to the transcription of the open genes into mRNA which is easily assayed by various techniques. However, situations exist where a "determined" gene does *not* express its mRNA. This is for instance the case of *Xenopus* liver cells which are determined to express vitellogenin genes but do not do so in the absence of steroid hormones (Brock and Shapiro, 1983; Burch and Weintraub, 1983; see also Yaniv and Cereghini, 1985).

These definitions are obviously valid in the case of the neuron where the repertoire of "open" genes include, but is not necessarily identical to, that of the actively transcribed ones. Nerve cells exhibit an extreme diversity of shape, biochemical composition, and connectivity. This diversification is particularly large compared to the total number of cells in the nervous system of invertebrates such as *Aplysia* [Castellucci et al.] or *Caenorhabditis* (Sulston, 1983). By contrast, in the central nervous system of vertebrates, *categories* of neurons which regroup populations of cells possessing a similar morphology and a similar function have been distinguished for years by anatomists and physiologists. The number of categories is rather limited (possibly hundreds) but that of individual neurons within a given category can be very large and increases in the course of evolution (for instance, the number of cerebellar Purkinje cells increases from 0.35 million in rat to about 15 million in man). Tentatively, one may propose to extend to the molecular level the definition of a "category" as the smallest group of cells possessing the same "determined" state or *repertoire of open specific genes* (see Changeux, 1983a,b).

Of course, different categories of neurons may share sets of open specific genes. This could be the case for the APUD system where almost 40 different categories of neuroendocrine cells have been grouped together by Pearse [this volume] on the basis of their *potential* expression of common "primary markers" which include among many others amine production, amine precursor uptake, endocrine "granules", specific peptide immunochemistry, neuron specific enolase. These cells however do not have a common embryological origin. For instance, some of them derive from the neural crest (adrenal medulla), others (parathyroid, pituitary) from ectodermal placodes [Pearse].

This raises a general question, which equally holds for neurons, whether the markers expressed in common by cells from different regions of the brain (or even of the body) belong or not to the *same* structural genes. Two alternative situations are plausible [Bloom]: (1) a set of distinct structural genes codes for the same (or homologous) protein but with different tissue specific promoters; (2) a single structural gene with several (at least two) promoters is *alternatively* transcribed in different tissue specific mRNA. The powerful methods of molecular genetics [Bloom] have demonstrated that both situations do occur for example in the case of the amylases in the pancreas, parotid gland or liver (see Schibler et al., 1983). Alternative RNA processing leading to different tissue specific polypeptide products has also been demonstrated in the case of the [calcitonin] [calcitonin-gene-related-peptide] gene in thyroid cells and brain (Rosenfeld et al., 1984).

It would be of interest to carry out this kind of analysis with specific marker genes and cells from different members of the APUD system or neurons exhibiting similar messenger phenotype in different areas of the brain or regions of the body. The possibility that common DNA sequences identify brain specific proteins (I.D. sequences) and serve as "enhancers" of their structural genes has been suggested (Sutcliffe et al., 1984) but recently challenged (Owens et al., 1985).

Variability and regulation of the chemical messengers phenotype

By their microculture technique, Potter et al. [this volume] have shown that, in addition to the fact that each single neuron may release several physiologically active messengers, the pattern of different messengers released *varies* from one neuron to the other. Among 217 cells studied, 20 different combinations of four coexisting messengers were identified [Potter et al.]. Also, within a given combination the relative amount of each messenger released varies in a *graded* manner. Serial recordings from the same neuron for several weeks further show that the balance between coexisting messengers may change with time, usually from a dominant adrenergic to a relatively more cholinergic direction through a dual status as it actually occurs during normal post-natal development (Landis, 1983). This flexibility persists in *adult* neurons derived from adult sympathetic ganglia [Potter et al.], but becomes evanescent with ageing [Black et al.]. It has also been reported in other systems such as adult rat iris innervation [Hökfelt et al.].

Another particularly elegant method to demonstrate the variability of messenger phenotype is the transplantation of neurons (as solid grafts or cell suspensions) into mammalian central nervous system [Schultzberg et al.]. For example, 5-HT neurons from the mesencephalic raphe nucleus express an additional messenger, substance P, when transplanted into rat hippocampus and striatum but not in the spinal cord, thus suggesting an influence of the *local tissue environment* on the expression of the transmitter phenotype [Schultzberg et al.].

Factors which regulate the patterns of coexisting messengers have been identified in the case of the parvo cellular neurosecretory neurons of rat hypothalamus [Swanson et al.]. There, the *steroid hormones* from the adrenal cortex (glucocorticoids) exert a negative feedback on CRF, vasopressin and angiotensin II production but do not significantly affect the levels of enkephalin and neurotensin. Yet it remains to be shown whether this regulation operates at the level of mRNA transcription or/and of post-translational processing or peptide turnover. In situ hybridization shows that levels of vasopressin mRNA increase after adrenalectomy (Wolfson et al., 1985). The molecular target(s) of the glucocorticoids involved in this regulation remain to be identified. Another example, based on quantitative measurement of neuronal messengers in situ, is the marked reduction of neuropeptide Y/phenyl-ethanolamine-*N*-methyl transferase ratio following chronic treatment with glucocorticoid steroids in adrenalectomized male rats [Fuxe].

Another important category of "epigenetic" factor which may differentially regulate coexisting transmitters is the *electrical activity,* spontaneous and/or evoked, of the nerve cell. For instance, in neonatal and mature rat superior cervical sympathetic ganglion [Black et al.], presynaptic impulse activity, acetylcholine or depolarization by veratridine, *suppress* the net synthesis of substance P. On the other hand, the same impulse activity has the opposite effect on the biosynthesis of the catecholamine enzyme tyrosine hydroxylase and can cause up to a 3-fold rise of its mRNA. Similarly, inactivity of rat chromaffin cells associated for example with explantation into cultures increases the content of the opiate peptide leucine enkephalin (up to 50-fold) and of the pre-proenkephalin mRNA (up to 74-fold) without affecting the activity of the colocalised catecholamine enzyme and depolarization by veratridine reverses this effect. In these two systems impulse activity thus differentially regulates levels of mRNA coding for coexisting messengers most likely at the transcription level (although an effect on mRNA stability may, alternatively or in addition, take place).

Chemical messengers selection: a plausible model for the development of the biochemical "singularity" of nerve cells

A point-to-point precise assembly of predetermined neurons into a hardwired, chemically rigid network does not hold for at least the terminal stages of development of the connectivity in vertebrate nervous system. As already mentioned, an important trend of the evolution of the central nervous system in higher vertebrates is *not* the increase of neuronal categories but that of individual neurons within a fixed number of categories. Such a process is of low gene cost but may result in a transiently redundant system. This is avoided in the adult by "epigenetic" processes of diversification which give to each individual neuron a particular connectivity or "singularity". The proposal made here is that the selectionist model suggested in the case of the connectivity (Changeux et al., 1973; Changeux and Danchin, 1976) extends to the chemical messenger phenotype.

The example of the sympathetic and of the hypothalamic CRF neurons and the transplantation experiments support the view that within a given category any individual neuron may *potentially* express a large number of chemical messengers. But at any given time and/or at any given position it synthesizes only a few of them. The genes for *all* these potential messengers may thus be considered as "open" and their repertoire used as an "identification card" of the considered category. The acquisition of the terminal phenotype would then result from the selective "activation" and/or "repression" of a *particular set* among all the specific genes open. For instance, in the case of the sympathetic ganglion, if one takes five as being the number of well-identified messengers, selection would take place among 25 or 31 combinations plus a null state [Potter et al.] but this number might be much larger since in vivo a dozen [Potter et al.] messengers may coexist.

Tentatively, one may hypothesize that at a "critical" stage (or stages) which possibly corresponds to that of the maximal diversity and transient redundancy of the connectivity, the neurons express, i.e. translate into active proteins, the maximal repertoire of open genes, though in variable amounts and at a lower rate. The nerve cell thus serves as a "generator of internal *diversity*" here expressed as patterns of messengers synthesized. These messengers are released onto the available targets which may respond by retrograde signalling. In addition, these neurons may be the target of developing afferent fibres. Evoked impulse activity may thus be superimposed on the spontaneous one, and retrograde signals and other diffusible messengers such as circulating hormones and/or local "ambient" signal may intervene. "Computation" of these "external" signals by the neuron via "internal" signals and regulatory proteins may produce changes in the pattern of protein biosynthesis, leading to the *selection* of the particular biochemical phenotype of each individual neuron of the category (Fig. 1).

This selection of the transmitter phenotype may coincide with the selective stabilisation and elimination of synapses, thereby yielding a "matching" or "fit" of the pattern of transmitters produced by each individual neuron with its connectivity and thus account for the regional variability mentioned in the section on Anatomical evidence for coexistence of neuronal messengers, p. 376. As a consequence, "biochemical maps" may superimpose onto the "connectivity maps" for instance via nearest-neighbour interactions by collateral coupling (see Fraser, 1985). This Selectionist model can be contrasted with a strictly Empiricist scheme which would not be constrained by the limits of the repertoire of open genes which characterizes the category and with a strictly Nativist one which would assume a developmentally programmed chemical differentiation of the individual neurons *prior to* the establishment of their connections and would then involve specific point-to-point mechanisms of recognition.

The Selectionist model assumes that the stabilisation of the phenotype will take place *in the course* of the establishment of the connectivity. It is thus an incentive to follow the evolution of the transmitter status in parallel with the development of the

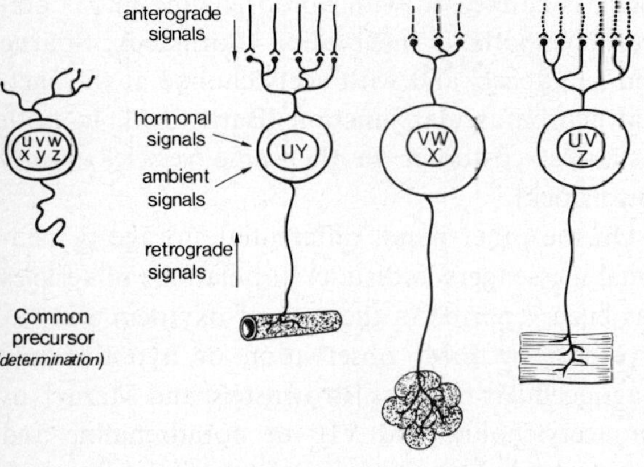

Fig. 1. Model of messenger phenotype selection. The different adult phenotypes shown on the right correspond to individual neurons belonging to the same *category*. Their biochemical "singularity" is characterized by the actual expression of a combination of peptide messengers or messenger biosynthetic enzymes indicated by capital letters UY, VWX and UVZ. Each individual neuron is assumed to derive from a common "determined" precursor, or stem cell, characterized by a set of "open" chromosomic genes indicated by lower case letters (u, v, w, x, y, z) which include *all* the genes actually expressed in the diverse adult phenotypes. The selection of the adult combination of messengers is assumed to take place in the course of the selective stabilization of the adult connectivity and is determined in particular by the activity of the cell, by anterograde and retrograde signals originating respectively from the afferent innervation and from the target cells and by hormonal and "local" signals. For discussion, see text.

connectivity and, for instance, look for a transient stage of maximal chemical diversity preceding the more restricted adult, phenotype. Interestingly, examples of central neurons that transiently produce a neuropeptide at early gestational stages and then cease to do it later have been reported [Schultzberg et al.] (see also Landis, 1983; [Black et al.]).

The model also points to factors which regulate gene expression and may plausibly account for the selection of the phenotype. It underlines the role of activity, in particular the *spontaneous* one (Hamburger, 1970; Harris, 1981) as an internal signalling system for neuronal differentiation (Changeux and Danchin, 1974, 1976; Changeux, 1983a,b) but also that of circulating hormones. In addition, if selection affects the *rate* of *expression* of already open genes rather than the opening of genes, i.e. differentiation rather than determination, then the chromosomic structures and regulatory proteins involved should differ from those which account for the determination of the category to which the individual neurons considered belong. This prediction can be tested by mapping the diverse DNA sequences (promoters, enhancers ...) which regulate in *cis* the structural genes coding for the messengers and/or their biosynthetic enzymes and identifying the different proteins which bind to each of them (see Yaniv, 1985). Also, the model predicts that the total number of open structural genes concerned by coexistence should be larger than that of actually transcribed ones. This "messenger elimination" (by analogy with synapse elimination) can be tested, for instance, by comparing the patterns of DNAse I hypersensitive genes with those of transcribed mRNA species.

Corelease or differential release of coexisting neuronal messengers?

Evidence for release of multiple functional messengers

From the anatomical fact that several chemical "messengers" coexist in the same neuronal soma or even in the same nerve endings, it does not a priori follow that these substances are released in a physiologically significant manner. Several converging reports [Hökfelt et al.; Lundberg and Hökfelt; Stjärne and Lundberg; Burnstock; Branton et al.; Bartfaï et al; Potter et al.; Skirboll et al.] however, show that the neurons which synthesize and accumulate multiple putative messengers also liberate them under conditions where they serve as intercellular communication signals. As pointed out by Stjärne and Lundberg [this volume] it becomes inappropriate, or even misleading, to label neurons or nerve fibres with the suffix *-ergic* (e.g. adrenergic or cholinergic) since a given sympathetic neuron may liberate altogether noradrenaline, neuropeptide Y and ATP. Instead of qualifying an anatomical feature, the suffix *-ergic* would better be used to specify a particular physiological *effect* on the target cell. This raises of course the critical issue of the liberation mechanism of multiple messengers. Are all of them rigidly coreleased in fixed amounts or does a more subtle and flexible differential liberation occur, at least in some privileged instances?

Problems of storage

A "classical" neurotransmitter is in general the product of a biosynthetic pathway composed of several enzymes; its enzymatic synthesis takes place in the nerve endings as in the cell soma and its reuptake (or that of a degradation product) may occur after release in the extracellular space. On the other hand, peptides are synthesized and packed into vesicles in the soma and the vesicles are transported to the nerve endings where no reuptake mechanisms have ever been identified. The peptides released by the nerve endings must thus be directly replaced by axonal transport from the cell soma and this raises the possibility of a differential storage of peptides and classical transmitters (Hökfelt et al., 1980).

The case of the chromaffin cells from adrenal medulla is simple. According to Viveros [this volume], the catecholamine and opioid peptides synthesized by these cells are costored in the same vesicles and coreleased by nicotinic agonists via a calcium-dependent mechanism. When one modifies their relative intracellular content, they are released in amounts which parallel the cell content. In this system, peptides and "classical" messengers are stored in the same compartment and coreleased by the same exocytotic mechanism, a feature compatible with the endocrine function of the adrenal medulla. Nevertheless, analysis of the release of ascorbic acid points to the possible existence in the same cells of a non-vesicular compartment parallel to the vesicular one.

Similarly, storage of several messengers in the same vesicular compartment and their corelease exists in nerve cells. For instance, ATP which tends to become a bona fide neurotransmitter [Burnstock], is coreleased with noradrenaline in vas deferens sympathetic innervation [Burnstock; Stjärne and Lundberg] and with acetylcholine at the skeletal neuromuscular junction [Burnstock]. In both instances, costorage in the same vesicles occurs [Burnstock].

On the other hand, differential storage of neuronal messengers in distinct populations of vesicles has been reported in the case of oxytocin and vasopressin by E.M. observation of hypothalamic magnocellular neurons [Brownstein and Mezey], or for acetylcholine and VIP or noradrenaline and neuropeptide Y on the basis of subcellular fractionation studies of cat salivary gland or rat vas deferens [Hökfelt et al.; Lundberg and Hökfelt; Stjärne and Lundberg]. In these last two instances the amines were found in both small (500 Å diameter) and large (1000 Å diameter) vesicles, while the peptide was mostly present in a heavy fraction composed of large vesicles. Stjärne and Lundberg [this volume] have tentatively proposed that a sympathetic nerve varicosity of mouse vas deferens contains some *450 small* vesicles, each with approximately 1000 molecules of noradrenaline and 20 molecules of ATP and *25 large* vesicles, each with up to 15,000 molecules of noradrenaline, 350 molecules of ATP and 150 molecules of neuropeptide Y. In other words, storage of multiple messengers in distinct populations of vesicles appears, at least for the conventional transmitters, differential rather than exclusive.

Problems of release

Even when it is partial, the segregation of different messengers into distinct vesicular compartments makes possible a selective regulation of their release. Transmitter release has been investigated in great detail by electro-physiological recordings at the neuromuscular junction under the explicit premise of a single-transmitter status of the motor neuron. Release of acetylcholine takes place in discrete "paquets" or quanta, which coincide with the acetylcholine content (Kuffler and Yoshikami, 1975) of a single presynaptic vesicle (Katz, 1966).

During physiological transmission several hundreds of quanta are released by a given motor nerve ending. Under resting conditions, single quanta are spontaneously released giving the well known miniature endplate potentials; meanwhile, acetylcholine steadily leaks from the nerve terminal into the cleft and yields an important loss of presynaptic acetylcholine (approximately 10^6 molecules per second) (Katz and Miledi, 1977). In the central nervous system quantal release of neurotransmitter also takes place, but miniature potentials have never been recorded as such. According to Korn and collaborators (1982, 1985), during transmission, a *single* quantum — rather than hundreds — at the most, would be released from a bouton by a presynaptic impulse. Moreover, not all the impulses elicit transmitter release, on average only one third of them do [Eccles]. Then, if in the same varicosity or bouton two populations of vesicles coexist, the probability of release of each kind of vesicle will be directly (but not exclusively) related to the relative abundance of the two categories of vesicles and of their biophysical properties including their size (Llinas and Heuser, 1977). On this basis alone, release of a neuropeptide is expected to occur "less frequently" than that of the "classical" messengers contained in the more abundant small vesicles.

An important outcome of the meeting was in agreement with these reasonings, the demonstration by several groups [Lundberg and Hökfelt; Hökfelt et al.; Potter et al.; Stjärne and Lundberg; Burnstock; Bartfai et al.] with different experimental systems that the firing rate of a neuron regulates the pattern of neurotransmitters released by its nerve endings. In at least three cases, cat salivary gland, pig spleen and mouse vas deferens, bursts of increasing frequency augment the secretion of peptides (VIP, NPY) to a quantity greater than that of conventional transmitters (acetylcholine, noradrenaline) [Lundberg and Hökfelt; Stjärne and Lundberg]. Moreover the firing frequencies used in the stimulation programme to release the peptides ($\sim$4 Hz) are in the range of those occurring in vivo [Stjärne and Lundberg]. Thus the considered nerve terminals are able to *translate* a frequency code into a chemical one [Lundberg and Hökfelt; Hökfelt et al.; Bartfai et al.]. A rather novel and powerful mechanism of information transfer in the nervous system thus results from the coexistence of neuronal messengers.

Dale metabolic unity of the neuron challenged?

Up to this point, all the data presented are consistent with Dale "metabolic unity" of the neuron. Even in the case of the last example discussed, the unity is saved as long as one assumes that the firing of the neuron affects to the same extent, the pattern of transmitters released by all its axonal terminals. But, is this assumption general or are there exceptions?

For the sake of the discussion and in a purely speculative manner, one may consider a neuron having both a highly branched terminal arborisation of its axon and short collaterals proximal to the cell body. At each branch point the probability of a failure in the propagation of the impulse increases and an attenuation may also occur. The "firing" rates at the distal tip of the axonal arborisation and at the end of the proximal collaterals may differ and one may thus hypothesize, that, assuming an even distribution of small and large vesicles throughout the axon, the proximal collaterals will liberate patterns of messengers richer in peptides than the distal branches. Yet, no evidence for such a possibility exists.

Along the same lines, one may further contest, still on strictly theoretical grounds, the assumption just made of an even distribution of the diverse categories of vesicles throughout the different branches of the axon. Without postulating any "traffic policeman" several plausible mechanisms can be envisaged which would lead to their anisotropic distribution. For instance, one may reasonably consider different "retrograde" effects of the diverse target organs on the various sets of axon terminals. Even if they utilize the same neurotransmitter, the axon terminals of the spinal cord motor neurons are expected to differ by their shape and by their mode of transmitter release on the Renshaw cells and on the skeletal muscle fibres. Why not by the relative proportion of the different categories of vesicles? In this system or in analogous ones with multiple targets, retrograde trans-synaptic signals could indeed differentially regulate the turnover and/or local supply of particular categories of vesicles as they affect the number of axon endings during development (see Changeux and Danchin, 1976; Gouzé et al., 1983; Cowan et al., 1984). Differential axonal transport per se may also contribute to an anisotropic distribution of vesicles in proximal and distal branches of the axon (see Ochs et al., 1978). None of these still strictly hypothetical alternatives has yet received experimental support but deserves a closer look.

Cybernetics of multiple signalling by coexisting neuronal messengers

Diversity of intercellular signalling

A straightforward consequence of the coexistence of multiple messengers in a given neuron is an increase of its abilities to communicate with other cells and, eventually, with itself. As long as complementary "receptors" exist on the target cells, the disposal of a large repertoire of chemical species multiplies its coding facilities. A priori, the more messengers a neuron produces, the more exchanges of information and thus computations become accessible to the network to which it belongs. An important limit, however, comes from the fact that even if some anisotropy exists in the patterns of messengers released (for instance between proximal and distal branches) most of them are usually coreleased by the same terminal and thus, at least at the level of the nerve ending, "chemical addressing" [Iversen] will largely coincide with "anatomical addressing". As a consequence, an unlimited growth of the number of messengers in the *same* synaptic channel will soon result in a chemical "noise" (or "soup"! [Iversen]) rather than in an enrichment of coding means. An "optimal" number of coexisting messengers may thus exist but, of course, looks difficult to evaluate in the present state of understanding communications in the nervous system.

Furthermore, the action of chemical messengers as relays of electrical signals imposes specific physical constraints on them. Once emitted, a chemical signal propagates by *diffusion*. As a consequence, its local concentration sharply declines with distance and its diffusion rate decreases as the inverse of the molecular weight square root. Peptides will thus reach their target slower than conventional transmitters (e.g. approximately three times between substance P and acetylcholine).

Moreover, the kinetics of the intrinsic response of the post-synaptic target cell may vary sometimes by several *orders of magnitude* between coreleased messengers, even with the same messenger [Stjärne and Lundberg; Branton et al.]. For instance, in frog sympathetic ganglion, acetylcholine elicits fast excitatory (30–50 msec), slow excitatory (30–60 sec) and slow inhibitory (1–2 sec) post-synaptic potentials while a LHRH-like peptide mediates a late slow (several minutes) excitatory post-synaptic potential [Branton et al.].

The coreleased messengers may thus contribute to distinct *modes* of communication:

In one extreme case or *"synaptic mode"* (e.g. acetylcholine at the neuromuscular junction or GABA and the amino-acid transmitters in central synapses), the confinement of the transmitter in the synaptic cleft is such that its local concentration rises very quickly (<1 msec) to high molar concentration (10^{-4}–10^{-3} M for acetylcholine) resulting in a fast and reversible transmission with short synaptic delay (0.3–0.5 msec) and no refractory period. The surface of the responsive post-synaptic target is also expected to coincide with that of the nerve ending.

In the other extreme case or *"endocrine mode"* (e.g. peptide hormones), the target sites are localised at large distances from the emission point and dispersed throughout the organism and the messengers reach them after seconds or minutes, there acting at concentrations in the nano to picomolar range.

In between, we have the case of the catecholamines, peptides and many other messengers which are released by multiple *"varicosities"* scattered in a diffuse manner among groups of target cells. Local diffusion at the scale of the cell (or tissue) then plays an important role in signal transfer (see Faber et al., 1985). This is for instance the case of the LHRH-like peptide released by sympathetic fibres in frog ganglion which does not act on the closely apposed C cells but on the nearby B cells to which it freely diffuses over tens of microns [Branton et al.].

As pointed out by Iversen [this volume], depending on the system, the same compound may contribute to different modes of signalling and for a given nerve ending, the different messengers coreleased may serve as signals operating via distinct transmission modes. The topological and functional relationships between the point of emission of the coexisting messengers and their targets, consequently follows a variety of schemes.

A first simple one, in principle, is that of *divergent and independent* "transmission lines" where the coreleased messengers affect diverse target cells or organs where they interact with distinct and independent receptors. This may occur — without being the rule — in the endocrine mode of signal transmission, e.g. from the adrenal medulla [Viveros] or from the neurosecretory neurons of the hypothalamus [Swanson et al.].

A more frequently encountered scheme is that of *convergent and interacting* paths *within* a given synapse or "varicose" contact ("homosynaptic" interaction) or *between* different synapses or varicosities ("heterosynaptic" interaction). Figure 2 illustrates some of the regulatory circuits which might plausibly be involved in these interactions.

(1) At the *pre-synaptic level,* the coexisting messengers once released may exert feedback inhibition on their own liberation by acting on "autoreceptors" (6, 8, Fig. 2) but also cross-inhibition on that of their coexisting partners (9, Fig. 2). This is, for instance, the case of NPY which inhibits vas deferens neurally evoked contractions most probably by blocking noradrenaline and ATP release [Lundberg and Hökfelt; Hökfelt et al.; Stjärne and Lundberg; Håkanson] or of acetylcholine and VIP which both auto- and cross-inhibit each others release in cat submandibular gland [Lundberg and Hökfelt; Hökfelt et al.; Bartfai et al.].

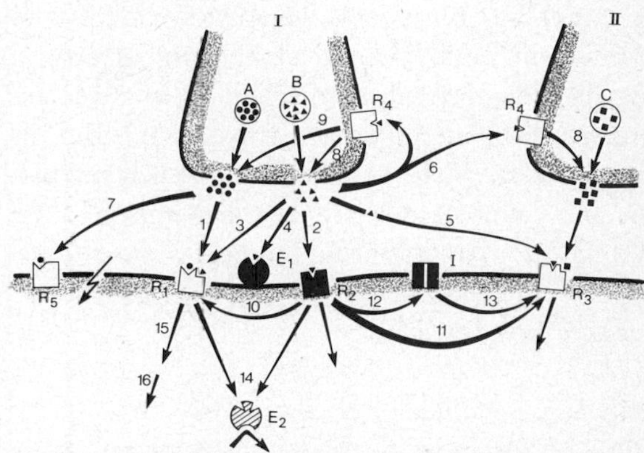

Fig. 2. Diagrammatic representation of signalization pathways possibly associated with neuronal messengers coexistence. Many of them are still largely hypothetical. A, B and C are the coexisting messengers represented here (for clarity) as stored independently in separate populations of vesicles (which is *not* necessarily the rule). Also, messenger B is arbitrarily shown as eliciting more regulatory interactions (2, 3, 4, 5, 6, 10, 11, 12, 14) than B (1, 7, 14, 15, 16), again, to simplify the picture. R_1 to R_5 are receptors for the messengers which are either subsynaptic (R_1–R_3), non-synaptic (R_5) and presynaptic (R_4). I is an ion channel, E_1 a messenger degradative enzyme and E_2 an allosteric cytoplasmic enzyme. For discussion, see text.

(2) At the level of a *degradative enzyme* (4, Fig. 2) one coexisting messenger may inhibit the degradation of the other. This is possibly the case for the calcitonin-gene-related-peptide which inhibits the degradation of substance P by an enzyme isolated, however, from the cerebrospinal fluid (Le Greves et al., 1985) [Hökfelt et al.].

(3) At the *post-synaptic level* (1–3, 5, 7, 10, 14, Fig. 2), many examples of functional interactions between coexisting messengers have been reported [see Hökfelt et al.; Fuxe et al.; Agnati et al.]. In general, they are "co-operative" or "synergistic" such as between acetylcholine and neuropeptide Y in cat blood vessels [Lundberg and Hökfelt], noradrenaline, ATP and neuropeptide Y in mouse or rat vas deferens [Lundberg and Hökfelt; Stjärne

and Lundberg; Burnstock; Håkanson], CCK and dopamine in brain [Agnati et al.] and in several other physiological situations said to involve "receptor-receptor interactions" [Fuxe et al.]. But, as pointed out by V. Mutt [discussion], such interactions may not necessarily be "synergistic" and could adopt an antagonistic mode.

Molecular cybernetics

Elementary regulatory interactions

One of the most positive consequences of coexistence is, thus, the possibility of creating interactions between communication lines both within a given synapse and between synapses and on both the pre- and post-synaptic sides. At the molecular level, these interactions are expected to take place between a minimum of two distinct categories of components:

(1) *The regulatory signals,* which carry and propagate the information and may consist, on the outside of the cells, of the coexisting messengers (classical neurotransmitters, peptides, ATP, ions ...), within the membrane, of the electrical potential and, inside the cell, of *intracellular second "messengers",* such as cyclic nucleotides (cAMP, cGMP), Ca^{2+} ions, diacylglycerol and phosphatidyl-inositol etc. [Iversen]. In this intracellular signalling, phosphorylation-dephosphorylation reactions may play a fundamental role [Agnati et al.] (Krebs and Beavo, 1983; Nestler and Greengard, 1984).

(2) *Specialized proteins* which act as "transducers", recognize, (or are sensitive to) the various kinds of regulatory signals, possess a biological activity, and mediate the interaction between the sites for the regulatory signals and the biologically active site. Models of such regulatory proteins are "classical" allosteric proteins such as haemoglobin (Baldwin and Chothia, 1979), regulatory enzymes such as phosphorylase b (Fletterick and Madsen, 1980) or aspartate transcarbamylase (Krause et al., 1985) and DNA binding proteins like gene repressors (Anderson et al., 1984) or activators (de Combrugghe et al., 1984) or hormone receptors (Ullrich et al., 1985), where the interactions between topographically distinct sites (Changeux, 1961; Monod et al., 1963, 1965) are mediated by conformational transitions of the protein molecule usually between a small number of discrete states (Monod et al., 1965). In general, these proteins exhibit "threshold responses" due to positive cooperative interactions for ligand binding, which are assigned to the cooperative assembly of their constitutive subunits into symmetrical oligomers (Monod et al., 1965).

These concepts have been extended to the proteins involved in intercellular communication typified, in the nervous system, by the receptors for neurotransmitters (Changeux, 1966; Changeux et al., 1967, 1984a; Karlin, 1967; Changeux, 1981) which bind transmitters on their external face, intracellular signals on their cytoplasmic face, can be sensitive to electric fields and can possess, as biologically active site, either a transmembrane ion channel (ionotropic action), or an enzyme catalytic site (metabotropic action) oriented towards the inside of the cell (review Changeux et al., 1984a; Snyder, 1984) [Eccles]. Yet, only a few membrane receptors have been studied at the molecular level. They include among others the acetylcholine receptor (see Changeux et al., 1984a; Popot and Changeux, 1984; Lindström, 1984; Karlin, 1983; see also Cold Spring Habor Symp. Quant. Biol. 47, 1983), the receptors for GABA (Barnard et al., 1983) and glycine (Pfeiffer et al., 1984), the acetylcholine muscarinic receptor (Sokolovsky, 1984) and the receptors for the low density lipoprotein (Yamamoto et al., 1984) and insulin (Ullrich et al., 1985). Thus, the interpretation in terms of allosteric effects of the data reported at the Symposium at the level of receptors for coexisting neuronal messengers is, at this stage, speculative and should only be taken as a plausible working hypothesis.

Direct allosteric interactions

Agnati, Fuxe and collaborators [this volume] have reported several examples of changes in the equilibrium binding affinity and/or maximum binding capacity of various radioactive "classical" neurotransmitters or related compounds in the presence of coexisting peptides. They include among many examples the effect of substance P on [^{3}H]serotonine binding to spinal cord membranes, of CCK-8 on [^{3}H]spiperone binding to dopamine D_2 receptors in striatal membranes among many others (see also [Hökfelt et al., Olasmaa and Terenius, Goldstein et al., Bartfai et al.]). Such "receptor-receptor interactions" can be altered in pathological states such as genetic hypertension, 6-OH dopamine denervated striatum and in the aged rat [Agnati et al.]. They may represent a basic mechanism for "heterostatic" regulation of synaptic transmission.

These interactions, to a certain extent, recall the allosteric effects of the "non-competitive blockers" on the equilibrium binding of [^{3}H]acetylcholine to the nicotinic receptor (Fig. 3) (Cohen et al., 1974; Heidmann et al., 1983; Changeux et al., 1984a) which take place in vitro in the absence of additional energy source, and are mediated by reversible conformational transitions of the receptor molecule. Two types of structural relationships can thus be envisaged concerning the binding sites involved.

Model 1: the sites are carried by the same oligomeric protein which resists solubilisation by non-denaturing detergents;

Model 2: they belong to distinct protein species which interact directly with the membrane, possibly via the lipid phase, and are dispersed by non-denaturing detergents.

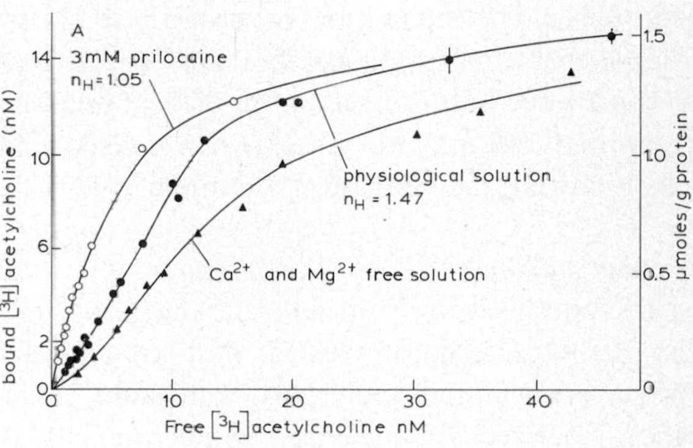

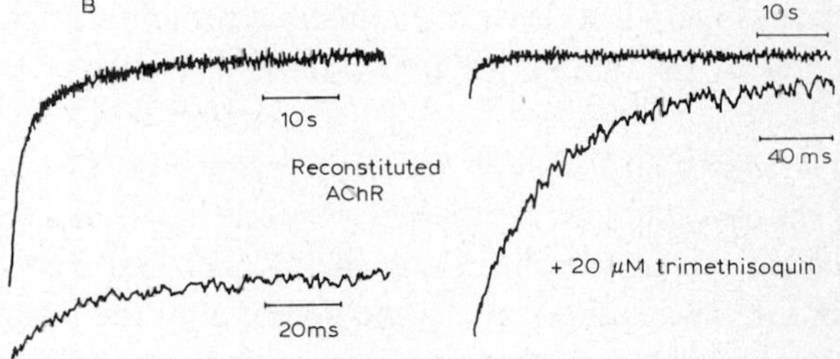

Fig. 3. Allosteric effects of two non-competitive blockers (prilocaïne and trimethisoquin) and of Ca^{2+} ions on the binding properties of the membrane bound (A) and purified lipid reconstituted (B) acetylcholine receptor. (A) The *equilibrium* binding curve of acetylcholine is shifted to higher affinities without change in the total number of sites by divalent cations and prilocaïne; in the presence of prilocaïne the Hill coefficient (n_H) decreases from 1.47 to 1.05. (From Cohen et al., 1974.) (B) *Rapid binding kinetics* of the fluorescent agonist DNS C6 Cho (dansyl-choline) (Waksman et al., 1976) to the lipid reconstituted receptor *before* (left) and *after* (right) equilibration with trimethisoquin; the traces are shown at two time scales; the fast binding takes place at the level of the high affinity conformation of the receptor which corresponds to about 20% of the receptor mole cules at rest. This fraction becomes larger than 90% in the presence of trimethisoquin. (From Changeux et al., 1979.)

Model 1 applies to the nicotinic receptor (Changeux et al., 1984a) and to the GABA-benzodiazepine receptor [E. Costa et al.]. In this last system, the benzodiazepines increase, in an allosteric manner, the apparent number of sites (B_{max}) for high affinity GABA binding and this effect is blocked by an endogenous peptide which also displaces benzodiazepines from their recognition sites. The covalent structure of the peptide is known [E. Costa et al.] and it has been located in GABAergic neurons though not exclusively. The benzodiazepine and GABA binding sites copurify until homogeneity and are thus carried by a single protein species to which the colocalized peptide also binds.

Model 2 fits the data reported by Olasmaa and Terenius [this volume] about the receptors for VIP and for neuropeptide Y and the β-adrenoreceptor which make transmembrane complexes with adenylate cyclase and the excitatory GTP binding protein N_S. The interaction between these diverse components from frontal cerebral cortex have been "reconstituted" after inactivation of the cyclase by membrane fusion with Friend erythroleukaemia cells following the method of Schramm (1979).

Indirect coupling

The alternative to a structural "allosteric" coupling between receptor sites for multiple neuronal messengers is an intermolecular "à distance" interaction mediated, for instance, by electric fields or internal second messengers, but such systems nevertheless include at least one allosteric protein to "integrate" the coupling signals.

(a) Electrical coupling (broken arrow Fig. 2) occurs in a standard manner as a simple consequence of the integrative properties of the neuronal membrane. The changes of electric potential of the post-synaptic cell may then regulate the properties of its receptors. In the case of the acetylcholine receptor, electric fields do affect both channel opening and desensitization (Takeyasu et al., 1983; Hess et al., 1983) and have been shown to cause short-term changes of efficacy mostly by regulating desensitization (Magleby and Pallota, 1981) in vivo, at the motor endplate and under near to physiological conditions.

(b) Chemical coupling. The secund messengers produced by the activation of ion-channels and/or receptors may mediate interactions between receptors and/or ion channels (10, 11, 12, 13, Fig. 2) in a rapidly reversible (Ca^{2+}) or covalent (phosphorylation) manner. Kandel and collaborators (refs. in [Castellucci et al.]) have offered experimental evidence for such coupling in *Aplysia* neurons. According to their views, the basic elementary mechanism which underlies classical conditioning is the enhanced release of transmitter from the sensory nerve endings which results from the joint firing of the sensory neuron and activation of a serotonin-sensitive adenylate cyclase present in the same nerve endings. Abrams et al. (1983) have proposed that a "synergism" occurs at the level of the serotonine-sensitive adenylate cyclase. There, the intracellular calcium ions which enter the nerve terminal by the Na^+ channel during the action potential would augment the production of cAMP via Ca^{2+}-calmodulin binding to adenylate cyclase. As a result, the cyclase now responds more efficiently to the neurotransmitter (serotonin?) by means of the GTP binding protein.
In the same system [Castellucci et al.], serotonin, as just mentioned, facilitates the release of transmitter from the sensory neuron by increasing the level of cAMP. A similar increase results from the binding of two distinct peptides SCPA and SCPB to their receptors on the sensory neuron. The cAMP produced in these three instances activates a common cAMP-dependent protein-kinase which itself phosphorylates a specific K^+ channel or S channel and thereby blocks it.

A similar, though more complex and still less detailed model, has been suggested by Iversen [this volume] to account for the secretory response of pancreatic acinar cells to multiple classes of secretagogues. Acting through distinct cell surface receptors, some agonists (acetylcholine, CCK, bombesin, substance P) regulate secretion by mobilising intracellular calcium, others (VIP, glucagon) by increasing cAMP. The two pathways converge onto a common secreting mechanism but their actual common target molecule is not known yet (14, Fig. 2).

A molecular model for multiple signals integration based on the allosteric properties of the acetylcholine receptor

In the network of interactions mediated by coexisting messengers, allosteric proteins and particularly receptors play the role of "critical knots". One of them, the nicotinic receptor from the electric organ of fishes and vertebrate neuromuscular junction has been studied in great detail (its complete primary structure is known in *Torpedo californica*; Noda et al., 1983a,b,c) and may serve as model for the transduction and integration of multiple signals at the *sub-molecular* level (Changeux et al., 1984a, 1983).

This heterologous pentamer ($\alpha_2\ \beta\ \gamma\ \delta$) of four different, though homologous, subunits (of exact protein molecular weight α = 50,116; β = 53,279; γ = 56,279; δ = 57,565; Noda et al., 1982, 1983a,b,c) make a transmembrane "bundle" with a rotational axis of quasi-symmetry perpendicular to the plane of the membrane (Bon et al., 1984; Brisson and Unwin, 1985). The molecule contains, in all, the ion channel and the structural elements required for the regulation of its opening by acetylcholine (see Schindler et al., 1984; Mishina et al., 1984; Popot and Changeux, 1984). It carries the two main acetylcholine binding sites at the level of the α subunits but, in addition, *other* categories of *"allosteric sites"* which affect the properties of the acetylcholine binding sites and/or the opening of the ion channel. These sites might, *potentially* be used as regulatory sites for coexisting messengers, yet such a physiological role has not been demonstrated. Some of them bind the already mentioned (Fig. 3) "non-competitive blockers" which include local anaesthetics, chlorpromazine, phencyclidine, the frog toxin histrionicotoxin ... (review Changeux, 1981; Heidmann et al., 1983), others bind Ca^{2+} and multivalent cations (Fig. 3) (see Rübsammen et al., 1978; Heidmann and Changeux, 1979; Oswald, 1983), other opiate-like substances (Oswald et al., 1984) (in *Torpedo* receptor). Substance P also affects the response to acetylcholine of cells derived from the neural crest (Stallcup and Patrick, 1980; Clapham and Neher, 1984). The δ, γ and α chains, and possibly all of the chains, contribute to the binding of these allosteric ligands (see Changeux et al., 1984a for discussion).

Rapid mixing experiments and an extensive series of biophysical measurements with the membrane-bound and/or purified receptor have led to the resolution in vitro of a cascade of conformational transitions which regulate the ability of the receptor molecule to be activated and are referred to as "desensitization": (a *fast* one, at the rate of 2–75 per sec and a *slow* one at the rate of 0.01–0.1 per sec; review Changeux et al., 1984a; Hess et al., 1983). The agonists, including acetylcholine, the non-competitive blockers, Ca^{2+}, ions electric fields affect these transitions (Takeyasu et al., 1983) and the experimental data are accounted for by a "four-state" model (Neubig and Cohen, 1980; Heidmann and Changeux, 1980) which is an adapted version of the concerted model for allosteric transitions of globular regulatory proteins (Monod et al., 1965) and of that proposed in a different context by Katz and Thesleff (1957) for pharmacological desensitization. According to this *minimal* scheme, the activation reaction, which corresponds to the fast opening of the ion channel, would concern low affinity states, with a K_d which fits with the *high local concentration* of acetylcholine in the synaptic cleft during transmission (0.1–1 mM). The desensitization reaction on the other hand, would be mediated by higher affinity states with the channel closed, some of them with a K_d in the range of the non-quantal *leak concentration* of acetylcholine in the cleft (10 nM) (Katz and Miledi, 1977).

This scheme has been simplified and presented as a possible mechanism of regulation of efficacy of central receptors (Heidmann and Changeux, 1982; Changeux and Heidmann, 1985; Fig. 4). The basic postulate is that the response efficacy of central receptors is governed by the ratio of a minimum of two conformations of the receptor: an activable A and an inactivable (desensitized) I which are discrete, present before ligand binding, and interconvertible within a time scale several orders of magnitude longer than that of the activation reaction. They differ by their relative affinities for the various classes of ligands binding to the receptor, by the oriented electrical dipolar moment of the protein, and, of course, by the biological activity which characterizes the A state (channel opening, enzyme activation). Binding of the different categories of ligands shifts the $A \rightleftharpoons I$ equilibrium to an extent determined by their relative affinities to the A and I states, and electric fields affect the transition as a function of the difference in dipole moment between the states. The regulatory signals would thus *select* a conformational state pre-existent to the interaction.

Signals distinct from the principal transmitter, in particular coexisting messengers released from the same or neighbouring nerve ending (or varicosity),

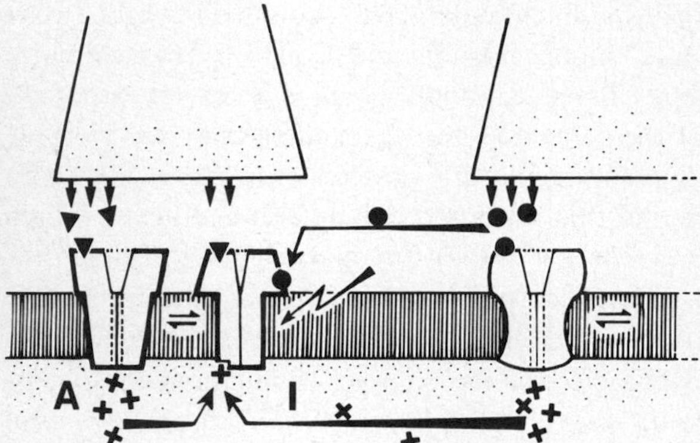

Fig. 4. A model for the regulation of receptor efficacy at the post-synaptic level. The ratio of the unresponsive, or desensitized (I), to the activable, resting (A) conformations determines the "efficacy" and can be regulated by the neurotransmitters from the same (▲) or different (●) synapse or by internal chemical signals (×). (From Changeux et al., 1983.)

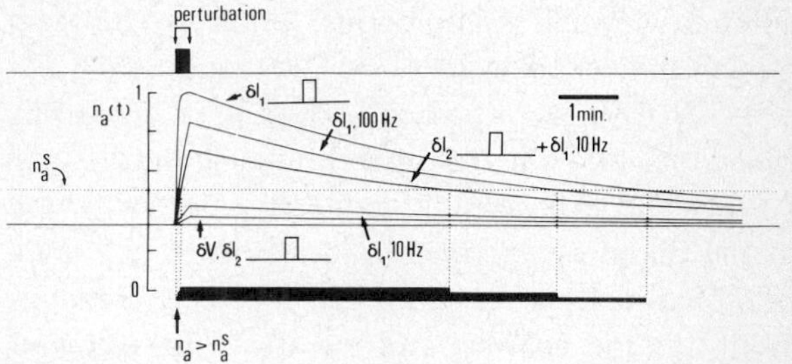

Fig. 5. Computer simulation of the two-state model or regulation of receptor efficacy illustrating the "synergistic" effect of two signals $\delta 1_1$ 10 Hz and $\delta 1_2$ square pulse. The ratio of I to A (n_a) is plotted as a function of time using for the rate constants the values actually measured with the acetylcholine receptor. The perturbation is applied at the indicated time for each signal, independently or simultaneously ($\delta 1_2$ square pulse + $\delta 1_1$ 10 Hz); the independent signals elicit a response which remains under threshold (n_a^s broken line) while their *joint* application triggers a response which lasts about 5 min *beyond* threshold. (From Heidmann and Changeux, 1982.)

internal second messengers produced by nearly located synapses and the electrical potential of the post-synaptic cell would then be able to regulate, in a concerted manner, the efficacy of the considered receptors. The model thus accounts for multiple-signals integration. It has been formalized and computer simulation carried out under different situations of heterosynaptic regulation, which include "classical conditioning" (Heidmann and Changeux, 1982; Changeux and Heidmann, 1985). One feature of the model relevant to the problem of coexisting messengers is that it predicts both the synergistic (Fig. 5) and antagonistic interactions noticed between coexisting messengers.

The model can be adapted to the relatively more complex case of the multi-protein receptor systems (see Schramm and Selinger, 1984). The short-term and reversible regulation of receptor properties may also be extended to longer time scales by covalent modifications (such as phosphorylation). It might equally be applied to "ion channels" which are not always viewed as typical allosteric proteins despite the fact that they share many structural and functional properties with channel-linked receptors for neurotransmitters (see Catterall, 1980; Talvenheimo et al., 1983; Noda et al., 1984).

The allosteric transitions of receptors and ion channels, in addition to that of cytoplasmic enzymes, may thus mediate the integration in space and time of multiple signals from both the inside and the outside of the neuron thereby making possible the association of neurons into "assemblies" (see Hebb, 1949) as a consequence, for instance, of a higher level selection by "resonance" (Changeux, 1983a,b; Changeux et al., 1984b; Heidmann et al., 1984; see also Edelman and Finkel, 1984 [Agnati et al.]). Such regulations would themselves involve mechanisms of molecular selection via the stabilisation by neuronal messengers, especially coexisting ones, of particular conformations accessible to diverse though specific allosteric proteins.

Long-term selection of receptor topology

Anisotropy of surface receptors distribution

Few, if any commentator of the Dale model has ever understood in literal sense the statement that "any one class of nerve cells operates at all its *synapses* by the same *chemical transmission* mechanism" [Eccles]. In this sentence, the word "synapses" means axon terminal and "chemical transmission mechanism" means neurotransmitter. But, if "synapse" is replaced by post-synaptic membrane and "chemical transmission" by receptor for neurotransmitter, then the proposition is no longer valid and, by the same token, the metabolic unity of the neuron loses its generality. Viewed from its "reception" rather than from its "emission" side, the surface of the neuron is, indeed, compartimented into vast domains (dendritic, somatic, axonal) with different chemical specificities and these domains are themselves fragmented into patches which correspond to the post-synaptic areas of the many different synapses converging on the neuron. In other words, *the surface of the neuron is highly anisotropic* (see Ramon y Cajal, 1909–1911).

The anisotropy of receptor distribution has been investigated by quantitative autoradiography at the E.M. level in the case of the electromotor synapse (Bourgeois et al., 1972, 1973, 1978) and of the motor endplate (review Salpeter et al., 1984). There, the surface density of the acetylcholine receptor reaches 5–15,000 molecules (with 2 α-bungarotoxin sites) per μm^2 under the nerve terminal and abruptly falls 100 to 1000-fold, at a distance of less than a μm from the nerve endings. A similar highly anisotropic distribution has been reported in peripheral and central neurons using microphysiological mapping (Kuffler et al., 1970; Roper et al., 1975) or immunocytochemical methods at the E.M. level (Triller et al., 1985). In the case of the electromotor synapse and in that of the neuromuscular junction, the absolute density of receptor coincides almost exactly with a monolayer of closely packed receptor molecules. If this disposition still holds for central synapses, then how does it account for the complex post-synaptic responses to multiple cotransmitters.

Several possibilities may be envisaged:

(1) The post-synaptic membrane is, as in the case of the motor endplate, a *one-protein* membrane, but the receptor protein carries multiple classes of allosteric sites with different specificities as in the case of the acetylcholine or GABA receptors (despite the fact that in these systems the functional relationship of these sites with coexisting messengers remains speculative) (see section on Corelease or differential release of coexisting neuronal messengers, p. 381).

(2) The post-synaptic membrane is a dense mosaic of *different* species of receptor molecules with pharmacological specificities complementary to that of the coexisting messengers. This raises the question of the assembly mechanism of this heterogeneous population of molecules.

(3) The nerve endings engaged in the functional release of multiple messengers form "loose" synaptic contacts or varicosities which let neuronal messengers diffuse over areas which extend beyond the surface of the nerve endings to uncovered areas of the neuronal surface containing multiple species of receptors (see [Hökfelt et al.; Agnati et al.; Castellucci et al.]), and even up to the post-synaptic membrane of neighbouring synapses (see [Branton et al.] and Faber et al., 1985).

Presence of multiple receptor species diffusely distributed over non-synaptic areas has indeed been reported in several systems such as the giant somas of *Aplysia* neurons (Tauc and Gerschenfeld, 1961, 1962; review Kandel, 1976), nerve cells in culture and central neurons [Hökfelt et al.]. More intriguing from a molecular point of view are situations (1) and (2) of highly localized and dense accumulations of receptors with different specificities. In the simple case of the peripheral nicotinic synapse, several classes of components have been claimed to play a role in the maintenance of the post-synaptic membrane architecture:

(1) On the cleft side, the *basal lamina* which in regeneration experiments, may elicit the clustering of the acetylcholine receptor in the absence of nerve (Nitkin et al., 1983; Sanes and Chiu, 1983).

(2) On the cytoplasmic side, a peripheral protein of molecular weight 43,000 v_1 which binds in stoichiometric amounts to the inner face of the ace-

tylcholine receptor (Sobel et al., 1977; Cartaud et al., 1981; Nghiêm et al., 1983; review in Changeux, 1981 and Cartaud et al., 1983). The 43,000 protein immobilizes the receptor, stabilizes it against thermal denaturation and may serve as an intermediate piece for the attachment of the cytoskeleton (Cartaud et al., 1983; Kordeli et al., 1986).

(3) Cell adhesion molecules (or CAM) (Edelman, 1985) which might possibly "bridge" the pre- and post-synaptic membranes (Rieger et al., 1985; Covault and Sanes, 1985).

The equivalent, in central synapses, could be the complex "densities" which underlie the post-synaptic membrane (see Carlin and Siekevitz, 1983) despite their rather complex chemical composition.

Assemblage of the post-synaptic membrane during motor endplate development

The genesis of the post-synaptic membrane has been investigated in detail, in the case of the motor endplate both in situ and in cell cultures (review Fambrough, 1979; Changeux, 1981; Reiness and Weinberg, 1981; Bennett, 1983; Merlie and Sanes, 1985). Before the arrival of the exploratory axons, the acetylcholine receptor is uniformly distributed on the myotube surface, exhibits significant lateral motion and is metabolically labile (half life: 18 h). Immediately after the growth cone contact, the density of receptors rises under the developing motor nerve ending and progressively becomes immobilized and metabolically stable (half life 11 days in the adult). Meanwhile, the extra junctional receptor disappears, acetylcholinesterase accumulates in the cleft and the channel mean open time of the receptor shortens from about 3 to 1 msec (except in birds) (review Changeux, 1981). The precise contribution of the basal lamina (Sanes and Chiu, 1983), of the 43,000 protein and of a newly discovered epsilon-subunit of the acetylcholine receptor (Takai et al., 1985) in this developmental process remains to be established.

Models have been proposed to account for both the formation of focal aggregates of acetylcholine receptor and the establishment of regular patterns of patches of receptors (as in the case of slow muscles such as avian ALD) (see Stent, 1973; Changeux and Danchin, 1976; Changeux et al., 1981; Fraser and Poo, 1982; Fraser, 1985; Schmidt, 1985). All of them are based on the management of a *fixed and limited stock* of embryonic receptors via lateral diffusion and aggregation-stabilization reaction of the receptor. The Stent model assumes that the degradation rate of the receptor is controlled by electric fields: "clamping" by the post-synaptic potential would protect against the "nocive" effect of the muscle action potential. Despite its elegance, this model has not received experimental support. The other models are based either on the electro-migration of the receptor (Fraser and Poo, 1982) or on chemical modification (phosphorylation) and/or association with the already mentioned peripheral proteins (basal lamina, 43,000 protein) elicited by "anterograde" signals (Changeux and Danchin, 1976; Changeux et al., 1981) released by the developing axon terminal in conjunction with "tangential" signals produced by neighbouring endplates and propagated either within the muscle membrane or via the cytoplasm. Selection operates among diverse and transient patterns of receptor *topologies*. Disappearance of the non-junctional receptor then results from exhaustion of the stock of receptors associated with its incorporation into the competing endplates in development.

A large body of experimental evidence further shows that, after a rapid onset, the biosynthesis of the non-junctional acetylcholine receptor stops at the moment the developing endplates become functional (review Fambrough, 1979; Klarsfeld and Changeux, 1985). This repression of acetylcholine receptor biosynthesis by the electrical activity of the muscle cell creates "the fixed and limited stock" of receptor mentioned above and can be reproduced in vitro. It manifests itself by an up to 15-fold difference in mRNA content between electrically active and silent chick muscle cells (Klarsfeld and Changeux, 1985) (Fig. 6). But, in adult muscle fibres, incorporation of acetylcholine receptor

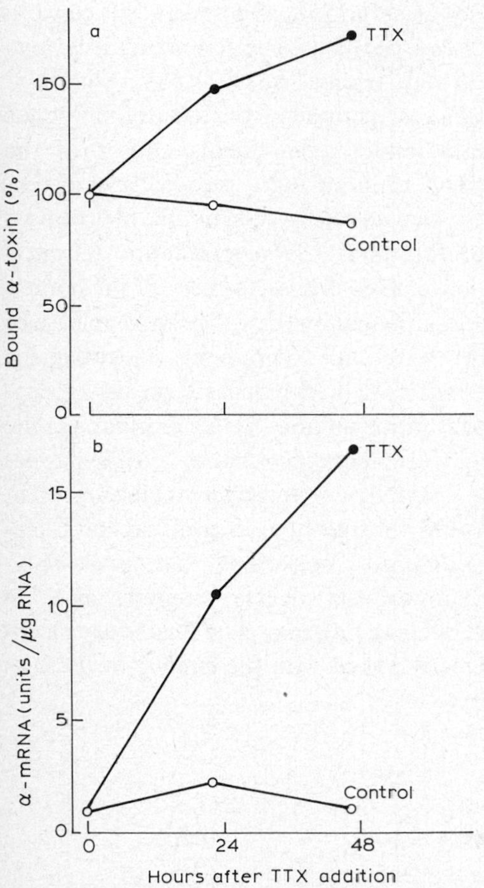

Fig. 6. Consequences of blocking the spontaneous activity of chick skeletal muscle cells in culture by tetrodotoxin (TTX) on the levels of acetylcholine receptor *protein* (assayed with α-[^{125}I]bungarotoxin) (a) and or α-subunit *mRNA* (assayed by hybridization on Northern blots) (b). (From Klarsfeld and Changeux, 1985.)

molecules persist in the mature endplates and accumulation of specific acetylcholine receptor mRNA has been detected at their level (Merlie and Sanes, 1985) raising the possibility of a differential transcription of receptor subunit genes by nuclei near to and far from the endplates.

Another important epigenetic regulation concerns acetylcholinesterase which does not accumulate at the endplate when the synapse is blocked by a curare-like agent (Giacobini et al., 1973; review Massoulié and Bon, 1982).

Ca^{2+} ions and/or cyclic nucleotides have been proposed as internal second messengers in these regulations (see Betz and Changeux, 1979; Rubin et al., 1980; Birnbaum et al., 1980) and may (or not) be identical with those which take part in the regulation of expression of the transmitter phenotype [Black et al.] (see section on Coexistence as a selected state of neuronal differentiation, p. 377).

A model for the long-term selection of receptor distribution in neurons

The extension of the mechanisms investigated with the motor endplate to the development of the neurono-neuronal synapse still remains speculative (see Kuffler et al., 1971 *but* Dunn and Marshall, 1985). The situation is, from the beginning, far more complex than at the motor endplate since *several species of receptors* are, in general, synthesized by the same neuron and because the nerve cell receives multiple nerve endings with different patterns of coexisting messengers. The setting up of a highly *anisotropic* distribution of the receptor species with, in addition, a *complementarity* with the coexisting transmitters further requires the intervention of highly sophisticated (but still unknown) epigenetic regulatory mechanisms.

Here again, one may hypothesize that mechanisms of molecular selection play a role but in a long-term time range:

(1) As in the case of the biosynthesis of coexisting messengers, the neurons may synthesize a pattern of receptor molecules which, in the adult state, corresponds to the selective transcription of a restricted set of genes among a larger group of "open genes" which characterizes the determined state of the considered category (see section on Coexistence as a selected state of neuronal differentiation, p. 377). The regulation of gene expression involved might as well be under the command of the state of activity of the nerve cell (see Kuffler et al., 1971; Schwartz et al., 1983 *but* Dunn and Marshall, 1985 [Agnati et al.]) and of hormonal and "ambient" signals. In other words, the selection of the adult phen-

otype will include the pattern of receptors (and eventually degradative enzymes, see Dunn and Marshall, 1985) synthesized. In all these cases, the regulation will concern the genes present in the *unique* nucleus of the neuron and thus affect the ability of the *whole cell* to synthesize a given pattern of receptors;

(2) The "patchy" distribution of a particular species of receptor on the surface of the neuron, hence, results from *post-transcriptional* processes of local segregation. The model proposed is, that at a critical stage of development of the neuron an additional step of molecular selection, a *topological selection,* takes place at the level of the cytoplasmic membrane and concerns several species of receptors synthesized and incorporated into the membrane. The mechanisms involved might be similar to those proposed for the motor endplate but, of course, require additional hypotheses (see Fig. 7)

A first series of additional hypotheses will concern the factors engaged in this selection. At least two possibilities may be envisaged: (1) there exist multigene *families* of peripheral proteins homologous of the basal lamina components and/or of the 43,000 protein, each having a specificity which coincides with that of the post-synaptic neurotransmitter receptor; then, the post-synaptic selection would simply consist in the assembly of the matching molecules initiated by the *anterograde* release of some of the "external" components (including the neurotransmitter itself and eventual coexisting peptides) present in the afferent nerve terminal; (2) the "peripheral" proteins (pre- and/or post-synaptic) are largely *ubiquitous,* coded by a small number of genes and thus "shared" by different receptor species; but "consensus" sequences exist on the polypeptide chains of the diverse receptors and are recognized by these proteins; then regulatory mechanisms, directly linked with the *binding of the neu-*

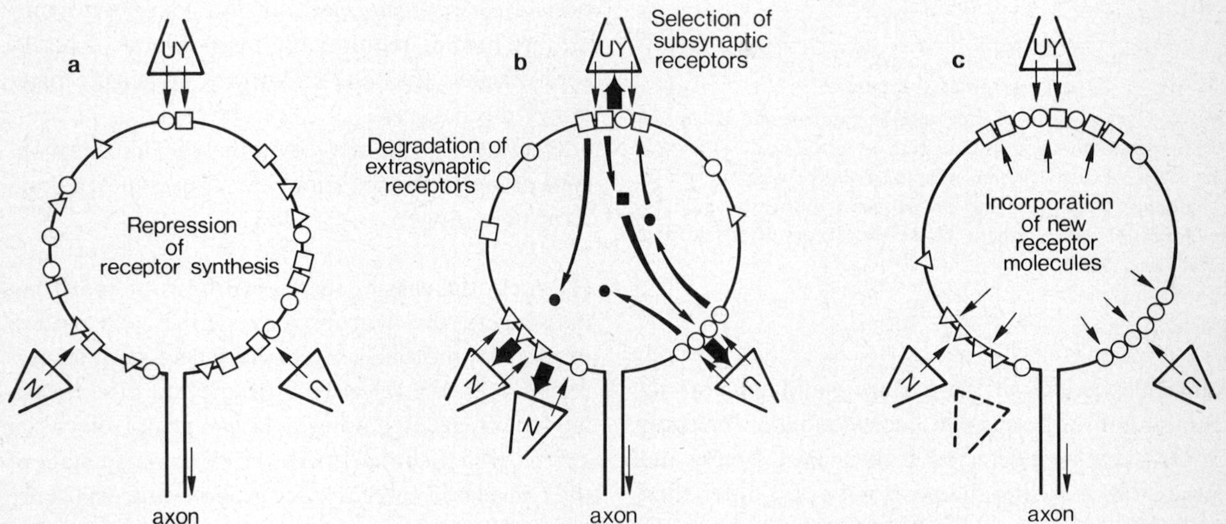

Fig. 7. A model for the selection of complementary receptor topology. Three pre-synaptic messengers (U, Y, Z) are considered. Their complementary post-synaptic receptors (○ for U, □ for Y and △ for N) are spread all over the neuronal soma in the initial stage a, become segregated by selection at the critical stage b and disappear from non-synaptic areas. The neuronal messengers liberated by the nerve endings and/or other anterograde factors may play a role in this process. Later on, in the adulte stage c, new receptor molecules may become incorporated into the areas selected at stage b. Meanwhile the selective stabilization of the afferent nerve endings is assumed to take place via a competition for retrograde signals (thick arrows). (Modified from Changeux and Danchin, 1976.)

rotransmitter to its specific receptor, will determine the local aggregation and stabilization of "activated" or "bound" receptor species.

Tangential signals may also play a role in regulating the development of *patterns* of receptor clusters with the same or different specificities (see Changeux et al., 1981). An interplay between these diverse regulatory signals and assembly processes may then result either in the segregation of one-receptor (or a few receptors) patches or, even, in the absence of their segregation.

A *second series* of hypotheses deals with the maintenance, through turnover, of the subsynaptic membrane with a given receptor specificity in the developing and adult neurons. The metabolic stability of receptors in the mature synapse is expected to be longer (half life: 11 days at the motor endplate) than that of the embryonic receptor but shorter than that of the synapse itself (3 weeks to several months; see Barker and Ip, 1966; Cotman and Nieto-Sampedro, 1984). A local replacement of the degraded receptor molecules with conservation of the transmitter specificity thus takes place in situ. Several models of self-perpetuating organisations have been discussed on the basis of covalent modifications (Crick, 1984) or assembly with peripheral proteins (for discussion see Yéramian and Changeux, 1986). Yet, the mechanisms involved are not known. Does a "channelled" *transport* of specific mRNA (see Steward, 1983) or of already assembled receptor species take place between the neuronal soma and particular dendritic (or even axonal) subsynaptic receptor patches? Does a change of *stability* for a specific receptor mRNA occur near the synapse which utilises the corresponding transmitter? Does a *selection* among *cotransported receptor proteins* occur locally, at the level of the post-synaptic membrane? All these questions are still without any answer.

Finally, to complement post-synaptic receptor selection by autograde signals one may also evoke the possibility of retrograde *trans-synaptic* signalling from the post-synaptic membrane to the nerve endings which would result in the persistence of the particular nerve terminal which matches the receptor specificity of the post-synaptic membrane (Fig. 7 thick arrows). As already mentioned (see p. 392), mechanisms of this type have been proposed, in the case of the neuromuscular junction, to account for the evolution of its motor innervation (Gouzé et al., 1983; Cowan et al., 1984). There again, the mechanisms suggested rely on a competition for the uptake by the active nerve endings of a limited stock of diffusible "retrograde factor". Attempts to isolate the factors involved are being made in chick (see Henderson et al., 1981, 1983). Interestingly, preliminary data suggest that, as for the acetylcholine receptor, the activity of the muscle cell inhibits the production of these factors (Henderson et al., 1986). Also, denervation and paralysis enhance the production by the muscle cells of the cell adhesion molecules N-CAM (Riéger et al., 1985; Covault and Sanes, 1985).

NGF (Levi-Montalcini, 1975; Thoenen and Barde, 1980), and various brain (Barde et al., 1982) and muscle-derived (Manthorpe and Varon, 1985) factors have been extensively investigated for their "neurotrophic" properties and, for some of them, a regulation by activity suggested (see Ebendal et al., 1980 and Henderson, 1986 for discussion). These remarks further extend the suggestion that some of the compounds synthesized by the neuron and here referred to as coexisting "messengers" may exert long-term autograde and retrograde effects.

Phylogenetic origins of the neuronal messengers

Many of the messengers synthesized in the brain are found in the peripheral nervous system where most of them were in fact first discovered and many of the neuronal messengers are synthesized by non--neural cells such as gland cells [Pearse; Roth et al.]. Even more surprising is the observation that an increasing number of them, or closely related molecules, also exist in microbes [Roth et al.] where receptors for these substances may also be found. Some of these microorganisms in particular yeasts and molds utilise peptide messengers or steroid-like molecules for intercellular communication between sex types. Higher plants also produce material related to vertebrate peptide hormones in particular insulin-like and somatostatin-like peptides in spinach [Roth et al.]. These observations raise the question of the functional significance of these messengers in such organisms deprived of nervous system. *A contrario,* would the presence of some of them in higher animal species correspond to the persistence of messengers which played an important role at early stages of the Evolution but, subsequently, became "vestigial organs" or "silent passengers" [Hökfelt et al.]?

In any case, these findings illustrate the remarkable evolutionary *stability* of these messenger molecules and further suggest, that in the course of Evolution their structure and number did not change much but rather their mode of utilization as communication signals. A possibility mentioned by V. Mutt [discussion] is that the molecules first used in "external" communication between microbes subsequently became "internalized" and served as intercellular or even intracellular signals in multicellular organisms (e.g. cAMP) (see also Tomkins, 1975). Such a possibility, among others, suggests that the phylogenesis of the systems of *intra* and *inter*cellular signalling of brain neurons took place with a remarkable *economy* of genetic information. Despite some variability among the different groups and even species of vertebrates noticed in the patterns of coexisting messengers [Hökfelt et al.], this economy looks general. As a counterpart, the development of coexistence of multiple neuronal messengers in the course of Evolution increased the number of coding possibilities for interneuronal signalling (both during morphogenesis and in the adult) thus contributing to make less paradoxical the *remarkable* divergence — particularly striking in mammals — existing between the increase in complexity of the brain and the relative stability of the genome (see Changeux, 1983a,b).

Conclusions

Two main conclusions emerge from the communications presented at the meeting:

(1) The classic view, of the neuron as a rather rigid entity with a unique neurotransmitter, an all-or-none behaviour and a uniform biochemistry has, to a large extent, to be amended. Instead, despite the regularity of many characteristic features, the neuron appears as a flexible and adaptable system, with variable patterns of several messengers synthesized and liberated, with diverse graded responses and a rather "anisotropic" cell surface.

(2) The synthesis and release of multiple coexisting messengers by the neurons increase their possibilities of communicating with each other and with other classes of cells and, in particular, offer opportunities of interactions and cross-regulations between, and within, communication lines.

This novel view of the neuron which justifies the general title of the Symposium points to molecular mechanisms which might be worth further investigating in the near future. They include among others:

(1) The *regulation* of *gene expression* during development and maturation of the neuron and in particular of the genes coding for the neuronal messengers and/or their biosynthetic enzymes, for their release devices, for their receptors and for various "retrograde" neurite growth and differentiation factors.

(2) The network of intracellular and membrane *signals* involved in the regulation of gene expression, at the transcriptional level but also at the level of all the subsequent steps which lead to the final localisation of the messengers release sites in the diverse branches of the axon (and perhaps of the dendrites) and of their receptors on the whole surface of the neuron. Elucidation of the role played by the activity (electrical and chemical, spontaneous and evoked) of the neurons and of their target cells in these processes may have important implications for the "epigenesis" of neuronal networks and as eventual long-term "learning" mechanisms during development and in the adult.

(3) The elementary regulatory interactions, covalent or not, mediated by *allosteric proteins* throughout these networks at the gene level (repressors, transcription factors), at the membrane level (receptors for neurotransmitters, peptides, growth factors ...) and in between (protein kinases, enzymes of intracellular metabolism ...).

The analysis of these mechanisms might possibly receive some impetus from the models of *molecular selection* presented in several chapters of this Synthesis keeping in mind that these models should always be considered as "provisional" hypotheses at this stage of the research. If the suggested extension of the Selectionist or Darwinist views to the molecular mechanisms involved in the development of the "singularity" of nerve cells have some truth, it is worth noting that they will concern *both* the pattern of messengers *liberated* by the neuron, their biosynthetic enzymes, their storage and release devices *and* the pattern of receptors for the messengers *recognized* by the same neuron which often differ from the former ones (with the notable exception of the "auto-receptors"). In other words, molecular selection will differentially affect the "emission" pole (release of messengers) from the "reception" pole (recognition and transduction of chemical signals) of the neuron considered as an information processing device with a dynamic functional polarity (Ramon y Cajal, 1909–1911). Connection of the two at the level of the unique nucleus and cell soma will insure the adjustment of the biochemical properties of the neuron with its *afferent* and *efferent connectivities* and thus contribute to its higher level of *integration* within the chain or network of cells to which it belongs.

The driving forces for selection at the molecular and subcellular level are still largely unknown. Yet, one may hypothesize that the selection of a particular pattern of chemical messengers synthesized and released by a given neuron is such that the communication networks to which it belongs is "optimized" for: (1) the *coordination* between organs and/or centers within the organism and (2) the *relationships* of the organism with its physical (and eventually social) environment.

Finally, the coexistence of several messengers in populations of neurons critically involved in neurological and/or mental diseases has already important implications in their understanding and their therapy [Hökfelt et al.; Fuxe et al.; Agnati et al.; Bartfai et al.].

Before closing, one should not forget that this Symposium is dedicated to the memory of Ulf Von Euler and Nils-Ake Hillarp who, in many instances, pioneered the field, the first by the identification of several new neuronal messengers, the second by tracing the paths of neurons which produce and liberate some of them. Listening to the presentations at the meeting and reading the chapters of this book convincingly illustrate the liveliness of the tradition of excellence they created in Sweden and the widespread impact of the work they inspired throughout the World.

Acknowledgements

I thank Odile Heidmann, André Klarsfeld and Henri Korn for pertinent remarks and constructive criticisms and Jacqueline Gex and Jocelyne Mesner for carefully typing the manuscript.

References

Abrams, T. W., Carew, T. J., Hawkins, R. D. and Kandel, E. R. (1983) Aspects of the cellular mechanisms of temporal specificity in conditioning in *Aplysia:* preliminary evidence for Ca^{2+} influx as a signal of activity. *Soc. Neurosci. Abstr.*, 9: 168.

Anderson, J., Ptashne, M. and Harrison, S. C. (1984) Cocrystals of the DNA binding domain of phage 434 repressor and a synthetic phage 434 operator. *Proc. nat. Acad. Sci. USA*, 81: 1307–1311.

Baldwin, J. and Chothia, C. (1979) Haemoglobin: the structural changes related to ligand binding and its allosteric mechanism. *J. Mol. Biol.*, 129: 175–220.

Barde, Y. A., Edgar, D. and Thoenen, H. (1982) Purification of a new neurotrophic factor from mammalian brain. *EMBO J.*, 1: 549–553.

Barker, D. and Ip, M. C. (1966) Sprouting and degenerations of mammalian motor axons in normal and deafferented skeletal muscle. *Proc. roy. Soc. Lond. (Biol.)*, 163: 538–554.

Barnard, E. A., Beeson, D., Bilbe, G., Brown, D. A., Constanti, A., Conti-Tronconi, B. M., Dolly, J. O., Dunn, S. M. J., Mehraban, F., Richards, B. M. and Smart, T. G. (1983) Acetylcholine and GABA receptors: Subunits of central and peripheral receptors and their encoding nucleic acids. *Cold Spring Harb. Symp. Quant. Biol.*, 48: 109–124.

Bennett, M. R. (1981) Development of neuromuscular synapses. *Physiol. Rev.*, 63: 915–1048.

Berzelius, J. J. (1835) *Théorie des Proportions Chimiques,* 2ème édition, Didot, Paris.

Betz, H. and Changeux, J. P. (1979) Regulation of muscle acetylcholine receptor synthesis in vitro by derivatives of cyclic nucleotides. *Nature (Lond.)*, 278: 749–752.

Birnbaum, M., Reiss, M. and Shainberg, A. (1980) Role of calcium in the regulation of acetylcholine receptor synthesis in cultured muscle cell. *Pflueger's Arch.*, 385: 37–43.

Bon, F., Lebrun, E., Gomel, J., Van Rappenbusch, R., Cartaud, J., Popot, J. L. and Changeux, J. P. (1984) Image analysis of the heavy form of the acetylcholine receptor from *Torpedo marmorata. J. Mol. Biol.*, 176: 205–237.

Bourgeois, J. P., Ryter, A. M., Menez, A., Fromageot, P., Boquet, P. and Changeux, J. P. (1972) Localisation of the cholinergic receptor protein in eel electroplax by high resolution autoradiography. *FEBS Lett.*, 25: 127–133.

Bourgeois, J. P. Popot, J. L., Ryter, A. and Changeux, J. P. (1973) Consequences of denervation on the distribution of the cholinergic (nicotinic) receptor sites from *Electrophorus electricus* revealed by high resolution autoradiography. *Brain Res.*, 62: 557–563.

Bourgeois, J. P. Popot, J. L., Ryter, A. and Changeux, J. P. (1978) Quantitative studies on the localization of the cholinergic receptor protein in the normal and denervated electroplaque from *Electrophorus electricus. J. Cell. Biol.*, 79: 200–216.

Brahic, M., Haase, A. and Cash, E. (1984) Simultaneous detection of viral RNA and antigens. *Proc. nat. Acad. Sci. USA*, 81: 5445–5448.

Breathnach, R. and Chambon, P. (1981) Organization and expression of eucaryotic split genes coding for proteins. *Ann. Rev. Biochem.*, 50: 349–383.

Brisson, A. and Unwin, P. N. T. (1985) Quaternary structure of the acetylcholine receptor. *Nature (Lond.)*, 315: 474–477.

Brock, M. L. and Shapiro, P. J. (1983) Estrogen regulates the absolute rate of transcription of the *Xenopus laevis* vitellogenin genes. *J. Biol. Chem.*, 258: 5449–5455.

Brown, D. (1984) The role of stable complexes that repress and activate eucaryotic genes. *Cell,* 37: 359–365.

Burch, J. B. and Weintraub, H. (1983) Temporal order of chromatin structural changes associated with activation of the major chicken vitellogenin gene. *Cell,* 33: 65–68.

Carlin, R. and Siekewitz, P. (1983) Plasticity in the central nervous system: do synapses divide? *Proc. nat. Acad. Sci. USA*, 80: 3517–3521.

Carlsson, A., Falck, B. and Hillarp, N. A. (1962) Demonstration of catecholamines with a histochemical fluorescence method. *Acta physiol. Scand.*, 56, suppl. 56: 1–28.

Cartaud, J., Sobel, A., Rousselet, A., Devaux, P. E. and Changeux, J. P. (1981) Consequences of alkaline treatment for the ultrastructure of the acetylcholine-receptor-rich membranes from *Torpedo marmorata* electric organ. *J. Cell. Biol.*, 90: 418–426.

Cartaud, J., Kordeli, C., Nghiêm, H. O. and Changeux, J. P. (1983) La proteine 43,000 daltons: pièce intermédiaire assurant l'ancrage du récepteur cholinergique au cytosquelette sous-neural? *C.R. Acad. Sci. (Paris)*, 297: 285–289.

Catterall, W. A. (1980) Neurotoxins that act on voltage-sensitive sodium channels. *Ann. Rev. Pharmacol. Toxicol.*, 20: 15–43.

Changeux, J. P. (1961) The feedback control mechanism of biosynthetic L-threonine deaminase by L-isoleucine. *Cold Spring Harbor Symp. Quant. Biol.*, 26: 313–318.

Changeux, J. P. (1966) Responses of acetylcholinesterase from *Torpedo marmorata* to salts and curarizing drugs. *Mol. Pharmacol.*, 2: 369–392.

Changeux, J. P. (1972) Le cerveau et l'évènement. *Communications,* 18: 37–47.

Changeux, J. P. (1981) The acetylcholine receptor: An "allosteric" membrane protein. In *Harvey Lectures,* Academic Press Inc., 75, pp. 85–254, New York.

Changeux, J. P. (1983a) *L'Homme Neuronal,* Fayard, Paris. English edition: *Neuronal Man* (1985), Panthéon, New York, 419 pp.

Changeux, P. J. (1983b) Concluding remarks: on the "singularity" of nerve cells and its ontogenesis. *Prog. Brain Res.*, 58: 465–478.

Changeux, J. P. and Danchin, A. (1974) Apprendre par stabilisation sélective de synapses en cours de développement. In: "L'Unité de l'homme". E. Morin and M. Piatteli (Eds.), *Centre Royaumont pour une science de l'homme,* Le Seuil, Paris, pp. 320–357. Ed. E. Morin et M. Piatelli.

Changeux, J. P. and Danchin, A. (1976) Selective stabilization of developing synapses as a mechanism for the specification of neuronal networks. *Nature (Lond.)*, 264: 705–712.

Changeux, J. P. and Heidmann, T. (1985) Allosteric receptors and molecular models of learning. In G. Edelman, W. E. Gall and W. M. Cowan (Eds.), *New Insights into Synaptic Function,* John Wiley Publ., New York (in press).

Changeux, J. P., Thiéry, J., Tung, Y. and Kittel, C. (1967) On the cooperativity of biological membranes. *Proc. nat. Acad. Sci. USA*, 57: 335–341.

Changeux, J. P., Courrège, P. and Danchin, A. (1973) A theory of the epigenesis of neuronal networks by selective stabilization of synapses. *Proc. nat. Acad. Sci. USA,* 70: 2974–2978.

Changeux, J. P., Heidmann, T., Popot, J. L. and Sobel, A. (1979) Reconstitution of a functional acetylcholine regulator under defined conditions. *FEBS Lett.*, 105: 181–187.

Changeux, J. P., Courrège, Ph., Danchin, A. and Lasry, J. M.

(1981) Un mécanisme biochimique pour l'épigénèse de la jonction neuromusculaire. *C.R. Acad. Sci. (Paris)*, 292: 449–453.

Changeux, J. P., Bon, F., Cartaud, J., Devillers-Thiéry, A., Giraudat, J., Heidmann, T., Holton, B., Nghiêm, H. O., Popot, J. L., Van Rapenbusch, R. and Tzartos, S. (1983) Allosteric properties of the acetylcholine receptor protein from *Torpedo marmorata. Cold Spring Harbor Symp. Quant. Biol.*, 48: 35–52.

Changeux, J. P., Devillers-Thiéry, A. and Chemouilli, P. (1984a) The acetylcholine receptor: an allosteric protein engaged in intercellular communication. *Science*, 225: 1335–1345.

Changeux, J. P., Heidmann, T. and Patte, P. (1984b) Learning by selection. In P. Marler and H. S. Terrace (Eds.), *The Biology of Learning*, Springer-Verlag, Berlin, pp. 115–133.

Clapham, D. E. and Neher, E. (1984) Substance P reduces acetylcholine-induced current in isolated bovine chromaffin cells. *J. Physiol. (Lond.)*, 347: 255–277.

Cohen, J. B., Weber, M. and Changeux, J. P. (1974) Effects of local anesthetics and calcium on the interaction of cholinergic ligands with the nicotinic receptor protein from *Torpedo marmorata. Mol. Pharmacol.*, 10: 904–932.

Cotman, C. W. and Nieto-Sampedro, M. (1984) Cell biology of synaptic plasticity. *Science*, 225: 1287–1294.

Covault, J. and Sanes, J. (1985) Neural cell adhesion molecule (N-CAM) accumulates in denervated and paralyzed skeletal muscles. *Proc. nat. Acad. Sci. USA*, 82: 4544–4548.

Cowan, W. M., Fawcett, J. W., O'Leary, D. D. and Stanfield, B. B. (1984) Regressive phenomena in the development of the vertebrate nervous system. *Science*, 225: 1258–1265.

Crick, F. (1984) Memory and molecular turnover. *Nature (Lond.)*, 312: 101.

Dahlström, A. and Fuxe, K. (1964) Evidence for the existence of monoamine containing neurons in the central nervous system. I. Demonstration of monoamines in the cell bodies of brain stem neurons. *Acta Physiol. Scand.*, 62, Suppl. 232: 1–55.

Dahlström, A. and Fuxe, K. (1965) Evidence for the existence of monoamine containing neurons in the central nervous system. II. Experimentally induced changes in the intraneuronal levels of bulbo spinal neuron system. *Acta physiol. Scand.*, 64, Suppl. 247: 5–36.

De Combrugghe, B., Busby, S. and Buc, H. (1984) Activation of transcription by the cyclic AMP receptor protein. In R. Goldberger and T. Yamamoto, *Biological Regulation and Development*, Plenum Press, New York, pp. 129–167.

Dunn, P. M. and Marshall, L. M. (1985) Lack of nicotinic supersensitivity in frogs sympathetic neurons following denervation. *J. Physiol. (Lond.)*, 363: 211–225.

Ebendal, T., Olson, L., Seiger, A. and Hedlund, K. O. (1980) Nerve growth factors in the rat iris. *Nature (Lond.)*, 286: 25–28.

Eccles, J. C. (1957) *The Physiology of Nerve Cells*, Johns Hopkins Press, Baltimore.

Eccles, J. C. (1962) Spinal neurons: synaptic connections in relation to chemical transmitters and pharmacological responses. In B. Uvnäs (Ed.), *Proc. First Inter. Pharmacol. Meeting*, 8: 157–182. Pergamon Press, Oxford.

Edelman, G. M. (1978) The mindful brain. Cortical organization and the group-selective theory of higher brain function. MIT Press, Cambridge, Mass.

Edelman, G. M. (1985) Molecular regulation of neural morphogenes. In G. Edelman, W. E. Gall and W. M. Cowan (Eds.), *Molecular Bases of Neural Development*, John Wiley, New York, pp. 35–60.

Edelman, G. M. and Finkel, L. (1984) Neuronal group selection in the cerebral cortex. In G. Edelman, W. E. Gall and W. M. Cowan (Eds.), *Dynamic Aspects of Neocortical Function*, John Wiley, New York, pp. 653–695.

Faber, D. S., Funch, P. D. and Korn, H. (1985) Evidence that receptors mediating central synaptic potentials extend beyond the postsynaptic density. *Proc. nat. Acad. Sci. USA*, 82: 3504–3508.

Fambrough, D. (1979) Control of acetylcholine receptors in skeletal muscle. *Physiol. Rev.*, 59: 165–227.

Finkel, L. and Edelman, G. M. (1985) Interaction of synaptic modification rules within populations of neurons. *Proc. nat. Acad. Sci. USA*, 82: 1291–1295.

Fletterick, R. J. and Madsen, N. B. (1980) The structures and related functions of phosphorylase a. *Ann. Rev. Biochem.*, 49: 31–61.

Fraser, S. E. (1985) Cell interactions involved in neuronal patterning: an experimental and theoretical approach. In G. M. Edelman, W. E. Gall and W. M. Cowan (Eds.), *Molecular Bases of Neural Development*, John Wiley, New York, pp. 481–508.

Fraser, S. E. and Poo, M. M. (1982) Development, maintenance and modulation of patterned membrane topography: model based on the acetylcholine receptor. *Curr. Top. Dev. Biol.*, 17: 77–100.

Freeman, W. J. (1983) The physiological basis of mental images. *Biol. Psychiatry*, 18: 1107–1125.

Fuxe, K. (1965) Evidence for the existence on monoamine neurons in the central nervous system. IV. The distribution of monoamine nerve terminals in the central nervous system. *Acta physiol. Scand.*, 64, Suppl. 247: 39–85.

Giacobini, G., Filogamo, G., Weber, M., Boquet, P. and Changeux, J. P. (1973) Effects of a snake-neurotoxin on the development of innervated motor muscles in chick embryo. *Proc. nat. Acad. Sci. USA*, 70: 1708–1712.

Gouzé, J. L., Lasry, J. M. and Changeux, J. P. (1983) Selective stabilisation of muscle innervation during development: a mathematical model. *Biol. Cybern.*, 46: 207–215.

Groudine, M. and Weintraub, H. (1981) Activation of globin genes during chicken development. *Cell*, 24: 393–401.

Hamburger, V. (1970) Embryonic motility in vertebrates. In F. O. Schmidt (Ed.), *Neurosciences: Second Study Program*, Rockefeller University Press, New York, pp. 141–151.

Harris, W. A. (1981) Neural activity and development. *Ann. Rev. Physiol.*, 43: 689–710.

Hebb, D. O. (1949) *The Organization of Behavior: A Neuropsychological Theory*, Wiley, New York.

Heidmann, A., Heidmann, T. and Changeux, J. P. (1984) Stabilisation sélective de représentations neuronales par résonance entre 'pré-représentation' spontanées du réseau cérébral et 'percepts' évoqués par interaction avec le monde extérieur. *C.R. Acad. Sci. (Paris)*, 299: Série III, no. 20, 839–844.

Heidmann, T. and Changeux, J. P. (1979) Fast kinetic studies on the interaction of a fluorescent agonist with the membrane-bound acetylcholine receptor from *Torpedo marmorata*. *Europ. J. Biochem.*, 94: 281–296.

Heidmann, T. and Changeux, J. P. (1980) Interaction of a fluorescent agonist with the membrane-bound acetylcholine receptor from *Torpedo marmorata* in the millisecond time range: resolution of an "intermediate" conformational transition and evidence for positive cooperative effects. *Biochem. Biophys. Res. Commun.*, 97: 889–896.

Heidmann, T. and Changeux, J. P. (1982) Un modèle moléculaire de régulation d'efficacité d'un synapse chimique au niveau postsynaptique. *C.R. Acad. Sci. (Paris)*, 295: 665–670.

Heidmann, T., Oswald, R. E. and Changeux, J. P. (1983) Multiple sites of action for non competitive blockers on acetylcholine receptor rich membrane fragments from *Torpedo marmorata. Biochemistry*, 22: 3112–3127.

Henderson, C. E. (1986) Activity and the regulation of neuronal growth factor metabolism. Dahlem Conference on Neural and molecular bases of learning (in press).

Henderson, C. E., Huchet, M. and Changeux, J. P. (1981) Neurite outgrowth from embryonic chicken spinal neurons is promoted by media conditioned by muscle cells. *Proc. nat. Acad. Sci. USA*, 78: 2625–2629.

Henderson, C. E., Huchet, M. and Changeux, J. P. (1983) Denervation increases the neurite-promoting activity in extracts of skeletal muscle. *Nature (Lond.)*, 302: 609–611.

Henderson, C. E., Benoit, P., Guénet, J. L., Huchet, M. and Changeux, J. P. (1986) Increased levels of neurite-promoting activity for spinal neurons in muscles of "paralysé" mice and tenotomised rats. *Devel. Brain Res.*, 25: 65–70.

Hess, G. P., Cash, D. J. and Aoshima, H. (1983) Acetylcholine receptor-controlled ion translocation: chemical kinetic investigations of the mechanism. *Ann. Rev. Biophys. Bioeng.*, 12: 443–473.

Hökfelt, T., Johansson, O., Ljungdahl, A., Lundberg, J. M. and Schultzberg, M. (1980) Peptidergic neurons. *Nature (Lond.)*, 284: 515–521.

Hopfield, J. (1982) Neural networks and physical systems with emergent collective computational abilities. *Proc. nat. Acad. Sci. USA*, 79: 2554–2558.

Jerne, N. (1967) Antibodies and learning: selection versus instruction. In G. C. Quarton, T. Melnechuck and F. O. Schmitt (Eds.), *The Neurosciences*, Rockefeller University Press, New York, pp. 200–205.

Jerne, N. (1985) The generative grammar of the immune system. *EMBO J.*, 4: 847–852.

Johnson, M. H., McConnell, J. and Van Blerkom, J. (1984) Programmed development in the mouse embryo. *J. Embryol. Exp. Morphol.*, 83, Suppl. 197–231.

Kandel, E. (1976) *Cellular Basis of Behavior*, Freeman, San Francisco.

Karlin, A. (1967) On the application of "a plausible model" of allosteric proteins to the receptor for acetylcholine. *J. Theoret. Biol.*, 16: 306–320.

Karlin, A. (1983) Anatomy of a receptor. *Neurosci. Commentaries*, 1: 111–123.

Katz, B. (1966) *Nerve Muscle and Synapse*, McGraw Hill, New York.

Katz, B. and Miledi, R. (1977) Transmitter leakage from motor nerve endings. *Proc. Soc. Lond. B.*, 196: 59–72.

Katz, B. and Thesleff, S. (1957) A study of the "desensitization" produced by acetylcholine at the motor end-plate. *J. Physiol. (Lond.)*, 138: 63–80.

Klarsfeld, A. and Changeux, J. P. (1985) Activity regulates the level of acetylcholine receptor alpha-subunit mRNA in cultured chick myotubes. *Proc. nat. Acad. Sci. USA*, 82: 4558–4562.

Kordeli, C., Cartaud, J., Nghiêm, O. H., Pradel, L. A., Dubreuil, C., Paulin, D. and Changeux, J. P. (1986) Evidence for a polarity in the distribution of proteins from the cytoskeleton in *T. marmorata* electrocytes. *J. Cell. Biol.*, 102: 748–761.

Korn, H. and Faber, D. S. (1985) Regulation and significance of probabilistic release mechanisms at central synapses. In G. M. Edelman, W. E. Gall and W. M. Cowan (Eds.), *New Insights into Synaptic Function*, Wiley, New York (in press).

Korn, H., Mallet, A., Triller, A. and Faber, D. S. (1982) Transmission at a central inhibitory synapse. II. Quantal description of release with a physical correlate for the binominal. *J. Neurophysiol.*, 48: 679–707.

Korn, H., Faber, D. S. and Triller, A. (1985) Probabilistic determination of synaptic strength. *J. Neurophysiol.*, 101: 683–688.

Krause, K., Volz, K. and Lipscomb, W. (1985) Structure at 2.9 A resolution of aspartate carbamoyl transferase complexed with the bisubstrate analogue N-(phosphon-acetyl)-L-aspartate. *Proc. nat. Acad. Sci. USA*, 82: 1643–1647.

Kuffler, S. W. and Yoshikami, D. (1975) The number of transmitter molecules in a quantum: an estimate from iontophoretic application of acetylcholine at the neuromuscular synapse. *J. Physiol. (Lond.)*, 251: 465–482.

Kuffler, S. W., Dennis, M. J. and Harris, A. J. (1971) The development of chemosensitivity in extrasynaptic areas of the neuronal surface after denervation of parasympathetic ganglion cells in the heart of the frog. *Proc. roy. Soc. B.*, 177: 555.

Landis, S. C. (1983) Development of cholinergic sympathetic neurons: evidence for neurotransmitter plasticity in vivo. *Fed. Proc.*, 42: 1633–1638.

Le Greves, P., Nyberg, F., Terenius, L. and Hökfelt, T. (1985) Calcitonin gene related peptide is a potent inhibitor of substance P degradation. *Europ. J. Pharmacol.* (in press).

Levi-Montalcini, R. (1975) NGF: an unchartered route. In *The Neurosciences: Paths of Discovery*, MIT Press, Cambridge, Mass.

Lindström, J. (1984) Nicotinic receptors: use of monoclonal antibodies to study synthesis, structure, function and auto-immune response. In *Monoclonal Antibodies and Anti-idiotypic Antibodies Probes for Receptor Structures and Function*, Liss, New York, pp. 21–57.

Lindström, J., Merlie, J. P. and Yogeeswaran, G. (1979) Biochemical properties of acetylcholine receptor subunits from *Torpedo californica. Biochemistry*, 18: 4465–4470.

Lindström, J., Tzartos, S., Gullick, W., Hochschwender, S., Swanson, L., Sargent, P., Jacob, M. and Montal, M. (1983) Use of monoclonal antibodies to study acetylcholine receptors from electric organs, muscle, and brain and the autoimmune response to receptor in *Myasthenia Gravis. Cold Spring Harbor. Symp. Quant. Biol.*, 48: 89–99.

Llinas, R. R. and Heuser, J. E. (1977) In R. R. Llinas and J. E. Heuser (Eds.), *Depolarization-release Coupling System in Neurons. Neurosci. Res. Prog. Bull.*, 15: 4, MIT Press, Boston, Mass.

Magleby, K. L. and Pallotta, B. S. (1981) A study of desensitization of acetylcholine receptors using nerve-released transmitter in the frog. *J. Physiol. (Lond.)*, 316: 225–250.

Manthorpe, M. and Varon, S. (1985) Regulation of neuronal survival and neuritic growth in the avian ciliary ganglion by trophic factors. In G. Guroff (Ed.), *Growth and Maturation Factors, Vol. 3*, John Wiley, New York, pp. 77–117.

Marler, P. and Terrace, H. S. (1984) *The Biology of Learning*, Springer-Verlag, Berlin.

Massoulié, J. and Bon, S. (1982) The molecular forms of cholinesterase and acetylcholinesterase in vertebrates. *Ann. Rev. Neurosci.*, 5: 57–106.

Merlie, J. and Sanes, J. (1985) Concentration of acetylcholine receptor mRNA in synaptic regions of adult muscle fibers. *Nature (Lond.)*, 317: 66–68.

Mishina, M., Kurosaki, T., Tobimatsu, T., Morimoto, Y., Noda, M., Yamamoto, T., Terao, M., Lindström, J., Takahashi, T., Kuno, M. and Numa, S. (1984) Expression of functional acetylcholine receptor from cloned cDNAs. *Nature (Lond.)*, 307: 604–608.

Monod, J., Changeux, J. P. and Jacob, F. (1963) Allosteric proteins and cellular control systems. *J. Mol. Biol.*, 6: 306–328.

Monod, J., Wyman, J. and Changeux, J. P. (1965) On the nature of allosteric transitions: a plausible model. *J. Mol. Biol.*, 12: 88–118.

Neubig, R. R. and Cohen, J. B. (1980) Permeability control by cholinergic receptors in *Torpedo* postsynaptic membranes: Agonist dose response relations measured at second and millisecond times. *Biochemistry*, 19: 2770–2779.

Nghiêm, H. O., Cartaud, J., Dubreuil, C., Kordeli, C., Buttin, G. and Changeux, J. P. (1983) Production and characterization of a monoclonal antibody directed against the 43,000 M.W. nu 1 polypeptide from *Torpedo marmorata* electric organ. *Proc. nat. Acad. Sci. USA*, 80: 6403–6407.

Nitkin, R. M., Wallace, B. G., Spira, M. E., Godfrey, E. W. and McMahan, U. J. (1983) Molecular components of the synaptic basal lamina that direct differentiation of regenerating neuromuscular junctions. *Cold Spring Harbor Symp. Quant. Biol.*, 48: 653–666.

Noda, M., Takahashi, H., Tanabe, T., Toyosato, M., Furutani, Y., Hirose, T., Asai, M., Inayama, S., Miyata, T. and Numa, S. (1982) Primary structure of alpha subunit precursor of *Torpedo californica* acetylcholine receptor deduced from cDNA sequence. *Nature (Lond.)*, 299: 793–797.

Noda, M., Takahashi, H., Tanabe, T., Toyosato, M., Kikyotani, S., Hirose, T., Asai, M., Takashima, H., Inayama, S., Miyata, T. and Numa, S. (1983a) Primary structures of beta and delta subunit precursors of *Torpedo californica* acetylcholine receptor deduced from cDNA sequences. *Nature (Lond.)*, 301: 251–255.

Noda, M., Takahashi, H., Tanabe, T., Toyosato, M., Kikyotani, S., Furutani, Y., Hirose, T., Takashima, H., Inayama, S., Miyata, T. and Numa, S. (1983b) Structural homology of *Torpedo californica* acetylcholine receptor subunits. *Nature (Lond.)*, 302: 528–532.

Noda, M., Furutani, Y., Takahashi, H., Toyosato, M., Tanabe, T., Shimizu, S., Kikyotani, S., Kayano, T., Hirose, T., Inayama, S. and Numa, S. (1983c) Cloning and sequence analysis of calf cDNA and human genomic DNA encoding alpha subunit precursor of muscle acetylcholine receptor. *Nature (Lond.)*, 305: 818–823.

Noda, M., Schimizu, S., Tanabe, T., Takai, T., Kayano, T., Ikeda, T., Takahashi, H., Nakayama, H., Kanaoka, Y., Minamino, N., Kangawa, R., Matsuo, H., Raftery, M. A., Hirose, T., Inayama, S., Hayashida, H., Miyata, T. and Numa, S. (1984) Primary structure of *Electrophorus electricus* sodium channel deduced from cDNA sequence. *Nature (Lond.)*, 312: 121–127.

Ochs, S., Erdman, J., Jersild, R. A. and McAdoo, V. (1978) Routing of transported material in the dorsal root and nerve fiber branches of the dorsal root ganglion. *J. Neurobiol.*, 9: 465–481.

Oswald, R. E. (1983) Effects of calcium on the binding of phencyclidine to acetylcholine receptor-rich membrane fragments from *Torpedo californica* electroplaque. *J. Neurochem.*, 41: 1077.

Oswald, R. E., Pennow, N. N. and McLaughlin, J. T. (1984) Demonstration and affinity labeling of a stereoselective binding site for a benzomorphan opiate on acetylcholine receptor-rich membranes from *Torpedo* electroplaque. *Proc. nat. Acad. Sci. USA*, 82: 940–944.

Owens, G. P., Chaudhari, N. and Hahn, W. E. (1985) Brain "identifier sequence" is not restricted to transcripts in brain: similar abundance in nuclear RNA of other organs. *Science*, 229: 1263–1265.

Peng, H. B. and Frochner, S. (1985) Association of the postsynaptic 43 K protein with newly formed acetylcholine receptor clusters in cultured muscle cells. *J. Cell Biol.*, 100: 1698–1705.

Pfeiffer, K., Simler, R., Grenningloh, G. and Betz, H. (1984) Monoclonal antibodies and peptide mapping reveal structural similarities between the subunits of the glycine receptor of rat spinal cord. *Proc. nat. Acad. Sci. USA*, 81: 7224–7227.

Popot, J. L. and Changeux, J. P. (1984) The nicotinic acetylcholine receptor: structure of an oligomeric integral membrane protein. *Physiol. Rev.*, 64: 1162–1184.

Potter, D. D., Furshpan, E. J. and Landis, S. C. (1981) Multiple transmitter status and "Dale's principle". *Neurosci. Commentaries*, 1: 1–9.

Reiness, C. G. and Weinberg, C. B. (1981) Metabolic stabilization of acetylcholine receptors at newly formed neuromuscular junction in rat. *Dev. Biol.*, 84: 247–254.

Rescorla, R. and Wagner, A. R. (1972) A theory of Pavlovian conditioning: variations in the effectiveness of reinforcement and non reinforcement. In A. Black and W. F. Prokasy (Eds.), *Classical Conditioning: II: Current Research and Theory*, Appleton, New York, pp. 64–99.

Reynolds, J. A. and Karlin, A. (1978) Molecular weight in detergent solution of acetylcholine receptor from *Torpedo californica. Biochemistry*, 17: 2035–2038.

Rieger, F., Grumet, M. and Edelman, G. (1985) N-CAM at the vertebrate neuromuscular junction. *J. Cell. Biol.*, 101: 285–293.

Roper, S., Purves, D. and McMahan, U. J. (1975) Synaptic organization and acetylcholine sensitivity of multiply innervated autonomic ganglion cells. *Cold Spring Harbor Symp. Quant. Biol.*, 40: 283–296.

Rosenfeld, M. G., Amara, D. G. and Evans, R. M. (1984) Alternative RNA processing determining neuronal phenotype. *Science*, 225: 1315–1320.

Rubin, L. L., Schuetze, S. M., Weill, C. L. and Fischbach, G. D. (1980) Regulation of acetylcholinesterase appearance at neuromuscular junction in vitro. *Nature (Lond.)*, 283: 264–267.

Rübsamen, H., Eldefrawi, A. T., Eldefrawi, M. E. and Hess, G. P. (1978) Characterization of the calcium-binding sites of the purified acetylcholine receptor and identification of the calcium binding subunit. *Biochemistry*, 17: 3818–3825.

Salpeter, M., Smith, C. and Matthews-Bellinger, J. A. (1984) Acetylcholine receptor and neuro-muscular junctions by E.M. autoradiography using mask analysis and linear source. *J. Electr. Microsc. Techn.*, 1: 63–81.

Samuelsson, B. (1983) Leukotrienes: mediators of immediate hypersensitivity reaction and inflammation. *Science*, 220: 568–575.

Sanes, J. R. and Chiu, A. Y. (1983) The basal lamina of the neuromuscular junction. *Cold Spring Harbor Symp. Quant. Biol.*, 48: 667–678.

Schibler, U., Hagenbüchle, O., Wellaver, P. K. and Pittet, A. C. (1983) Two promoters of different strengths control the transcription of the mouse alpha-amylase gene *Amy* 1 a in the parotid gland and the liver. *Cell*, 33: 501–508.

Schindler, H., Spillecke, F. and Neumann, E. (1984) Different channel properties of *Torpedo* acetylcholine receptor monomers and dimers reconstituted in planar membranes. *Proc. nat. Acad. Sci. USA*, 81: 6222–6226.

Schmidt, J. T. (1985) Factors involved in retinotopic map formation: complementary roles for membrane recognition and activity dependent synaptic stabilisation. In G. M. Edelman, W. E. Gall and W. M. Cowan (Eds.), *Molecular Bases of Neural Development*, Wiley, New York, pp. 453–480.

Schramm, M. (1979) Transfer of glucagon receptor from liver membranes to a foreign adenylate cyclase by a membrane fusion procedure. *Proc. nat. Acad. Sci. USA*, 76: 1174–1178.

Schramm, M. and Selinger, Z. (1984) Message transmission: receptor controlled adenylate cyclase system. *Science*, 225: 1350–1356.

Schwarts, J. C., Llorens Cortes, C., Rose, C., Quach, T. T. and Pollard, H. (1983) Adaptive changes of neurotransmitter mechanisms in the central nervous system. *Prog. Brain Res.*, 58: 117–130.

Snyder, S. (1984) Drug and neurotransmitter receptors in the brain. *Science*, 224: 22–31.

Sobel, A., Weber, M. and Changeux, J. P. (1977) Large scale purification of the acetylcholine receptor protein in its membrane-bound and detergent extracted forms from *Torpedo marmorata* electric organ. *Europ. J. Biochem.*, 80: 215–224.

Sokolowsky, M. (1984) Muscarinic receptors in the central nervous system. *Int. Rev. Neurobiol.*, 25: 139–183.

Stallcup, W. B. and Patrick, J. (1980) Substance P enhances cholinergic receptor desensitization in a clonal nerve cell line. *Proc. nat. Acad. Sci. USA*, 77: 634–638.

Stent, G. (1973) A physiological mechanism for Hebb's postulate of learning. *Proc. nat. Acad. Sci. USA*, 70: 997–1001.

Steward, O. (1983) Polyribosomes at the base of dendritic spines of central nervous system neurons: possible role in synapse construction and modification. *Cold Spring Harbor Symp. Quant. Biol.*, 48: 745–760.

Sulston, J. E. (1983) Neuronal cell lineage in the nematode *Caenorhabditis elegans. Cold Spring Harbor Symp. Quant. Biol.*, 48: 443–452.

Sutcliffe, J. G., Milner, R. J., Gottesfeld, J. M. and Reynolds, W. (1984) Control of neuronal gene expression. *Science*, 225: 1308–1315.

Takai, T., Noda, M., Mishina, M., Shimizu, S., Furutani, Y., Kayano, T., Ikeda, T., Kubo, T., Takahashi, H., Takahashi, T., Kuno, M. and Numa, S. (1985) Cloning sequencing and expression of cDNA for a novel subunit of acetylcholine receptor from calf muscle. *Nature (Lond.)*, 315: 761–764.

Takeyasu, K., Udgoankar, J. B. and Hess, G. P. (1983) Acetylcholine receptor: Evidence for a voltage-dependent regulatory site for acetylcholine. Chemical kinetic measurements in membrane vesicles using a voltage clamp. *Biochemistry*, 22: 5973–5978.

Talvenheimo, J. A., Tamkun, M. M., Hartshorne, R. P., Messner, D. J., Sharkey, R. G., Costa, M. R. C. and Catterall, W. A. (1983) Structure and functional reconstitution of the voltage-sensitive sodium channel from rat brain. *Cold Spring Harbor Symp. Quant. Biol.*, 48: 155–164.

Tauc, L. and Gerschenfeld, H. (1961) Cholinergic transmission mechanisms for both excitation and inhibition in molluscan central synapses. *Nature (Lond.)*, 192: 366–367.

Tauc, L. and Gerschenfeld, H. (1962) A cholinergic mechanism of inhibitory synaptic transmission in a molluscan nervous system. *J. Neurophysiol.*, 25: 236–262.

Thoenen, H. and Barde, Y. A. (1980) Physiology of nerve growth factor. *Physiol. Rev.*, 60: 1284–1335.

Tomkins, G. (1975) The metabolic code. *Science*, 189: 760–763.

Toulouse, G., Dehaene, S. and Changeux, J.-P. (1986) A spin glass model of learning by selection. *Proc. nat. Acad. Sci. USA*, 83: 1695–1699.

Triller, A., Cluzeaud, F., Pfeiffer, F., Betz, H. and Korn, H. (1985) Distribution of glycine receptors at central synapses: immunoelectron microscopy study. *J. Cell Biol.*, 101: 683–688.

Ullrich, A., Bell, J. R., Chen, E. Y., Herrera, R., Petruzzelli, L. M., Dull, T. J., Gray, A., Conssens, L., Liao, Y. C., Tsubokawa, M., Mason, A., Seeburg, P. H., Grunfeld, C., Rosen, O. M. and Ramachandran, J. (1985) Human insulin receptor and its relationship to the tyrosine kinase family of oncogenes. *Nature (Lond.)*, 313: 756–761.

Waksman, G., Fournié-Zaluski, M. C., Roques, B., Heidmann, T., Grünhagen, H. H. and Changeux, J. P. (1976) Synthesis of fluorescent acyl-choline with agonistic properties: pharmacological activity on *Electrophorus* electroplaque and interaction in vitro with *Torpedo* receptor-rich membrane fragments. *FEBS Lett.*, 67: 335–342.

Weintraub, H., Larsen, A. and Groudine, M. (1981) Alpha-globin gene switching during the development of chicken embryo: expression and chromosome structure. *Cell*, 24: 333–344.

Wolfson, B., Manning, R. W., Davis, L. G., Arentzen, R. and Baldino, F. (1985) Colocalisation of corticotropin releasing factor and vasopressin mRNA in neurons after adrenalectomy. *Nature (Lond.)*, 315: 59–61.

Yamamoto, T., Geoffrey Davis, C., Brown, M. S., Sneider, W. J., Casey, M. K. L., Goldstein, J. L. and Russel, D. W. (1984) The Human LDL receptor: a cysteine rich protein with multiple alu sequences in its mRNA. *Cell*, 39: 27–38.

Yaniv, M. (1984) Regulation of eucaryotic gene expression by transactivating proteins and *Cis* acting DNA elements. *Biol. Cell.*, 50: 203–216.

Yaniv, M. and Cereghini, S. (1986) Structure of transcriptionally active chromatin. *Crit. Rev. Biochem.* (in press).

Yeramian, E. and Changeux, J. P. (1986) Un modèle de changement d'efficacité synaptique à long terme fondé sur l'interaction du récepteur de l'acetylcholine avec la protéine sous-synaptique de 43 000 daltons. *C.R. Acad. Sci. Paris*, 302: 609–616.

Subject Index

Acetylcholine, 6, 10, 15, 16, 33, 41, 44, 45, 48, 83, 103, 106, 113, 121, 157, 193, 233, 241, 323, 379
Acetylcholinesterase, 392
Acinar cells, 18, 20
Actinomycin D, 95, 124
Activating signals, 284
Active zones (synapses), 92
Adenosine, 103, 194
Adenosine deaminase, 114
Adenosine triphosphate (ATP), 9, 10, 40, 114, 193–199, 250, 263–276, 382
Adenylate cyclase, 6, 14, 18, 90, 307, 337, 364, 388
Adrenal gland, 169
Adrenal medulla, 29, 121, 123, 346, 382, 385
Adrenalectomy, 177, 185, 235
Adrenaline (epinephrine), 6, 180, 183, 246, 280, 303
Adrenergic, 111, 234
Adrenoceptor antagonists, 193, 245, 251, 303
Adrenocorticotropic hormone (ACTH), 45, 73, 76, 164, 169, 337
After hyperpolarization, 233
Aging, 122, 291, 379
Airways, 256
Alaproclate, 326
Allosteric, 386
Amine precursor, 25
Amino acid decaboxylase, 6, 25
p-Aminoclonidine, 303
p-Aminopyridine, 11
Amoeba, 72
Amphetamine, 358
Amplifier, 275
Amphibia, 214
Anaphylactic challenge, 257
Anatomical unit, 374
Anterograde signals, 392
Antidepressant, 326
Anisotropic, 321, 384, 395
Antidromic activation, 234
Antipsychotic, 327
Anxiogen, 345
Apamine, 220
Aplysia, 84, 325, 378, 388, 391
Apomorphine, 358
APUD theory, 25, 28, 378
Arachidonic acid, 40
Arcuate nucleus, 45
Argyrophilia, 25, 26
Aspartate, 6
ATPase, 197
Atrial natriuretic factor (ANF), 165
Atropine, 51, 106, 111, 195, 252, 323
Autapse, 107
Autocontrol, 272
Autoinhibition, 269, 308, 322
Autonomic neurons, 217
Autoreceptor, 16, 34, 315, 322, 385
Avidin-biotin, 226
Avoidance behaviour, 255
Angiotensin, 165, 170, 173, 181, 379
Axonal transport, 5, 246, 327, 382
Axotomy, 113

Bacteria, 72, 73
Baroreceptor, 170, 182
Basal lamina, 391, 394
Behavior, 83
Benzodiazepine, 344, 351, 387
Benzotript, 364
Bicuculline, 344
Bipolar cells, 323, 338
Bladder, 197
Blood brain barrier, 359
Blood flow, 242
Blood pressure, 303
Blood vessels, 195, 247, 279–286
Blood volume, 242
Body water regulation, 169
Bombesin, 165

Caeruletide, 367
Calcitonin gene-related peptide (CGRP), 57, 59, 115, 150, 157, 226, 255, 282, 378

Capsaicin, 254
β-Carboline, 345
Cardiovascular region, 303
Carotid body, 28
Catalytic unit, 337
cDNA, 123, 346
Cell adhesion molecule (CAM), 392
Cerebellum, 347
Cerebral cortex, 155, 310, 326, 331, 339, 347
Channel blocker, 194, 345, 352
Chemical coding, 17, 217, 234, 241, 252, 322
Chemical coupling, 388
Chemical heterogeneity, 45
Chemical lesion, 221
Chemogenic irritation, 256
Chimaera, 28, 111
Chlorisondamine, 246
p-Chloroamphetamine, 325
Chlorpromazine, 327, 389
Cholecystokinin (CCK), 38, 42, 43, 46, 129, 133, 150, 164, 218, 226, 313, 343, 357–367, 377
Cholera toxin, 18, 196
Choline acetyltransferase, 49, 226
Cholinergic, 103, 111, 218, 233, 241
Cholinergic-link, 113
Cholinomimetic, 19
Chorionic gonadotropin, 75
Chromaffin cells, 195, 379
Chromaffin granules, 321
Chromogranin A, 26, 28
Chronotropic, 249
Cigartette smoke, 256
Clonidine, 268, 305
Cloning, 151
Cocaine, 282
Cockroach, 99
Co-distribution, 295
Coeliac ganglion, 4, 227
Co-existence, 18, 20, 25, 29, 33, 38, 76, 97, 99, 130, 149, 157, 195, 207, 213, 217, 241, 279, 295, 314, 321, 339, 343, 357, 373, 391
Colchicine, 38, 152, 224, 350
Collateral coupling, 380
Co-localization, 123, 129, 161
Co-modulation, 314
Computer assisted morphometry, 303
Conditioning, 84, 388
Conflict situation, 351
Connectivity, 380
Co-operativity, 51, 56, 84, 270, 385
Co-produce, 27
Co-reception, 97
Co-release, 10, 97, 123, 242, 381
Co-secretion, 9, 10, 18, 26, 97, 103, 113, 263, 269, 279
Corticosterone, 75, 185, 316
Corticotropin-releasing factor (CRF), 150, 164, 169, 173–186, 235, 377, 379
Co-storing, 30, 114, 303, 314
Co-transmission, 193, 291, 303, 343
Co-transmitter, 166, 193
Coupling system, 343
Cross-reactivity, 38, 224
Cross-regulation, 328
Cybernetics, 384
Cyclic AMP, 18, 20, 75, 83, 84, 87, 292, 325, 340, 386, 388
Cyclic GMP, 344, 386
Cyclic nucleotide, 16
Cytosine-arabinoside, 124
Cytoskeleton, 392

Dale's principle, 3, 108, 322, 373, 383
dbGMP, 364
Decentralization, 247
Defense reflex, 84
Degradative enzyme, 385
Dendritic site, 322
Dense-cored vesicles, 47, 242, 252, 264
Desensitization, 388, 389
Determination, 377
Diacylglycerol, 16, 386
Diaphragm, 197
Diazepam binding inhibitor (DBI), 345–354
Differential release, 47
Differentiation, 377, 381
Diffuse neuroendocrine system (DNES), 27
Diffusion, 384
Disinhibition, 323
Division, 377
DNA, 374
DNAse, 378
DNA technology, 20
DOPAC, 327
Double staining, 35, 37, 221, 235, 376
Drosophila, 77
Drugs, 321
Dopamine, 6, 28, 40, 130, 133, 166, 173, 234, 292, 313, 343, 357–367
Dopamine β-hydroxylase, 113, 165, 234, 242, 279, 321
Dorsal root ganglion, 5
Double-staining, 37
Dual function, 103
Dynorphin, 157, 162, 218, 227

E. coli, 151
Ectoenzyme, 194
Egg-laying hormone (ELH), 99

Electrical coupling, 387
Electric organ, 196, 388
Electro-chemical transmission, 299
Electron microscopy, 7, 47, 105
Electrophysiology, 4, 86, 105, 233, 265, 352, 357
Electrogenic, 116
Electro-mechanical coupling, 194
Elution-restaining, 37, 357
Embryology, 71
Endplate potential, 283
Endocoid, 346
Endocrine cells, 25, 72
Endorphin, 150
Enkephalin, 115, 117, 123, 129, 157, 162, 173, 218, 225, 338, 377, 379
Enteric neurons, 217
Enteric projections, 227
Epicenter, 346
Epigenetic, 374
Estrogen, 75
Evolution, 48, 71, 157, 378
Excitation, 361
Exocrine, 255
Exon, 157
Exocytosis, 6, 8, 9, 11, 195, 197, 282
Explantation, 122, 379
Exploratory behavior, 359
Extrajunctional, 276, 392
Extrasynaptic, 312, 314
Extravasation, 59, 254

Facilitation, 85, 96, 322, 344, 361
Fast signalling, 16
Fluorescein isothiocyanate (FITC), 37, 223
Flunitrazepam, 344
Fluorophores, 223, 235
FMRF, 165
Frequency coding, 48, 241, 322, 383
Frog skin, 76, 150
Frog sympathetic ganglia, 205
Fungi, 72
Fusion transfer, 339

GABA, 6, 16, 33, 38, 40, 45, 83, 218, 343–346, 351–354, 376
Galanin, 44, 45, 164, 218
Ganglia, sympathetic, 44, 51, 359
Gastrin-releasing peptide, 218
Gastro-intestinal, 25, 217, 256
Gene, 98
Gene activation, 380, 386
Gene repression, 377, 380, 386
Genetic, 374
Genome, 151, 157, 185, 375
Glandulocentric, 71, 74
Glial cell, 20, 27, 348
Glucagon, 164
Glucocorticoid, 177, 184, 379
Glucocorticoid receptor, 316
Glycosylation, 152
Glutamate, 6, 16, 33, 83, 99, 358
Glutamic acid, 26
Glutamic acid decarboxylase (GAD), 38, 351
α-Glycerophosphate dehydrogenase, 25
Glycine, 6, 16, 33, 83
Gonadotrophin releasing hormone (GnRH), 74
Graft, 129
Granular vesicle, 9, 11
Grooming, 363
Group selection, 375
Growth cone, 392
Growth hormone releasing factor (GRF), 45, 150, 314
GTP-binding protein, 337, 388
Guanethidine, 195, 242, 264
Guanylate-regulated protein (Gi protein), 307

Habituation, 84
Haloperiodol, 327
Heart, 195, 246, 255
Heart rate, 317
Hemorrhage, 169
Heterostatic regulation, 314, 385
Hexamethonium, 113
Hippocampus, 139, 349
Histamine, 40, 166, 249
Homeostatic regulation, 315, 385
Hormones, 25, 29, 71, 72, 73
Human brain, 346
Hybridization, 125, 151, 161
Hydra, 77
5-Hydroxydopamine, 109
6-Hydroxydopamine, 130, 242, 263, 279, 292, 357
5-Hydroxytryptamine (5-HT), 6, 10, 17, 27, 28, 42, 51, 86, 103, 114, 129, 136–140, 166, 280, 324, 376
Hypertension, 56, 295, 338, 387
Hypothalamus, 45, 61, 161, 169, 326, 333, 347
Hypoxanthine, 346

Image analysis, 304
Imipramine, 326
Immunohistochemistry, 25, 34, 86, 130, 152, 206, 210, 218, 347, 357, 376
  specificity, 38, 235
  sensitivity, 38
Information transfer, 373
Inosine, 346
Inositol phosphate, 16

In situ hybridization, 161, 376, 379
Insulin, 73, 76
Insulin-like growth factor, 76
Intercellular communication, 71, 73, 286
Interferon, 75
Intermediolateral cell column, 213
Interneurons, 213
Intersynaptic, 314
Intestinofugal, 220
Intrajunctionally, 276
Intramembrane feedback, 296, 314
Intrasynaptic, 314
Intracisternal, 307
Intrathecal, 59
Invertebrates, 34, 81, 94, 376
Ion channels, 6, 15, 34, 83, 88, 298, 388
Ionophore, 343
Ionophoresis, 360
Ionotropic, 6, 249
Iris, 51
Isoprenaline, 19, 328
Isoreceptor, 297

Junction potentials, 193, 233, 251, 263, 268

Ketanserin, 325

Lateral diffusion, 392
Learning, 84, 97
Learning theory, 375
Ligand binding, 309
Leukotriene, 41, 61, 376
Local anaesthetics, 389
Local circuit, 298, 313
Locus coeruleus, 42
Locomotor activity, 292, 358, 363
Luteinizing hormone (LH), 61
Luteinizing hormone releasing hormone (LHRH), 10, 41, 74, 150, 205–214, 384

Magnocellular neurons, 40, 161, 170, 382
Mauthner cell, 9
Median eminence, 161, 170
Medulla oblongata, 305, 360
Membrane fusion, 338, 388
Memory, 85, 90, 95
Metabolic response, 297
Metabolic unity, 3, 374
Metabotropic, 6
Metachromasia, 26
Metamorphosis, 209
Methylene blue, 218
Methysergide, 114
Microbe, 72, 395
Microculture, 103, 376
Microdensitometry, 292, 303
Mineralocorticoids, 177
Miniaturization, 297, 304
Mismatch, 56
Modulation, 84, 90, 194, 234, 294, 313, 337, 345, 361
Molecular biology, 149, 185, 378
Molecular selection, 373
Molluscs, 72
Monosodium glutamate, 164
Morphometry, 292, 303
Motoneuron, 8, 52, 99, 116, 344, 382
Motor endplate, 198, 391
mRNA 98, 121, 123, 150, 324, 344, 376, 379
mRNA processing, 157
Multiple coding, 232
Multiple signals, 322
Muscle derived factor, 395
Myenteric ganglia, 220, 232
Myocytes, 105
Myotubes, 197, 392

Nerve growth factor, 105, 395
Nerve stimulation, 265
Neural crest, 27, 111
Neuro-effector junction, 285
Neuroendocrine, 25, 29, 45, 169
Neurohemal, 170
Neurohormones, 6
Neurohumors, 6
Neurokinin, 254
Neuromodulation, 16
Neuromodulators, 6, 16, 343
Neuromuscular junction, 15, 83, 382
Neuromuscular transmission, 264
Neuronal map, 322, 375
Neurone-specific enolase (NSE), 26, 378
Neuronocentric, 71, 74
Neuron theory, 374
Neuropeptide K, 254
Neuropeptide Y, 38, 113, 115, 129, 132, 150, 180, 183, 218, 226, 241–252, 263–276, 279–286, 303–314, 337–340, 376, 379, 381
Neuroregulators, 6
Neurosecretory, 38, 161, 169, 385
Neurotensin, 42, 73, 115, 129, 165, 173, 292, 313, 377
Neurotoxin, 50
Neurotransmitter quanta, 268
Nicotinamide, 346
Nictitating membrane, 194
Nifedipine, 247, 280
Non-adenergic, non-cholinergic, 194
Non-competitive blockers, 389

Non-junctional receptors, 392
Non-synaptic transmission, 9, 299
Noradrenaline (norepinephrine), 6, 15, 20, 33, 103, 106, 113, 180, 183, 193, 234, 241–250, 263–276, 279–286, 323, 337, 376, 382
Normotensive, 305
Noxious, 84
N-protein, 337
Nucleus accumbens, 292, 363
Nucleus basalis, 44
Nucleus caudatus (striatum), 55, 133, 140, 293, 363
Nucleus paraventricularis, 161, 170–186
Nucleus supraopticus, 161
Nucleus tractus solitarii, 42, 56, 305–315, 359

Occlusion method, 304
Octopamine, 40
Octadecaneuropeptide (ODN), 346
Olfactory bulb, 154
Ontogeny, 48, 129
Oocytes, 344
Open genes, 378
Opioid peptides, 75
Operant behavior, 345
Oubain, 291
Oxytocin, 150, 161, 170, 377

Postjunctional receptor, 235
Postsynaptic potential, 8, 206, 213, 256, 384
Post-translational modification, 152, 185
Potentiation, 282, 286, 364
Prazosin, 269
Preautonomic cell, 182
Prejunctional action, 196, 250, 264, 279
Pre-proenkephalin, 125, 379
Presynaptic, 55, 361, 385
Presynaptic facilitation, 85, 90
Presynaptic feedback, 10, 11
Presynaptic inhibition, 54, 246, 344
Presynaptic receptor, 11, 16, 55, 253
Prevertebral ganglia, 232
Proctolin, 99
Proglumide, 364
Prohormone, 150, 156
Promotor, 378
Pro-opiomelanocortin (POMC), 157
Prostaglandin, 249, 280, 339
Proteolytic processing, 151
Protozoa, 73
1B236 Protein, 151
Protein kinase, 83, 87, 388
Protein S-100, 27
Protein synthesis, 95
Punishment, 351

Purine, 193
Purinergic, 11, 111, 195
Purinoceptor, 193
Purkinje cells, 351, 377

Quantal emission, 6, 382
Quinacrine, 195

Rauwolscine, 303
Raphe nucleus, 42, 136
Receptor
  acetylcholine, muscarinic, 6, 18, 323, 338, 386
  acetylcholine, nicotinic, 6, 15, 83, 113, 121, 386, 388
  α-adrenoceptor, 34, 56, 245, 269, 303, 323
  β-adrenoceptor, 34, 338, 387
  benzodiazepine, 344, 387
  bombesin, 18
  cholecystokinin/gastrin, 18, 317, 359
  dopamine, 18, 295, 339, 366, 387
  GABA, 344, 386
  glycine, 386
  histamine, 18
  5-hydroxytryptamine, 18, 52, 87, 323, 387
  insulin, 386
  intrinsic, 83
  LHRH, 213
  neuropeptide tyrosine (NPY), 317, 323, 339, 387
  neurotensin, 18
  noradrenaline, 18, 34, 340
  secretin/VIP, 18, 323, 339, 387
  steroid, 180, 185
  tachykinin, 18
  vasopressin, 18
Receptor autoradiography, 56, 61, 294, 307, 362
Receptor binding, 249, 292
Receptopr biosynthesis, 392
Receptor clustering, 391
Receptor distribution, 391
Receptor domaine, 345
Receptor-effector coupling, 337
Receptor-receptor interaction, 55, 291, 303, 337, 343, 386
Receptor subunit, 338
Recognition site, 83, 309, 344
Recombinant DNA, 57, 150
Redundancy, 380
Regulatory peptide, 6
Regulatory proteins, 381
Regulatory signals, 386
Relaxin, 73
Release, 6, 9, 17, 19, 47, 62, 85, 379, 381, 385
Releasable pool, 327
Release site, 274
Remote receptor, 83

Renshaw cells, 4, 116, 384
Reputable, 282, 382
Reserpine, 114, 193, 242, 263, 268, 325
Respiratory frequency, 317
Retrograd tracing, 44, 173, 180, 206
Rhodamine (TRITC), 37, 223
Ribosomes, 323
RNA processing, 378
RNA synthesis, 122

Salivary gland, 18, 51, 234, 241, 252, 323, 338, 382
Satiety, 359
Schizophrenia, 327, 366
Second messenger, 6, 16, 83, 386, 393
Secretagogue, 18, 179, 388
Secretin, 164
Secretomotor neuron, 217, 233
Selection, 375, 390, 395
Sensitization, 84
Sensory ganglia, 27, 49
Sensory neuron, 57, 85, 87, 113, 217, 241, 254
Sensory relay, 359
Serotonin, 6, 9, 84, 218, 234, 325
Sexual behaviour, 52
Signal expansion, 337
Signal recognition site, 343
Singularity, 377
Skeletal muscle, 197
Slow signalling, 16
Small cardioactive peptide (SCP), 86
Sniffing, 363
Somatostatin, 20, 44, 45, 73, 75, 115, 129, 150, 173, 218, 226, 231, 337
Spinal cord, 51, 59, 137, 295, 324
Spinal injury, 54
Spinal trigeminal nucleus, 56
Spiperone, 366
Spleen, 245
Sponges, 72
Stereotypy, 364
Steroid, 74
Stimulation frequency, 252
Storage vesicle, 26, 40, 263, 264
Striatum (nucleus caudatus), 55, 133, 140, 293, 363
Stress, 169
Stretch reflex, 51
Subcellular fractionation, 48, 242, 382
Subfornical organ, 182
Submucous ganglia, 220, 232
Substance K, 218, 254, 324
Substance P, 6, 10, 18, 19, 27, 33, 42, 54, 56, 57, 59, 115, 121, 123, 129, 136–141, 150, 218, 226, 231, 254, 324, 358, 376, 379
Substance P antagonist, 54, 256
Substantia nigra, 42, 358
Subsynaptic membrane, 395
Sudomotor nerve, 235
Supersensitive, 296, 327
Sweat gland, 109, 111, 241
Sympathectomy, 51, 195
Sympathetic neuron (ganglia), 44, 103, 105, 121, 129, 193, 195, 205, 218, 232, 241, 263, 279, 376
Synapse, 7, 52, 84
Synapse stabilization, 375, 380
Synaptic communication, 337, 343
Synaptic contact, 9, 15, 377
Synaptic potential, 207, 233
Synaptic vesicle, 5, 7, 9, 10, 11, 47, 93, 108, 113, 161, 196, 357, 383
Synaptosome, 196
Synergism, 18, 19, 179, 323, 385, 390

Tachykinin, 59, 254, 324
Teleost, 208
Texas red, 223
Theory, 374
Therapy, 316
Thirst, 169, 183
Thyroid gland, 28, 72
Thyroid-stimulating hormone (TSH), 72
Thyrotropin-releasing hormone (TRH), 6, 10, 42, 51, 54, 75, 136–141, 149, 324, 376
Tissue culture, 103, 195
Transducer, 343, 386
Transplantation, 48, 129, 133–141, 379
Trophic effect, 62
Tryptophan hydroxylase, 323
Tolerance, 323
Topological selection, 394
Torpedo, 197, 389
Transcription, 95, 186, 377, 379
Translation, 378
Transmembrane complex, 387
Transmission line, 298, 315, 385
Transmural nerve stimulation (TNS), 250
Trans-synaptic, 123, 126, 384, 395
Trigger mechanism, 273
Tyrosine hydroxylase, 43, 50, 113, 120, 132, 133, 165, 242, 266, 297, 323, 357, 379

Unicellular organism, 72
Upregulation, 298
Uptake, 20, 326

Vagotomy, 358
Vas deferens, 54, 196, 250, 263–276, 284, 382
Vasoactive intestinal polypeptide (VIP), 20, 45, 48, 51, 115, 165, 218, 225, 252, 337–340, 343

Vasoconstriction, 59, 247, 251, 264, 279
Vasodilator, 251
Vasomotor neuron, 217
Vasopressin, 150, 161, 170, 182, 377, 379
Ventral tegmental area, 42, 133, 358
Verapamil, 280
Veratridine, 122, 126, 150
Vesicle, 321, 382
Vesicular grid, 7, 9

Whole mount, 50, 218
Withdrawal reflex, 84

Yeast, 73
Yohimbine, 250, 268

Zimelidine, 326